THE HUMAN GENOME PROJECT

Deciphering the Blueprint of Heredity

THE HUMAN GENOME PROJECT

Deciphering the Blueprint of Heredity

Edited by NECIA GRANT COOPER

LOS ALAMOS NATIONAL LABORATORY

Foreword by PAUL BERG

BECKMAN CENTER FOR MOLECULAR AND GENETIC MEDICINE
STANFORD UNIVERSITY SCHOOL OF MEDICINE

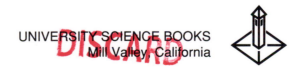

UNIVERSITY SCIENCE BOOKS
Mill Valley, California

University Science Books
20 Edgehill Road
Mill Valley, CA 94941
Fax (415) 383-3167

Production manager: *Susanna Tadlock*
Science writers: *Steve Elder, Gerald Friedman, Richard Reichelt, Nancy K. Shera*
Editor's assistant: *Nadine Shea*
Technical illustration: *Andrea Kron*
Original art: *Jim Cruz, David R. Delano, Steve Elder, Mel Prueitt, Gloria Sharp*
Production: *Nadine Shea*
Photography: *John Flower*
Jacket and cover designer: *Robert Ishi*
Printer: *Palace Press*

Library of Congress Catalog Number: 93-085290
ISBN 0-935702-29-6

Printed in Hong Kong

10 9 8 7 6 5 4 3 2 1

Contents

Foreword *by Paul Berg*   vii

A Guide to This Book *by David Dressler*   ix

Understanding Inheritance: An Introduction to Classical and Molecular Genetics   1
by Robert P. Wagner

BOXES

Early Ideas about Heredity   3
The Variety of Cells   6
Components of Eukaryotic Cells   8
The Eukaryotic Cell Cycle   9
Chromosomes: The Sites of Hereditary Information   10
Mitosis   14
Meiosis   15
Mendelian Genetics   22
Inheritance of Mendelian Disorders   26
Crossing Over: A Special Type of Recombination   32
Determining a Genetic Distance   34
DNA: Its Structure and Components   40
DNA Replication   42
Protein Synthesis   45
The Genetic Code   48
Restriction Enzymes   54
Gel Electrophoresis   55
Hybridization Techniques   63
The Anatomy of a Eukaryotic Protein Gene   64

Mapping the Genome: The Vision, the Science, the Implementation   68
a round table with David Baltimore, David Botstein, David R. Cox, David J. Galas, Leroy Hood, Robert K. Moyzis, Maynard V. Olson, Nancy S. Wexler, and Norton D. Zinder

Part I: What Is the Genome Project?   71

Classical Linkage Mapping   86
Modern Linkage Mapping with Polymorphic DNA Markers—A Tool for Finding Genes   94
Informativeness of Polymorphic DNA Markers
  by Carl E. Hildebrand, David C. Torney, and Robert P. Wagner   100

Part II: Maps, Markers, and the Five-Year Goals   103

Physical Mapping—A One-Dimensional Jigsaw Puzzle   112
The Polymerase Chain Reaction and Sequence-tagged Sites
  by Norman A. Doggett   128
YAC Library Pooling Scheme for PCR-based Screening
  by David J. Balding and David C. Torney   135
cDNAs and Expressed Genes   138

Part III: Technological Challenges in the Genome Project   142

DNA Sequencing   151

Part IV: Implications for Biology and Society   164

Unraveling the Chromosome
  by E. Morton Bradbury   168

The Mapping of Chromosome 16   182
by Norman A. Doggett

> **Various Classes of Human Repetitive DNA Sequences**   186
>
> **Collaborations on the Isolation of Disease Genes on Chromosome 16**   207
>
> **What's Different about Chromosome 16?**
> by Raymond L. Stallings and Norman A. Doggett   211
>
> **Mapping Chromosome 5**
> by Deborah Grady   216

DNA Libraries: Recombinant Clones for Mapping and Sequencing   218
by Larry L. Deaven

> **Libraries from Flow-sorted Chromosomes**
> by Larry L. Deaven   236

Computation and the Genome Project—A Shotgun Wedding   250
by James W. Fickett

> **Decades of Nonlinearity: The Growth of DNA Sequence Data**
> by Christian Burks, Michael J. Cinkosky, and Paul Gilna   254
>
> **SCORE: A Program for Computer-Assisted Scoring of Southern Blots**
> by T. Michael Cannon, Rebecca J. Koskela, Christian Burks, Raymond L.
> Stallings, Amanda A. Ford, Philip E. Hempfner, Henry T. Brown, and James W.
> Fickett   258
>
> **SIGMA: A System for Integrated Genome Map Assembly**
> by Michael J. Cinkosky, James W. Fickett, William M. Barber, Michael A.
> Bridgers, and Charles D. Troup   267
>
> **Electronic Data Publishing in GenBank**
> by Michael J. Cinkosky, James W. Fickett, Paul Gilna, and Christian Burks   270

Rapid DNA Sequencing Based on Single-Molecule Detection   280
by Lloyd M. Davis, Frederick R. Fairfield, Mark L. Hammond, Carol A. Harger, James H. Jett,
Richard A. Keller, Jong Hoong Hahn, Letitia A. Krakowski, Babetta Marrone, John C. Martin,
Harvey L. Nutter, Robert R. Ratliff, E. Brooks Shera, Daniel J. Simpson, Steven A. Soper, and
Charles W. Wilkerson

> **Single-Molecule Spectroscopy in Solution**
> by Steven A. Soper, Lloyd M. Davis, and E. Brooks Shera   286

ELSI: Ethical, Legal, and Social Implications   302
by Gerald Friedman and Richard Reichelt

An Invitation to Genetics in the Twenty-first Century   314
a round table with David Baltimore, David Botstein, Leon Botstein, Robert K. Moyzis, James D.
Watson, and Nancy S. Wexler

Glossary   330

Index   339

Foreword

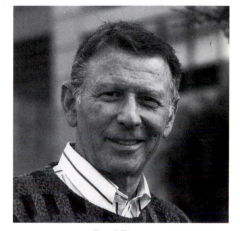

Paul Berg

THE HUMAN GENOME PROJECT is the first internationally coordinated effort in the history of biological research. It aims to determine the complete sequence of the nearly 3 billion base pairs that constitute the human genome, and, in its course, to identify the 100 thousand or so genes that define the human species. A subsidiary but essential goal is to learn the base-pair sequences of several model experimental organisms: the bacterium *Escherichia coli* (3 million base pairs), the yeast *Saccharomyces cerevisiae* (14 million base pairs), the nematode *Caenorhabditis elegans* (80 million base pairs), the invertebrate *Drosophila melanogaster* or fruit fly (165 million base pairs), and the mammal *Mus musculus* or house mouse (3 billion base pairs). The purpose of this unprecedented effort is to learn the DNA sequences that determine each organism's phenotypic characteristics and guide its development. This information is critical for expanding and refining our understanding of cellular and organismal functions.

In the course of these analyses, we are sure to identify genes governing a variety of human diseases and, thereby, to develop new strategies for their diagnosis, prevention, and therapy—and, we hope, for their cure. Thus, completing the Human Genome Project will not be the endpoint of our effort. Rather, it will provide us with a new beginning in our quest for understanding life on our planet: its origins; its evolution; the wonders of its development, capabilities, and maintenance; and its vulnerability to the stresses and challenges of the environment.

This highly readable volume summarizes the strategies for proceeding with the project, and it describes the tools that have been developed, and those that still need to be developed, in order to accomplish this formidable task. Thus, the ways in which genetic-linkage, physical, and sequence maps are being constructed are clearly explained. Especially interesting are the discussions by the founders of the discipline and its leading participants concerning the project's implications with regard to human health and the ethics of dealing with the diagnostic and predictive capabilities that will follow.

Paul Berg

Director, Beckman Center
for Molecular and Genetic Medicine,
Stanford University

Studying the Human Genome is one of the great enterprises of 20th Century science—and one that will carry modern molecular biology well into the 21st Century.

The Human Genome Project rests firmly on the foundation of a half-century of research into the fundamental nature of the gene. This epoch-making progress in molecular biology is chronicled in the first 64 pages of this book. Here the gene is progressively defined—from Mendel's invisible particle of inheritance to Watson and Crick's informational DNA molecule, with its Morse code-like message for the synthesis of enzymes and other proteins. A series of well-illustrated diagrams lays out the Genetic Code and the mechanism for the retrieval and use of the information stored in DNA to manufacture various proteins (pages 45–48).

The section of the book that establishes the DNA → RNA → protein dialectic of classical molecular biology is followed by a discussion of the new and powerful recombinant DNA techniques upon which the Human Genome Project rests. These enable one to dissect the huge cellular chromosomes, with their thousands of adjacent genes, into smaller DNA segments whose individual genes can then be analyzed. Here Restriction Enzymes are introduced as the tools for cleaving large DNA molecules at specfic nucleotide sequences, along with the electrophoretic technology for separating individual gene-size DNA pieces according to size (pages 52–58). The introductory chapter concludes by explaining how the isolated DNA segments can be individually transplanted ("cloned") into self-duplicating minichromosomes in order to maintain them in living bacterial cells. Collectively these cells form a "library" of the human genetic information, with each bacterium corresponding to one volume of the library. Ultimately, individual bacterial cells can be grown and processed to generate the large amounts of purified human DNA necessary for analysis at the molecular level (pages 58–64).

A series of Nobel Prizes recognizes the importance of this pioneering work—

- To Watson, Crick, and Wilkins in 1962 for their discovery of the structure of DNA.

- To Nirenberg, Khorana, and Holley in 1968 for their elucidation of the Genetic Code.

- To Arber, Smith, and Nathans in 1978 for their discovery of Restriction Enzymes.

- To Sanger and Gilbert in 1980 for their development of methods for determining the nucleotide sequence of DNA molecules.

- To Berg in 1980 for developing the first methods for cloning genes.

- To Bishop and Varmus in 1989 for the use of recombinant DNA techniques to identify several of the genes involved in cancer.

- To Sharp and Roberts in 1993 for their discovery of RNA Splicing and Split Genes.

- To Mullis and Smith in 1993 for the Polymerase Chain Reaction, which allows one to selectively amplify chosen DNA molecules, and for methods that allow the production of biologically useful mutant DNA molecules.

The analysis of human genes in which mutation has led to disease is a primary objective of the Human Genome Project.

In recent years hundreds of human diseases have been identified that have a genetic basis. Some are as mild as red-green color blindness, while others are as severe as the defects in lipid metabolism that lead to cardio-vascular disease. The recombinant DNA analysis of mutant genes from affected individuals has shown that these diseases generally result from simple, interpretable changes of one or a few of the three billion base pairs that constitute the human genome. An immediate practical consequence of identifying such genetic lesions is that it becomes possible to devise prenatal DNA tests to determine whether an individual has inherited two recessive defective genes—or one dominant gene—and is therefore at risk for the disease.

One of the first steps in the Human Genome Project is to develop a rough map of the whole human genome, which can then, by ever expanding effort, be increased in resolution until finally every base pair is assigned its own particular location. As a case study for exploring human chromosomes and their genes, the middle section of the book focuses on the molecular analysis of Chromosome 16 carried out at the Los Alamos National Laboratory. Chromosome 16—some 100,000,000 base pairs in length and about 3% of the human genome—contains a number of important genes, including several involved in disease. For example, the chromosome contains the metallothionein gene family that gives rise to a set of proteins that bind to heavy metals such as mercury, and thus play a role in the body's defense against these toxic environ-mental agents. Among the other important genes on Chromosome 16 are the hemoglobin gene, where mutations are associated with severe anemia, a gene involved in kidney disease, one associated with a neurodegenerative disorder known as Batten's disease, and a gene where DNA rearrangements lead to a form of leukemia (pages 184–185).

The chapter on "The Mapping of Chromosome 16" explains the general strategy by which the Los Alamos National Laboratory has defined the molecular architecture of this chromosome. The discussion traces the purification of Chromosome 16 by a process called Flow Sorting, in which the chromosome to be isolated is first marked by the binding of a fluorescent targeting molecule (pages 182, 236–246). The purified chromosome then becomes the source of material for thousands of specific DNA fragments generated by restriction enzymes. Collectively these restriction fragments represent the individual gene areas of the chromosome. Step by step the Los Alamos researchers explain how the various restriction fragments are ordered into a linear array—a series of adjacencies determined by virtue of overlapping DNA information. In the end a continuous DNA map is constructed in much the same way as the word Biochemistry can be constructed from the overlapping terms biochem and chemistry.

An interesting aspect of the analysis of Chromosome 16 is the discussion of the chromosome's various classes of repeated DNA elements. These multiply-reiterated short sequences not only serve as important landmarks along the length of the chromosome, aiding in the mapping of other genes, but are often interesting in their own right. For instance, one such repeated element, Alu, is a defective version of the gene that codes for an RNA molecule important in the transfer of enzymes and other proteins between the cytoplasm and other cellular compartments (page 186).

The pioneering methods used to map Chromosome 16 are already being extended to the construction of molecular maps for other human chromosomes, en route to a full understanding of the three billion base pair human genome.

Engineers will be fascinated to see the extent to which modern molecular biology has been automated.

The massive effort required to identify, clone, and sequence the entire human genome is not merely a matter of organizing many technicians to work repetitively until finally the three billion base pairs are put together. In fact, techniques available only in the last 5–10 years and ones currently being developed, especially in computer-controlled automation and data analysis, are essential to the Human Genome Project.

One of the most innovative techniques to have been developed and mechanized in the last few years is called the Polymerase Chain Reaction (PCR). This is a way to obtain large amounts of a specific DNA segment by repeatedly amplifying a very small amount of starting material. The technique is so sensitive that a single cell containing two copies of a particular sequence can, after amplification, yield sufficient DNA to allow all of the standard molecular analyses, such as cloning, restriction mapping, and sequencing.

Ultimately, the order of nucleotides in the pieces of DNA that have been mapped onto the human genome must be determined. As with many techniques, the DNA sequencing procedure (pages 151–159) has undergone a continuing revolution. When Greg Sutcliffe in Gilbert's lab sequenced the first plasmid, pBR322—about 40 nucleotides at a time—it took three years and over $100,000 to determine the 4,361 base pair sequence. Modern techniques have been so significantly improved by the introduction of DNA sequencing machines that all of pBR322 could now be sequenced in a few days for under $1000. Indeed, researchers are rapidly generating hundreds of thousands of base pairs of sequence information monthly, which are read directly into computers, where the data can be accessed by other researchers and subjected to detailed comparative analysis using sophisticated computer programs (pages 250–295).

This unusual book integrates the basic science, the specific research goals, and the public policy considerations that are involved in the Human Genome Project. The understanding gained in this project will have profound effects both in our lifetime and beyond. For the information that will be collected about the human genome will permanently reshape our understanding of human disease and indeed of human diversity.

David Dressler
HARVARD MEDICAL SCHOOL

THE HUMAN GENOME PROJECT

Deciphering the Blueprint of Heredity

Understanding

Over the past 125 years, humankind has made great progress in unraveling the mysteries of inheritance. The story of that progress naturally includes the researchers who made discoveries, but it also includes an odd assortment of organisms—starting with Mendel's garden peas. Other unwitting objects of scientific curiosity include fruit flies, maize, the house mouse, the transparent roundworm

Inheritance

Robert P. Wagner

Caenorhabditis elegans, baker's yeast, the rod-shaped bacterium *E. coli*, the cress *Arabidopsis thaliana*, and the tiny, machine-like viruses that infect bacteria. Each of these organisms has contributed to our understanding of molecular interactions among DNA, RNA, and proteins. Each has helped scientists reveal the genetic unity underlying the tremendous diversity of life on Earth.

Delano '92

That like begets like—that what is now called a species begets offspring of the same species—must have been evident to the earliest humans. Recognition of the inheritance of variations within a species must also have come early, since domestication of animals undoubtedly involved elimination of individuals with undesirable characteristics (a penchant for human flesh, for example). The first animals to be domesticated may well have been members of the dog family, which were used as food, and domestication of canines may have started even before the advent of *Homo sapiens*. The remains of an old hominid relative of ours, *Homo erectus* (also known as Java or Peking man), have been found associated with those of a dog-like animal in 500,000-year-old fossils. The earliest canine remains associated with our own species are a mere 12,000 years old. The domestication of food plants probably began between 8000 and 9000 years ago, although some authorities contend that the domestication of cereals preceded that of most animals.

Humans must also have very early related mating between "male" and "female" animals, including humans, with the subsequent issuance of offspring. Sexual reproduction in plants was probably recognized much later—many plants, after all, are discreetly bisexual—but at least 4000 years ago, as evidenced by the Babylonians' selective breeding, through controlled pollination, of the date palm (*Phoenix dactylifera*), which occurs as separate male and female trees. (The dates borne by a female tree result from fertilization of its eggs by sperm-containing pollen from male trees.)

The oldest recorded thoughts about heredity appear in the religious writings of the ancient Hindus and Jews, which reveal recognition of the heritability of disease, health, and mental and physical characteristics. The caste system of the Hindus, the hereditary priesthood among the Jews of the tribe of Levi, and later, in Homer's time, the inheritance of the gift of prophecy are a few reflections of ancient thinking about the link between successive generations of humans. Some of those ideas, which of necessity were based primarily on philosophical outlook rather than scientific fact, are discussed briefly in "Early Ideas about Heredity."

The Dawn

The first significant advances toward our current understanding of inheritance came in the late Renaissance with the work of the English physician William Harvey (1578–1657) and the invention of the microscope (circa 1600). Harvey is best known for his discovery of the dynamics of the circulation of the blood, but he also propounded a new view about the relative importance of the contributions of male and female animals to the creation of offspring. Previously, the female contribution, the egg, had been regarded as mere matter, matter that assumes a form dictated entirely by the male's semen. But Harvey proposed that both egg and semen guide the development of an offspring. His observation of the eggs of many species led him to conclude (in *De generatione animalium*, 1651) that "*ex ovo omnia*." That everything arises from an egg was meant to apply to humans also, even though Harvey had never seen the eggs of humans or any other live-bearing creature.

EARLY IDEAS ABOUT HEREDITY

Ancient beliefs about heredity included the idea that inborn characteristics are inherited from parents, as well as the idea that they could be affected by external influences on the parents at conception or during pregnancy. The biblical story of Jacob's wages (Genesis, chapter 30) combines both. Jacob had agreed to tend the flock of his uncle and father-in-law, Laban, if he could take when he left all the unusually colored animals: the sheep with dark wool and the goats with white streaks or speckles. But Laban, a deceitful and greedy man, took his few such animals three days' journey away. The remaining stock he assumed would not produce offspring of the colorations Jacob had named. However, Jacob peeled tree

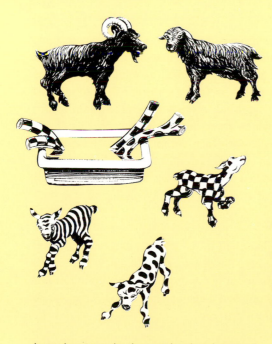

branches to make them striped and spotted and stood them in the watering troughs when the stronger goats were mating nearby. The kids from those matings, unlike their parents, had the markings that made them his, and they were more vigorous than the offspring of the weaker goats. He herded the sheep so they faced Laban's dark-colored goats; they then bore dark-colored lambs. Today the appearance in offspring

of characteristics different from those of either parent can be attributed to the combined effects of the genetic contributions of each parent (see "Mendelian Genetics").

The ancient Greeks gave considerable attention to human inheritance in their writings. Plato, for example, made cogent statements about human traits being determined by both parents. He emphasized that people are not completely equal in physical and mental characteristics and that each person inherits a nature suited to fulfilling only certain societal functions. Also prominent in the thinking of the early Greeks was the inheritance of acquired characteristics. Aristotle, for example, wrote that

> children are born resembling their parents in their whole body and their individual parts. Moreover this resemblance is true not only of inherited but also of acquired characters. For it has happened that the children of parents who bore scars are also scarred in just the same way in just the same place. In Chalcedon, for example, a man who had been branded on the arm had a child who showed the same brand letter, though it was not so distinctly marked and had become blurred.

The idea that external influences play a role in heredity persisted even until the early part of the twentieth century. We now know that the idea contains some truth. For example, ionizing radiation, many chemicals, and infection by some viruses can cause heritable changes, or mutations, but generally those changes are entirely random and cannot be directed toward specific outcomes.

One of the more remarkable theories about human inheritance, pangenesis, was developed in about the fifth century B.C. and espoused by Hippocrates and his followers. According to that theory, semen was formed in every part of the male body and traveled through the blood vessels to the testicles, which were merely repositories. Variations of the theory lasted well into the ninteenth

century A.D. and were even accepted by Charles Darwin. Pangenesis was for some reason dominant in the thinking of the philosophers and theologians of the Middle Ages. Albertus Magnus (1193–1280), his pupil Thomas Aquinas (1225–1274), and the naturalist Roger Bacon (circa 1220–1294) all accepted pangenesis as a fact. One variant of the theory was the idea that both male and female produced semen. According to Paracelsus (1493–1541), semen was an extract of the human body containing all the human organs in an ideal form and was thus a physical link between successive generations.

Also prevalent during the Middle Ages was the concept of entelechy, the Aristotelian idea that the way an individual develops is determined by a vital, inner force. The determining force is provided by the male and transmitted in his semen. The female provides no semen but only, so to speak, raw material. Aristotle compared the roles of male and female in the creation of an offspring with the roles of sculptor and stone in the creation of a sculpture.

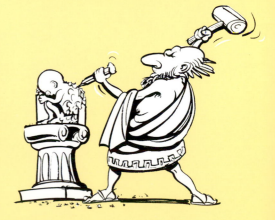

Other forms of vitalism continued to be popular even up to the beginning of the twentieth century primarily because people lacked knowledge about the nature of the physical connection between generations of animals and plants.

3

With his naked eye Harvey could see no form in a newly laid, fertilized chicken egg. But he assumed the form that did appear later arose epigenetically from matter that has some sort of inherent, though invisible, organization. The theory of epigenesis—that an organism arises from structural elaboration of formless matter rather than by enlargement of a preformed entity—dates back to Aristotle, but Harvey differed from Aristotle in seriously doubting that the living can arise from the nonliving. Experimental justification for his doubt came about a century later.

Thoughts about heredity would probably not have advanced beyond Harvey's had it not been for the compound microscope, an invention credited sometimes to Zaccharias Janssen and sometimes to Galileo. Other Renaissance men noted for their discoveries with the microscope and improvements to its design are regarded as the founders of microscopy: Nehemiah Grew (1641–1712), Robert Hooke (1635–1703), Antoni van Leeuwenhoek (1632–1723), Marcello Malpighi (1628–1694), and Jan Swammerdam (1637–1680). Their observations—among which were sperms in semen and structural elements, dubbed cells by Hooke, in plant and animal tissues—formed the foundations of the science now called cell biology.

Users of the early, low-resolution microscopes could (and did) let their imaginations run wild. Some thought they saw miniature humans, homunculi, preformed in human sperms; others saw tiny animals, animalcula, preformed in animal eggs. Those apparitions led to resurrection of the theory of preformation originally propounded by Democritus and other Greeks. In the eighteenth century the preformation theory developed into the encapsulation theory, which stated that, at the time of creation, all future generations were packaged, one inside the other, within the primordial egg or sperm. Logically, all life would come to an end when the last homunculus or animalculum was born. The encapsulation theory died—because it was ridiculous—although many eminent biologists were its fierce advocates up to the beginning of the nineteenth century.

The higher-resolution microscopes of the later half of the eighteenth century allowed Caspar Friedrich Wolff (1734–1794) to observe the development of chicken embryos. His work clearly showed that the components of a new organism are not preformed but, as stated two millenia before by Aristotle and a century before by Harvey, arise from the undifferentiated matter of the fertilized egg.

The Great Awakening

Modern biology may be said to have been born in the nineteenth century, several hundred years after the beginnings of modern chemistry and physics. Earlier biologists were either physicians or naturalists (what we now call botanists and zoologists), and their work focused on structure, physiology, and classification. But the nineteenth century brought several developments that were basic to emergence of the newer branches of biology, including cell biology and genetics.

The Rise of Cell Biology. During the first half of the nineteenth century, evidence accumulated for the so-called cell theory, which states that the cell is the structural and functional unit of all organisms. The diversity of cell shapes and sizes was noted (see "The Variety of Cells"), and various intracellular structures were observed (see "Components of Eukaryotic Cells"). Of particular importance to genetics is the membrane-bound intracellular structure called the nucleus, which was found to be a common feature of the cells of all organisms more complex than bacteria and blue-green algae. Organisms possessing a nucleus were classified as eukaryotes, and organisms lacking a nucleus were classified as prokaryotes.

Later, during the early 1850s, came the momentous finding, embraced in the aphorism *omnis cellula e cellula*, that cells divide to form new cells. A leading proponent of the idea that all cells come from cells was the German physician Rudolph Virchow (1821–1902). A cancer specialist, among other things, Virchow asserted that cancer cells arise from cells pre-existing in the body and do not, as earlier physicians had thought, arise by spontaneous generation from unorganized matter.

Another development was the realization that gametes (sperms and eggs) are also cells, in particular cells specialized for transmitting information from one generation of a sexually reproducing organism to the next. The remarkable difference in size between sperms and eggs was found to be due to cell components other than their nuclei, and that observation, coupled with the belief that sperms and eggs contain the same amount of hereditary information, indicated that hereditary information resides in the nuclei of gametes. The nucleus was found to be the site also of the information transmitted from one cellular generation to the next.

The above developments led to formulation of the law of genetic continuity, which succinctly summarizes what was probably the most important advance toward the understanding of living systems up to that time: Life comes only from life through the medium of cells.

By the late 1880s hereditary information had been localized further to intranuclear elements that can be seen with the microscope during the mitotic phase of the cell cycle, the phase that culminates in cell division (see "The Eukaryotic Cell Cycle"). The elements, which were named chromosomes because they can be stained (selectively colored) with certain dyes, are most easily observed during the portion of the mitotic phase called metaphase. (We now know that each "metaphase chromosome" consists of two duplicates of a single chromosome bound together along a more or less central region.)

Facts accumulated about chromosomes (see "Chromosomes: The Sites of Hereditary Information"). All the somatic cells (cells other than gametes) of a sexually reproducing organism have the same even number of chromosomes, the so-called diploid number, whereas all its gametes have the same so-called haploid number of chromosomes, which is exactly one-half the diploid number. Furthermore, the diploid and

THE VARIETY OF CELLS

Cells vary in shape from the
most simple to the indescribably
complex. Shown here are electron
micrographs of a few examples
from nature's cornucopia.

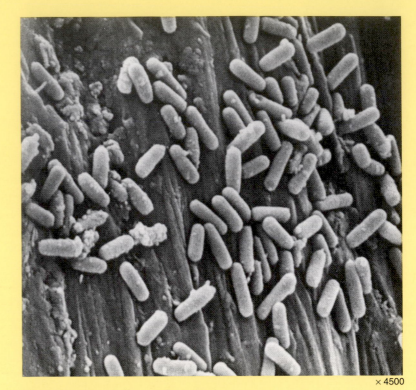

× 4500

Escherichia coli, **the most studied
of all bacteria**

From *Molecular Biology of the Cell,* second
edition, by Bruce Alberts et al. Copyright 1989
by Garland Publishing, Inc. Reprinted with
permission. Courtesy of Tony Brain and
the Science Photo Library.

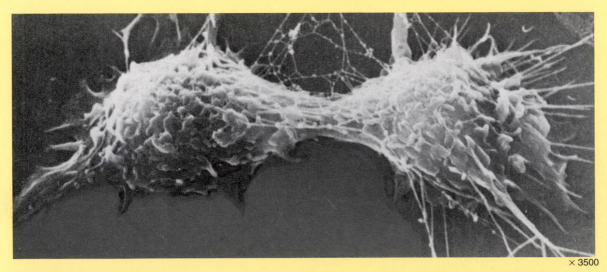

× 3500

**Mouse fibroblast during the
final stage of cell division**

From *Molecular Biology of the Cell,*
second edition, by Bruce Alberts et al.
Copyright 1989 by Garland Publishing, Inc.
Reprinted with permission. Courtesy of
Guenter Albrecht-Buehler.

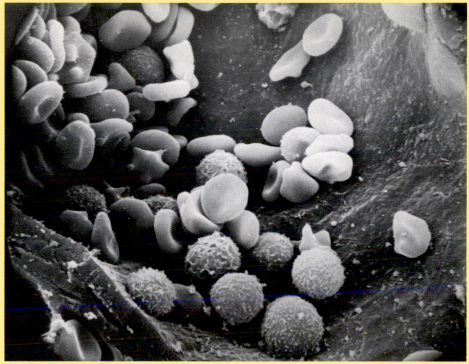

Human red blood cells (biconcave) and white blood cells (rounded)

From *Tissues and Organs: A Text-Atlas of Scanning Electron Microscopy* by Richard G. Kessel and Randy H. Kardon. Copyright 1979 by W. H. Freeman and Company. Reprinted with permission. Courtesy of Richard G. Kessel.

× 3000

× 450

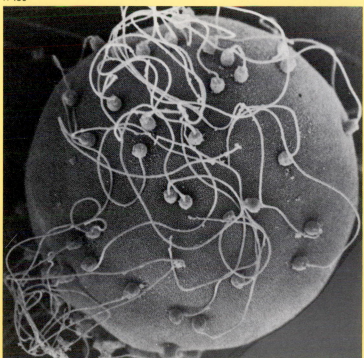

A clam egg with many sperms bound to its surface

From *Molecular Biology of the Cell*, second edition, by Bruce Alberts et al. Copyright 1989 by Garland Publishing, Inc. Reprinted with permission. Courtesy of David Epel.

COMPONENTS OF EUKARYOTIC CELLS

Eukaryotic cells, unlike prokaryotic cells, possess membrane-bound internal structures called organelles. The organelles common to eukaryotic plant and animal cells include mitochondria (the sites of energy production by oxidation of nutrients), a Golgi apparatus (where various macromolecules are modified, sorted, and packaged for secretion from the cell or for distribution to other organelles), an endoplasmic reticulum (the principal site of protein synthesis), and a nucleus (the residence of chromosomes and the site of DNA replication and transcription). The nucleolus is the site of ribosomal-RNA synthesis. The organelles unique to plant cells are chloroplasts (the sites of photosynthesis in green plants) and vacuoles (water-filled compartments that serve as space fillers and as storage vessels). Plant cells differ from animal cells also in being surrounded by a cellulose cell wall, a much more rigid form of the extracellular matrix that surrounds animal cells.

Figure adapted (with permission) from an illustration in *Genes and Genomes* by Maxine Singer and Paul Berg (University Science Books, 1991).

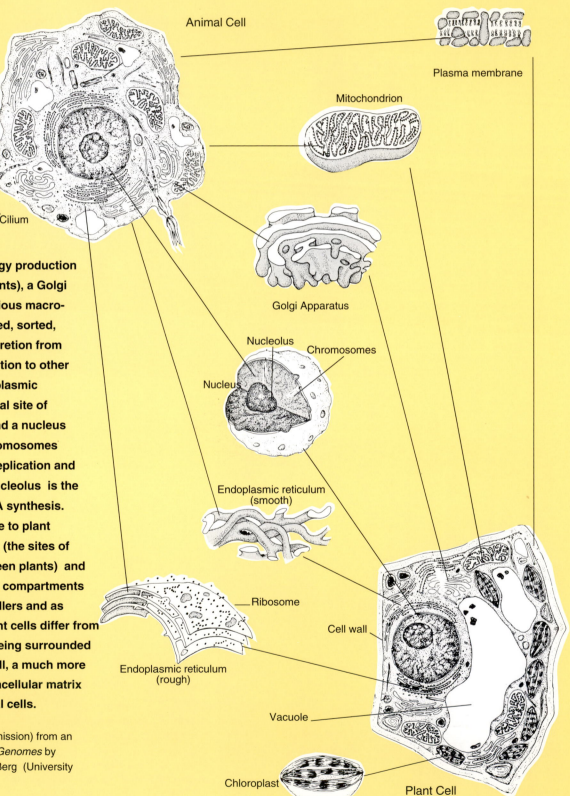

Animal Cell

Plasma membrane

Mitochondrion

Golgi Apparatus

Nucleolus

Chromosomes

Nucleus

Endoplasmic reticulum (smooth)

Cilium

Ribosome

Cell wall

Endoplasmic reticulum (rough)

Vacuole

Chloroplast

Plant Cell

THE EUKARYOTIC CELL CYCLE

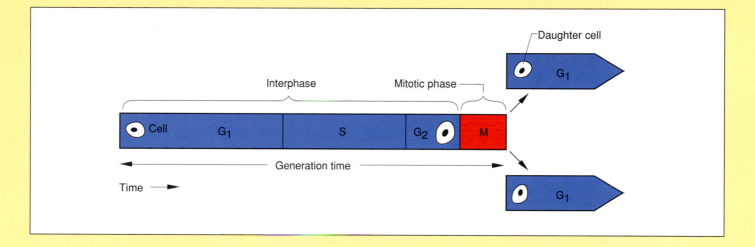

The term "cell cycle" refers collectively to the events that occur within a eukaryotic cell between its birth by mitosis and its division, again by mitosis, into two daughter cells. The cell may be either a one-celled organism such as baker's yeast (*Saccharomyces cerevisiae*) or a somatic cell of a multicellular organism. Early studies of the eukaryotic cell cycle concentrated on the microscopically visible and dramatic physical events of the cell-division, or mitotic, phase (M). Onset of the mitotic phase is signaled by the appearance of microscopically visible worm-like bodies within the nucleus, that is, by the condensation of duplicated chromosomes into a much less diffuse configuration. The mitotic phase ends when the cell separates into two daughter cellls, each of which then embarks on its own cycle. (Details of the mitotic phase are presented in "Mitosis.")

Because the early microscopic studies revealed little physical activity during the portion of the cell cycle that precedes the mitotic phase (other than a relatively small increase in cell size), that portion was inappropriately named the resting phase, or interphase. We now know that most of the biosynthetic activity required of a cell—both for its own maintenance and reproduction and for its function or functions as a constituent of a multicellular organism—occurs during interphase.

Most of the biochemicals produced by a cell are synthesized throughout interphase. DNA is a notable and easily detected exception, and for that reason interphase is subdivided into the period between cell birth and the onset of DNA synthesis (G_1), the period of DNA synthesis (S), which ends when all the nuclear DNA has been replicated and hence the number of chromosomes has doubled, and the period between the end of DNA synthesis and the beginning of the mitotic phase (G_2). After a cell has entered S, it is committed to completing the cell cycle, even when environmental conditions are extremely adverse.

The length of the cell cycle, the generation time, varies with environmental conditions and among species and cell types. For example, epithelial cells, the cells that line the interior and exterior surfaces of the human body, have relatively short generation times (about eight hours); fibroblasts, cells that assist in healing wounds, complete their cell cycle only on demand; mature red blood cells never undergo mitosis; and embryonic cells divide very rapidly. Observed generation times for those cells that do have a regular cycle range from about a few minutes to a few months. The variation in generation time is due mainly to a variation in the length of G_1 and of G_2. The mitotic phase of most species and most cell types occupies only about 10 percent of the generation time.

The cell cycle of bacteria, in addition to being shorter (typically less than an hour), is also less complex. In particular, DNA is synthesized continuously, the two copies of the single bacterial chromosome do not undergo extensive condensation before cell division, and a mechanism simpler than the one illustrated in "Mitosis" assures parceling out of one chromosome copy to each daughter cell.

CHROMOSOMES: the sites of hereditary information

Within the nucleus of each cell of a eukaryotic organism are a number of chromosomes, each composed of a single molecule of DNA (see "DNA: Its Structure and Components") and a roughly equal mass of proteins (primarily the proteins called histones). The DNA molecule carries hereditary information; the proteins help effect the ordered condensation, or compaction, of the very long, very thin DNA molecule. During most of a cell's life, its chromosomes are too decondensed to be visible with an optical microscope. However, during metaphase, a phase preparatory to cell division (see "Mitosis" and "Meiosis"), the chromosomes become highly condensed and hence easily visible. Most studies of chromosomes are therefore carried out on chromosomes extracted from cells arrested at metaphase. Each such "metaphase chromosome" consists in reality of two duplicates of a single chromosome bound together along a somewhat constricted region called a centromere. The three micrographs of metaphase chromosomes shown here illustrate some general facts about chromosomes.

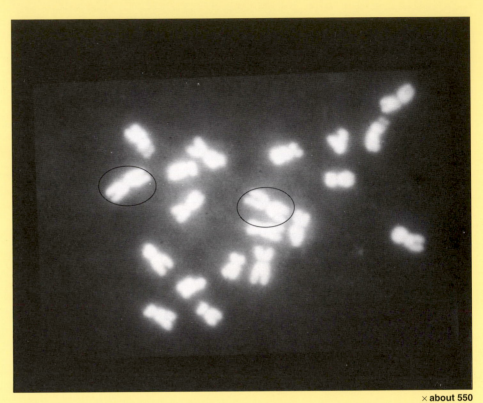

× **about 550**

Shown above are the metaphase chromosomes extracted from a root-tip cell of maize (*Zea mays*). The chromosomes were stained with a fluorescent dye and photographed through an optical microscope while being illuminated by a laser that excites the dye's fluorescence. (The chromosomes could have been stained instead with a nonfluorescent dye.) A total of twenty metaphase chromosomes is visible in the micrograph, and any somatic cell (any cell other than an egg or a sperm) of any *Zea mays* plant possesses that same number of metaphase chromosomes. In general, all the somatic cells of all the members of a species possess the same even number of metaphase chromosomes, called the diploid chromosome number. The diploid chromosome number varies erratically from species to species: the known values range from 2 to many hundreds. (Note that the diploid chromosome number is not a measure of a species' evolutionary status.) The twenty metaphase chromosomes of *Zea mays* obviously exhibit different morphologies, that is, different sizes and centromere positions. However, even the untrained observer might notice that the two highlighted metaphase chromosomes look very much alike. In fact, the twenty metaphase chromosomes of *Zea mays* can be grouped into ten homologous, or morphologically indistinguishable, pairs. The metaphase chromosomes of all eukaryotic species occur as homologous pairs, and that general fact is due to the occurrence of chromosomes themselves as homologous pairs. Furthermore, the homology of a pair of chromosomes is due to a high degree of similarity between the base sequences of their constituent DNA molecules. (Micrograph courtesy of Paul Jackson and Jérôme Conia.)

Shown at right are the metaphase chromosomes extracted from a somatic cell of a house mouse (*Mus musculus*). To help identify homologous pairs, the chromosomes were stained with a dye called Giemsa that produces a pattern of dark and light bands, a pattern that varies from one homologous pair to another. The chromosome images have been grouped in homologous pairs and arranged in order of decreasing size. Such a display of metaphase chromosomes is called a karyotype. The last entry in the karyotype is the pair of chromosomes that are involved in determining sex. Because this particular mouse cell posseses two *homologous* sex chromosomes, it is a cell from a female mouse. Cells of a male mouse possess two nonhomologous sex chromosomes, one X chromosome and a smaller Y chromosome.

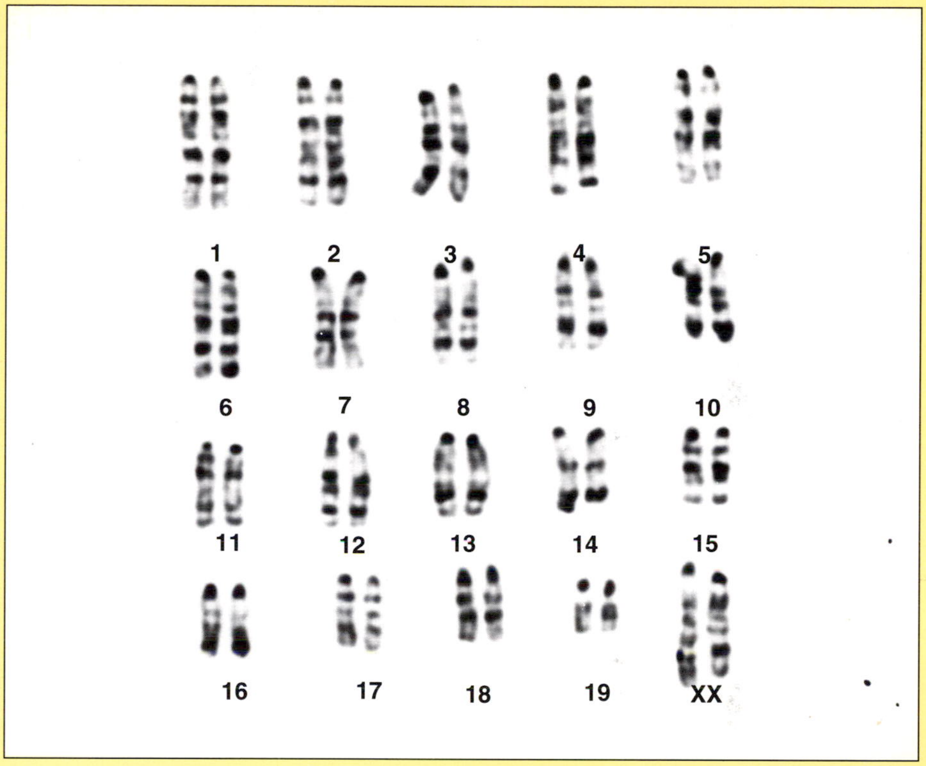

× **about 750**

× **about 650**

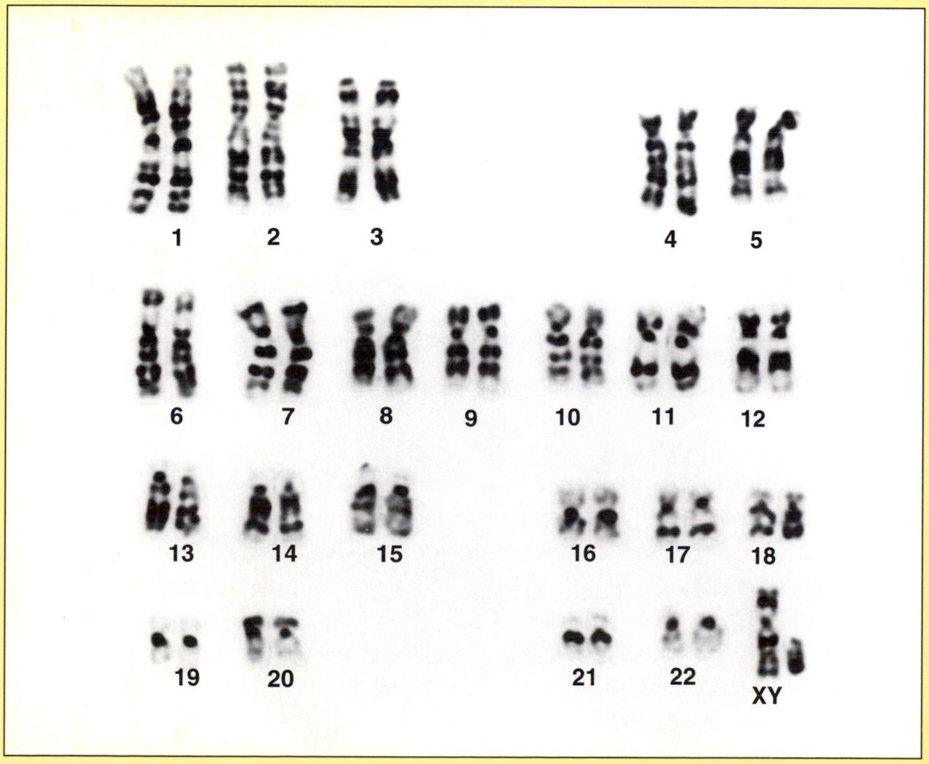

Shown at left is the karyotype of a human prepared from the Giemsa-stained metaphase chromosomes of a lymphocyte. Note the twenty-two homologous pairs of autosomes (chromosomes other than sex chromosomes) and the two nonhomologous sex chromosomes. The nonhomology of the sex chromosomes indicates that this is the karyotype of a male human, namely of the well-known cytogeneticist T. C. Hsu of the University of Texas System Cancer Center. (Both of the karyotypes on this page were provided by T. C. Hsu.)

haploid chromosome numbers are constant among different members of the same species but vary among different species. For example, all somatic cells of all members of the species *Homo sapiens* contain forty-six chromosomes, all somatic cells of all members of the species *Drosophila melanogaster* (a fruit fly) contain eight chromosomes, all somatic cells of all members of the species *Pisum sativum* (the garden pea) contain fourteen chromosomes, and all somatic cells of all members of the species *Mus musculus* (the house mouse) contain forty chromosomes. And all the gametes of all members of each of the above species contain twenty-three, four, seven, and twenty chromosomes, respectively. Second, the metaphase chromosomes within a single cell vary morphologically (in size and shape), but the variations remain constant among all cells of all members of a single species. (We now know that exceptions to the above generalizations occur and that the exceptions are often causes or symptoms of disease.)

The morphological differences among the metaphase chromosomes of a species led to recognition that metaphase chromosomes occur as morphologically indistinguishable (homologous) pairs. Although the members of a pair of homologous metaphase chromosomes are indistinguishable by any low-resolution physical technique, they do differ, as we now know, in fine details of the nucleotide sequences of their constituent DNA molecules. The occurrence of metaphase chromosomes as morphologically indistinguishable pairs is due to the occurrence of chromosomes themselves as homologous pairs, pairs whose constituent DNA molecules have nearly identical nucleotide sequences.

An exception to the occurrence of chromosomes as homologous pairs should be noted. Males of some species, including all mammals and *Drosophila melanogaster*, possess two chromosomes, called the X and Y chromosomes, that do not form a homologous pair, the Y chromosome generally being much smaller than the X chromosome. Females of such species possess two X chromosomes, each of which is homologous to the other and to the X chromosome of the male. Collectively, the X and Y chromosomes are called sex chromosomes; the remaining chromosomes are called autosomes. In the case of humans and other placental mammals, the presence of a Y chromosome is necessary for maleness (the presence of testes), but in the case of other species, including *D. melanogaster*, the presence of a Y chromosome, although necessary for fertility, is not necessary for maleness.

Also observed during the late nineteenth century were microscopic details of cell division and the effect of cell division on chromosomes. Mitosis, the type of cell division undergone by all somatic cells other than the immediate precursors of gametes, was found to yield two daughter somatic cells with the same diploid number of chromosomes as the mother cell (see "Mitosis"). Furthermore, the German zoologist Theodor Heinrich Boveri (1862–1915) found that the metaphase chromosomes of a mother cell and a daughter cell had the same morphologies. Those observations indicated that each chromosome in the mother cell is somehow duplicated before the cell undergoes mitosis.

Meiosis, the type of cell division undergone by the precursors of gametes, was found to be a much more complex process than mitosis. It involves two successive cell divisions and can yield four gametes each containing one-half the number of chromosomes as the precursor cell. (Thus meiosis also must be preceded by chromosome duplication.) Furthermore, the haploid set of chromosomes in each gamete is not a haphazard selection from the diploid set of the mother cell. Instead each gamete is endowed with a randomly selected member of each pair of homologous chromosomes in the mother cell (see "Meiosis"). That is, the probability of a gamete's being endowed with one member of a pair of homologous chromosomes is the same as the probability of its being endowed with the other member, and, equally important, the outcome of its endowment with a member of one pair of homologous chromosomes has no effect on the outcome of its endowment with a member of another pair. In other (and more arcane) words, meiosis equally segregates each pair of homologous chromosomes and independently assorts the complete set of homologous chromosomes.

The X chromosome and the Y chromosome of a male also were found to segregate equally during meiosis, even though they are not homologous in the sense of being physically indistinguishable. That fact implies that a male produces two equally probable sperm types, one containing a Y chromosome and the other an X chromosome. Thus fertilization of an egg by a sperm results in two equally probable combinations of sex chromosomes, XY and XX.

The equal segregation and independent assortment of chromosomes during meiosis leads to diversity among the chromosome sets of the offspring of sexually reproducing organisms. Consider, for example, an organism that possesses but two pairs of homologous chromosomes denoted by 1 and 1' and 2 and 2'. Such an organism produces, with equal probability, four types of gametes, those containing 1 and 2, 1 and 2', 1' and 2, and 1' and 2'. If the organism is self-fertilizing (as are many plants and lower animals), then of the sixteen possible types of offspring, only four possess a set of chromosomes identical to the parental set. In contrast, bacteria reproduce asexually by a type of cell division that, like mitosis, yields only genetic replicas of the mother cell. (Bacteria are not, however, genetically immutable, since various mechanisms can effect changes in their genetic material, which are then transmitted to their offspring.) In general, if a sexually reproducing organism has N pairs of homologous chromosomes, it can produce 2^N types of gametes, and if it is self-fertilizing, only 2^N of the 2^{2N} possible types of offspring possess a set of chromosomes identical to the parental set. In other words, the probability of an offspring's possessing a set of chromosomes identical to the parental set is $1/2^N$. When N equals twenty-three, that probability equals 1/8,388,608, a very small number. The probability of human parents producing an offspring with a set of chromosomes identical to that of either parent is even closer to zero, since although humans do possess twenty-three pairs of equally segregating and independently assorting chromosomes, they are not of course self-fertilizing. Discussed later is a process that leads to even more differences among the chromosome sets of sexually

MITOSIS

Mitosis is the type of cell division that produces two daughter cells from a single mother cell. Each daughter cell has a set of chromosomes identical to the set possessed by the mother cell. Mitosis is the mechanism whereby a multicellular organism increases in size and replaces dead cells and whereby single-celled eukaryotic organisms reproduce asexually. The interested reader can find a striking series of photomicrographs of mitosis in the lily *Haemanthus katherinae* on page 7 of *Genes and Genomes: A Changing Perspective* by Maxine Singer and Paul Berg (University Science Books, 1991).

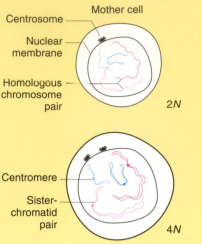

Centrosome
Mother cell
Nuclear membrane
Homologous chromosome pair
2N

Centromere
Sister-chromatid pair
4N

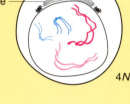
Mitotic spindle
Microtubule
4N

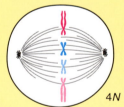
4N

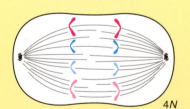
4N

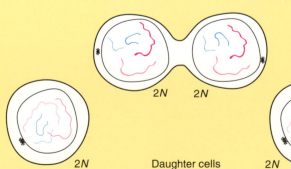
2N   2N

2N   Daughter cells   2N

INTERPHASE

G_1—During G_1 (see "The Eukaryotic Cell Cycle") the chromosomes of the mother cell are very long and very thin. Only two of the cell's *N* pairs of homologous chromosomes are shown, and the members of each homologous pair are depicted in different shades of the same color. The centrosome is the source of fibrous proteins called microtubules. One function of microtubules is to direct the motion of chromosomes during mitosis (and meiosis).

G_2—The mother cell has replicated its complement of chromosomes (during the preceding S phase) and all other cellular material required for cell division, including the centrosome. The two identical copies of each chromosome are bound together along their centromeres into a so-called sister-chromatid pair.

MITOTIC PHASE

Prophase
The onset of mitosis is signaled by the ordered compaction, or condensation, of chromosomes into microscopically visible threads. Microtubules radiating from the two centrosomes collectively compose the mitotic spindle.

Prometaphase
The chromosomes have condensed further, and the centrosomes have migrated to opposite sides of the cell. Disintegration of the nuclear membrane has allowed microtubules to bind to each chromosome at a region within its centromere.

Metaphase
The chromosomes have assumed their most condensed configuration, and the sister-chromatid pairs have assumed the familiar X shape. Under the influence of opposing forces exerted by microtubules radiating from both centrosomes, each sister-chromatid pair has become aligned along the midplane of the cell.

Anaphase
The bond joining each sister-chromatid pair has broken, and the members of each former sister-chromatid pair have begun moving toward opposite sides of the cell. As a result, a set of chromosomes identical to the set initially possessed by the mother cell becomes segregated in each side of the cell. The cell has begun to elongate and narrow at the midplane.

Telophase
A new nuclear membrane has formed around each segregated set of chromosomes, the chromosomes have begun to decondense, and the cell has begun to divide.

INTERPHASE

G_1—Cleavage of the extranuclear cellular material has produced two daughter cells, and the chromosomes in each have decondensed further in preparation for the biosynthetic activities of G_1.

MEIOSIS

Meiosis is the type of cell division that produces the gametes (eggs and sperms) whose union is the first step in the creation of a new human or other sexually reproducing organism. Only so-called germ-line cells undergo meiosis, and each gamete contains a haploid set of chromosomes—a set composed of one member of each of the N pairs of homologous chromosomes possessed by the diploid germ-line cell. The transition from diploidy to haploidy is accomplished by two successive partitions of nuclear material. During each partition the motions of the chromosomes are directed, as they are during mitosis, by microtubules radiating from two centrosomes.

PREMEIOTIC PHASE

The germ-line cell, whch may be an oogonium in an ovary or a spermatogonium in a testis, appears little different from a somatic cell in G_i. Only two of the germ-line cell's N pairs of homologous chromosomes are shown, and the members of each homologous pair are depicted in different shades of the same color.

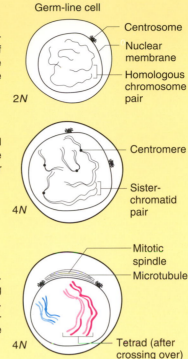

Germ-line cell
- Centrosome
- Nuclear membrane
- Homologous chromosome pair

2N

The germ-line cell has replicated its complement of chromosomes and all other cellular material required for cell division, including the centrosome. The two identical copies of each chromosome are bound together along their centromeres into a sister-chromotid pair.

- Centromere
- Sister-chromatid pair

4N

MEIOTIC PHASE

Prophase I

The onset of meiosis is signaled by a limited condensation of chromosomes. Homologous sister-chromatid pairs have become closely associated, forming N tetrads and allowing "crossing over" to occur, here within both tetrads. Crossing over results in the exchange of corresponding portions of homologous chromosomes. The germ-line cell now lingers in prophase I for a time that ranges, depending on the species, from a few days to many years.

- Mitotic spindle
- Microtubule

4N

- Tetrad (after crossing over)

Metaphase I

The germ-line cell has passed through prometaphase I (not shown) and has entered metaphase I. The chromosomes have fully condensed, and the tetrads have become aligned along the midplane of the cell.

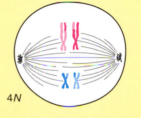

4N

Anaphase I

The members of each tetrad have separated and begun moving toward opposite sides of the cell. Depicted here is but one of the $2N$ possible outcomes of the motion of the members of the N tetrads. The equal probability of each possible outcome is the physical basis for Mendel's laws of equal segregation and independent assortment.

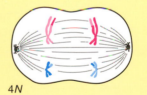

4N

Prophase II

The germ-line cell has passed through telophase I (not shown) and has divided into two cells, each of which has entered prophase II. Note that the products of the first meiotic division, like the products of mitosis, have the same number of chromosomes as the original cell. However, a product of mitosis contains N homologous chromosome pairs, whereas a product of the first meiotic division contains two identical copies of each of N nonhomologous chromosomes.

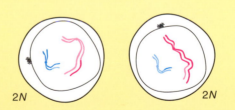

2N   2N

Anaphase II

Both cells have passed through prometaphase II and metaphase II (not shown). Each sister-chromatid pair has separated, and the members of each former sister-chromatid pair have begun migrating to opposite sides of the cell.

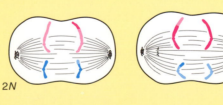

2N   2N

POSTMEIOTIC PHASE

Each cell has passed through telophase II (not shown) and divided into two gametes. Thus each meiosis can yield four gametes. However, meiosis of an oogonium usually yields only one egg because each division of extranuclear material usually yields only one cell that survives because it receives most of the extranuclear material.

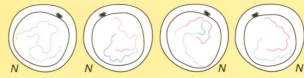

N   N   N   N

Gametes

reproducing organisms and their offspring: the "crossing over" that occurs between homologous chromosomes during the first stage of meiosis (see "Meiosis"). Together, crossing over and equal segregation and independent assortment essentially guarantee that in the whole history of *Homo sapiens*, no two individuals (except the pairs of identical twins arising from single fertilized eggs) have been alike genetically.

The facts that accumulated about chromosomes and their behavior during mitosis and meiosis suggested that the link between generations (of cells or organisms) was a substance present in chromosomes. In 1896 the American cell biologist Edmund Beecher Wilson (1856–1939) suggested that the substance of inheritance was the "nuclein" isolated in 1874 by the Swiss chemist Johann Friedrich Miescher (1844–1895) from the nuclei of human pus cells and salmon sperms. Nuclein was found to be composed of two types of chemicals, a nucleic acid and various "albumins," or proteins. By the end of the century, the most advanced thinkers about the mechanism of inheritance, such as Wilson, Boveri, and August Friedrich Leopold Weismann (1834–1915), were of the opinion that nuclein was the stuff of inheritance.

A Theory of Inheritance. The nineteenth century was the setting also for the elegant work of the Austrian Gregor Johann Mendel (1822–1884), an Augustinian monk better versed in mathematics and physics than in biology. In 1865 Mendel published visionary explanations for the results of his plant-breeding experiments. Among them was the notion that discrete units of heredity (which he called *Merkmale* and we call genes) are passed unchanged from generation to generation even though each unit is not necessarily expressed as an observable trait in every generation. He also proposed that each plant possesses two such units for each observable trait, one inherited from its male parent and the other from its female parent. Mendel developed statistical laws for predicting how the paired units of heredity are parceled out to offspring. The laws are now known to be applicable (within certain limits) to all sexually reproducing organisms. Furthermore, Mendel's laws parallel the behavior of homologous chromosome pairs during meiosis (the equal segregation of a single chromosome pair and the independent assortment of different chromosome pairs) because, as we now know, Mendel's units of heredity reside on chromosomes. Remarkably, Mendel deduced his theory *before* chromosomes were identified as the probable carriers of genetic information. His proposals are discussed here out of chronological order because their significance to the emerging science of genetics was not grasped—and probably could not have been grasped—until after the observed behavior of chromosomes during meiosis could provide a physical basis for his abstract theory. Mendel's publication remained unknown, in fact, until 1900 when, working independently, the German botanist Karl Erich Correns (1864–1933), the Dutch botanist Hugo De Vries (1848–1935), and the Austrian botanist Erich Tschermak von Seysenegg (1871–1962) performed similar experiments, arrived at similar explanations, and brought Mendel's publication to light, garnering him well-deserved albeit posthumous fame.

To best appreciate Mendel's work, one needs to know something about the successes and shortcomings of previous efforts at selective breeding of plants and animals. Selective breeding was certainly well under way in the Neolithic period, and numerous early successes produced most of the strains of domestic plants and animals now in existence. Some of the plant-breeding efforts led to plants so different from their ancestral relatives that they can be considered human-made species. Notable examples are today's *Zea mays* (maize, or corn) and *Solanum tuberosum* (the potato plant). Natives of present-day Mexico began developing maize from tiny-eared relatives between 4000 and 5000 years ago, and the pre-Columbian inhabitants of present-day Peru and Bolivia developed a plant producing palatable tubers from relatives producing tubers so bitter as to be inedible. When introduced into the Old World in the sixteenth century, maize and the potato had a tremendous influence on the world's economy. The potato, for example, replaced wheat and rye in the cool areas of northern Europe as a staple food because it produces more calories per acre. (Only rice is as efficient a calorie-producer as the potato, and rice is a warm-climate plant.) The introduction of maize and the potato is thought by some historians to have significantly accelerated the great increase in the rate of population growth of western Europe that began in about the fourteenth century.

Successful as the early breeding efforts were, and those of the noted eighteenth-century plant breeders Josef Gottlieb Koelreuter (1733–1806) and Joseph Gaertner (1732–1791), they certainly were not what we would now call scientific, since in general the outcomes of breedings were quite unpredictable. In contrast, Mendel's aim at the outset of his eight-year effort was to ascertain the statistical rules governing the inheritance of variable traits. Both his methodology and his theoretical conclusions are the foundation for all future studies in genetics.

Mendel chose to work with a plant that exhibits distinct variants of a number of traits, the garden pea (*Pisum sativum*). He concentrated on two variants of each of seven traits, including pod color (green and yellow) and flower color (violet and white). His unique experimental approach began by allowing plants that bore, say, green pods to self-pollinate for a sufficient number of generations to assure that each new generation of self-pollinated plants would also bear only green pods. Since each of the fourteen purebred strains consistently bore only one variant of each of a single trait, the purebred strains were advantageous to Mendel's work, providing a certain and observable starting point and amounting, essentially, to a control on his experiments. Mendel proceeded to study the inheritance of each of the seven traits, first one at a time and then in pairs. All of the experiments on the inheritance of single traits followed the same pattern as that described here for pod color.

First, Mendel cross-pollinated the two strains purebred for pod color, the strain bred true for green pods and the strain bred true for yellow pods. (Together the two purebred strains are called the parental generation.) Regardless of which strain he used as the male (pollen-contributing) parent, all the resulting offspring (called here hybrids or members of the first generation) bore only green pods. Today we would say that all members of the first generation exhibited the same phenotype, a term introduced in 1909 by the Danish botanist Wilhelm Ludwig Johannsen (1857–1927). Symbolically,

$$\text{parental generation} \rightarrow \text{first generation,}$$

and in particular,

$$\text{purebred green} \times \text{purebred yellow} \rightarrow \text{hybrids, all green.}$$

The natural question to ask is: Has the capacity to produce the yellow-pod phenotype disappeared altogether, or is it still present but somehow suppressed in the first-generation hybrids? To find out, Mendel selfed the hybrids (that is, he allowed them to self-pollinate), and he observed that the yellow-pod phenotype reappeared among the resulting offspring (the second generation). When Mendel counted the number of second-generation offspring exhibiting each phenotype (a novel procedure at the time), he found that the ratio of green-podded plants to yellow-podded plants was approximately 3 to 1. Symbolically,

$$\text{first generation} \rightarrow \text{second generation}$$

and in particular,

$$\text{green hybrid} \times \text{green hybrid} \rightarrow \text{3 green : 1 yellow.}$$

To find out whether any members of the second generation had the capacity to produce offspring with the phenotype they themselves did not exhibit, Mendel selfed the members of the second generation. He found that all the yellow-podded members behaved like plants purebred for yellow pod color; that is, they produced only yellow-podded offspring. In contrast, only one-third of the green-podded members of the second generation behaved like plants purebred for green pod color, whereas the remaining two-thirds behaved like the first-generation hybrids, producing both green- and yellow-podded progeny in the ratio of 3 to 1. In other words, the ratio 3 green:1 yellow exhibited by the second generation is more accurately described as the ratio 1 pure green:2 hybrid green:1 pure yellow. Mendel continued selfing the green-podded members of successive generations and always found that approximately two-thirds of the green-podded progeny of green hybrids were again green hybrids, behaving just like the first-generation hybrids. That is, when those two-thirds were allowed to self-pollinate, they produced green- and yellow-podded progeny in the approximate ratio of 3 to 1.

To explain the mathematical regularity of his results, Mendel advanced a theoretical model of inheritance. First, and most basic, is the idea that the fertilized egg (zygote) from which a plant develops contains two genes, or units of heredity, for pod color, one contributed by the egg and the other contributed by the sperm. ("Gene" is another term coined by Johannsen.) Mendel also proposed that there were two distinct genes for pod color, one for green and one for yellow. The gene for green pod color he called dominant (and designated it by a capital letter, say P) because any plant that carried that gene bore green pods. The gene for yellow pod color he called recessive (and designated it by a lowercase letter, *p*). Today we say *P* and *p* are different forms, or alleles, of the gene for pod color. Since the egg and sperm each contain only one allele, a fertilized egg contains one of three possible allele pairs (or possesses one of three possible genotypes, another word coined by Johanssen): *PP, Pp,* or *pp.* Mendel proposed that the plants purebred for green pod color contained the pair *PP*, those purebred for yellow pod color contained the pair *pp*, and the hybrid plants, which bore only green pods but produced both green- and yellow-podded progeny when allowed to self-pollinate, contained the pair *Pp.* In modern terminology plants possessing the genotype *PP* are said to be homozygous dominant; those possessing the genotype *pp* are homozygous recessive; and those with the genotype *Pp* are heterozygous. This terminology and other nomenclature of genetics is illustrated in the table.

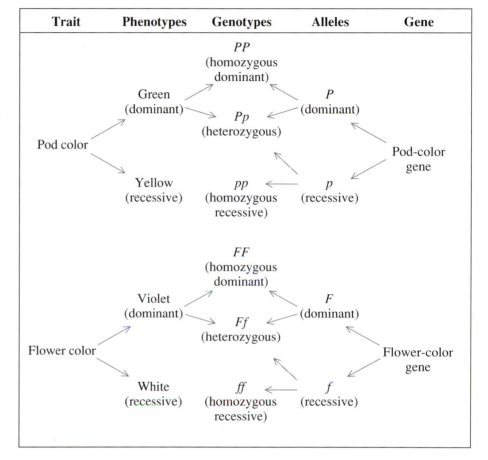

Trait	Phenotypes	Genotypes	Alleles	Gene
Pod color	Green (dominant)	*PP* (homozygous dominant), *Pp* (heterozygous)	*P* (dominant)	Pod-color gene
	Yellow (recessive)	*pp* (homozygous recessive)	*p* (recessive)	
Flower color	Violet (dominant)	*FF* (homozygous dominant), *Ff* (heterozygous)	*F* (dominant)	Flower-color gene
	White (recessive)	*ff* (homozygous recessive)	*f* (recessive)	

With those hypotheses and the laws of probability Mendel constructed a probabilistic model that explained the results of his experiments. The model is shown in "Mendelian Genetics." The element of chance is operative in both the formation of gametes (eggs and sperms) and in the formation of zygotes (fertilized eggs). Mendel assumed that during the formation of gametes, the pair of alleles for pod color separates (or segregates) equally; in other words, the probability that a gamete will receive one or the other of the pair is equal to one-half. He therefore predicted correctly that among the gametes produced by a green hybrid (a plant heterozygous for pod color), approximately one-half would contain *P* and the remainder would contain *p*. Because, as is now known, each member of the allele pair for a given trait resides at the same location on one or the other of a pair of homologous, equally segregating chromosomes, only one allele enters each gamete. Therefore, the behavior of a single allele pair during meiosis is known as Mendel's law of equal segregation.

The element of chance is also operative in the random union of an egg and a sperm to form a zygote with a particular genotype. For example, in the formation of offspring of the green hybrids, the probability of forming a zygote with the genotype *PP*, call it Pr(*PP*), is the joint probability of two independent events, namely, the probability that an egg contains P, and the probability that a sperm contains P. Since the joint probability is the product of the probabilities of the two independent events, we can write $\Pr(PP) = \Pr(P)\Pr(P)$.

Mendel applied this rule to predict the probability of finding a given genotype among the progeny of the green hybrids. Since green hybrids produce gametes containing P or p, each with a probability of 1/2, the eggs and sperms combine in four equally probable ways to produce offspring with the genotypes PP, Pp, pP, or pp, and the probability of each of those genotypes is 1/2 times 1/2, or 1/4. Since Pp and pP are equivalent genotypes (it doesn't matter whether a particular allele arrived with the sperm or the egg), the probabilities for Pp and pP are added to predict that the probability of an offspring's having the genotype Pp is 1/2. In other words, the three possible genotypes occur in the ratio 1 PP:2 Pp:1pp. Translating the genotypes into phenotypes yields the ratio 3 green:1 yellow in agreement with Mendel's observations.

Having explained the 3 green:1 yellow ratio by advancing a general model, Mendel went on to test the model by crossing green hybrids (genotype Pp) with plants purebred for yellow pod color (genotype pp). He predicted that the offspring would have the genotypes Pp and pp in the ratio 1 Pp:1 pp and found, in agreement with the model, that approximately one-half the progeny bore green pods and the remainder bore yellow pods.

Mendel obtained similar results for all seven traits. In other words, he inferred the existence of two alleles for each trait, one dominant and one recessive. However, we now know that the alleles of a gene do not always exhibit a dominant-recessive relationship. Sometimes the pairing of different alleles leads to a blend (for example, pairing of the snapdragon alleles that specify white and red flowers leads to pink flowers); sometimes it leads to simultaneous exhibition of both phenotypes (for example, pairing of the human alleles that specify A and B blood types, which are characterized by the presence of the antigens A and B, respectively, on the surface of red blood cells, leads to AB blood type, which is characterized by the presence of both antigens). However, the validity of Mendel's research and theoretical conclusions is unaffected by the fact that he focused, presumably by chance, on traits controlled by alleles that do exhibit the phenomenon of dominance.

Mendel next proceeded to study the co-inheritance of two traits, say pod color (specified by dominant and recessive alleles P and p, respectively) and flower color (specified by dominant and recessive alleles F and f, respectively). Again, he first developed two purebred strains, one purebred for green pod color and violet flower color (genotype $PPFF$) and the other purebred for yellow pod color and white flower color (genotype $ppff$).

As before, Mendel cross-pollinated the purebred strains, thus producing dihybrid offspring, each heterozygous for both traits. He selfed the resulting first dihybrid generation to produce the second dihybrid generation. Each member of the first dihybrid generation exhibited both dominant phenotypes; that is, they bore green pods and violet flowers. Members of the second dihybrid generation exhibited four composite phenotypes in a 9:3:3:1 ratio, as shown below.

Possible Phenotypes among Second Dihybrid Generation	Fraction Exhibiting Phenotype
green pods, violet flowers	$\frac{9}{16}$
green pods, white flowers	$\frac{3}{16}$
yellow pods, violet flowers	$\frac{3}{16}$
yellow pods, white flowers	$\frac{1}{16}$

Note that the ratio of green- to yellow-podded members of the second dihybrid generation was still 3 to 1, just as it was in the second generation produced by the experiments on pod color alone. The ratio of violet- to white-flowered members of the second dihybrid generation also was 3 to 1. Mendel realized that the 9:3:3:1 ratio resulted from multiplicative combinations of the two 3:1 ratios. He therefore concluded that the phenotypes for the two traits are inherited independently. In other words, the probability of each composite phenotype is the product of the probabilities of the two "component" (single-trait) phenotypes. For example, the probability that a second-dihybrid-generation member will bear green pods and white flowers (3/16) is the product of the probability of its bearing green pods (3/4) and the probability of its bearing white flowers (1/4).

The independent inheritance of the two traits implies that when members of the first dihybrid generation produce gametes, segregation of the alleles for pod color is independent of the segregation of the alleles for flower color. In other words, the two allele pairs assort independently. The members of the first dihybrid generation have the genotype $PpFf$, so each gamete receives P or p with a probability of 1/2 and F or f with a probability of 1/2. Since the segregation of each allele pair is an independent event, the individual probabilities are multiplied to predict that the probability of forming each of the four possible types of gametes, those containing PF, Pf, pF, or pf, is 1/2 times 1/2, or 1/4.

Random fertilization of eggs by sperms produces the sixteen genotypes shown in the probability table for the second dihybrid generation in "Mendelian Genetics." Each has a probability of 1/4 times 1/4, or 1/16. The composite phenotype corresponding to each genotype is also shown. Counting the number of times each phenotype appears yields the 9:3:3:1 ratio observed by Mendel.

The physical basis for Mendel's law of independent assortment is the independent assortment of the various different pairs of homologous chromosomes during meiosis.

MENDELIAN GENETICS

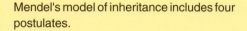

Mendel's experiments on the inheritance of single traits and pairs of traits, illustrated here, led him to postulate the concept of discrete, particulate units of heredity that pass unchanged from generation to generation. He studied seven traits (characteristics) of the garden pea, each of which exhibited two alternative forms. For example, pod color could be either green or yellow, and flower color could be either violet or white. As described in the main text, Mendel found that one form of each trait was dominant and the other recessive and that the progeny of controlled breedings exhibited one form or the other in definite ratios. The observed mathematical regularities led to the model of inheritance described here. Mendel knew that his plants reproduced sexually, but he did not know that chromosomes exist nor that the number of chromosomes was reduced by one-half during the formation of gametes. As a result his terminology was rather imprecise. He did not clearly distinguish the form of a trait from the units of heredity whose actions determine the trait. That distinction was made almost half a century later by Johannsen, who coined the term gene for the particulate units of heredity, the term genotype for the genes whose action determines a trait, and the term phenotype for the form of the trait determined by the genotype. The more precise terminology is used in the following description of Mendel's model and in the accompanying figures.

Mendel's model of inheritance includes four postulates.

1. Each plant contains a pair of genes for each trait; that is, the genotype for a trait is specified by a pair of genes.

2. During the formation of gametes, the gene pair for a trait segregates equally; that is, the genes in the pair are parceled out to the gametes in a fashion such that each gamete receives only one member of the pair and has an equal chance of receiving either member of the pair (the law of equal segregation).

3. A gene has two forms, or alleles, designated by, say, *A* and *a*. Only plants with the genotype *aa* (homozygous for *a*) exhibit the recessive phenotype. A plant with the genotype *AA* (homozygous for *A*) or the genotype *Aa* (heterozygous) exhibits the dominant phenotype.

4. During the formation of gametes, segregation of the gene pair for any one trait is independent of the segregation of the other gene pairs. Consequently a plant heterozygous for two traits (genotype *AaBb*) produces gametes containing *AB, Ab, aB,* and *ab* with equal probability (the law of independent assortment). Note that the law of independent assortment holds only if the genes for the different traits are on different pairs of homologous chromosomes.

Mendel's laws of equal segregation and independent assortment can be applied in two ways. If one knows the genotypes of both parents, one can predict the probability of the genotype of a future offspring. Or, working backward, if one observes in existing offspring the approximate ratios of phenotypes predicted by Mendel's laws, one can often infer the genotypes of the parents, just as Mendel did.

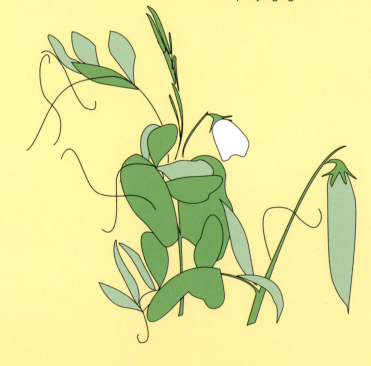

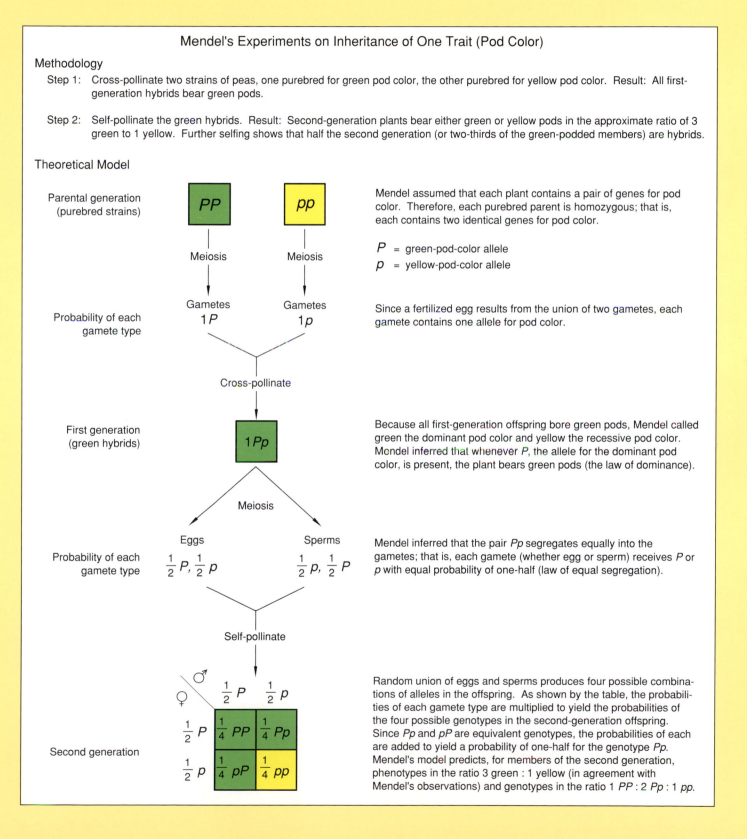

Mendel's Experiments on Inheritance of One Trait (Pod Color)

Methodology

Step 1:   Cross-pollinate two strains of peas, one purebred for green pod color, the other purebred for yellow pod color. Result: All first-generation hybrids bear green pods.

Step 2:   Self-pollinate the green hybrids. Result: Second-generation plants bear either green or yellow pods in the approximate ratio of 3 green to 1 yellow. Further selfing shows that half the second generation (or two-thirds of the green-podded members) are hybrids.

Theoretical Model

Parental generation
(purebred strains)

PP pp

Mendel assumed that each plant contains a pair of genes for pod color. Therefore, each purebred parent is homozygous; that is, each contains two identical genes for pod color.

Meiosis   Meiosis

P = green-pod-color allele

p = yellow-pod-color allele

Gametes   Gametes

Probability of each
gamete type $1P$ $1p$

Since a fertilized egg results from the union of two gametes, each gamete contains one allele for pod color.

Cross-pollinate

First generation
(green hybrids)

$1Pp$

Because all first-generation offspring bore green pods, Mendel called green the dominant pod color and yellow the recessive pod color. Mendel inferred that whenever P, the allele for the dominant pod color, is present, the plant bears green pods (the law of dominance).

Meiosis

Eggs   Sperms

Probability of each
gamete type $\frac{1}{2}P, \frac{1}{2}p$ $\frac{1}{2}p, \frac{1}{2}P$

Mendel inferred that the pair Pp segregates equally into the gametes; that is, each gamete (whether egg or sperm) receives P or p with equal probability of one-half (law of equal segregation).

Self-pollinate

	♂ $\frac{1}{2}P$	$\frac{1}{2}p$
♀ $\frac{1}{2}P$	$\frac{1}{4}PP$	$\frac{1}{4}Pp$
$\frac{1}{2}p$	$\frac{1}{4}pP$	$\frac{1}{4}pp$

Second generation

Random union of eggs and sperms produces four possible combinations of alleles in the offspring. As shown by the table, the probabilities of each gamete type are multiplied to yield the probabilities of the four possible genotypes in the second-generation offspring. Since Pp and pP are equivalent genotypes, the probabilities of each are added to yield a probability of one-half for the genotype Pp. Mendel's model predicts, for members of the second generation, phenotypes in the ratio 3 green : 1 yellow (in agreement with Mendel's observations) and genotypes in the ratio 1 PP : 2 Pp : 1 pp.

Mendel's Experiments on Inheritance of Two Traits (Pod Color and Flower Color)

Methodology

Step 1: Cross-pollinate two strains of peas, one purebred for the two dominant phenotypes (green pods and violet flowers), the other purebred for the two recessive phenotypes (yellow pods and white flowers). Result: All first-generation dihybrids bear green pods and violet flowers.

Step 2: Self-pollinate the first-generation dihybrids. Result: Second-generation plants exhibit four composite phenotypes (pod color, flower color) in the ratio of 9 (green, violet) : 3 (yellow, violet) : 3 (green, white) : 1 (yellow, white).

Theoretical Model

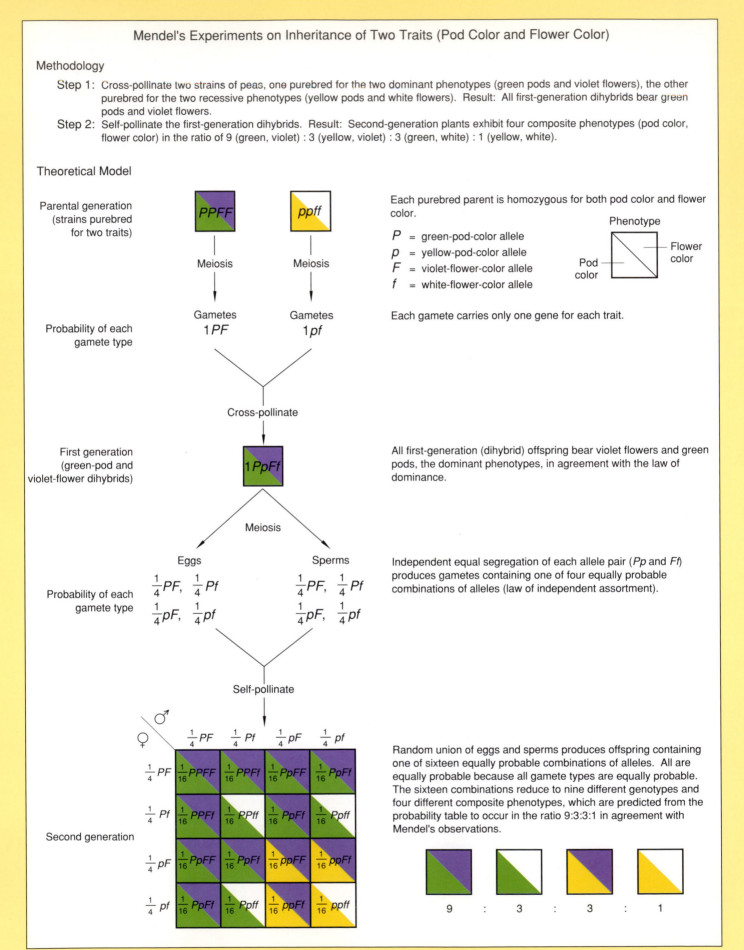

Parental generation (strains purebred for two traits)

PPFF   *ppff*

Meiosis   Meiosis

Gametes   Gametes
$1PF$ $1pf$

Probability of each gamete type

Cross-pollinate

First generation (green-pod and violet-flower dihybrids)

$1PpFf$

Meiosis

Eggs   Sperms

Probability of each gamete type

$\frac{1}{4}PF, \ \frac{1}{4}Pf$ $\frac{1}{4}PF, \ \frac{1}{4}Pf$

$\frac{1}{4}pF, \ \frac{1}{4}pf$ $\frac{1}{4}pF, \ \frac{1}{4}pf$

Self-pollinate

Each purebred parent is homozygous for both pod color and flower color.

P = green-pod-color allele
p = yellow-pod-color allele
F = violet-flower-color allele
f = white-flower-color allele

Phenotype — Pod color / Flower color

Each gamete carries only one gene for each trait.

All first-generation (dihybrid) offspring bear violet flowers and green pods, the dominant phenotypes, in agreement with the law of dominance.

Independent equal segregation of each allele pair (*Pp* and *Ff*) produces gametes containing one of four equally probable combinations of alleles (law of independent assortment).

Second generation

♀ \ ♂	$\frac{1}{4}PF$	$\frac{1}{4}Pf$	$\frac{1}{4}pF$	$\frac{1}{4}pf$
$\frac{1}{4}PF$	$\frac{1}{16}PPFF$	$\frac{1}{16}PPFf$	$\frac{1}{16}PpFF$	$\frac{1}{16}PpFf$
$\frac{1}{4}Pf$	$\frac{1}{16}PPFf$	$\frac{1}{16}PPff$	$\frac{1}{16}PpFf$	$\frac{1}{16}Ppff$
$\frac{1}{4}pF$	$\frac{1}{16}PpFF$	$\frac{1}{16}PpFf$	$\frac{1}{16}ppFF$	$\frac{1}{16}ppFf$
$\frac{1}{4}pf$	$\frac{1}{16}PpFf$	$\frac{1}{16}Ppff$	$\frac{1}{16}ppFf$	$\frac{1}{16}ppff$

Random union of eggs and sperms produces offspring containing one of sixteen equally probable combinations of alleles. All are equally probable because all gamete types are equally probable. The sixteen combinations reduce to nine different genotypes and four different composite phenotypes, which are predicted from the probability table to occur in the ratio 9:3:3:1 in agreement with Mendel's observations.

9 : 3 : 3 : 1

Therefore, the law applies *only* if the allele pairs for the two traits reside on different pairs of homologous chromosomes. In fact, deviations from Mendelian predictions for the co-inheritance of two traits is evidence that the two traits are specified by allele pairs that reside on the same pair of homologous chromosomes.

This discussion of Mendel's theory of inheritance ends with two points of note. First, although the theory is now known to be applicable to humans as well as to pea plants, it is unlikely that it could have been deduced from data about the outcomes of human breedings. As subjects of inheritance studies, humans pose several disadvantages: The controlled breeding of humans is generally regarded as inappropriate and would be difficult to achieve even if it were not; each pair of human parents typically produces too few data (offspring) for analysis of the sort required; and the rate at which humans produce offspring is too slow to suit most experimenters' taste. Moreover, many human traits are specified not by a single allele pair but by many allele pairs.

The second point of note concerns the utility of Mendel's theory as a predictive tool, particularly for human breedings. The theory can be applied directly only to traits determined by a single allele pair. Such traits are called Mendelian traits because they are inherited in accordance with Mendel's laws. Most Mendelian traits of humans are disorders—some mild, some grave—caused by the presence of a defective allele. To determine the probability that an offspring will be affected by a Mendelian disorder requires knowing the parental genotypes for the disorder and whether the disorder is caused by a dominant or a recessive allele. The required genotypic information for the parents can often be inferred from the phenotypes of their existing offspring and of their parents, and information about whether the defective allele is dominant or recessive can often be inferred from the pattern of inheritance of the disorder in other families (see "Inheritance of Mendelian Disorders"). More than three thousand human Mendelian disorders have been identified. One of the goals of the Human Genome Project is to supply the tools necessary to isolate the causative alleles from the vast quantity of human genetic material and to identify the defects in the alleles.

A Theory of Evolution. The nineteenth century brought not only the rise of cell biology and the work of Mendel but also a growing acceptance of the fact of evolution, of the creation of extant organisms by changes in the life forms that first populated this planet. Belief in the ancient principle of the invariability of species waned, and in its place came the conviction that new species had been and are being formed. (A notable holdout to the idea of evolution was the eminent Harvard zoologist Jean Louis Rudolphe Agassiz (1807–1873), who was what we would today call a creationist.) The veering of scientific opinion toward evolution led to development of a theory of evolution based on natural selection. Formulated independently by Charles Robert Darwin (1809–1882) and Alfred Russell Wallace (1823–1913), the theory was presented to the world first in a jointly authored short publication (1858) and later in Darwin's classic book *On the Origin of Species* (1859). Crucial to development of the theory were the observations that offspring resembled their parents

INHERITANCE OF MENDELIAN DISORDERS

Although some inherited disorders of humans are due to the combined effects of multiple genes (multigenic disorders) or to the combined effects of genes and the environment (multifactorial disorders), a so-called Mendelian disorder is caused by a single defective allele. Over 3000 Mendelian disorders are known. They range from mild conditions such as red-green color blindness to life-threatening diseases such as cystic fibrosis. Because the defective allele can be either dominant or recessive and can reside on either an autosome or a sex chromosome (in particular, the X chromosome–very few genes reside on the small human Y chromosome), four types of Mendelian disorders are possible: autosomal dominant, autosomal recessive, X-linked dominant, and X-linked recessive. Each type of disorder reveals itself through a distinctive pattern of inheritance in a family pedigree. Illustrated here are the patterns for three of the four types of Mendelian disorders.

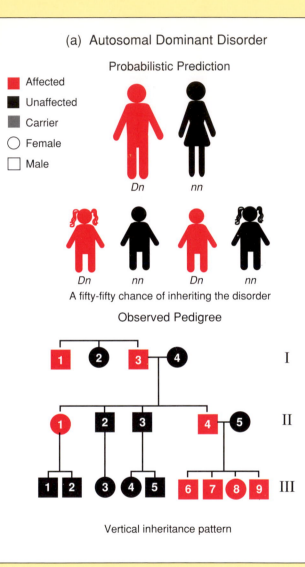

(a) Autosomal Dominant Disorder

Probabilistic Prediction

■ Affected
■ Unaffected
■ Carrier
○ Female
□ Male

Dn   *nn*

Dn   *nn*   *Dn*   *nn*

A fifty-fifty chance of inheriting the disorder

Observed Pedigree

I

II

III

Vertical inheritance pattern

Consider first the inheritance of an autosomal dominant Mendelian disorder. Many such disorders are expressed only in adulthood, including Huntington's disease, neurofibromatosis, and polycystic kidney disease. Shown in (a) are the equally probable genotypes and the phenotypes of the offspring of an affected father and an unaffected mother (or of an affected mother and an unaffected father). The genotype of the affected father can be either *DD* or *Dn*, where *n* is the nondefective recessive version of the defective dominant allele *D*. Because the father's having the genotype *DD* is the less typical and less interesting situation (all his offspring would be affected), it is assumed in (a) that the father has the genotype *Dn*. Because the mother is unaffected, her genotype must be *nn*. The equal segregation of chromosomes during meiosis implies that the offspring of such a mating can have one of two equally probable genotypes: *Dn* or *nn*. Therefore the probability of an offspring's being affected is 1/2. Note carefully, though, that only in the limit of an infinite number of offspring will the ratio of affected to unaffected offspring be

equal to 1. Also shown in (a) is the pedigree of a family afflicted with hypercholesterolemia, a dominant disorder that causes excess levels of cholesterol in the blood. A thirty-year-old white male (II-4) suffered a myocardial infarction, a type of heart blockage, and was then found to test positively for hypercholesterolemia. Further tests indicated that his sister (II-1) and his four children (III-6, III-7, III-8, III-9) also had hypercholesterolemia. In addition, a family history revealed that the man's father (I-3) and uncle (I-1) both died of myocardial infarctions before reaching the age of fifty-five. Note that all of II-4's children are affected by the disorder, an outcome that is not inconsistent (although it may appear to be) with the probabilistic predictions based on the chromosome theory of heredity. Note also that the disease appears in all three generations of the pedigree; such a "vertical" pattern is characteristic of dominant disorders.

Shown in (b) is the inheritance of an autosomal recessive Mendelian disorder, examples of which include Tay-Sachs disease, cystic fibrosis, and sickle-cell anemia. Assume a typical situation: Both parents are carriers, or, in other words, are unaffected but have the genotype *Nd*, where *N* is the nondefective dominant version of *d*. The equal segregation of chromosomes during meiosis implies that the probability of an offspring's having the genotype *dd* and therefore of being affected is 1/4. In addition, the probability of an offspring's having the genotype *Nd* or *dN* (and of being a

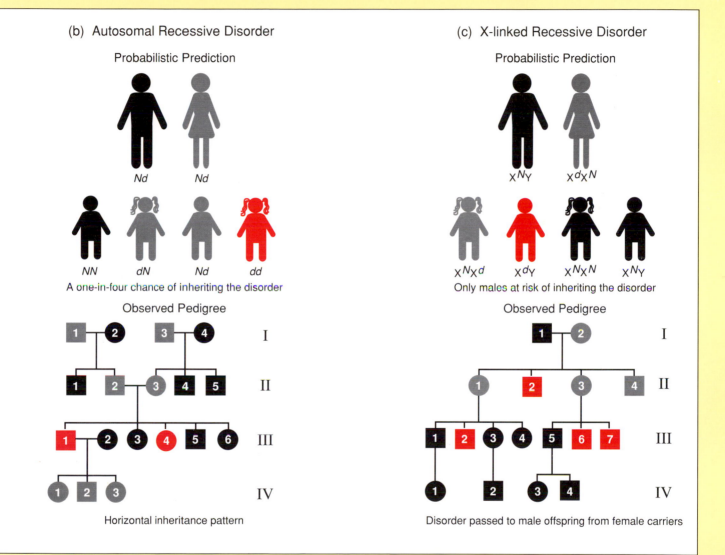

(b) Autosomal Recessive Disorder

Probabilistic Prediction

Nd   Nd

NN   dN   Nd   dd

A one-in-four chance of inheriting the disorder

Observed Pedigree

I   II   III   IV

Horizontal inheritance pattern

(c) X-linked Recessive Disorder

Probabilistic Prediction

$X^N Y$ $X^d X^N$

$X^N X^d$ $X^d Y$ $X^N X^N$ $X^N Y$

Only males at risk of inheriting the disorder

Observed Pedigree

I   II   III   IV

Disorder passed to male offspring from female carriers

carrier) is 1/2 and of having the genotype *NN* (and of being unaffected) is 1/4. Also shown in (b) is the pedigree of a family with an autosomal recessive Mendelian disorder. Only two individuals, both in the third generation (III-1 and III-4), are affected. All the other individuals listed are either carriers or unaffected. Since typically siblings in only a single generation are affected by a recessive Mendelian disorder, its inheritance pattern is referred to as horizontal.

Shown in (c) is the inheritance of an X-linked recessive Mendelian disorder. Such disorders include hemophilia, which is the result of a lack of an essential blood-clotting factor, and Duchenne muscular dystrophy, which causes progressive muscle weakness and death in early adulthood from respiratory problems. Again assume a typical situation: The mother is a carrier and therefore has the genotype $X^d X^N$, and the father is unaffected and therefore has the genotype $X^N Y$. Any male offspring has a probability of 1/2 of being affected, and any female offspring has a probability of 1/2 of being a carrier. Also shown in (c) is a pedigree of a family with Duchenne muscular dystrophy. One son (II-2) and two daughters (II-1 and II-3) inherited the maternal X chromosome on which the defective allele resides. The son, possessing only one X chromosome, is affected. On the other hand, the daughters are unaffected carriers, but their sons (III-2, III-6, and III-7) inherited the defective allele. The pedigree illustrates the typical pattern of inheritance of an X-linked recessive disorder: transmission from an affected male through his daughters to his grandsons. Females can inherit the disease if the father is affected and the mother is either affected or a carrier.

only incompletely and that selective breeding had produced plants and animals quite different from the ancestral strains. Darwin arrived at his conclusions in large part by doing a *Gedankenexperiment*, much as Albert Einstein later arrived at his theory of relativity. It should be noted that not all of Darwin's thinking was as forward-looking as his theory of evolution. He was an exponent of a form of pangenesis (see "Early Ideas about Heredity") and of blending inheritance (the notion that the characteristics of offspring are the result of a melding of the parental characteristics). Darwin's cousin Francis Galton (1822–1911), in his own way also a genius, tried to point out to Darwin, without success, that neither theory of inheritance made much sense. In doing so Galton came very close to developing the same theory of particulate inheritance as had Mendel, although like Darwin, he was unaware of Mendel's work. Like Mendel, Galton was cognizant of probability and statistics. He can be considered the founder of modern biostatistical theory, which has been an immensely powerful tool in the development of genetic theory.

The cell biologists, Mendel, and Darwin and Wallace made basic contributions to the foundations of modern genetics, but they did so essentially in isolation from each other. Mendel was influenced to some extent by the findings of the cell biologists and of the evolutionists, but neither of the latter were influenced by him or by each other. Such isolation among different fields of science, though detrimental to progress, is still today not uncommon.

Things Come Together

The science of genetics was born in the first decade of the twentieth century through fusion of Mendel's theory of inheritance and the cell biologists' knowledge about chromosomes. In 1902 a student of Wilson's, Walter Stanborough Sutton (1877–1916), and Boveri independently recognized the parallels between the real objects called chromosomes and the theoretical constructs called genes—the occurrence of both as pairs, their separation in a similar fashion during gamete formation, and their re-pairing during fertilization—and proposed that each member of a pair of alleles is located on one or the other member of a pair of homologous chromosomes. Thus was born the chromosome theory of heredity. The theory was soon proved, and during the period between 1910 and 1940—the heyday of classical genetics—many allele pairs were localized to particular homologous chromosome pairs.

Classical Genetics. The term "classical genetics" refers to those aspects of genetics that can be studied without reference to the molecular details of genes. The early stars of classical genetics were the American Thomas Hunt Morgan (1866–1945), his students Calvin Blackman Bridges (1889–1938), Hermann Joseph Muller (1890–1967), and Alfred Henry Sturtevant (1891–1970), and last but not least members of the genus *Drosophila*, most notably the common fruit fly *Drosophila melanogaster*. Morgan's interest lay (initially at least) in determining whether the changes that result in new species occur gradually or abruptly. He chose to study changes in *D. melanogaster* because it reaches sexual maturity so rapidly, produces so many offspring, and is so easily and cheaply raised in the laboratory. The discovery, in the spring of 1910, of a lone white-eyed male fly among thousands upon thousands of red-eyed flies in the Fly Room at Columbia University was a momentous event, leading not only to proof of the chromosome theory of heredity but also to knowledge of previously unknown aspects of meiosis.

Now is an appropriate time to emphasize the critical role of mutants in genetics. (A mutant is a member of a species that exhibits a phenotype different from the "wild-type" phenotype exhibited by most members of a natural population of the species.) Even knowledge of the existence of a gene is usually inferred from the existence of a mutant. When faced, for example, with a vast population of only red-eyed flies, how could anyone suspect that eye color is a manifestation of genes in operation? To be discussed later is another invaluable role of mutants—as tools for learning more specifically what genes do. (That genes determine physically observable traits is certainly true but remarkably vague.)

An early outcome of the discovery of the white-eyed fly was Morgan's proposal that alleles for red and white eye color in *D. melanogaster* are located on its X chromosomes. Morgan arrived at that proposal by observing the eye colors of the progeny resulting from a series of breedings, a series that began with matings between the white-eyed male and wild-type red-eyed females. (Note that mutants must not only be discovered but also be allowed to survive and breed.) Because all the progeny were red-eyed, Morgan concluded that the red-eye-color allele is dominant. Next he interbred the progeny and found, just as Mendel would have predicted, that three-quarters of the resulting second-generation progeny were red-eyed and one-quarter were white-eyed. However, among neither the red-eyed nor the white-eyed second-generation flies did he find an equal number of males and females, as would be predicted if the observed segregation of sex chromosomes was independent of the presumed segregation of red-and white-eye-color alleles. Instead two-thirds of the red-eyed second-generation flies were females and all of the white-eyed flies were males. Morgan continued by mating red-eyed males to white-eyed females, a breeding that is the "reciprocal" of the original breeding of the lone white-eyed male. He found that half of the progeny were female and red-eyed and the other half were male and white-eyed, whereas Mendel would have predicted that all of the progeny would be red-eyed, just as all of the progeny resulting from the original breeding were red-eyed. To explain those deviations from Mendelian predictions, Morgan proposed that the red- and white-eye-color alleles are X-linked, or in other words that they are located on the X chromosomes.

The reader can more easily verify that Morgan's hypothesis explains the outcomes of the breedings he carried out by using some symbolism. Let w and W denote, respectively, the recessive white-eye-color allele and the dominant red-eye-color allele. Denote an X chromosome containing w by X^w and an X chromosome containing W by X^W. Then the first breeding Morgan carried out, the breeding between wild-type red-eyed females and the white-eyed male, is denoted by $X^W X^W \times X^w Y$. The progeny of such a breeding contain one of two equally probable combinations of sex chromosomes: $X^W X^w$ and $X^W Y$. In other words, half the progeny are female and red-eyed and half are male and red-eyed. The reader is urged to verify that Morgan's proposal explains the outcomes of the other breedings he carried out, namely $X^W X^w \times X^W Y$ and $X^w X^w \times X^W Y$.

Morgan's experiments certainly supported the chromosome theory of heredity, but the work of Bridges provided more direct confirmation. Bridges started by repeating, on a large scale, one of the breedings Morgan had carried out, the breeding between white-eyed female flies and red-eyed male flies. If, as Morgan proposed, the w and W alleles reside on the X chromosomes, that breeding can be represented by $X^w X^w \times X^W Y$ and, as Morgan had observed, half of the resulting progeny would possess the sex-chromosome combination $X^w X^W$ (would be red-eyed females) and half would possess the sex-chromosome combination $X^w Y$ (would be white-eyed males). But Bridges' large-scale breeding produced a surprise: A very small fraction of the progeny (about one in every two thousand) were either white-eyed females or sterile red-eyed males. Bridges found, by direct microscopic observation of the chromosomes of the unusual progeny, that they possessed an anomolous number of sex chromosomes. The white-eyed females possessed two X chromosomes and one Y chromosome, and the sterile red-eyed males possessed a single X chromosome. Obviously the single X chromosome of a sterile red-eyed male must be the residence of the red-eye-color allele he must possess, and the pair of homologous X chromosomes of a white-eyed female must be the residences of the two white-eye-color alleles she must possess. Thus a combination of cytological data and genotypic and phenotypic data directly confirmed the chromosome theory of heredity. (Note that Bridges' "cytogenetic" evidence also indicated that the Y chromosome of *D. melanogaster* is involved in determining fertility rather than maleness.)

A question about Bridges' work remains: How could the abnormal numbers of sex chromosomes in the unusual progeny be explained? Bridges proposed that the homologous X chromosomes of a female fruit fly occasionally fail to segregate during meiosis. Meioses in which such "nondisjunctions" occur would yield two equally probable types of eggs: eggs containing two X chromosomes and eggs containing no X chromosomes. Fertilization of those two types of eggs by the two types of sperms produced by a male fruit fly would result in four types of fertilized eggs: those containing the combination of sex chromosomes $X_m X_m X_p$, the combination $X_m X_m Y$, the combination X_p, and the combination Y. (The subscript on each X chromosome denotes maternal origin or paternal origin.) The combinations $X_m X_m Y$ and X_p are the combinations Bridges observed in the unusual progeny; he attributed the absence of unusual progeny containing the $X_m X_m X_p$ and Y combinations to a lethal overdose and a lethal underdose of X chromosomes. Nondisjunction is now known to be a rare but medically significant feature of meiosis. The human disorder known as Down syndrome, for example, is caused by nondisjunction of chromosomes 21.

It is odd that proof for the existence of a rare meiotic glitch—nondisjunction—antedated clear evidence for the existence of what is now known to be a common feature of meiosis—crossing over. (Nondisjunction occurs once in about every hundred thousand human meioses, whereas crossing over occurs about thirty-three times per human meiosis, or on average more than once per homologous chromosome pair per human meiosis.) As proposed by Morgan, crossing over brings about an exchange, between two homologous chromosomes, of corresponding regions of the chromosomes. (An analogy is the exchange, between two nearly identical yardsticks, of, say, initial seven-inch regions.) Because homologous chromosomes differ from each other in details of their chemical composition, the products of a single crossover are two "recombinant" chromosomes, each different from (but still homologous to) the other and the chromosomes that participated in the crossover. In particular, if the exchanged regions contained different alleles of two genes, the recombinant chromosomes contain combinations of alleles that are different from the combinations of alleles possessed by the participants (see "Crossing Over: A Special Type of Recombination"). Thus crossing over, like independent assortment, increases the genetic diversity of sexually reproducing organisms. But whereas independent assortment merely creates new combinations of existing chromosomes, crossing over can create new chromosomes, ones containing new combinations of alleles.

Crossing over might today be regarded as merely another item in the phenomenology of meiosis were it not that it is the key element of a method for determining a measure of the distance between two genes (or, more precisely, two allele pairs) resident on the same chromosome (or, more precisely, on the same homologous chromosome pair). (Note that the method is applicable only to genes for which two or more alleles exist.) Called classical linkage analysis, the method is far from straightforward. The first step, of course, is to establish that two allele pairs are linked (are resident on the same homologous chromosome pair) by observing deviations from Mendelian predictions for the co-inheritance of the traits specified by the allele pairs. The next step is to measure the fraction of meioses in which crossing over leads to new combinations of alleles. The final step (and one not known to be necessary to the earliest linkage analysts) is to convert the measured "recombination fraction" to a "genetic distance" for the two allele pairs, which is defined as the probability of the occurrence of crossing over anywhere in the chromosomal region between the allele pairs. (Although a genetic distance is a dimensionless number, it is expressed in terms of a unit called a morgan or, more usually, in centimorgans.) The relationship between recombination fraction and genetic distance is complex (see "Classical Linkage Mapping" in "Mapping the Genome"), but a recombination fraction is approximately equal to its corresponding genetic distance when the recombination fraction is less than about 0.10. The significance of the genetic distance for two allele pairs is that the genetic distance is proportional to the physical distance between the loci of the allele pairs, provided crossing over occurs with equal probability at any point along the chromosome pair. Despite the fact that the stated proviso is not in general satisfied, genetic distance was until recently the only available measure of the physical distance between gene loci.

CROSSING OVER: a special type of recombination

DNA molecules, and hence chromosomes, are not immutable, even in the absence of external mutagenic agents. One of the natural mechanisms whereby DNA molecules can change is recombination, which rearranges genetic material by breaking and joining portions of the same DNA molecule or portions of different DNA molecules of the same organism. (Recombination can occur also between the DNA of an organism and the DNA of a virus that infects the organism.) Crossing over is the type of recombination undergone by the similar DNA molecules within two homologous chromosomes. It occurs almost exclusively during prophase I of meiosis, when homologous chromosomes are closely apposed. A single crossover between homologous chromosomes effects an exchange of corresponding chromosome regions and results in the formation of recombinant chromosomes, which differ in their content of hereditary information from the chromosomes that participated in the crossover. Crossing over also occurs between the identical DNA molecules within the chromosomes of a sister-chromatid pair, but because the recombinant chromosomes so formed are usually identical to the participants, such recombination has little genetic significance.

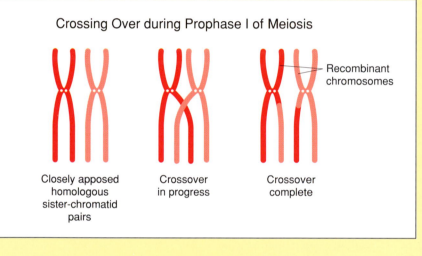

Crossing Over during Prophase I of Meiosis

Closely apposed homologous sister-chromatid pairs

Crossover in progress

Crossover complete

Recombinant chromosomes

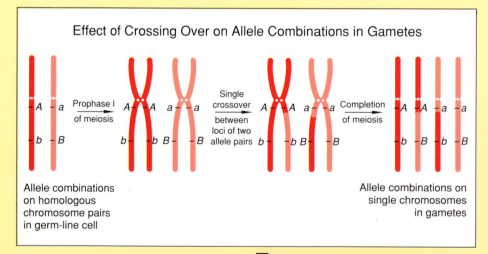

Effect of Crossing Over on Allele Combinations in Gametes

Allele combinations on homologous chromosome pairs in germ-line cell

A a

b B

Prophase I of meiosis

A A a a

b b B B

Single crossover between loci of two allele pairs

A A a a

b b B B

Completion of meiosis

A A a a

b B b B

Allele combinations on single chromosomes in gametes

The occurrence of a single crossover between the loci of two allele pairs, say A and a and B and b, resident on a homologous chromosome pair results in the formation of some gametes that possess combinations of alleles different from the combinations possessed by the parent germ-line cell. Crossing over is thus a mechanism for increasing genetic diversity. It also is the basis of a standard method for determining a "distance" between the locus of A and a and the locus of B and b. The first step in the method (see "Determining a Genetic Distance") is to carry out a certain breeding experiment and thereby measure, among a group of gametes produced by one parent, the fraction possessing the new allele combinations (the so-called recombination fraction). When the measured recombination fraction is relatively small (less than about 0.10), it is approximately equal to the "genetic distance" between the two loci, that is, to the average number of crossovers between the two loci per meiosis. The genetic distance between the two loci in turn is a rough measure of the physical distance (the distance along the DNA molecule) between the two loci.

As illustrated in "Determining a Genetic Distance," linkage analysis is facilitated by carrying out either one of two particular breedings. (Each breeding is a "test cross" involving one doubly heterozygous parent and one doubly recessive parent.) Morgan happened to carry out both breedings—between fruit flies, of course—in the early 1910s and thereby not only gathered the first clear evidence for the existence of crossing over but also measured the first recombination fractions.

Then in 1913 Sturtevant measured recombination fractions for various pairwise combinations of six allele pairs known to reside on the X chromosomes of *Drosophila*. By assuming that the loci of the six allele pairs dot the X chromosome as points dot a line and that the measured recombination fraction for, say, the allele pairs *A,a* and *B,b* is directly proportional to the length of the X-chromosome segment between the locus of *A,a* and the locus of *B,b*, Sturtevant constructed a diagram—the first "genetic-linkage map"—showing the relative locations of the six genes and their pairwise separations. Sturtevant then used his diagram to calculate the recombination fractions for those pairwise combinations of allele pairs that he had measured but not needed to construct the diagram. The approximate agreement between calculated and measured recombination fractions indicated that both of his assumptions were at least approximately valid. We now know that, although the genes of all eukaryotic organisms lie along linear DNA molecules, the genes of prokaryotic organisms lie instead along circular DNA molecules. Furthermore, as indicated above, recombination fractions are not in general proportional to physical distance.

As noted previously, genetic studies of an organism demand the availability of mutants, that is, of individuals possessing alleles different from those possessed by wild-type individuals. For many years, though, geneticists had to survive on the rare mutants provided by nature. (Fewer than ten out of every million members of a natural population of a species are phenotypically obvious mutants.) Then in 1927 Muller (one of Morgan's trio of brilliant students) demonstrated that x rays induce heritable mutations in the fruit fly, and a year later the American geneticist Lewis John Stadler (1896–1954) used x rays to create new alleles in barley. The availability of x-ray-induced mutants accelerated the pace of gene discovery and genetic-linkage mapping.

The demonstrated power of combining cytological data about the chromosomes of an organism with genotypic and phenotypic data led, in the 1930s, to emergence of cytogenetics as a separate field of biology. Crucial to cytogeneticists is the ability to distinguish one pair of homologous metaphase chromosomes from another. For distinguishing features, early cytogeneticists relied on sizes and shapes, which do not always provide unambiguous identification. (The word "shape" generally means centromere location, but it can also mean an unusual structural feature specific to only certain metaphase chromosomes of certain organisms. Chromosome 9 of a strain of *Zea mays*, for example, is sometimes blessed with a conspicuous knob at the end of its short arm, a feature that helped elucidate the mechanism of crossing over.) It was soon learned, however, that each homologous chromosome pair within a metaphase

DETERMINING A GENETIC DISTANCE

The classical method for determining the genetic distance between the loci of two allele pairs known to reside on the same homologous chromosome pair of an organism involves observing the phenotypes of the offspring of one of two particular breedings. During the course of Thomas Hunt Morgan's work on fruit flies, he happened to carry out both breedings and was rewarded not only with the first clear evidence of crossing over but also with the first unambiguous genetic-distance data. Morgan's experiments and data are used here to illustrate the procedure.

The allele pairs in question reside on one of the homologous autosome pairs of *Drosophila melanogaster*. One allele pair affects eye color: a dominant allele *A* that specifies red eye color and a recessive allele *a* that specifies purple eye color. The other allele pair affects wing length: a dominant allele *B* that specifies wild-type wings and a recessive allele *b* that specifies vestigial (very short) wings.

The participants in the first breeding are a female fruit fly that is heterozygous for both traits (and therefore has red eyes and normal wings) and a male fruit fly that is homozygous for both recessive trait variants (and therefore has purple eyes and vestigial wings). Furthermore, the female is known to be a product of the breeding $AABB \times aabb$. Therefore the distribution of the alleles *A, a, B,* and *b* on the homologous autosome pair of the female is known: Both dominant alleles (*A* and *B*) reside on one member of the homologous autosome pair, and both recessive alleles (*a* and *b*) reside on the other member. Such an allele distribution is denoted by writing the genotype of the female as *AB/ab*. The distribution of the alleles *a, a, b,* and *b* on the homologous autosome pair of the male is also known (because the male is homozygous for both traits) and is denoted in a similar fashion as *ab/ab*. Thus the first breeding can be symbolized by

$$AB/ab \text{ female} \times ab/ab \text{ male.} \qquad (1)$$

Meioses in the heterozygous female that involve no crossovers between the two loci yield two types of eggs: those possessing the chromosome with the allele combination *AB* and those possessing the chromosome with the allele combination *ab*. In other words, the two dominant alleles and the two recessive alleles remain linked (resident on the same chromosome), just as they are in the female herself. But those

meioses in the female that involve a single crossover between the two loci (or any odd number of crossovers) yield in addition two other types of eggs: those possessing a chromosome with the allele combination *Ab* and those possessing a chromosome with the allele combination *aB*. In other words, a single crossover between the two loci establishes linkage between one dominant and one recessive allele. On the other hand, meioses in the doubly homozygous male, whether or not they invove crossovers between the two loci, yield sperms possessing only the allele combination *ab*. Thus the offspring of breeding 1 possess four genotypes, each corresponding to one of the four possible phenotypes:

$$AB/ab \text{ female} \times ab/ab \text{ male} \longrightarrow$$
$$AB/ab + ab/ab + Ab/ab + aB/ab.$$

Morgan examined more than 2800 progeny of breeding 1 and found that 47.2 percent had red eyes and normal wings (*AB/ab*), 42.1 percent had purple eyes and vestigial wings (*ab/ab*), 5.3 percent had red eyes and vestigial wings (*Ab/ab*), and 5.4 percent had purple eyes and normal wings (*aB/ab*). All the offspring exhibiting the last two phenotypes (the combinations of one recessive trait variant and one dominant trait variant) result only from crossovers during meioses in the female parent. Thus the data indicate that the probability of new allele linkages being formed by crossing over is 0.107 = 0.053 + 0.054. That value for the so-called recombination fraction corresponds to a genetic distance of about 12 centimorgans. (The relationship between recombination fraction and genetic distance is presented in "Classical Linkage Mapping" in "Mapping the Genome.")

The participants in the other breeding that provides unambiguous recombination-fraction data are, like the participants in breeding 1, a doubly heterozygous female and a doubly homozygous-recessive male. However, the second female is known to be a product of the breeding $Ab/Ab \times aB/aB$ (rather than the breeding $AB/AB \times ab/ab$). Therefore the distribution of alleles on her homologous autosome pair is Ab/aB (rather than AB/ab). (The difference in allele distributions of the two doubly heterozygous females is often referred to as a difference in linkage phase.) The second breeding is thus symbolized by

$$Ab/aB \text{ female} \times ab/ab \text{ male.} \qquad (2)$$

Breeding 2 yields offspring that exhibit the same genotypes and phenotypes as breeding 1:

$$Ab/aB \text{ female} \times ab/ab \text{ male} \longrightarrow$$
$$Ab/ab + aB/ab + AB/ab + ab/ab.$$

Morgan examined more than 2300 progeny of breeding 2 and found that 41.3 percent had red eyes and vestigial wings (Ab/ab), 45.7 percent had purple eyes and normal wings (aB/ab), 6.7 percent had red eyes and normal wings (AB/ab), and 6.3 percent had purple eyes and vestigial wings (ab/ab). Again, all the offspring exhibiting the last two phenotypes result only from crossovers during meioses in the female parent. Thus the data indicate that the recombination fraction for the two allele pairs is 0.130, which corresponds to a genetic distance of about 15 centimorgans.

Note that the two data sets yield different values for the same genetic distance. However, the difference between the values is within the statistical uncertainties associated with measurements of probabilistic events. Note also that the same genetic distance could in principle be determined by carrying out the reciprocal of breeding 1 or breeding 2 (that is, a breeding between a doubly heterozygous male and a doubly homozygous-recessive female). Then, the crossovers detected are those that occur during meioses in the male parent rather than in the female parent. However, for some unknown reason crossing over simply does not occur in male fruit flies. But fruit flies are exceptional in that respect, and genetic distances for other species can be determined by carrying out either breeding 1, say, or its reciprocal.

Breedings 1 and 2 are those that provide unambiguous recombination-fraction data. As an example of the ambiguities that can arise, consider the fruit-fly breeding

$$AB/ab \text{ female} \times AB/ab \text{ male.} \qquad (3)$$

Assume first that crossing over between the two loci does not occur during meioses in the female parent. Then the offspring of breeding 3 exhibit two phenotypes: red eyes and normal wings (AB/AB and AB/ab) and purple eyes and vestigial wings (ab/ab). Now assume that crossing over does occur during meioses in the female parent. Then among the offspring of breeding 3 are some that exhibit the two other possible phenotypes: red eyes and vestigial wings (Ab/ab) and purple eyes and normal wings (aB/ab). All offspring that exhibit those two phenotypes result only from crossing over. However, crossing over also leads to offspring that exhibit one of the phenotypes produced in the absence of crossing over, namely, red eyes and normal wings (Ab/AB and aB/AB). In other words, whereas the offspring produced by breeding 1 or 2 can unambiguously be sorted by phenotype into two categories—those that are the result of crossovers and those that are not—the offspring resulting from breeding 3 cannot be so sorted because meioses that do and do not involve crossovers result in the doubly dominant phenotype.

The reader can accept on faith or verify personally that breedings 1 and 2 are the only breedings that provide unambiguous recombination-fraction and hence genetic-distance data. Note, in addition, that obtaining even ambiguous data requires that one parent be doubly heterozygous.

Determining a genetic distance is thus relatively easy when the breeding of the organism in question can be manipulated at will. But determining the genetic distance between the loci of two human allele pairs is much more difficult, since the breeding of humans cannot be manipulated, the genotypes and allele distributions of human parents are not always known, and human breedings generally produce so few offspring that the statistical uncertainty in the measured recombination fraction is large.

cell displays a characteristic pattern of dark and light bands when stained with an appropriate dye (see "Chromosomes: The Sites of Hereditary Information"). Because the banding pattern characteristic of a pair of homologous metaphase chromosomes varies along the length of the chromosomes, it can also be used to identify different regions of the chromosomes. The advent of chromosome banding led to recognition of the occasional occurrence of aberrant chromosomes. (The incidence of aberrant chromosomes, like the incidence of gene mutations, can be increased by exposure to x rays or other mutagenic agents.) Several types of chromosome aberrations, or rearrangements, were noted, including translocations (the exchange of chromosome regions between nonhomologous chromosomes) and inversions (the reversal of the orientation of a chromosome region).

Obviously a chromosome rearrangement can lead to changes in the complement of genes present on a chromosome or to changes in their relative locations. The gene (or genes) affected by a chromosome rearrangement (as determined from genetic data) can then be assigned a locus within the rearranged chromosome region. Although the locus so obtained is inexact, it is better than the alternative of knowing nothing at all about the locus. Knowledge of the whereabouts on a chromosome of a gene then serves to "anchor" a genetic-linkage map including that gene to the chromosome. (Recall that a linkage analysis provides only distances between genes on a chromosome; additional information is required to locate the genes relative to the chromosome itself.)

Chromosome rearrangements and gene mutations are but two examples of naturally rare phenomena that, once noted, are exploited to gain basic information about genes. Another example is the exceptional behavior of the cells that compose the salivary glands of *Drosophila* (and other insects of the order Diptera). In 1933 the American zoologist Theophilus Shickel Painter (1889–1969) and independently two German geneticists discovered that the chromosomes in those cells were microscopically visible during interphase. (Interphase chromosomes are usually not microscopically visible because they have not yet condensed in preparation for mitosis.) For some unknown reason the salivary cells of *Drosophila* undergo not a single round but many successive rounds of chromosome duplication during the S phase of interphase (see "The Eukaryotic Cell Cycle"). The numerous (on the order of a thousand) copies of each chromosome remain closely associated along their lengths, forming a fiber sufficiently thick to be microscopically visible. Because such "polytene" chromosomes are not condensed, sites of chromosome rearrangements can be pinpointed with much greater resolution.

The Rise of Molecular Genetics. By 1940 many genes were known to exist, and a goodly number of the known genes had been assigned to particular regions of particular chromosomes. But the gene remained an abstract concept. No one knew what genes do or even of what they are made. A speculation about what genes do had appeared as early as 1903, when the French geneticist Lucien Claude Cuénot (1866–1951) proposed that inherited coat-color differences in mice were due to the action of different genes. And in 1909 the English physician Archibald Edward Garrod (1857–1936) established that the human disease alkaptonuria was inherited as a recessive trait variant and proposed that the unmistakable symptom of the disease (urine that blackens after being excreted) was due to accumulation in the urine of a metabolic product that normally is degraded with the help of a certain enzyme. (An enzyme is a protein that catalyzes a biochemical reaction.) But Cuénot's and Garrod's proposals were regarded as mere speculation for many years. Then, in 1941, the American geneticist George Wells Beadle (1903–1989) and the American biochemist Edward Lawrie Tatum (1909–1975) clearly demonstrated the connection between the genes an organism possesses and the biochemicals it is able to synthesize.

Beadle and Tatum's work focused on the bread mold *Neurospora crassa*. Because wild-type spores of *N. crassa* can be cultured in the laboratory on a minimal growth medium (one containing only sucrose, inorganic salts, and the vitamin biotin), they reasoned that the mold must possess enzymes that help convert those simple molecules into all the other necessities of life. By exposing *N. crassa* to ultraviolet light, Beadle and Tatum produced a very few mutant spores that could not be cultured on a minimal growth medium but could be cultured on a growth medium containing a single additional nutrient (vitamin B_6, for example). They concluded that the x rays had caused a mutation in a gene that somehow directs the synthesis of an enzyme involved in the synthesis of the nutrient. Evidence in support of such a conclusion accumulated, and in 1948 the American geneticist and biochemist Norman Harold Horowitz (1915–) propounded the famous one gene–one enzyme hypothesis. Molecular genetics was born. Horowitz's hypothesis has since been modified to state that one gene directs the synthesis of one protein, or, more precisely, one polypeptide chain, since some proteins contain more than one polypeptide chain.

Beadle and Tatum's work on *N. crassa* demonstrated the value of studying such a simple organism. Attention soon turned to even simpler organisms—bacteria. The bacterium *Escherichia coli*, a tenant of the vertebrate gut, gained particular favor. As a result of studies begun soon after World War II by François Jacob (1920–), Joshua Lederberg (1925–), Jacques Lucien Monod (1910–1976), and Elie Leo Wollman (1917–), more is known about the genes of *E. coli*, including their regulation, than of any other living organism. Attention also focused on viruses, the simplest of all organisms, and in particular on the viruses that infect bacteria, known as bacteriophages or simply phages. (Viruses are composed of a nucleic acid core encased in a protein coat. They are not living organisms in the sense that they lack the machinery for biosynthesis. They can, however, reproduce—by usurping the biosynthetic machinery of the cells they infect—and pass their characteristics from generation to generation through the medium of genes just as cellular organisms do.) In the United States the so-called Phage Group, led by Max Delbruck (1906–1981), Alfred Day Hershey (1908–), and Salvador Edward Luria (1912–1991), aroused interest in the interaction between phages and bacteria as a model system for studying the fundamental mechanisms of heredity. Work by the Phage Group included developing quantitative methods for studying the life cycles of phages and later the discovery that phages can transfer bacterial genes from one bacterial strain to another, a process called transduction. (Transduction was to become a progenitor of recombinant-DNA technology.) The promiscuous exchange of genetic material between different strains of bacteria and between bacteria and their viruses facilitated the mapping of genes and the identification of their functions.

What genes are made of was the other big question about genes in the 1940s. In 1925 Wilson, reversing his previous stance, espoused protein as the genetic material. The idea of a proteinaceous genetic material was subsequently widely accepted for more than two decades, primarily because the nonproteinaceous component of chromosomes, DNA (deoxyribonucleic acid), was thought by chemists to have a structure that rendered it incapable of carrying any kind of message. However, in 1944 the American bacteriologists Oswald Theodore Avery (1877–1955) and his colleagues presented strong evidence that the genetic material was DNA. Their evidence was the ability of DNA extracted from dead members of a pathogenic strain of *Streptococcus pneumoniae* to impart the inherited characteristic of pathogenicity to live members of a nonpathogenic strain of the same bacterium. (We now know that the mechanism involved in the transformation from nonpathogenicity to pathogenicity is DNA recombination, of which crossing over is a specific example.) And in 1952 Hershey and another member of the Phage Group, the American geneticist Martha Chase (1927–), showed that DNA is the component of a phage that enters a bacterium and thus presumably directs the synthesis of new phages within the infected bacterium. Nevertheless, despite the accumulating evidence, DNA was not widely accepted as the genetic material.

Then in 1953 James Dewey Watson (1928–) and Francis Harry Compton Crick (1916–) proposed a structure for DNA that accounted for its ability to self-replicate and to direct the synthesis of proteins. The structure they proposed is of course the famous double helix, which, like two-ply embroidery floss, is composed of two strands coiled helically about a common axis. Each strand is a polymer of deoxyribonucleotides, and each deoxyribonucleotide contains a phosphate group, the residue of the sugar deoxyribose, and the residue of one of four nitrogenous organic bases (adenine, cytosine, guanine, and thymine). The deoxyribonucleotides are linked together in a manner such that alternating phosphate groups and sugar residues form a backbone off which the bases project. Hereditary information is encoded in the order, or sequence, of bases along the strands. The two strands are coiled about the helix axis in a manner such that the backbones form the boundaries of a space within which the bases are contained. Each base on one strand is linked by hydrogen bonds to a base on the other strand; the members of each "base pair" lie in a plane that is essentially perpendicular to the axis of the helix. Of the ten theoretically possible base pairs, only two so-called complementary pairs are found in DNA: the pair adenine and thymine and the pair cytosine and guanine. Thus the order of the bases on one strand is precisely related to the order of the bases on the other strand, and the two strands are said to be complementary. Further details are presented in "DNA: Its Structure and Components."

Watson and Crick arrived at their structure for DNA with the help of x-ray diffraction data for DNA fibers obtained by Maurice Hugh Frederick Wilkins (1916–) and Rosalind Franklin (1920–1957) and of the observation in 1950 by Erwin Chargaff (1905–) that the number of molecules of adenine in any of various DNA samples equals the number of molecules of thymine and that the number of molecules of cytosine equals the number of molecules of guanine. In addition, following the example of the American chemist Linus Carl Pauling (1901–), who in 1951 had worked out the details of a helical polypeptide structure (the so-called α helix), they made liberal use of ball-and-stick models.

Molecules of DNA are exceptional among biological macromolecules in two respects. First, they are very long relative to their width. If the diameter of the double helix could be increased to that of a strand of angel-hair pasta, the length of the DNA molecule in a typical human chromosome would be about 12 kilometers. Second, although single-helical configurations are not uncommon in biological macromolecules, the double-helical configuration of DNA is unique. One might wonder why DNA is double-stranded. After all, normally only one of the strands directs protein synthesis, the two strands are replicated separately, and some viruses manage quite nicely with only single-stranded DNA. The evolutionary advantage of double-stranded DNA is thought to lie in the fact that, if one strand is damaged, the other strand can provide the information required to repair the damaged strand.

The base-pairing feature of DNA immediately suggested that each strand of DNA could serve as the template for directing the synthesis of a complementary strand. The result would be two identical double-stranded DNA molecules, each containing one new and one old strand. The suggestion that DNA replication is "semiconservative" was proved correct (for the DNA of *E. coli* and a higher plant) several years after the double-helical DNA structure was proposed. The details of DNA replication, however, are very complex, involving a number of enzymes. One enzyme first uncoils a portion of the DNA molecule, and another separates the two strands. Then an enzyme called a DNA polymerase, using one of the separated DNA strands as a template, catalyzes the polymerization of free deoxyribonucleoside triphosphates into a strand that is complementary to the template. Some features of the process are detailed in "DNA Replication."

Now that genes were known to direct the synthesis of proteins and to be made of DNA, the next problem was to determine the relationship between DNA and proteins. The first clue about the relationship came in 1949 when Pauling presented evidence that the hemoglobin present in humans suffering from sickle-cell anemia differed *structurally* from the hemoglobin in humans not suffering from that inherited disease. (Hemoglobin is composed of two copies each of two polypeptides, the so-called α and β chains. The α chain contains 141 amino acids, and the β chain contains 150 amino acids.) What features of a protein affect its structure? By the 1940s biochemists were beginning to realize that the structure of a protein is determined not so much by which amino acids it contains but more by the sequence of the amino acids along the

DNA: its structure and components

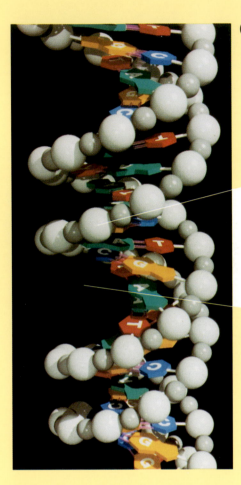

(a) Computer-generated
Image of DNA
(by Mel Prueitt)

(b) Uncoiled DNA Fragment

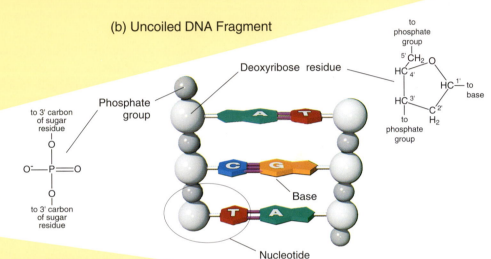

Deoxyribose residue

Phosphate group

to 3' carbon of sugar residue

to 3' carbon of sugar residue

to phosphate group

to base

to phosphate group

Base

Nucleotide

The usual configuration of DNA is shown in (a). Two chains, or strands, of repeated chemical units are coiled together into a double helix. Each strand has a "backbone" of alternating deoxyribose residues (larger spheres) and phosphate groups (smaller spheres). Free deoxyribose, $C_5O_4H_{10}$, is one of a class of organic compounds known as sugars; the phosphate group, $(PO_4)^{-3}$, is a component of many other biochemicals.

Attached to each sugar residue is one of four essentially planar nitrogenous organic bases: adenine (A), cytosine (C), guanine (G), or thymine (T). The plane of each base is essentially perpendicular to the helix axis. Encoded in the order of the bases along a strand is the hereditary information that distinguishes, say, a robin from a human and one robin from another.

As shown, the two strands coil about each other in a fashion such that all the bases project inward toward the helix axis. The two strands are held together by hydrogen bonds (pink rods) linking each base projecting from one backbone to its so-called complementary base projecting from the other backbone. The base A always bonds to T (A and T are complementary bases), and C is always linked to G (C and G are complementary bases). Thus the order of the bases along one strand is dictated by and can be inferred from the order of the bases along the other strand. (The two strands are said to be complementary.) The pairing of A only with T and of C only with G is the feature of DNA that allows it to serve as a template not only for its own replication but also for the synthesis of proteins (see "DNA Replication" and "Protein Synthesis"). Note that the members of a base pair are essentially coplanar.

All available evidence indicates that each eukaryotic chromosome contains a single long molecule of DNA, only a small portion of which is shown here. Furthermore, the ends of each DNA molecule, called telomeres, have a special base sequence and a somewhat different structure.

Shown in (b) is an uncoiled fragment of (a) containing three complementary base pairs. From the chemist's viewpoint, each strand of DNA is a polymer made up of four repeated units called deoxyribonucleotides, or simply nucleotides. The four nucleotides are regarded as the monomers of DNA (rather than the sugar residue, the phosphate group, and the four base residues) because the nucleotides are the units added as a strand of DNA is being synthesized (see "DNA Replication").

A particular nucleotide is commonly designated by the symbol for the base it contains. Thus T is a symbol not only for the base thymine (more precisely, the thymine residue) but also for the indicated nucleotide. Also shown are chemical and structural details of the backbone components. Note that four carbon atoms of the sugar residue and its one oxygen atom form a pentagon in a plane parallel to the helix axis, and that the fifth carbon atom of the sugar residue projects out of that plane.

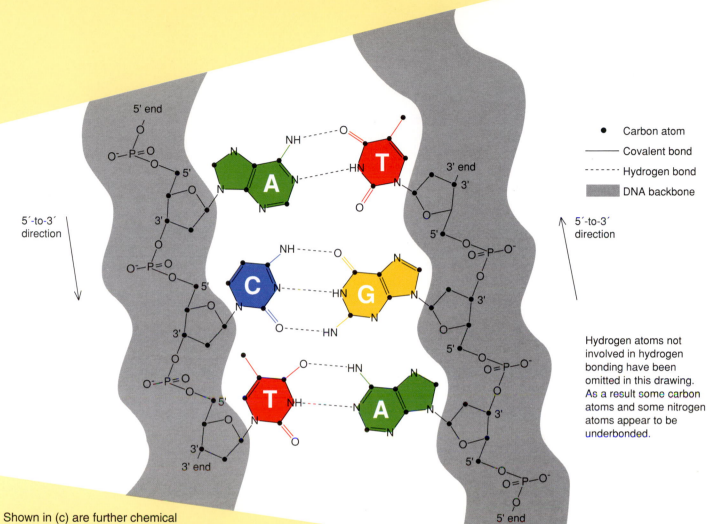

5' end

5'-to-3' direction

3' end

3' end

5' end

- Carbon atom
— Covalent bond
- - - Hydrogen bond
▨ DNA backbone

5'-to-3' direction

Hydrogen atoms not involved in hydrogen bonding have been omitted in this drawing. As a result some carbon atoms and some nitrogen atoms appear to be underbonded.

Shown in (c) are further chemical and structural details of the DNA segment shown in (b). The planes of the three base pairs have been rotated into the plane of the sugar residues. Details of particular note include the following.

Linking any two neighboring sugar residues is an -O–P–O- "bridge" between the 3' carbon atom of one of the sugars and the 5' carbon atom of the other sugar. (The designations 3' (three prime) and 5' (five prime) arise from a standard system for numbering atoms in organic molecules.) When a DNA molecule is broken into fragments, as it must be before it can be studied, the breaks usually occur at one of the four covalent bonds in each bridge.

Because deoxyribose has an asymmetric structure, the ends of each strand of a DNA fragment are different. At one end the terminal carbon atom in the backbone is the 5' carbon atom of the terminal sugar (the carbon atom that lies outside the planar portion of the sugar), whereas at the other end the terminal carbon atom is the 3' carbon atom of the terminal sugar (a carbon atom that lies within the planar portion of the sugar).

The two complementary strands of DNA are antiparallel. In other words, arrows drawn from, say, the 5' end to the 3' end of each strand have opposite directions. Most of the enzymes that move along a backbone in the course of catalyzing chemical reactions move in the 5'-to-3' direction. The composition of a DNA fragment is represented symbolically in a variety of ways. However, all of the representations focus on the order, or sequence, of the nucleotides (and hence the bases) along the strands of the fragment. For example, the most complete representation for the fragment shown above is

5'-ACT-3'
3'-TGA-5'.

The most abbreviated representation, ACT (or, equivalently, AGT), gives the sequence of only one strand (since the sequence of the complementary strand can be inferred from the given sequence) and follows the convention that the left-to-right direction corresponds to the 5'-to 3' direction.

DNA REPLICATION

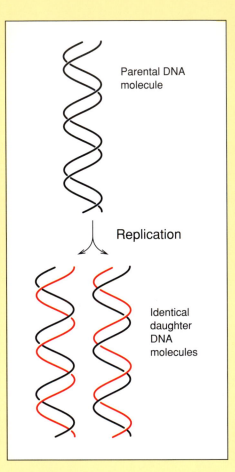

Parental DNA molecule

Replication

Identical daughter DNA molecules

An overall description of DNA replication is quite simple. Each strand of a parent DNA molecule serves as the template for synthesis of a complementary strand. The result is two daughter DNA molecules, each composed of one parental strand and one newly synthesized strand and each a duplicate of the parent molecule. But this overall simplicity, illustrated above, is misleading, since DNA replication involves the intricate and coordinated interplay of more than twenty enzymes. The most important general feature of DNA replication is its extremely high accuracy. A "proofreading" capability of DNA polymerase, the enzyme that catalyzes the basic chemical reaction involved in replication, guarantees that only about one per billion of the bases in a newly synthesized strand differs from the complement of the corresponding base in the template strand.

A more detailed description of DNA replication should note first that replication of a chromosomal DNA molecule does not begin at one end of the molecule and proceed uninterruptedly to the other end. Instead, scattered along the molecule are numerous occurrences of a particular base sequence, and each occurrence of that sequence serves as an "origin of replication" for a portion of the molecule. Thus different portions of a DNA molecule are replicated separately. Baker's yeast, *Saccharomyces cerevisiae*, is one of the few eukaryotes for which the base sequence of its origins of replication is now known. Knowledge of the base sequence of an organism's origins of replication is necessary in the creation of artificial chromosomes of the organism, synthetic entities that are treated by the organism`s cellular machinery just as its own chromosomes are treated. The cloning vectors known as YACs are an example of artificial chromosomes.

Replication of the portion of a DNA molecule flanked by two origins of replication begins with the action of enzymes that move along the parental DNA, progressively uncoiling and denaturing (separating into single strands) the double helix. Uncoiling and denaturation expose the bases in each parental strand and thereby enable the bases to direct the order in which deoxyribonucleotides are added by DNA polymerase to the strand being synthesized.

Because, as shown in the figure at right, DNA polymerase elongates a growing chain of deoxyribonucleotides only in the 5´-to-3´ direction (arrows), one of the new DNA strands can be synthesized continuously but the other strand must be synthesized in short pieces called Okazaki fragments. (The Okazaki fragments shown here are much shorter than they are in reality.) The discontinuous synthesis of one of the new strands is the source of additional complexities in replicating the very ends, the telomeres, of a DNA molecule.

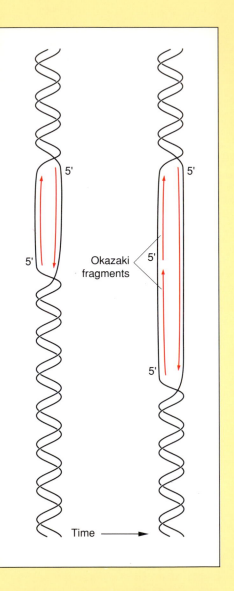

5'
5'
5'
Okazaki fragments
5'
5'
5'
Time

As shown in the figure on the next page, the participants in the chemical reaction by which each portion of a DNA strand is synthesized include a "primer," the enzyme DNA polymerase, a DNA template (a parental strand), and a supply of free deoxyribonucleoside triphosphates (dNTPs). The usual primer is a very short strand of RNA, generally containing between four and twelve ribonucleotides. (RNA is a single-stranded nucleic acid; its structure is very similar to that of a strand of DNA. Because the sugar residue in RNA is derived from ribose rather than deoxyribose, the repeated units in RNA are

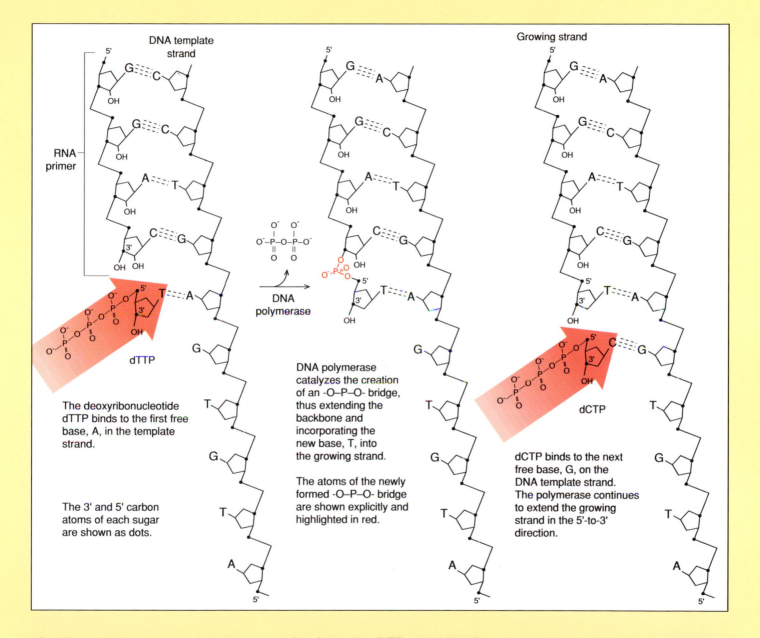

DNA template strand

Growing strand

RNA primer

The deoxyribonucleotide dTTP binds to the first free base, A, in the template strand.

The 3' and 5' carbon atoms of each sugar are shown as dots.

dTTP

DNA polymerase

DNA polymerase catalyzes the creation of an -O–P–O- bridge, thus extending the backbone and incorporating the new base, T, into the growing strand.

The atoms of the newly formed -O–P–O- bridge are shown explicitly and highlighted in red.

dCTP

dCTP binds to the next free base, G, on the DNA template strand. The polymerase continues to extend the growing strand in the 5'-to-3' direction.

called ribonucleotides rather than deoxyribonucleotides.) A primer is required because DNA polymerase catalyzes the addition of a deoxyribonucleotide to an existing chain of nucleotides (either ribonucleotides or deoxyribonucleotides) but not the de novo synthesis of a chain of deoxyribonucleotides. The action of each parental strand as a template is based on hydrogen bonding between complementary bases. In particular, a base in a parental strand hydro-

gen bonds to the dNTP containing the complementary base. As a result, the dNTP is fixed in a position such that the DNA polymerase can exert its catalytic action on the triphosphate group of the dNTP and the 3´ hydroxyl group of the 3´-terminal sugar of the primer. The result is the addition of a deoxyribonucleotide to the primer and the release of a pyrophosphate group, $(P_2O_7)^{-4}$. The next deoxyribonucleotide in the template strand fixes its complementary dNTP

into position, the DNA polymerase moves further along the chain being elongated, and addition of another deoxyribonucleotide is effected by action of the polymerase on the triphosphate group of the dNTP and the hydroxyl group of the sugar of the deoxyribonucleotide just previously added. Successive repetitions of the process and eventual replacement of the RNA primer with DNA lead to formation of double-stranded DNA identical to the parental DNA.

polypeptide chain. Then in 1957 Vernon Martin Ingram (1924–) demonstrated that the sixth amino acid in the β chain of normal hemoglobin is glutamic acid, whereas the sixth amino acid in the β chain of sickle hemoglobin is valine. Otherwise, the amino-acid sequences of both β chains are identical. Ingram's work suggested that the function of DNA was to determine the order in which amino acids are assembled into a protein, a process called translation. Details of transcription and translation are illustrated in "Protein Synthesis."

DNA itself could not, however, be the template for the synthesis of proteins, since DNA is sequestered in the nucleus of a eukaryotic cell, whereas proteins were known to be synthesized in the cytoplasm outside the nucleus. Perhaps an intermediary substance was involved, one that receives hereditary information from DNA in the nucleus and then moves to the cytoplasm, where it serves as the template for protein synthesis. A likely candidate for such an intermediary was the other known nucleic acid, namely ribonucleic acid, or RNA, which is found primarily in the cytoplasm. Like DNA, RNA is a polymer of four different nucleotides, but the nucleotides are ribonucleotides containing the sugar ribose, which differs from deoxyribose in possessing a hydroxyl group on its $2'$ carbon atom. Another difference is that the base thymine is absent from RNA, being replaced by the base uracil (U), which lacks the extra-ring methyl group of thymine but, like thymine, hydrogen bonds with adenine. The final difference between DNA and RNA is that RNA is usually single-stranded.

That RNA is the intermediary between DNA and proteins soon became the working hypothesis of biochemists, and the details of protein synthesis were worked out in the fifties and sixties. Briefly, a segment of DNA (a gene) serves as the template for the synthesis, in the nucleus, of so-called messenger RNA (mRNA), a process called transcription and similar to DNA replication. The mRNA then enters the cytoplasm, where it serves as the template for the ordered assembly of amino acids into a protein, a process called translation. Details of transcription and translation are illustrated "Protein Synthesis."

The last general problem about the relation between DNA and proteins was to crack the code relating the sequence of deoxyribonucleotides that constitutes a gene to the sequence of amino acids that constitutes a protein. Experiments performed in 1961 by Crick and the British molecular biologist Sydney Brenner (1927–) suggested that the code was a triplet code, or, in other words, that a sequence of three adjacent deoxyribonucleotides (a codon) specifies each amino acid. The genetic code was completely cracked by 1966, thanks primarily to the independent efforts of two groups, one led by Marshall Warren Nirenberg (1929–) and the other by Har Gobind Khorana (1922–). As shown in "The Genetic Code," eighteen of the twenty amino acids are specified by two or more codons. The redundancy of the code implies that gene mutations involving single-base substitutions do not necessarily result in a change in an amino acid.

Now that what seemed the major questions about the material and mechanisms of heredity had been answered, was anything fascinating left to learn? Or would

PROTEIN SYNTHESIS

(a) Protein Synthesis in Prokaryotic and Eukaryotic Cells

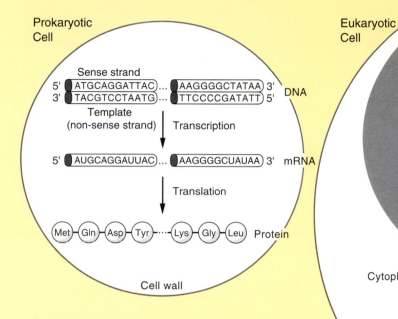

Prokaryotic Cell

Sense strand
5' ATGCAGGATTAC ... AAGGGGCTATAA 3' DNA
3' TACGTCCTAATG ... TTCCCCGATATT 5'
Template (non-sense strand) | Transcription

5' AUGCAGGAUUAC ... AAGGGGCUAUAA 3' mRNA

Translation

Met–Gln–Asp–Tyr ···· Lys–Gly–Leu Protein

Cell wall

Eukaryotic Cell

Nucleus
Exon Intron
DNA
Transcription
Primary RNA transcript
Splicing
mRNA
Cytoplasm
mRNA
Translation
Protein
Cell wall

Protein synthesis is the process by which information encoded in a gene is converted into a specific protein. In 1957 Francis Crick proposed two hypotheses about protein synthesis, which later became known as the central dogma of molecular biology. He proposed first that gene sequences are "collinear" with protein sequences. In other words, the linear arrangement of subunits (deoxyribonucleotides) composing a gene corresponds to the linear arrangement of subunits (amino acids) composing a protein. Second, Crick proposed that a segment of RNA (a ribonucleotide sequence) acts as an intermediate translator between the deoxyribonucleotide sequence and the amino-acid sequence, or, in other words, that genetic information flows from DNA to RNA to protein. Crick had no experimental evidence to support his hypotheses. But very shortly Charles Yanofsky and Seymour Benzer, working independently, provided the first evidence in support of the collinearity hypothesis. Their experiments showed that mutations in the genes of *E. coli* and of the T4 bacteriophage produced parallel changes in amino-acid sequences. And as details of protein synthesis were worked out, the role of RNA as an intermediary was also established.

Shown in (a) is an overview of protein synthesis in a prokaryotic cell. In the first stage, called transcription, a DNA segment, a gene, serves as a template for the synthesis of a single-stranded RNA segment called a messenger RNA (mRNA). The base sequence of the mRNA is complementary to the base sequence of one strand of the gene (the template, or "non-sense," strand) and is therefore identical to the base sequence of the other strand of the gene (the "sense" strand). The one exception to the identity is that the base U (uracil) replaces the base T. (Recall that in RNA uracil, rather than thymine, is the base complementary to adenine.)

In the second stage of protein synthesis, called translation, the mRNA serves as the template for the stringing together of amino acids into a protein. The protein is assembled according to the genetic code. That is, the

succession of codons (triplets of adjacent ribonucleotides) that compose the mRNA dictates the succession of amino acids that compose the protein. (A listing of codons and corresponding amino acids is presented in "The Genetic Code.") Although transcription and translation are depicted here as if they occurred at different times, translation of a prokaryotic mRNA often begins before its synthesis by transcription is complete.

Also shown in (a) is an overview of protein synthesis in a eukaryotic cell. Unlike prokaryotic genes, most eukaryotic genes are composed of stretches of protein-coding sequences (exons) interrupted by longer stretches of noncoding sequences (introns). Both the exons and introns within a eukaryotic gene are transcribed. The resulting primary transcript is then spliced; that is, each intron is removed and the adjacent exons are linked together.

The shortened RNA is now an mRNA, an RNA that contains only protein-coding sequences. The mRNA leaves the nucleus and in the cytoplasm is translated into a protein according to the genetic code. Thus transcription and translation are of necessity temporally separated in eukaryotic cells.

The overviews in (a) illustrate that, as Crick had postulated, genetic information flows from DNA to RNA to protein within both prokaryotic and eukaryotic cells. One important exception to the central dogma is the class of viruses known as retroviruses, of which the AIDS virus is an example. Retroviruses store genetic information in RNA and then convert the information to DNA—a reversal of the usual information flow that is known as reverse transcription.

Details of transcription and translation are shown in (b) and (c) respectively. Transcription begins when an enzyme, an RNA polymerase, binds to a particular segment of a gene called the promoter. The double helix then uncoils and separates into two strands, exposing a small number of bases. The RNA polymerase facilitates hydrogen bonding between an exposed base in the template strand and its complementary base in a free ribonucleoside triphosphate (NTP) and then between the next exposed base in

the template strand and its complementary base in another free NTP. While the two NTPs are held in proximity by the hydrogen bonds, the RNA polymerase catalyzes the formation of an -O–P–O- bridge between them, thus forming a chain of two covalently linked ribonucleotides. (See "DNA Replication" for details about formation of -O–P–O- bridges.) A third NTP is hydrogen-bonded to the third exposed base in the template strand and is covalently linked to the second ribonucleotide in the chain. The RNA polymerase moves along the template in the 3'-to-5' direction, continuing to unwind and separate the double helix and to elongate the RNA chain in the 5'-to-3' direction by catalyzing the addition of successive ribonucleotides. At the same time, the distorted DNA in the wake of the polymerase rewinds. After the gene is fully transcribed, the polymerase separates from the double helix. If the gene transcribed is a eukaryotic gene, the newly minted RNA is spliced and the resulting mRNA enters the cytoplasm through pores in the nuclear membrane.

As shown in (c), translation occurs with the help of transfer RNA molecules (tRNAs) and ribosomes. Each tRNA is a tiny, cloverleaf-shaped molecule that serves as an adapter: At one end it contains a triplet of ribonucleotides (an anticodon) that binds

with a complementary codon on the mRNA strand, and at the other end it has an attachment site for a single amino acid. Many varieties of tRNAs exist. An important difference between one tRNA and another is the presence of a different anticodon on the central cloverleaf stem. The number of different anticodons found in the various tRNAs is less than the number of codons in the genetic code. That is so because the base pairing between the third base of the mRNA codon and the first base of the tRNA anticodon can depart from the usual Watson-Crick rules. For example, G can pair with U in addition to C.

Ribosomes are very large molecules composed of ribosomal RNA (rRNA) and approximately fifty different proteins. As a ribosome travels along an mRNA it catalyzes the reactions that lead to synthesis of the protein encoded in the mRNA. Thousands of ribosomes exist within each cell.

Before a tRNA molecule participates in translation, it must be converted to an aminoacyl-tRNA (become attached to the amino acid corresponding to its anticodon). Each of the twenty amino acids found in proteins can be attached to at least one type of tRNA, and most can be attached to several. The binding between tRNA and amino acid is cata-

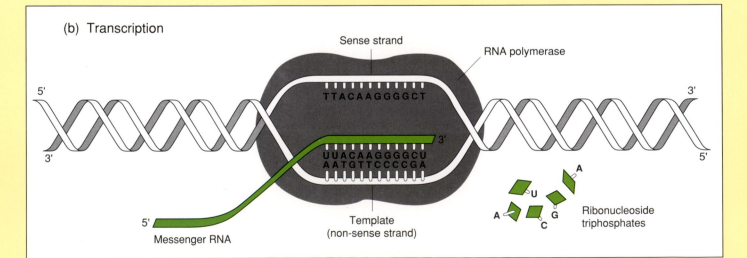

(b) Transcription

Sense strand

RNA polymerase

5'

3'

TTACAAGGGGCT

3'

3'

5'

UUACAAGGGGCU
AATGTTCCCCGA

A

U

A

G

C

Ribonucleoside
triphosphates

5'

Messenger RNA

Template
(non-sense strand)

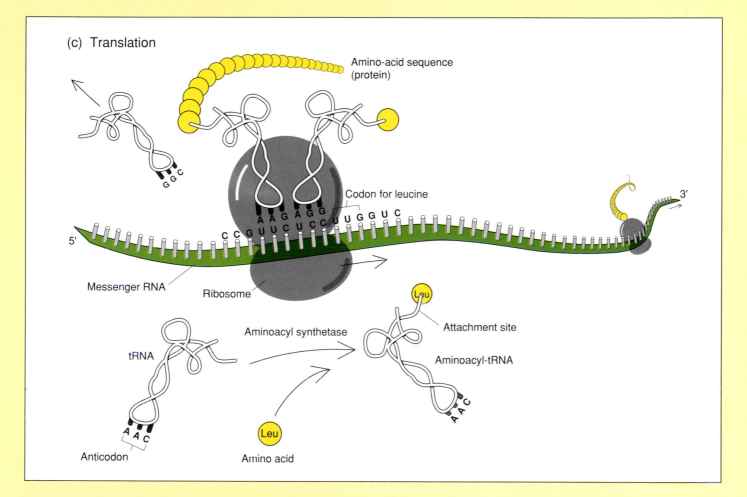

(c) Translation

Amino-acid sequence (protein)

Codon for leucine

Messenger RNA

Ribosome

tRNA

Aminoacyl synthetase

Attachment site

Aminoacyl-tRNA

Anticodon

Amino acid

lyzed by one of a group of enzymes. Those exquisitely specific enzymes, called aminoacyl synthetases, are in fact the agents by which the genetic information in mRNA is decoded.

Translation begins when an aminoacyl-tRNA containing the amino acid methionine and a ribosome bind to an initiation sequence near the 5´ end of the mRNA. The initiation sequence consists of the START codon AUG, to which the aminoacyl-tRNA binds through complementary base pairing. A second aminoacyl-tRNA, which contains an anticodon complementary to the second mRNA codon, binds to the mRNA. Then the amino acid on the first aminoacyl-tRNA is joined by a peptide bond to the amino acid on the second aminoacyl-tRNA, thus creat-

ing a chain of two amino acids dangling off the end of the second aminoacyl-tRNA. The process continues as the ribosome moves along the mRNA (in the 5´-to-3´ direction) and as peptide bonds are formed between successive amino acids. When the ribosome reaches a STOP codon within the mRNA, the ribosome detaches from the mRNA, and the completed protein is released into the cytoplasm.

The process of translation is fast: A single ribosome can translate up to fifty ribonucleotides per second. Furthermore, at any one time numerous ribosomes may be traveling along a single mRNA, each producing a molecule of the same protein. Thus a protein needed for diverse tasks within the cell can be quickly and efficiently produced.

Note: Published only recently (in June 1992) was strong evidence that the formation of peptide bonds between amino acids during translation is catalyzed not by some protein enzyme within a ribosome but instead by an RNA component of the ribosome. That news is exciting but not completely unexpected, since the ability of RNA to function as a catalyst in other situations had been demonstrated in the early 1980s. In particular, the primary transcript of a ribosomal-RNA gene of the protozoan *Tetrahymena thermophila* had been shown to effect its own splicing and the catalytic action of an RNA-protein complex that processes the primary transcripts of certain transfer-RNA genes had been ascribed to the RNA component of the complex rather than the protein component.

THE GENETIC CODE

What triplet of ribonucleotides directs the addition of, say, the amino acid alanine to a protein that is being synthesized? Of lysine? Of any one of the twenty amino acids found in proteins? That was the problem to be faced after advancement of the ideas that a gene is a string of deoxyribonucleotide triplets, that the string of deoxyribonucleotide triplets is transcribed into a string of ribonucleotide triplets, and that the string of ribonucleotide triplets is translated into a string of amino acids–a protein. The results of research on the problem is condensed in the genetic code, a listing of the sixty-four possible ribonucleotide triplets and the amino acid (or translation command) corresponding to each. Fortunately for those who worked on the problem, the genetic code is organism-independent. That is, the same genetic code is used by virtually all organisms.

Researchers began to crack the genetic code in the early 1960s. Marshall Nirenberg and his collaborators added a synthetic RNA, consisting entirely of repetitions of a single ribonucleotide, say U, to a bacterial extract that contained everything necessary for protein synthesis except RNA. The result was a string of the amino acid phenylalanine. They concluded that the ribonucleotide triplet UUU codes for phenylalanine. Other ribonucleotide triplets were decoded by performing similar experiments with synthetic RNAs containing only A's, C's, or G's or various combinations of ribonucleotides. By 1966 research teams led by Har Gobind Khorana and Marshall Nirenberg had cracked the entire genetic code.

(a) RNA Codons for the Twenty Amino Acids

			Second base			
		U	**C**	**A**	**G**	
U		Phe	Ser	Tyr	Cys	U
		Phe	Ser	Tyr	Cys	C
		Leu	Ser	STOP	STOP	A
		Leu	Ser	STOP	Trp	G
C		Leu	Pro	His	Arg	U
		Leu	Pro	His	Arg	C
		Leu	Pro	Gln	Arg	A
		Leu	Pro	Gln	Arg	G
A		Ile	Thr	Asn	Ser	U
		Ile	Thr	Asn	Ser	C
		Ile	Thr	Lys	Arg	A
		Met (start)	Thr	Lys	Arg	G
G		Val	Ala	Asp	Gly	U
		Val	Ala	Asp	Gly	C
		Val	Ala	Glu	Gly	A
		Val	Ala	Glu	Gly	G

(First base down the left side; Third base down the right side.)

Amino-acid abbreviations

Ala = Alanine
Arg = Arginine
Asp = Aspartic acid
Asn = Asparagine
Cys = Cysteine
Glu = Glutamic acid
Gln = Glutamine
Gly = Glycine
His = Histidine
Ile = Isoleucine
Leu = Leucine
Lys = Lysine
Met = Methionine
Phe = Phenylalanine
Pro = Proline
Ser = Serine
Thr = Threonine
Trp = Tryptophan
Tyr = Tyrosine
Val = Valine

Shown in (a) is the usual representation of the genetic code. The letters U, C, A, and G are symbols for the ribonucleotides containing the bases uracil, cytosine, adenine, and guanine, respectively. The symbols in the body of the table are three-letter abbreviations for the amino acids. To find the amino acid specified by a particular codon (say the codon CAG), locate the first nucleotide (C) along the left side of the table and the second nucleotide (A) along the top of the table. Their intersection pinpoints one of four amino acids. Of those four the one aligned with the third nucleotide (G) is the amino acid in question. Thus the amino acid glutamine (Gln) is specified by the three-nucleotide sequence CAG.

Shown in (b) is another version of the genetic code, one expressed in terms of DNA codons instead of RNA codons. Each single-stranded deoxyribonucleotide triplet listed in (b) is the sequence of the so-called sense strand of a DNA codon—the strand that does not serve as a template for synthesis of RNA. Note that most of the amino acids are specified by at least two codons. For example, phenylalanine is specified by two codons: TTT and TTC. Arginine is specified by a total of six codons: CGT, CGC, CGA, CGG, AGA, and AGG. In general, the more an amino acid is used in protein synthesis the likelier it is to be specified by more than one codon. Note also the start codon (ATG) and the three stop codons (TAA, TGA, and TAG) that are used to signal the beginning and end of protein synthesis. The substantive difference between the two versions of the genetic code is that in (b) the deoxyribonucleotide T replaces the ribonucleotide U.

(b) DNA Codons for the Twenty Amino Acids

Ala	Arg	Asp	Asn	Cys	Glu	Gln	Gly	His	Ileu	Leu	Lys	Met (START)	Phe	Pro	Ser	Thr	Trp	Tyr	Val	STOP
GCA	AGA	GAT	AAT	TGT	GAA	CAA	GGA	CAT	ATA	TTA	AAA	ATG	TTT	CCA	AGT	ACA	TGG	TAT	GTA	TAA
GCG	AGG	GAC	AAC	TGC	GAG	CAG	GGG	CAC	ATT	TTG	AAG		TTC	CCG	AGC	ACG		TAC	GTG	TAG
GCT	CGA						GGT		ATC	CTA				CCT	TCA	ACT			GTT	TGA
GCC	CGG						GGC			CTG				CCC	TCG	ACC			GTC	
	CGT									CTT					TCT					
	CGC									CTC					TCC					

molecular genetics degenerate into clearing up details here and details there? Some thought so, and bemoaned the passing of a golden age. But in reality another era, and one just as golden, was opening, thanks to development of techniques for manipulating and analyzing DNA.

The Techniques of Molecular Genetics

The late 1960s mark the beginning of the recombinant-DNA revolution. During the ensuing years it became possible to make billions of identical copies of segments of DNA by cloning (duplicating) each segment individually as a recombinant DNA molecule in the bacterium *Escherichia coli*. The significance of that breakthrough was enhanced by other new developments, including the ability to separate fragments of DNA that differ in length by only a few nucleotide pairs, to determine the nucleotide sequences of cloned segments of DNA, to create specific mutations in cloned genes, and to introduce cloned eukaryotic genes into experimental organisms.

Those startling developments arose from advances during the previous decade in nucleic-acid biochemistry and in bacterial and phage genetics. Basic features of the replication, repair, and recombination of DNA and of the synthesis of proteins had been elucidated, and identification and isolation of the enzymes that catalyze the chemical reactions involved had allowed those processes to be reproduced in vitro. The action of phages as carriers of genetic material between different strains of *E. coli* had been utilized to isolate individual *E. coli* genes. The rates of transcription of *E. coli* genes had been determined (by measuring the amounts of RNA transcribed from the different genes) and had been found to be regulated, that is, to vary from gene to gene and in response to external stimuli. The observed regulation of gene expression in *E. coli* had been traced to the interaction of certain proteins with regulatory sequences in its genome. By 1968 about a hundred genes had been ordered on the genetic maps of phages, and about fifteen hundred genes had been ordered on the genetic map of *E. coli*.

On the other hand, essentially nothing was known about the structure of eukaryotic genes, their regulation, or their organization in chromosomal DNA molecules. Even the major difference between prokaryotic and eukaryotic genes—the presence of introns in the latter—had not yet been discovered. Most frustrating was the lack of a methodology for studying eukaryotic genomes analogous to the phage-bacteria system for studying the organization, rearrangement, and functions of phage and bacterial genomes.

But in 1968 techniques began to be developed that exploit the cellular machinery and the biosynthetic products of bacteria to replicate, manipulate, and analyze eukaryotic genes and to manufacture eukaryotic proteins. Improvements during the past twenty years in recombinant-DNA techniques have produced an explosion of knowledge about eukaryotic genes and about the organization and rearrangements of DNA in eukaryotic genomes, including the human genome.

This section briefly describes some of the techniques that are employed in the study of DNA and points out some of the facts about DNA the techniques have helped to reveal. The chronological approach will be more or less abandoned, and none of the contributions will be attributed to their originators.

A description of the preparation of a sample of DNA is appropriate as a preliminary to this section. The usual preparation procedure involves treating a large number of cells (typically about 5 million) of the organism in question with a detergent, which dissolves cellular membranes and dissociates the proteinaceous component of the chromosomes from the DNA. Then the membrane components and the proteins are removed with an organic solvent such as a chloroform-phenol mixture, and the DNA is precipitated with ethanol as a highly viscous liquid. The mass of the DNA in such a sample is small, about 30 micrograms in the case of human DNA and correspondingly smaller in the case of DNA extracted from organisms with smaller genomes.

It is worth noting that no DNA sample prepared in the above manner contains intact DNA molecules. The mechanical aspects of sample preparation (such as stirring and pipetting) invariably break some of the covalent bonds of the DNA backbones. That accidental fragmentation is usually of little consequence, however, because most of the techniques employed to study DNA at the molecular level are applicable only to stretches of DNA shorter than the intact molecules found in chromosomes. In fact, deliberate fragmentation, by either mechanical or biochemical means, is the first step in many of the techniques to be described below.

The length of a DNA molecule or fragment is expressed in terms of the number of base pairs it contains. (Because the structure of DNA is regular, number of base pairs is directly proportional to physical length.) The average length of the intact DNA molecules within human chromosomes, for example, is about 130 million base pairs, which corresponds to a physical length of about 4.5 centimeters. The lengths of the known human genes are much shorter, ranging from less than a hundred base pairs for the transfer-RNA genes to over a million base pairs for the Duchenne muscular-dystrophy gene and the cystic-fibrosis gene.

We turn now to the means for manipulating and analyzing DNA.

Fractionation by Copy Number and Repetitive DNA. The mid 1960s brought to light a surprising feature of eukaryotic DNAs: their content of multiple identical or nearly identical copies of various sequences. The various repeated sequences are collectively called repetitive DNA, and, depending on the species, repetitive DNA is estimated to constitute between 3 and 80 percent of the total. (Between 25 and 35 percent of the human genome, and of other mammalian genomes, is repetitive DNA.) In contrast, the DNAs of viruses and prokaryotes contain no or very little repetitive DNA. The phenomenology of repetitive DNA is complex and not yet fully explored. A few of the repeated sequences are genes, but most have no known function. The multiple copies of some repeated sequences are situated one after the other; the known lengths of the repeated units in such tandem repeats range from two base pairs to several thousand base pairs. Some tandem repeats occur at only one location within a genome; others, called interspersed tandem repeats, occur at many locations. Like the multiple copies of an interspersed tandem repeat, the multiple copies of other repeated sequences are scattered here and there within a genome; the known lengths of such interspersed repeats range from about a hundred base pairs to seven thousand base pairs. And finally the copy numbers of the various repeated sequences range from less than ten to over a million. Two of the many repeated sequences found in the human genome are the GT sequence, an interspersed tandem repeat that consists of between fifteen and thirty tandem repetitions of the sequence 5'-GT and has a copy number on the order of a hundred thousand, and the *Alu* sequence, an interspersed repeat that is about three hundred base pairs in length and has a copy number close to 2 million.

The existence of repetitive DNA became known from comparison of the renaturation kinetics of prokaryotic and eukaryotic DNAs. Recall that the natural configuration of DNA is double-stranded. However, DNA can be separated into single strands (denatured) by, say, heating an aqueous solution of the DNA to about 100°C. When the temperature of a thermally denatured sample of DNA is lowered, random encounters among the single-stranded fragments lead to renaturation, or the re-establishment of hydrogen bonds between complementary fragments. The kinetics of the renaturation can be monitored by, for example, measuring the time dependence of the absorption of ultraviolet light by the sample, since single- and double-stranded DNA have different capacities to absorb ultraviolet light.

Consider the renaturation of two samples of denatured DNA, one prepared by breaking the genome of *E. coli* into equal-length fragments and the other prepared by breaking, into fragments of the same length as the *E. coli* fragments, a hypothetical DNA molecule of the same total length as the *E. coli* genome but composed of multiple repetitions of a single sequence. Each single-stranded *E. coli* fragment is complementary to only one of the many single-stranded fragments in the first sample, whereas each single-stranded hypothetical fragment is complementary to one-half of the equally numerous single-stranded fragments in the second sample. Obviously, then, the hypothetical sample renatures more rapidly, at least initially, than the *E. coli* sample, and therefore the graphs of fraction renatured versus time for the two samples are different. This example illustrates why renaturation-kinetics data are the source of information about the presence of repetitive DNA.

Other types of information can be extracted from renaturation-kinetics data. Consider the renaturation of the *E. coli* genome and the genome of the virus known as T4, each broken into fragments of the same length. Both genomes contain essentially no repetitive DNA, but the sample of *E. coli* DNA contains a greater number of fragments because the *E. coli* genome (which contains about 5,000,000 base pairs of DNA) is larger than the T4 genome (which contains about 170,000 base pairs of DNA). Therefore the *E. coli* genome renatures less rapidly than the T4 genome. In other words, renaturation kinetics provides information about the relative sizes of genomes. Furthermore, because the rate at which hydrogen bonds are established between fragments of single-stranded DNA that have similar but not identical base sequences depends on the degree of similarity of the base sequences of the fragments, the kinetics of the joint renaturation of samples of DNA from different species provides an estimate of the overall similarity of the base sequences of the DNAs.

Today renaturation is most often used to fractionate fragments of DNA by copy number, that is, to separate a DNA sample into components containing highly repetitive DNA, less highly repetitive DNA, and single-copy DNA. Such a separation narrows the search for genes, most of which occur only once within a genome and hence are contained in the single-copy fraction.

Fragmenting DNA with Restriction Enzymes. Until 1970 DNA molecules were of necessity fragmented by mechanical means, such as forcing a sample through a syringe. Mechanical fragmentation has disadvantages: Identical pieces of DNA are not fragmented at the same points, and the lengths of the resulting fragments vary widely. Then came discovery of restriction enzymes (or, more precisely, type II restriction endonucleases), biochemicals capable of "cutting" double-stranded DNA not only in a reproducible manner but also into less widely varying lengths. In particular, a restriction enzyme recognizes and binds to an enzyme-specific, very short sequence within a DNA segment and catalyzes the breaking of two particular oxygen-phosphorus-oxygen (-O–P–O-) bridges, one in each backbone of the segment. The locations along a stretch of DNA of the sequence recognized by a restriction enzyme are called restriction sites.

The -O–P–O- bridges broken by a restriction enzyme usually lie within the recognition sequence of the enzyme. For example, the restriction enzyme *Eco*RI recognizes and binds to the sequence

$$5'\text{-GAATTC-}3'$$
$$3'\text{-CTTAAG-}5'$$

and, if allowed to interact with a sample of DNA for a sufficiently long time (to completely "digest" the DNA), cuts the DNA within every occurrence of that sequence. Note that the sequence recognized by *Eco*RI, like the sequences recognized by many other restriction enzymes, is palindromic; in other words, the $5'$-to-$3'$ sequence of one strand is identical to the $5'$-to-$3'$ sequence of the other strand.

The average length of the restriction fragments produced by *Eco*RI, a "6-base cutter" (a restriction enzyme that recognizes a 6-base-pair sequence), can be estimated to be about 4000 base pairs, since DNA is approximately a random sequence of four base pairs and any given sequence of six base pairs occurs on average every $4^6 = 4096$

base pairs within such a sequence. (Note, however, that the observed average length of the fragments produced by an N-base cutter sometimes differs considerably from the estimate of 4^N.) Fragments with a shorter average length can be obtained by complete digestion with, say, a 4-base cutter, and fragments with a longer average length can be obtained by complete digestion with a restriction enzyme that recognizes a sequence longer than 6 base pairs or by partial digestion with a 6-base cutter, which leaves some of the restriction sites uncut.

A majority of the many restriction enzymes available today, including *Eco*RI, cut DNA in a fashion such that the resulting fragments terminate in a very short section of single-stranded DNA. For example *Eco*RI cuts the DNA segment

$$5'- \ldots \text{GAATTC} \ldots -3'$$
$$3'- \ldots \text{CTTAAG} \ldots -5'$$

into the fragments

$$5'- \ldots \text{G-}3'$$
$$3'- \ldots \text{CTTAA-}5'$$

and

$$5'\text{-AATTC} \ldots -3'$$
$$3'\text{-G} \ldots -5'$$

Note that the single-stranded ends of the two *Eco*RI restriction fragments are complementary. The utility of such "sticky" ends in the creation of recombinant DNA molecules will be described below.

A brief natural history of restriction enzymes is presented in "Restriction Enzymes," as well as a listing of a few of the many available.

Fractionating DNA Fragments by Length: Gel Electrophoresis. Because DNA fragments are negatively charged, they are subject to an electrical force when placed in an electric field. In particular, DNA fragments placed in a gel (a porous, semisolid material) move through the gel in a direction opposite to the direction of an applied electric field. Furthermore, the rate at which a fragment travels is approximately inversely proportional to the logarithm of its length. Therefore gel electrophoresis is a means for separating DNA fragments by length. Details of the technique are described in "Gel Electrophoresis."

But what is the point of separating fragments of DNA by length? After all, the lengths of the fragments obtained either by breaking a DNA molecule mechanically or by cutting it with a restriction enzyme bear no relation to the functioning of the molecule within a cell. Nevertheless, gel electrophoresis, particularly of restriction fragments, is of great utility in the study of DNA. For example, consider the genome of the phage known as λ (lambda), a double-stranded DNA molecule about 50,000 base pairs in length. When many copies of the λ genome are completely digested with *Eco*RI and the resulting restriction fragments are subjected to gel electrophoresis, groups of

RESTRICTION ENZYMES

Like the immune systems of vertebrate eukaryotes, the restriction enzymes of bacteria combat foreign substances. In particular, restriction enzymes render the DNA of, say, an invading bacteriophage harmless by catalyzing its fragmentation, or, more precisely, by catalyzing the breaking of certain -O–P–O- bridges in the backbones of each DNA strand. The evolution of restriction enzymes helped many species of bacteria to survive; their discovery by humans helped precipitate the recombinant-DNA revolution.

Three types of restriction enzymes are known, but the term "restriction enzyme" refers here and elsewhere in this issue to type II restriction endonucleases, the only type commonly used in the study of DNA. (A nuclease is an enzyme that catalyzes the breaking of -O–P–O- bridges in a string of deoxyribonucleotides or ribonucleotides; an endonuclease catalyzes the breaking of internal rather than terminal -O–P–O- bridges.) Many restriction enzymes have been isolated; more than seventy are available commercially. Each somehow recognizes and binds to its own restriction sites, short stretches of double-stranded DNA with a specific base sequence. Having bound to one of its restriction sites, the enzyme catalyzes the breaking of one particular -O--P–O- bridge in each DNA strand.

The accompanying table lists a few of the more commonly used restriction enzymes and the organism in which each is found. The first three letters of the name of a restriction enzyme are an abbreviation for the species of the source organism and are therefore customarily italicized. The next letter(s) of the name designates the strain of the source organism, and the terminal Ro-

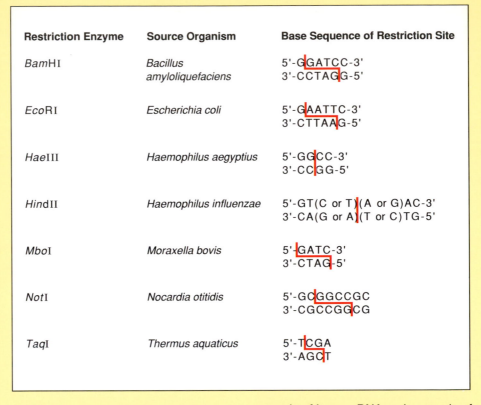

Restriction Enzyme	Source Organism	Base Sequence of Restriction Site
BamHI	Bacillus amyloliquefaciens	5'-G GATCC-3' 3'-CCTAG G-5'
EcoRI	Escherichia coli	5'-G AATTC-3' 3'-CTTAA G-5'
HaeIII	Haemophilus aegyptius	5'-GG CC-3' 3'-CC GG-5'
HindII	Haemophilus influenzae	5'-GT(C or T) (A or G)AC-3' 3'-CA(G or A) (T or C)TG-5'
MboI	Moraxella bovis	5'- GATC-3' 3'-CTAG -5'
NotI	Nocardia otitidis	5'-GC GGCCGC 3'-CGCCGG CG
TaqI	Thermus aquaticus	5'-T CGA 3'-AGC T

man numeral denotes the order of its discovery in the source organism.

Also listed in the table are the base sequences of the restriction sites of the enzymes. The red line separates the ends of the resulting fragments. The restriction sites of many of the known restriction enzymes and of all the restriction enzymes listed in the table have palindromic base sequences. That is, the 5´-to-3´ base sequence of one strand is the same as the 5´-to-3´ base sequence of its complementary strand. Both the bridges broken by a restriction enzyme that recognizes a palindromic sequence lie within or at the ends of the sequence.

Note that most of the restriction enzymes in the table make "staggered" cuts; that is, they produce fragments with protruding single-stranded ends. Those "cohesive," or "sticky," ends are very useful. Suppose that

a sample of human DNA and a sample of phage DNA are both fragmented with the same restriction enzyme, one that makes staggered cuts. When the resulting fragments are mixed, they will tend to hydrogen bond with each other because of the complementarity of their sticky ends. In particular, some human DNA fragments will hydrogen bond to some phage DNA fragments. And that bonding is the first step in the creation of a recombinant DNA molecule.

A final point about restriction enzymes is the problem of how the DNA of a bacterium avoids being chopped up by the friendly fire of the restriction enzyme(s) it produces. Evolution has solved that problem also. A bacterium that produces a type II restriction endonuclease produces in addition another enzyme that catalyzes the modification of restriction sites in its own DNA in a manner such that they cannot serve as binding sites for the restriction enzyme.

GEL ELECTROPHORESIS

Historically gel electrophoresis was first applied to separating proteins essentially according to mass, but the technique was adapted to separating fragments of DNA (or RNA) essentially according to fragment length. The technique works on DNA because the phosphate groups of a DNA fragment are negatively charged, and therefore, under the influence of an electric field, the fragment migrates through a gel (a porous, semisolid medium) in a direction opposite to that of the field. Furthermore, the rate at which the fragment migrates through the gel is approximately inversely proportional to the logarithm of its length.

Gel electrophoresis of DNA is carried out with two types of electric field. Conventional gel electrophoresis employs a field that is temporally constant in both direction and magnitude. In contrast, pulsed-field gel electrophoresis employs a field that is created by pulses of current and therefore varies periodically from zero to some set value. More important, the direction of the electric field also varies because different pulses flow through pairs of electrodes at different locations. (Note, however, that the time-averaged direction of the electric field is along the length of the gel.) The advantage of such a pulsed field is that it prevents long DNA fragments, fragments longer than about 50,000 base pairs, from jackknifing within the structural framework of the gel and thus allows the long fragments to migrate through the gel in a length-dependent manner, just as shorter fragments migrate in a constant electric field.

The gel employed is usually a solidified aqueous solution of agarose, a purified form of agar. By varying the concentration of agarose in the gel, conventional gel electrophoresis can be applied to samples containing DNA fragments with average lengths between a few hundred base pairs and tens of thousands of base pairs. (Another gel used for conventional electrophoresis is polyacrylamide, which is particularly suited

(a) Conventional Gel Electrophoresis

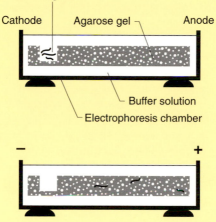

to separating fragments with lengths less than about a thousand base pairs and is therefore the gel of choice for sequencing.) Conventional gel electrophoresis in an agarose gel is illustrated in (a); details of the technique are as follows.

Agarose is dissolved in a hot buffer solution, and the gel solution is allowed to solidify into a thin slab in a casting tray in which the teeth of a comb-like device are suspended. After the gel has solidified, the comb is removed. The "wells" formed by the teeth of the comb are the receptacles into which the samples of DNA are loaded. The thickness of the gel is about 5 millimeters; its length and width are much greater and vary with the purpose of the electrophoresis. Before being loaded with the DNA sample(s), the gel is immersed in a conducting buffer solution in an electrophoresis chamber.

Before a DNA sample is loaded into a well, it is mixed with a dense solution of sucrose or glycerol to prevent the DNA from escaping into the buffer solution. Into one well is

loaded a gel-calibration sample, a sample containing fragments of known lengths. As shown in (a), the flow of electricity through the gel causes the fragments to migrate toward the positive electrode. The shorter fragments move more easily through the gel and therefore travel farther.

The positions of the fragments after electrophoresis can be detected by soaking the gel in a solution of ethidium bromide, which binds strongly to DNA and emits visible light when illuminated with ultraviolet light. In a photograph of the ultraviolet-illuminated gel, the fragments appear as light bands. The ethidium-bromide visualization technique makes the positions of all the fragments in the gel visible. An alternative visualization technique detects only certain fragments (see "Hybridization Techniques").

The above description of gel electrophoresis might suggest that the sample of DNA contains but one copy of each fragment. In reality the sample must contain many copies of each fragment, and each band seen in the image of the length-separated fragments contains many fragments, all of which have the same length but not necessarily the same sequence.

(b) Conventional Gel Electrophoresis of Fragmented Human DNA Segments

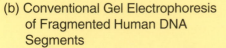

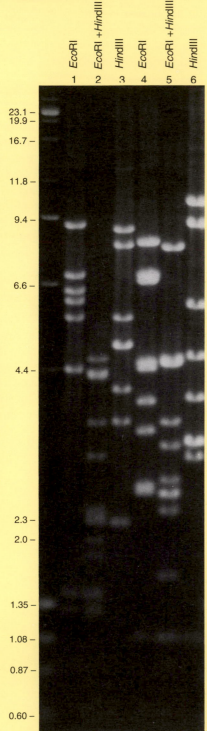

Fragment length (thousands of base pairs)

Lane	Enzyme
1	EcoRI
2	EcoRI + HindIII
3	HindIII
4	EcoRI
5	EcoRI + HindIII
6	HindIII

23.1 –
19.9 –
16.7 –
11.8 –
9.4 –
6.6 –
4.4 –
2.3 –
2.0 –
1.35 –
1.08 –
0.87 –
0.60 –

Shown in (b) are the results of conventional gel electrophoresis of six different samples of human DNA. Samples 1, 2, and 3 consisted of the restriction fragments produced by cutting the same cloned segment of human DNA with EcoRI alone (a 6-base cutter), with both EcoRI and HindIII (another 6-base cutter), and with HindIII alone, respectively. Samples 4, 5, and 6 consisted of the restriction fragments produced by cutting a different cloned segment of human DNA again with EcoRI alone, with both EcoRI and HindIII, and with HindIII alone, respectively. The leftmost lane of the gel contains fragments of the lengths indicated. Note that all the restriction fragments are well resolved.

Shown in (c) are the results of pulsed-field gel electrophoresis of three identical samples, each containing all sixteen of the intact DNA molecules that compose the genome of the yeast *Saccharomyces cerevisiae*. The four longest chromosomal DNA molecules are not resolved; all four are located in the topmost band. The remaining twelve chromosomal DNA molecules, however, are well resolved. The indicated lengths of the resolved DNA molecules were determined from the positions, in the rightmost lane of the gel, of the fragments in a calibration sample. Even longer fragments, fragments with lengths up to about 5 million base pairs, can be separated by increasing the duration of the pulses.

(c) Pulsed-field Electrophoresis of Intact DNA Molecules of *Saccharomyces cerevisiae*

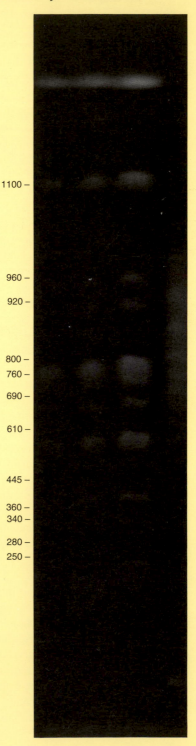

Fragment length (thousands of base pairs)

1100 –
960 –
920 –
800 –
760 –
690 –
610 –
445 –
360 –
340 –
280 –
250 –

DNA fragments are found in the gel at locations corresponding to lengths of 3400, 4900, 5300, 6000, 7900, and 22,000 base pairs. That set of six *Eco*RI restriction-fragment lengths is unique to the λ genome and hence can be used as an identifying characteristic of the genome, a characteristic called its *Eco*RI restriction-fragment fingerprint. Only viral genomes can be fingerprinted with a 6-base cutter such as *Eco*RI. Complete digestion of the much larger bacterial and eukaryotic genomes with a 6-base cutter yields so many restriction fragments that gel electrophoresis produces an essentially continuous smear of fragments rather than a relatively small number of well-separated fragments. However, a short segment of a large genome can be fingerprinted with a 6-base cutter, provided many copies of the segment are available.

Note that the *Eco*RI restriction-fragment fingerprint of the λ genome provides no information about the order of the restriction fragments along the λ genome. More information is needed to order the fragments and thereby construct an *Eco*RI restriction-site map of the λ genome, a map showing the distances between its *Eco*RI restriction sites. One way to get the additional information is to carry out two digestions, one of which is complete and the other only partial. The complete digestion produces fragments such that the length of each is equal to the distance between some two adjacent restriction sites; the partial digestion produces some fragments such that the length of each is equal to the distance spanned by three or more adjacent restriction sites. Together the length data obtained from the two digestions provide sufficient information to order the fragments and construct the restriction-site map.

The restriction-fragment fingerprints of cloned segments of a large genome have found application in the efforts to "map" the segments, that is, to arrange the segments in the order in which they appear along the genome. The principle behind this application is as follows. Suppose that the restriction-fragment fingerprints of two segments of a genome include a number of restriction-fragment lengths in common. Calculations based on the distribution of restriction sites along the genome and on the number of restriction-fragment lengths in common lead to a value for the probability that the two fragments overlap and therefore contain pieces of DNA that are contiguous along a chromosomal DNA molecule. (See "Physical Mapping—A One-Dimensional Jigsaw Puzzle" in "Mapping the Genome.")

This discussion of gel electrophoresis concludes by noting that the electric field used to carry out the procedure is usually a constant electric field. However, in such a field long DNA fragments (fragments longer than about 50,000 base pairs) tend to become trapped at arbitrary locations in the gel and thus do not migrate through the gel in a length-dependent manner. But fragments that long or longer are of interest, and separating them by length is sometimes desirable. For example, making a *Not*I restriction-site map of a human chromosome involves gel electrophoresis of restriction fragments that are on average 1,000,000 base pairs long. (*Not*I is an 8-base cutter; the estimated average length of the fragments it produces, namely $4^8 = 65,536$ base pairs, differs considerably from the observed average length because the recognition sequence of that restriction enzyme includes several occurrences of the dinucleotide sequence 5'-CG, which happens to be rare in mammalian genomes. *Not*I is one of a group of "infrequent cutters," all of which contain at least one occurrence of the sequence 5'-CG and produce fragments with average lengths ranging from 100,000 base pairs to 1 million base pairs.) Length separation of long fragments can be accomplished by using an electric field that varies intermittently in direction but has a time-averaged direction along the length of the gel. Such a "pulsed" field allows long DNA fragments to wind their way through the molecular framework of the gel. As shown in "Gel Electrophoresis," pulsed-field electrophoresis can separate even the very long DNA molecules extracted intact from yeast chromosomes. (Note that pulsed-field gel electrophoresis of long fragments requires preparation of the DNA sample by special methods because the accidental fragmentation involved in the method described at the beginning of this section cannot be tolerated when DNA molecules are to be studied either intact or as the long, reproducibly cut fragments produced by a restriction enzyme such as *Not*I.)

Amplifying DNA. Most of the techniques currently used to analyze a segment of DNA require the availability of many copies of the segment. Two methods for "amplifying" a DNA segment are now at hand: molecular cloning, which was developed in the 1970s, and the polymerase chain reaction (PCR), which was developed less than a decade ago.

Amplification by Molecular Cloning. Molecular cloning involves replication of a foreign DNA segment by a host organism, usually the bacterium *E. coli*. However, a segment of DNA that has entered an *E. coli* cell will not be replicated by the cell unless the segment has first been combined with a cloning "vector," a DNA molecule that the cell does replicate. The combination of the segment to be cloned, the "insert," and the vector is called a recombinant DNA molecule.

The phenomenon of transduction, discovered in 1952, had shown that DNA from the genome of one strain of *E. coli* is sometimes incorporated into the genome of a phage without affecting the ability of the phage to be replicated in another strain of *E. coli*. In other words, the phage genome was known to act as a vector, a DNA molecule that carries foreign DNA into a host cell, where it is then replicated. Nevertheless, the earliest cloning vectors were plasmids, small DNA molecules found in and replicated by bacteria. (Plasmids, like the genomes of bacteria, are circular DNA molecules. They are, however, much smaller than bacterial genomes. Some plasmids are replicated only when their hosts replicate and occur as single copies. The replication of other plasmids is not coordinated with host-cell replication; such plasmids occur as multiple copies.) The plasmid first used was one of a number that had been studied intensively because they contain genes that confer on the bacteria in which they reside the ability to survive in the presence of antibiotics. Today two vectors in addition to phage genomes and plasmids are also widely used: cosmids, which are replicated in *E. coli*, and yeast artificial chromosomes (YACs), which are replicated in the single-celled eukaryotic organism *Saccharomyces cerevisiae* (baker's yeast). Both cosmids and YACs are synthetic rather than naturally occurring DNA molecules.

The first step in molecular cloning is to make the recombinant DNA molecules in vitro. The following is a description of the procedure employed when the vector is a plasmid that contains a single restriction site for *Eco*RI embedded within a gene for resistance to ampicillin. Digestion of a population of such plasmids with *Eco*RI produces "linearized" plasmids with sticky ends. Inserts with identical sticky ends are formed by digesting the DNA to be cloned also with *Eco*RI. When the linearized plasmids and the inserts are mixed together, along with an enzyme called a DNA ligase, the sticky ends of some inserts hydrogen bond to the sticky ends of the linearized plasmids. The backbones of such hydrogen-bonding products are then covalently linked by the DNA ligase into recombinant DNA molecules (here recombinant plasmids). Note that the ligation mixture also contains some nonrecombinant plasmids because some linearized plasmids simply recyclize.

A more detailed description of the making of recombinant DNA molecules with plasmids and other vectors is presented in the article "DNA Libraries." Here we point out only that different vectors are used to clone inserts of different lengths. Plasmids carry inserts that are usually about 4000 base pairs long, λ phages carry inserts that are usually four to five times longer, and YACs carry inserts that are usually more than one hundred times longer. (The great lengths of the inserts carried by YACs implies that YAC cloning, like pulsed-field gel electrophoresis, requires a special method of DNA preparation.)

The next step in molecular cloning with plasmids is to expose a population of *E. coli* cells to the ligation mixture in the hope that one recombinant plasmid will enter each of a reasonable fraction of the cells. Entry of a plasmid into an *E. coli* cell is said to transform the cell, provided the plasmid is replicated by the cell. The mechanism by which a plasmid (or a YAC) enters a host cell is not completely understood, but several empirical methods have been found that increase the efficiency of transformation (number of cells transformed per unit mass of recombinant DNA molecules). In contrast, the mechanism by which a phage enters (infects) a host cell is fairly well understood and is inherently more efficient.

After the *E. coli* cells have been exposed to the ligation mixture, the solution containing the exposed cells is diluted, a small amount of the diluted solution is transferred to each of a number of culture dishes containing a solid growth medium, and the cells are allowed to divide. (Dilution of the exposed cells assures that only a relatively small number of cells is transferred to each culture dish.) The aggregate, or colony, of cells produced by successive divisions of a single cell is called a clone of the single cell. Each member of a clone that arises from a transformed cell contains at least one copy of the plasmid and, if the transforming plasmid was a recombinant plasmid, at least one copy of the insert.

Because the goal of molecular cloning is not only to obtain many copies of the insert within a recombinant DNA molecule but also to do so in as short a time as possible, one criterion for a host cell is a short generation time. The generation times of both *E. coli* and yeast are suitably short. For example, the generation time of *E. coli* is about 20 minutes. Thus a single *E. coli* cell can, under suitable conditions, multiply into more than a billion cells in about 10 hours.

The final step in plasmid cloning is to identify the clones arising from cells transformed by recombinant plasmids. Recall that the *Eco*RI restriction site of the plasmid used in this example lies within its ampicillin-resistance gene. Assume that each host cell itself contained a plasmid carrying a gene for resistance to ampicillin. Then only those clones that arose from cells transformed by a recombinant plasmid possess an *inoperative* ampicillin-resistance gene (because the insert interrupts the gene). Using that fact to identify the clones of interest involves transferring a portion of each clone from the culture dish to some other vessel in a manner that preserves the positions of the clones. Ampicillin is then added to the other vessel, and the positions of the clones that die are noted. The clones at the corresponding positions on the culture dish are the clones desired. Other ingenious tricks have been devised to identify the desired clones.

The sample of DNA to be cloned usually consists of many different fragments, all from the same source. Examples are the large sets of fragments obtained by cutting, say, the mouse genome or the human X chromosome with a restriction enzyme. Then each recombinant DNA molecule contains a different fragment of the source DNA, and each host cell entered by a recombinant DNA molecule gives rise to a clone of a different fragment. A collection of such clones is called a DNA library—a mouse-genome DNA library, say, or a human-X-chromosome DNA library. The article "DNA Libraries" describes molecular cloning more fully and discusses the problems it presents.

Amplification by PCR. Unlike cloning, the polymerase chain reaction is carried out entirely in vitro and, more important, is capable of amplifying a specific one of the many fragments that may be present in a DNA sample. The selectivity of the reaction implies that it is also a means for detecting the presence of the fragment being amplified. Details of the reaction are presented in "The Polymerase Chain Reaction and Sequence-tagged Sites" in "Mapping the Genome."

Sequencing DNA. The ultimate in detailed information about a fragment of DNA is its base sequence. The process of obtaining that information is called sequencing. Two sequencing methods were developed in 1977, both based on essentially the same principle but each realizing the goal in a different way. Let $b_1 b_2 b_3 \ldots b_N$ be the base sequence of the fragment to be sequenced. Consider the set of subfragments $\{b_1, b_1 b_2, b_1 b_2 b_3, \ldots, b_1 b_2 b_3 \ldots b_N\}$. Assume that such a set of subfragments can be generated and, equally important, can be separated into four subsets: the subset A consisting of those subfragments that end in the base A; the subset C consisting of those subfragments that end in C; the subset G consisting of those subfragments that ends in the base G; and the subset T consisting of those subfragments that end in the base T. Note that together the four subsets compose the set $\{b_1, b_1 b_2, b_1 b_2 b_3, \ldots, b_1 b_2 b_3 \ldots b_N\}$. The subsets A, C, G, and T are subjected to electrophoresis, each in a different "lane" of a gel (a different strip of gel parallel to the direction of the applied electric field). After electrophoresis each subfragment is located in one of the four lanes according to its length. Suppose that the shortest subfragment, b_1, appears in the A lane of the gel; that the next longer subfragment, $b_1 b_2$, appears in the T lane; that the next longer subfragment, $b_1 b_2 b_3$, appears in the G lane; . . . ; and that the longest subfragment, $b_1 b_2 b_3 \ldots b_N$, appears in the T lane. Then the base sequence of the fragment is ATG . . . T.

Obviously the above description of the principle of the two sequencing methods has avoided the question of how the four subsets of subfragments are generated. The procedures for doing so are described in "DNA Sequencing" in "Mapping the Genome."

Although sequencing is still a tedious and expensive process, the information so obtained is crucial to identification of the DNA mutations that cause inherited disorders and to a broad understanding of the functioning and evolution of genes and genomes. Much effort is being devoted to increasing the speed and decreasing the cost of current sequencing methods and to searching for new methods.

Hybridization: Detecting the Presence of Specific DNA Sequences. The two single-stranded DNA fragments produced by denaturation of a (double-stranded) DNA fragment will, under appropriate conditions, renature (form a double-stranded fragment by hydrogen bonding) because the single-stranded fragments are complementary along the entirety of their lengths. (Recall that two single-stranded fragments are complementary if and only if the 5′-to-3′ base sequence of one is the complement of the 3′-to-5′ base sequence of the other.) Similarly, hydrogen bonding between an RNA fragment and a complementary single-stranded DNA fragment will form a double-stranded DNA-RNA fragment, a phenomenon called hybridization. (Hybridization between the RNA transcript of an *E. coli* gene and the template strand of the gene was the technique used in the 1960s to measure the rates of transcription of various *E. coli* genes.) The term "hybridization" now also includes the hydrogen bonding that occurs between any two single-stranded nucleic-acid fragments that are complementary along only some portion (usually a relatively short portion) of their lengths.

Hybridization is widely used to detect the presence of a particular DNA segment in a sample of DNA. If the sample consists of a set of cloned DNA fragments, each cloned fragment is denatured and then allowed to interact with a solution containing many copies of a radioactively labeled "probe," a relatively short stretch of single-stranded DNA whose sequence is identical to or complementary to some unique portion of the segment of interest. Under the right conditions the probe hybridizes only to the cloned fragment (or fragments) that contains the segment of interest, and the radioactivity of the probe identifies the fragment to which the probe has hybridized. For example, suppose that the sample is a complete set of cloned human DNA fragments and the segment of interest is the interspersed tandem repeat $(5'\text{-GT})_n$. Examples of a probe for that segment are the single-stranded fragments with the sequences $(5'\text{-AC})_7$ and $(5'\text{-GT})_7$. Because the segment $(5'\text{-GT})_n$ appears at numerous locations in the human genome, such a probe hybridizes to numerous cloned fragments but only to those containing the interspersed tandem repeat (or a portion thereof). If the sample to be interrogated with a probe is instead a solution containing many different DNA fragments, the fragments must first be separated and immobilized, usually by gel electrophoresis. If the probe is sufficiently short, hybridization can be carried out directly on the gel. Usually, however, the length-separated fragments are first transferred from the gel to a nitrocellulose filter. The procedure, called Southern (or gel-transfer) hybridization, is illustrated in "Hybridization Techniques."

In-situ hybridization is a variation of hybridization in which the sample to be interrogated with a probe consists of the intact DNA molecules within metaphase chromosomes. The metaphase chromosomes are spread out on a microscope slide and partially denatured. The probe copies are labeled with a fluorescent molecule and allowed to interact with the denatured chromosomes. The presence of bound probe is detected by observing the chromosomes with a fluorescence microscope. An example of the fluorescence signal obtained by using the technique is shown in "Hybridization Techniques." In-situ hybridization provides information about which chromosome contains the segment of interest and its approximate location on the chromosome.

This section on the techniques of molecular genetics concludes with an application that not only requires the use of almost all the techniques described but also is of particular significance to the efforts to arrange cloned fragments of human DNA in the same order as they appear in the intact DNA molecules of human chromosomes. The application involves the use of long cloned fragments of human DNA to obtain an upper limit on the length of the segment of DNA that separates the chromosomal locations of any two short cloned fragments of human DNA (such as those provided by plasmid, phage, or cosmid cloning). The long fragments, which are produced by cutting human genomic DNA with an infrequent cutter, are subjected to pulsed-field gel electrophoresis and then to Southern hybridization. Two different probes are used separately in the hybridization; each is unique to one of the two short cloned fragments. If both probes hybridize to the same long fragment, then both short fragments lie within the long fragment. In other words, the chromosomal locations of the short fragments are separated by a length of DNA no longer than the length of the long fragment to which both probes hybridized.

HYBRIDIZATION TECHNIQUES

Southern hybridization is a technique for identifying, among a sample of many different DNA fragments, the fragment(s) containing a particular nucleotide sequence. As depicted in (a), the sample has typically been fragmented with a restriction enzyme. The restriction fragments are subjected to gel electrophoresis to separate them by length and immobilize them. The length-separated fragments are then transferred to a filter paper made of nitrocellulose, a procedure called blotting. (Note that blotting preserves the locations of the fragments.) The filter is washed first with a solution that denatures the fragments and then with a solution containing many copies of a radioactively labeled, single-stranded "probe" whose sequence is identical to or complementary to some unique portion of the sequence of interest. The probe hybridizes (hydrogen bonds) to only the denatured fragments containing the complement of its sequence and hence the sequence of interest. The unbound probe is washed away, and the filter is dried and placed in contact with x-ray film. The radioactivity of the bound probe exposes the film and creates an image, an autoradiogram, of the fragment(s) to which the probe has bound. Southern hybridization is particularly useful for detecting variations among different members of a species in the lengths of the restriction fragments originating from a particular region of the organism's genome (see "Modern Linkage Mapping with Polymorphic DNA Markers" in "Mapping the Genome").

The number of fragments "picked out" by a probe depends on the number of times the sequence of interest occurs in the sample DNA. If the sequence occurs only once (if a probe for, say, a single-copy gene is being used), the probe picks out one or at most two fragments (provided the probe is shorter than any of the fragments in the sample). On the other hand, if the sequence of interest occurs more than once (if a probe for a multiple-copy gene or a repeated sequence is being used), the probe picks out a larger number of fragments. Furthermore, the hybridization conditions (temperature and salinity of the probe solution) can be adjusted so that either exact complementarity or a lesser degree of complementarity is required for binding of the probe.

In-situ hybridization is a variation of hybridization in which the sample consists of the complement of chromosomes within a cell arrested at metaphase. The metaphase chromosomes are spread out and partially denatured on a microscope slide, the probe is labeled with a fluorescent dye, and the bound probe is imaged with a fluorescence microscope. Shown in (b) is the fluorescence signal resulting from in-situ hybridization of a probe for the human telomere to human metaphase chromosomes. (A telomere is a special sequence at each end of a eukaryotic DNA molecule that protects the molecule from enzymatic degradation and prevents shortening of the molecule as it is replicated. The sequence of the human telomere was discovered by Robert K. Moyzis and his colleagues, who also provided evidence that all vertebrates share the same telomeric sequence. Note that, as expected, the probe has bound only to the terminal regions of each chromosome. (Micrograph courtesy of Julie Meyne.)

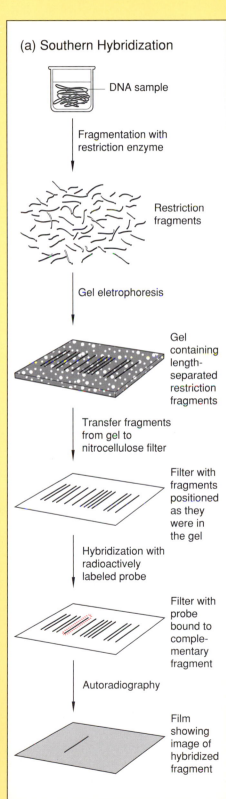

(a) Southern Hybridization

DNA sample

Fragmentation with restriction enzyme

Restriction fragments

Gel electrophoresis

Gel containing length-separated restriction fragments

Transfer fragments from gel to nitrocellulose filter

Filter with fragments positioned as they were in the gel

Hybridization with radioactively labeled probe

Filter with probe bound to complementary fragment

Autoradiography

Film showing image of hybridized fragment

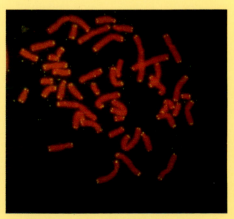

(b) Results of In-Situ Hybridization of Human-Telomere Probe to Human Chromosomes

THE ANATOMY OF A EUKARYOTIC PROTEIN GENE

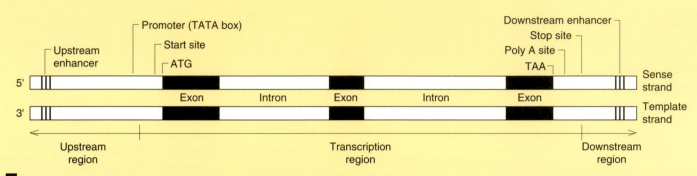

Each eukaryotic gene is placed in one of three classes according to which of the three eukaryotic RNA polymerases is involved in its transcription. The genes for RNAs are transcribed by RNA polymerases I and III. The genes for proteins, the class first brought to mind by the word "gene" and the class focused on here, are transcribed by RNA polymerase II (*pol* II).

Shown above are the components of a prototypic protein gene. By convention the sense strand of the gene, the strand with the sequence of DNA bases corresponding to the sequence of RNA bases in the primary RNA transcript, is depicted with its 5´-to-3´ direction coincident with the left-to-right direction. (Often only the sense strand of a gene is displayed.) The left-to-right direction thus coincides with the direction in which the template strand is transcribed. The terms "upstream" and "downstream" describe the location of one feature of a gene relative to that of another. Their meanings in that context are based on regarding transcription as a directional process analogous to the flow of water in a stream.

The start site is the location of the first deoxyribonucleotide in the template strand that happens to be transcribed. It defines the beginning of the transcription region of the gene. Note that the start site lies upstream of the DNA codon (ATG) corresponding to the RNA codon (AUG) that signals the start of translation of the transcribed RNA. The transcription region ends at some nonspecific deoxyribonucleotide between 500 and 2000 base pairs downstream of the poly A site. Within the poly A site are sequences that, when transcribed, signal the location at which the primary RNA transcript is cleaved and equipped with a "tail" composed of a succession of ribonucleotides containing the base A. (The poly A tail is thought to aid the transport of messenger RNA from the nucleus of a cell to the cytoplasm.) Note that the poly A site lies downstream of the DNA codon (here TAA) corresponding to one of the RNA codons (UAA) that signals the end of translation of the transcribed RNA.

Within the transcription region are exons and introns. Exons tend to be about 300 base pairs long; each is a succession of codons uninterrupted by stop codons. Introns, on the other hand, are not uninterruped successions of codons, and the RNA segments transcribed from introns are spliced out of the primary RNA transcript before translation. A few protein genes contain no introns (the human α–interferon gene is an example), most contain at least one, and some contain a large number (the human thyroglobulin gene contains about forty). Generally the amount of DNA composing the introns of a protein gene is far greater than the amount composing its exons.

Close upstream of the start site is a promoter sequence, where *pol* II binds and initiates transcription. A common promoter sequence in eukaryotic genes is the so-called TATA box, which has the consensus sequence 5´-TATAAA and is located at a variable short distance (about 30 base pairs) upstream of the start site.

The region upstream of the promoter and, less frequently, the downstream region or the transcription region itself contain sequences that control the rate of initiation of transcription. Although expression of a protein gene is regulated at a number of stages in the pathway from gene to protein, control of replication initiation is the dominant regulatory mechanism. (Primary among the other regulatory mechanisms is control of splicing.) The regulated expression of a gene (the when, where, and degree of expression) is the key to phenotypic differences between the various cells of a multicellular organism and also between organisms that possess similar genotypes.

Initiation of transcription is controlled mainly by DNA sequences (*cis* elements) and by certain proteins, many but not all of which are sequence-specific DNA-binding proteins (*trans*-acting transcription factors). Thus both temporal and cellular specificities of transcription control are governed by the availability of the different *trans*-acting transcription factors. Interactions of transcription factors with *cis* elements and with each other lead to formation of complex protein assemblies that control the ability of *pol* II to initiate transcription. Most of the complexes enhance transcription initiation, but some act as repressors. Enhancers and repressors can be located as far as 10,000 base pairs away from the transcription region.

Class I and class III genes differ from protein genes not only in their anatomies but also in the promoters, *cis* elements, and *trans*-acting factors involved in their transcription.

Genes and Genomes: What the Future Holds

The techniques described in the preceding section, and others not mentioned, have greatly increased our knowledge of the molecular anatomies of genes. Previously, a gene for a protein was defined narrowly as a segment of DNA that is transcribed into a messenger RNA, which in turn is translated into the protein. The definition considered more appropriate today includes not only the protein-coding segment of the gene (its transcription region) but also its sometimes far-flung regulatory regions (see "The Anatomy of a Eukaryotic Protein Gene"). The regulatory regions contain DNA sequences that help determine whether and at what rate the gene is expressed (or, equivalently, the protein is synthesized). Some of the genes of a multicellular organism, its "housekeeping" genes, are expressed at more or less the same level in essentially all of its cells, regardless of type. Others are expressed only in certain types of cells or only at certain times. Gene regulation is, in fact, the key not only to appropriate functioning of the organism but also to its development from a single cell. In addition, gene regulation may also be responsible for the striking phenotypic differences between higher apes and humans despite the negligible differences between the structures of their proteins. "The Anatomy of a Eukaryotic Protein Gene" presents also a few details about the mechanisms of gene regulation.

Despite the accumulating knowledge, it is safe to say that what is known about genes, particularly human genes, is far less than what remains to be learned. The total number of human genes can now be only crudely estimated, remarkably few have been localized to particular regions of particular chromosomes, and even fewer have been sequenced or studied in sufficient detail to understand their regulation. Other outstanding questions include the mechanisms by which the expression of genes is coordinated and the effects of gene mutations on morphology, physiology, and pathology.

The techniques of molecular genetics are also providing information about genomes as a whole, opening the way to comparative studies of genome anatomy, organization, and evolution. For example, the available evidence indicates remarkable similarities between the mouse genome and the human genome, despite the 60 million years that have elapsed since rodents and primates diverged from a common ancestor. The similarities lie not only in the base sequences of genes but also in their linkages. Perhaps the conserved linked genes represent units of some higher, as yet unknown operational feature. The same may be true also of repetitive DNA, about which we now know so little. In time, when those and other genomes have been sequenced in their entireties, the observed similarities and differences will be a rich source of answers and new questions about the operation and evolution of genomes. ■

Further Reading

James A. Peters, editor. 1964. *Classic Papers in Genetics.* Englewood Cliffs, New Jersey: Prentice-Hall, Inc.

J. Herbert Taylor, editor. 1965. *Selected Papers on Molecular Genetics.* New York: Academic Press.

John Cairns, Gunther S. Stent, and James D. Watson, editors. 1966. *Phage and the Origins of Molecular Biology.* Cold Spring Harbor, New York: Cold Spring Harbor Laboratory of Quantitative Biology.

John C. Kendrew. 1968. *The Thread of Life: An Introduction to Molecular Biology.* Cambridge, Massachusetts: Harvard University Press.

René J. Dubos. 1976. *The Professor, the Institute, and DNA.* New York: The Rockefeller University Press.

Franklin H. Porugal and Jack S. Cohen. 1977. *A Century of DNA: A History of the Discovery of the Structure and Function of the Genetic Substance.* Cambridge, Massachusetts: The MIT Press.

Horace Freeland Judson. 1979. *The Eighth Day of Creation.* New York: Simon and Schuster.

James D. Watson. 1980. *The Double Helix: A Personal Account of the Discovery of the Structure of DNA.* New York: W. W. Norton and Co.

James D. Watson and John Tooze. 1981. *The DNA Story: A Documentary History of Gene Cloning.* San Francisco: W. H. Freeman and Company.

James D. Watson, Nancy H. Hopkins, Jeffrey W. Roberts, Joan Argetsinger Steitz, and Alan M. Weiner. 1987. *Molecular Biology of the Gene.* Menlo Park, California: The Benjamin/Cummings Publishing Company, Inc.

David A. Micklos and Greg A. Freyer. 1990. *DNA Science: A First Course in Recombinant DNA Technology.* New York: Cold Spring Harbor Laboratory Press.

James Darnell, Harvey Lodish, and David Baltimore. 1990. *Molecular Cell Biology*, second edition. New York: W. H. Freeman and Company.

Maxine Singer and Paul Berg. 1991. *Genes & Genomes: A Changing Perspective.* Mill Valley, California: University Science Books.

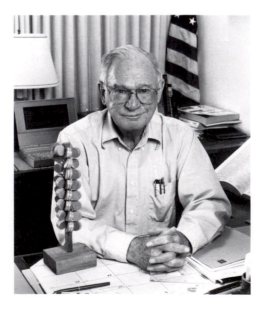

Robert P. Wagner is a consultant to the Laboratory's Life Sciences Division and Professor Emeritus of Zoology at the University of Texas, Austin, the institution from which he received his Ph.D. His work at the Laboratory focuses on the activities of the Center for Human Genome Studies. He has taught undergraduate and graduate genetics for over thiry-five years and has authored or co-authored six books and many research and review articles on various aspects of genetics. His numerous honors and awards include fellowships from the National Research Council and the Guggenheim Foundation and election as a fellow of the American Association for the Advancement of Science and as president of the Genetics Society of America.

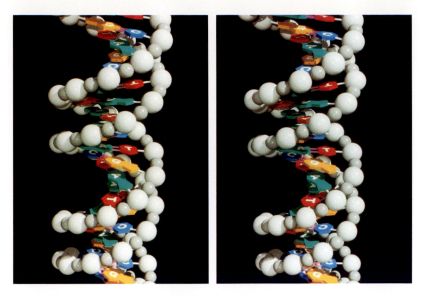

To create a stereoscopic image of DNA from the two images on this page, focus your eyes on a distant object above the page and then move the images up into your line of sight, holding the page 12 to 18 inches away and being careful to keep your eyes focused at infinity. If your eyes have not shifted, you should be aware of three images. Concentrate on the middle one, which is the desired stereoscopic image. You may have to practice a few times and should be sure the page and your head are vertical.

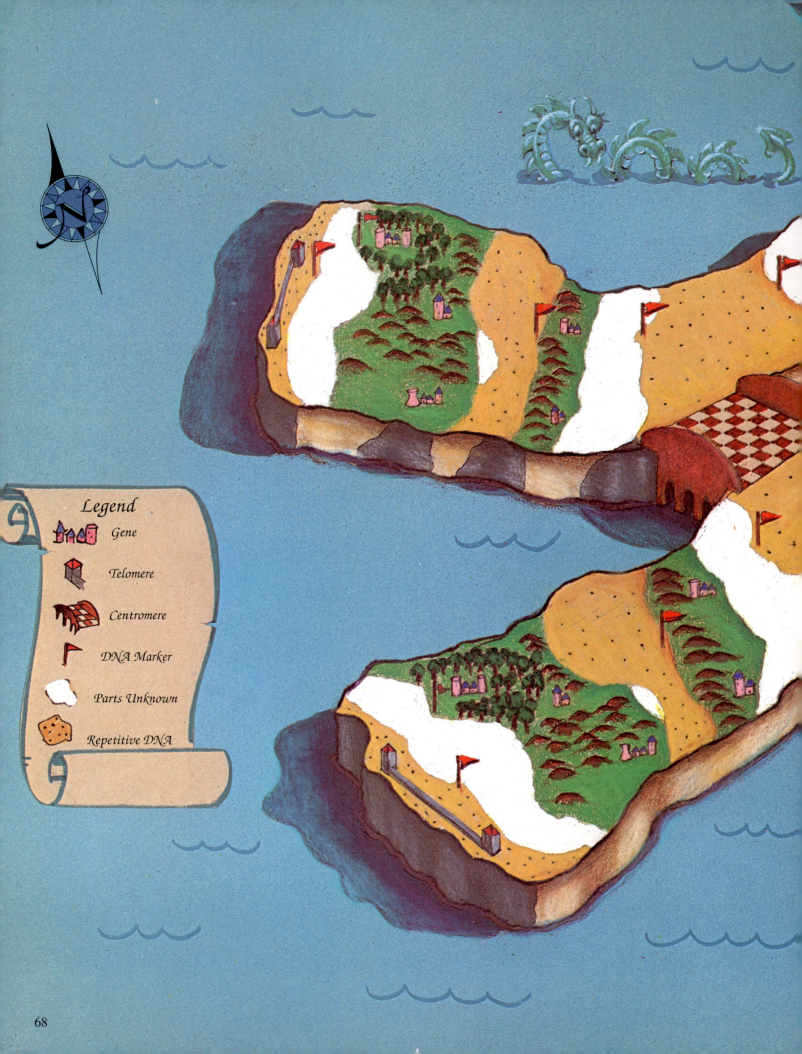

Legend

Gene

Telomere

Centromere

DNA Marker

Parts Unknown

Repetitive DNA

Mapping the Genome

the vision, the science, the implementation

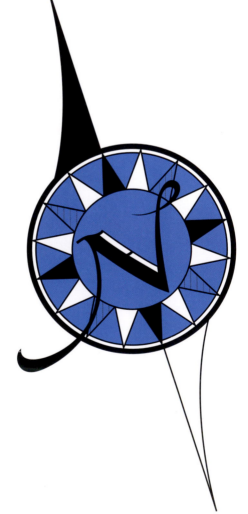

*T*he Human Genome Project is the first large coordinated effort in the history of biological research. The aim is to make a detailed map of human DNA—the hereditary instructions inscribed in DNA that guide the development of a human being from a fertilized egg cell.

Like sixteenth-century maps of the new world, present maps of the human genome contain few landmarks and many parts unknown. And like the explorers of the new world, the genome explorers are pushing forward into vast uncharted territory in the face of great uncertainties—both political and technological.

Some conservatives in the genetics community have expressed skepticism about the ultimate value of the project, and many biologists worry about the lack of funds for other projects. The project itself is fraught with technical uncertainties. But there is also a sense of creating a new order in biology, a revolution in which computers and automation are joined with advanced technologies in molecular biology to speed the process of DNA analysis. The far-reaching goal is to sequence not one human genome but many and routinely, to sequence the genomes of many other organisms and compare those sequences with the human sequence, to store all the data in computers and share them electronically, and to make cooperation the rule instead of the exception.

Egos are apparent in this ambitious enterprise—a self-consciousness of being part of a historic project and of having the chance to stake a claim in this wide-open territory. The goal is tantalizing. But to overcome the danger of promising too much, the disappointment of slow beginnings, the threat that dissension in the community will destroy the effort, the fear of centralization, the discomfort with quantitative analysis, the difficulty of the task, the inertia of the establishment—will require great determination and skill.

During 1991 and early 1992, we invited some of the modern-day explorers to discuss their vision, their answers to the skeptics, and their progress toward their goals. The following compilation of those discussions reveals a rapidly changing panorama of problems and priorities, as should be expected in this emerging field. It also reveals differences of opinion about strategies and timing. But the participants agree unanimously that this project is not only the culmination of the recombinant-DNA revolution of the 1970s but also the beginning of a new technological revolution enabling us to answer some of the great mysteries of evolution and human development. It promises to increase our understanding of our place among species and to reveal new limitations and new potential for shaping our individual destinies and those of future generations.

I: What Is the Genome Project?

Bob Moyzis: This discussion is meant to address scientists, particularly physical scientists, who know very little about the Human Genome Project and may have many misconceptions about it. Let's share our perceptions of how this project got started. Why are we doing it, and why did the idea of taking on the entire human genome gain support in the scientific community?

David Botstein: The answers are complicated because the human genome is largely unexplored territory. It's tremendously information-rich, and different people have had different ideas about the best way to go about finding out what's there. The initial proponents of the Genome Project, especially Charles DeLisi in the Department of Energy [DOE], said, "The human genome is the blueprint for the development of a single fertilized egg, into a complex organism of more than 10^{13} cells. The blueprint is written in a coded message given by the sequence of nucleotide bases—the As, Cs, Gs, and Ts that are strung along the DNA molecules in the genome. So let's read the entire sequence from one end to the other, put the whole thing in a computer, and give it to the theoreticians and computer analysts to decode the instructions." And what instructions does the human genome contain? Everyone who has taken high-school biology knows that DNA contains genes, that genes are the coded messages for making proteins, and that proteins carry out all of the functions of an organism. So why not begin by reading the sequence?

Now many of us, including me, thought the straight sequencing approach was crazy because it ignores biology. Yes, we can read the sequence, pick out a gene, and use the genetic code to translate the coding regions of the gene into the sequence of amino acids that composes the protein. But then we run into a big problem: How do we know what the protein does? At present we have no way to determine the function of a protein from its amino-acid sequence alone. Wally Gilbert likes to say that if we had a catalog of all the protein amino-acid sequences, we would be able to deduce protein functions. Some day we may get there, but right now that's science fiction, not science.

Bob Moyzis: Interpreting protein function is a problem. But the straight sequencing approach, as initially proposed, presented other serious difficulties. First and foremost, the technology to sequence the whole genome was just not available. That was the conclusion of the human genome workshop sponsored by the DOE in 1986 in Santa Fe, New Mexico, and it is true today. We're not too bad at reading stretches of DNA 10,000 bases long—the average length of a gene—but present technologies are still too labor-intensive and too expensive to think of sequencing the 6 billion bases in the human genome. However, the technology is changing rapidly, a point we'll return to later. We're also not certain how to pick out the genes from all the other DNA sequences in the genome or how to separate the gene sequences into protein-coding regions, or exons, and noncoding regions, or introns. We're making progress, but the problems are still unsolved. On the other hand, most participants at the 1986 meeting agreed that a major effort in genetic and physical mapping was appropriate. That conclusion was confirmed by the report, published in 1987, of the DOE's Health and Environment Research Advisory Committee. Many individuals with a physical-science background do not understand that a DNA sequence *without* a genetic map is nearly useless.

David Botstein: Most of us were unaware of the DOE workshop and report, but the idea of understanding the human genome stirred up so much interest that the National Research Council organized its own committee to assess the feasibility of the Project. Some members of that committee are here—Maynard Olson, Lee Hood, and I. We independently recommended that the Human Genome Project go ahead—but, as Bob pointed out, in an entirely different manner than originally proposed. We said, "Let's postpone sequencing the genome until we develop better sequencing technology and focus on developing the tools, the genetic and physical maps, needed to interpret the sequence once we have it. Let's build some biology into this effort."

Bob Moyzis: But we still have a problem of perception in the scientific community. The conclusion of every meeting and report on the Human Genome Project has been that the goal is *not* to immediately sequence the entire human genome. That idea died an early death. But every negative report about the Project says that we are going to be doing this mindless sequencing.

Maynard Olson: Critics often do not take the time to understand what they are criticizing.

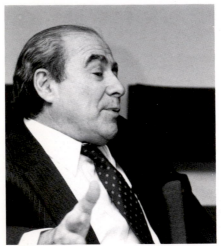

Norton Zinder

Until recently people tried to guess which protein from among the tens of thousands of human proteins was produced by the mutant gene . . . the new approach is to avoid playing around with lots of proteins and instead to find the responsible gene in the DNA.

Norton Zinder: I'd like to go back to an earlier point, that different people are interested in different aspects of the genome. The most ambitious interest is a very long-term goal—to understand the whole blueprint. But there's a large group of people, and maybe they're in the majority, who are more practical. They are interested in understanding human disease, and they support the Genome Project because the maps that will be developed are just the tools needed to find the genes responsible for inherited diseases. Victor McKusick has compiled a catalog of over 4000 such diseases and many of them are Mendelian, which means that they are each caused by a single mutant gene. People are very excited about the prospect of finding those genes.

Bob Moyzis: It's ironic that the genetic-mapping community had little to do, I feel, with initiating the Human Genome Project, recent books documenting the history of this project notwithstanding. Once the Project gained momentum, however, it was clear that the human genetic-mapping community would be a primary user of the maps, particularly in the search for the genes causing the Mendelian diseases that Norton just mentioned. Our audience may be surprised to learn that the method used to infer that a single gene is the cause of an inherited disease goes all the way back to Mendel. Despite all the advances we've made in molecular genetics, Mendel's laws and his indirect methods of inference still provide the basic methods for much of what is done in genetics.

David Botstein: Mendel identified the basic unit, the quantum, of heredity, which is the gene. Mendel's laws are the quantum mechanics of genetics. They provide a quantitative link between physical traits, the traits we see, and genetic traits, which are the unseen messages in the genetic material. In the case of humans, looking for Mendelian patterns of inheritance is often the only method we have for connecting phenotype with genotype.

Bob Moyzis: Mendel's laws apply only to discrete variable traits—for example having or not having unusually short fingers, a trait called brachydactyly. Because those traits [normal or short digits] are inherited according to the ratios predicted by Mendel, geneticists can infer a number of things. First, that digit length is determined by a single pair of genes, one inherited from each parent, and second that the brachydactyly gene has two versions, or alleles, say A and a, where A is the rare dominant allele that causes the anomalous digit length.

Most variable traits are not Mendelian. They result from the complex interaction of many genes. On the other hand, many inherited diseases *are* the result of a single mutant gene. How do we determine that? We can't do controlled-breeding experiments and analyze thousands of offspring as Mendel did. But if we trace the disease through the generations of families affected by the disease, we can use statistical analysis to infer from a relatively small sample whether a single gene-pair is involved, and if so, whether the mutant gene, the allele that causes the disease, is dominant or recessive. [For a discussion of Mendel's laws, see "Understanding Inheritance."]

Norton Zinder: Yes, but how do we go further toward understanding the disease? Until recently people tried to guess which protein from among the tens of thousands of human proteins was produced by the mutant gene. They would use various biochemical and cytological methods to compare normal and disease-affected tissues, but often the disease gives no clue as to what proteins might be involved. The new approach is to avoid playing around with lots of proteins and instead to find the responsible gene in the DNA, sequence the gene, determine its protein product, and then try to determine what the protein does.

How do we find the gene responsible for a Mendelian trait? Until 1980 we had no practical method. Then David Botstein came up with a brilliant idea that's been used successfully to locate several of the more common disease genes and given great impetus to the Genome Project. The idea is based on a very old method for inferring the order of and relative distances between genes that lie along a single chromosome, what we call genetic-linkage mapping.

David Cox: Methods for constructing classical linkage maps are basic to what we are doing in the Genome Project, and again, they are an extension of Mendelian inference. Suppose we focus on two different Mendelian, or single gene, traits and trace the pattern of their co-inheritance from one generation to the next just as Mendel did. We may find that the phenotypes of two traits don't follow Mendel's law of independent assortment, but rather, that specific forms of those traits are almost always co-inherited. Statistically, that means the gene pairs for the two traits are linked and therefore lie on the same chromosome pair.

If we had a blackboard, we could show the particular type of mating, called the test cross, that reveals linkage between two different gene pairs. The gist of it is that if one parent is heterozygous for both traits—has the genotype *AaBb*—and the other parent is homozygous recessive for both traits—has the genotype *aabb*—then

the combinations of the two traits in the offspring tell us whether or not the two gene pairs are on the same chromosome pair. [See "Classical Linkage Mapping."]

The interesting thing is that some fraction of the time the alleles—particular forms of the two genes—on a given chromosome are *not* co-inherited. How do they break apart? During the formation of either eggs or sperms, a pair of homologous, or matching, chromosomes can exchange corresponding chunks of DNA in a process called crossing over and thereby produce chromosomes containing new combinations of alleles. The recombinant chromosomes can then be inherited by an offspring.

How often do two alleles get separated by crossing over? It depends on how far apart they are. And that's the key to estimating the distance separating the two alleles. That distance is called the genetic distance. People have done many such linkage studies and constructed linkage maps giving the order of and genetic distances between genes that specify Mendelian traits and that lie on the same chromosome. The problem is that linkage analysis provides no way of locating genes on the chromosome itself.

Norton Zinder: The breakthrough in finding human genes was Botstein's idea to apply the methods of linkage not to variable physical traits that we see with our eyes but to variations in the base sequence of the DNA, that is, to variations in the spelling of the DNA. Variations in spelling are called polymorphisms, and they may occur anywhere along the genome—not only in the genes. The important point is that if the variations at some locus, some region, of a chromosome can be detected by a DNA probe, the region

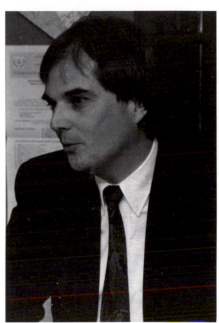

Bob Moyzis

We are asked frequently whether the isolation of a disease gene immediately leads to a cure. Of course it does not, but without isolation of the gene, finding a cure is almost impossible.

becomes a DNA marker, that is, a variable DNA trait that can be traced through families in the same way we trace variable physical traits. [See "Modern Linkage Mapping with Polymorphic DNA Markers—A Tool for Finding Genes."]

In fact, we can construct a linkage map of DNA markers spaced throughout the genome provided we can find the appropriate probes. The search for DNA probes that detect variable loci is done at random and is very time-consuming. Once a probe for a DNA marker is found, however, not only can the marker be used in linkage analysis but also the probe can be used to find the physical location of the marker on the genome. And then we have a way of locating disease genes on the genome. Because if a disease is co-inherited most of the time with some marker, then the disease gene must be physically close to the site of the marker.

Bob Moyzis: There's a tremendous amount of effort involved in this approach, but it works. It's been used to find a number of disease genes, including the genes for cystic fibrosis and neurofibromatosis. That's why the first priority of the Genome Project, as outlined in the joint DOE/NIH five-year plan, is to construct linkage maps of polymorphic markers and furthermore to include enough markers on the linkage maps so that no two are very far apart. At the same time we will build physical maps consisting of cloned DNA fragments that cover the genome in a more or less continuous way, so we can locate the markers from the linkage maps on the DNA itself.

And once we integrate the physical maps and the linkage maps, we'll be able to find the genes related to virtually all inherited diseases, including

multigenic diseases such as cancer and neurological disorders. That's the plan, and it's what we're doing right now. We're also developing more efficient technology for sequencing and applying that technology to the sequencing of million-base stretches of DNA.

Norton Zinder: Most people don't see this project the way we do. That's why there are so many misconceptions about it. This Project is creating an infrastructure for doing science; it's not the doing of the science per se. It will provide the biological community with the basic materials for doing research on human biology.

> *This Project is creating an infrastructure for doing science; it's not the doing of science per se. It will provide the biological community with the basic materials for doing their research on human biology. And the whole endeavor is technology-driven because getting 6 billion of anything is a hard job. At every level it is a bootstrapping operation.*

The whole endeavor is technology-driven because getting 6 billion of anything is a hard job. At every level it is a bootstrapping operation. First, we

have to improve the technology to do mapping and sequencing on a large scale, and then we have to do the mapping and sequencing.

Bob Moyzis: Norton, why don't you expand on what you mean by *creating an infrastructure for doing science.*

Norton Zinder: There are two kinds of biological science. The one most of us like to talk about—synthetic science—concerns topics like physiology, biochemistry, and biological function. The second is analytical science, which many of us take for granted. Analytical science answers questions such as: What is hemoglobin made of? How many disulfide bridges are in that protein? Does it have two amino-acid chains or just one? And answering such questions generates the technical means for doing synthetic science.

Now the Genome Project is analytical science. It will determine the structure of the genome down to the order of the nucleotide bases along the DNA molecule in each chromosome. Some biologists complain that not every base is important and that we are doing analysis for the sake of doing analysis. But careful analysis often leads to surprises.

Let me give you one beautiful example. No one knew that many proteins are initially made with a sequence of amino acids, called the signal sequence, that allows those proteins to be transported from the membrane where they are made—the endoplasmic reticulum—to other locations in the cell. The signal sequence is usually removed after the protein reaches its destination, so its existence was not detected. But when the RNA template for the protein hemoglobin was sequenced, we discovered that it coded for this extra sequence of amino acids not found in mature hemoglobin. This one fact led to the whole theory of protein translocation, and it is the kind of discovery that will almost certainly come from sequencing the human genome.

Maynard Olson: Wally Gilbert is among those who say that the Genome Project isn't science because it's about improving the technology for doing things we already know how to do rather than about new ideas. But that's a rather naive view of what science is. As Sydney Brenner once said, "In molecular biology there are technical advances, discoveries, and ideas, and they usually occur in that order." Was von Leeuwenhoek doing science when he developed the microscope and realized how to use it for biology?

For more than a hundred years advances in biology correlated more closely with advances in optics than with anything else that was happening. As biologists could see better, they made discoveries about organisms, cells, and subcellular structures, and from these came more powerful ideas. We know science doesn't always work that way. Darwinism and Mendelism are counterexamples, where abstract ideas really led the way. But most of the time biology is driven forward by new technology.

Norton Zinder: I'm known to be overly cautious about predicting new technological developments, and at the moment we need new technology to meet the goals of the Genome Project. But during my forty years in molecular biology, I've learned to have great faith that when people start thinking about doing something, they're going to come through with a means of doing it and that means invariably opens up a whole world of new possibilities. Back in 1969 Gunther Stent wrote a book saying that we were at the end

of the great discoveries in molecular biology. At that point we knew the genetic code and we knew that DNA was the genetic material. The next step was to learn how to manipulate DNA so we could study just how it really works, but there seemed to be no way of doing that because DNA molecules are so chemically monotonous—they are just long strings of four different nucleotides. Then came the discovery of restriction enzymes, enzymes that recognize specific nucleotide sequences and cut DNA at just those sites. And that changed everything because we had a way to break up DNA molecules in a reproducible way. Questions we couldn't conceive of even asking suddenly became accessible to study.

Bob Moyzis: The discovery of restriction enzymes started the recombinant-DNA revolution in the 1970s. I was a graduate student at Johns Hopkins University when pioneers like Hamilton Smith isolated the first restriction enzymes. Smith later received the Nobel Prize for his work, and this was an incredibly exciting time at Hopkins.

Using restriction enzymes, it became possible to cut pieces of DNA from, say, mouse, and combine them with a piece of bacterial DNA. One could then propagate that recombinant DNA molecule in a host organism, usually the bacterium *E. coli*, and then either harvest the recombinant clones for further analysis or study the expression of the foreign DNA insert in the host organism. So restriction enzymes turned out to be a tremendous breakthrough.

Norton Zinder: I had the good fortune to experience the impact of a technological breakthrough firsthand because it was a breakthrough in which I actually participated. It was 1948, and I was a graduate student working on the genetics

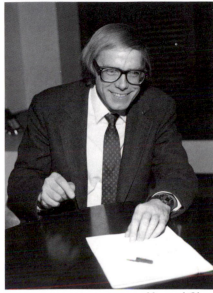

Maynard Olson

For more than a hundred years advances in biology correlated more closely with advances in optics than with anything else that was happening . . . We know science doesn't always work that way. Darwinism and Mendelism are counterexamples, where abstract ideas really led the way. But most of the time biology is driven forward by new technology.

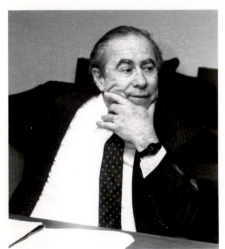

Norton Zinder

During my forty years in molecular biology, I've learned to have great faith that when people start thinking about doing something, they're going to come through with a means of doing it and that means invariably opens up a whole world of new possibilities.

of *E. coli*. At that time it was almost impossible to make new bacterial mutants, and without new mutants, geneticists can't work. The standard practice was to irradiate the bacteria and test them, one at a time, for some new trait. The type of trait we were looking for was a biochemical defect that would affect their ability to grow in the absence of some growth factor. Unfortunately, almost all the bacteria would die, and in a month's work, you would find maybe one mutant. Well, the day after Joshua Lederberg and I thought of using penicillin as a negative selection factor for mutants, we had more mutants than we could ever analyze in our lifetimes.

Maynard Olson: Let me fill in Norton's story. The idea was to deprive the bacteria of a growth factor, say a certain amino acid. Since normal, or wild-type, bacteria manufacture all the amino acids, they would continue to grow. But penicillin was known to kill only growing cells. So when you apply penicillin to the culture, it kills the wild-type bacteria, whereas the mutants that stopped growing because they didn't manufacture the amino acid would sit there in a latent state, unaffected by the penicillin. Then you washed the penicillin away and isolated the new mutants.

Norton Zinder: From that moment on all of the intermediary metabolisms of *E. coli*, that is, all the biochemical steps needed to synthesize important chemical compounds, became accessible to study, and bacterial genetics moved forward in ways that led us to understand a great deal about how genes really work. It led, for example, to my discovery of bacterial transduction, which is the introduction of genes from one bacterial mutant into another by a bacterial virus. Bacterial transduction is a natural progenitor of recombinant-DNA technology.

Maynard Olson: We need to remind ourselves that when Norton was doing those experiments, molecular biology was barely a field. Only a few people like Norton, with eclectic interests in microbiology, biochemistry, physiology, and so on, were thinking about biological processes in a new way and trying to understand their origins in the genetic material. But recombinant-DNA technology has had a huge impact on the way biologists work because it enables almost anyone to study DNA. The field of molecular biology is now defined by a certain experimental paradigm, and people interested in population genetics, developmental biology, protein chemistry, or whatever are all, in a sense, molecular biologists. They all search for answers at the level of the DNA. And they all use more or less the same experimental techniques. You take DNA out of cells, find out something about it, change it, put it back into cells, and then you see how the cells work differently. That's the basic paradigm.

Norton Zinder: Molecular biology is a powerful approach because all of biology starts from genes. I'm not saying genes are everything, but without them you don't get very far. That's why our colleagues, whether they are molecular biologists, neurobiologists, or students of African killer bees are all trying to locate and clone the genes relevant to their interests. When the Genome Project delivers these global maps of the human genome, the search for human genes at least will be a lot easier.

David Botstein: It's worth expanding that point. Our recent success in isolating human disease genes has made everybody optimistic about the usefulness of the Human Genome Project. But those genes were found one at a time. Once we have the linkage maps of highly polymorphic markers and the physical maps of ordered, cloned DNA fragments, the search for disease genes will become routine.

The first step in isolating a disease gene will be to trace the markers one at a time through several generations of a family or families affected by the disease. The markers that are inherited most often with the disease are physically closest to the causative gene. After identifying markers that flank the region containing the gene, you find the markers on the physical map, pick out the DNA between the markers, find the gene in the DNA, read the sequence, and use the genetic code to translate the base sequence of the gene into the amino-acid sequence of the protein.

Now I said earlier that we have no way of deducing the function of a protein from its amino-acid sequence. But sometimes there is an empirical way. The sequence may be similar to the sequence of another protein whose function is known, and almost without exception that other protein is in a simpler model system—either yeast, or *Drosophila*, or something else that you can study in the laboratory. That is the reason mapping and sequencing the genomes of nonhuman organisms are part of the Human Genome Project.

We can figure out the function of a human gene by analogy with the function of a similar, or homologous, gene in an experimental organism. For example, we found that the gene responsible for muscular dystrophy codes for a protein that is similar to certain cytoskeletal proteins that have been well studied in a number of organisms. The gene for cystic fibrosis is similar to the multidrug-resistance gene, which had been studied to death in some systems and could be recognized immediately. The gene for neurofibromatosis codes

for a gap protein that had been studied even more than the preceding two and whose mechanism of action is quite well understood.

Bob Moyzis: Before those genes were found, little was known about the causes of the diseases at the molecular or biochemical level. But after isolating a disease gene, finding another gene of known function, and identifying the mutation in the DNA responsible for the disease, one can then begin to identify the molecular mechanism of the disease and begin to design a therapy to counteract the defect caused by the mutant gene.

We are asked frequently whether the isolation of a disease gene immediately leads to a cure for the disease. Of course it does not, but *without* isolation of the gene, finding a cure is almost impossible. For example, our chances of combating the AIDS virus would be very slim if its genome had not been isolated and sequenced. With that information in hand, rational drug treatments to inhibit viral replication can be devised and tested.

Another informative example is muscular dystrophy. For over twenty years various drug treatments were tested on what was considered an animal model system for muscular dystrophy, namely, mutant chickens that exhibited similar muscle degeneration. Once the muscular-dystrophy gene was identified, it was discovered that the physical defect in the chickens was completely unrelated to the physical defect in humans. Hence, all those years of drug research were of little value. A mouse mutant with the mouse homolog of the muscular-dystrophy gene, however, has now been identified. Ironically, that mutant had been known for years, but it was unrecognized as a muscular-dystrophy

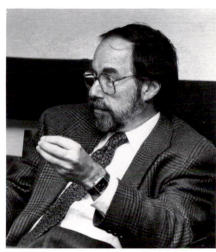

David Baltimore

The only way to study the genetics of the higher perceptual and integrative human functions is by studying human beings. We can't study the genetics of human beings in the way biologists like because you can't mate them in a controlled way. So we have to get the information we need out of natural matings. The linkage and physical maps will help us do that.

77

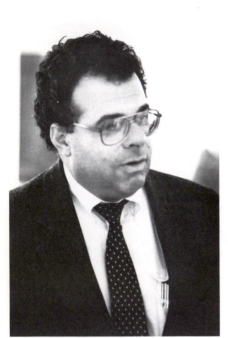

David Botstein

There just isn't enough information in noncontrolled crosses between humans to pinpoint the genes involved in very complex traits. For that you need model systems. And that's precisely why mapping and sequencing the genomes of model organisms is an integral part of the Human Genome Project.

mutant until the human gene was isolated. Now, because the underlying molecular defect is known, rational drug regimes can be tested on the new animal model system.

David Baltimore: I'd like to point out that investigators were searching for disease genes and finding them long before the Genome Project existed. We were looking at homologies between DNA from humans and model organisms. No one needed a new Project to continue doing what we were doing before.

But the Genome Project is something quite different because it will allow us to examine human variability, for example, variations in mathematical ability or in what we call intelligence. Those variations are caused by the interaction of many genes. And certainly the best way that biologists have to unravel which genes are involved in complex traits is to find a set of markers that are linked to the disease and then find the genes associated with those markers. In other words, we need the linkage maps and the physical maps that will be generated by the Human Genome Project. Those maps will allow us to do new kinds of science.

I am particularly *uninterested* in the sequence of the entire human genome because I believe that level of detail is not very useful. But I'm very interested in studying the genome at a level where we can get at multigenic traits and at subtle aspects of human genetics. That is why we are mapping the human genome rather than the mouse genome, and the rationale for doing so should not be to find human disease genes, because we're doing moderately well at finding them right now.

But the only way to study the genetics of the higher perceptual and integrative

human functions is by studying human beings. We can't study the genetics of human beings in the way biologists like because you can't mate them in a controlled way. So we have to get the information we need out of natural matings. The linkage and physical maps will help us do that. So I believe that the Human Genome Project will open up an entirely new level of human biology. To my mind that is the only reasonable rationale for the whole program.

David Botstein: With some claim to proprietorship of the method you are describing for studying multigenic traits, let me say that without some organized effort like the Genome Project, we can't even find the genes for single-gene diseases in an efficient way. But because the Human Genome Project exists and the maps are being made, people are having the courage to set up relatively simply experiments on multigenic traits.

One experiment, proposed by Jasper Rine of the Berkeley Genome Center, involves selecting dogs with different behavioral characteristics, treating those characteristics as multigenic traits, and figuring out by experimental matings what genes are involved. Human genes similar to those genes will be identified and studied to see whether they are involved in determining similar behavioral characteristics in humans. We can't do that without the experimental work on model organisms. There just isn't enough information in noncontrolled crosses between humans to pinpoint the genes involved in very complicated traits. For that you need the model systems. And that's precisely why mapping and sequencing the genomes of model organisms is an integral part of the Human Genome Project.

David Baltimore: I'm not arguing against model systems. My point is that the Genome Project will allow us to study complex traits that are specific to human beings, something we couldn't do before.

David Galas: Yes, the Genome Project will allow us to examine human variability and complex human traits, but that's only one of the reasons for doing this project. Although human disease genes are only a small fraction of the information in the human genome, they are very important to society, and the time has now come when it doesn't make sense to continue chasing individual genes. Just look at the funding history of cystic fibrosis. It cost over $100 million to find that one gene and took eight years of prodigious effort.

David Cox: The others we've found have been just as time-consuming and expensive. Each one has cost many, many millions of dollars. So to say we're doing moderately well with disease genes misses the point.

David Galas: We would spend much more money trying to find disease genes one at a time than we are going to spend on the entire Genome Project.

Bob Moyzis: I agree. Having participated in both the cloning of single genes and the mapping of entire chromosomes, I would estimate that the Human Genome Project is a hundred times more efficient. Further, the Genome Project will result in the identification of very rare disease genes. Such orphan genes, like orphan drugs, will never receive the funding needed for their isolation. But a *complete* map will make it possible to isolate all disease genes efficiently, including orphan genes.

David Galas: We're going from targeted hunts for individual genes to a search for all the genes, which can then be studied one by one. It's a change in the paradigm for gathering information about genes, and it's much more efficient. If you're a guy who wants to study a particular gene, you won't have to first map the region, find the gene and sequence it. Instead, all that information will already be available.

Bob Moyzis: It's a paradigm shift, however, that's threatening to some investigators. They do not like the *perceived* loss of control. They should realize, however, that the tools that will come out of the Genome Project will serve to liberate their research.

David Cox: Of course! Then people will be able to spend their time studying the biology, not isolating the genes. The Genome Project will provide the maps and the sequences, and those raw materials will be used not only to understand human diseases, but also to study much more global biological questions about complex disorders involving many genes and about the interaction of genes with their environment. We'll be able to study how different genes are turned on and off in different tissues and at different times, and we'll study the developmental processes that turn a fertilized egg into a mature organism. But first we have to get the raw materials.

David Botstein: Everybody agrees that the physical maps and the linkage maps will revolutionize a certain kind of genetics, and the major emphasis of the Genome Project during its first five years is to make those maps. But if we get only that far and don't go down to the level of the DNA sequence, we will have missed a great fraction of the possible benefit of the Project.

We need to know the sequences of many, many genes if we are ever to be able to predict the function of a protein from

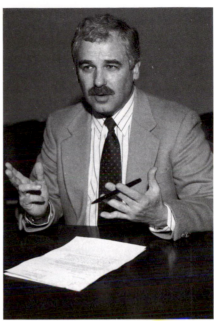

David Galas

Although human disease genes are only a small fraction of the information in the human genome, they are very important to society, and the time has come when it doesn't make sense to continue chasing individual genes. Just look at the funding history of cystic fibrosis. It cost over $100 million to find that one gene and took eight years of prodigious effort.

its DNA sequence or to understand the bigger picture of how genes are organized and regulated.

My favorite analogy with physics is spectroscopy. We're now cataloguing genes just like Fraunhofer catalogued atomic spectra. He had no idea what the lines meant in physical terms, but he knew they were important. And people made their living measuring fine structure, and hyperfine structure, and *superhyperfine* structure—not that such a thing exists—for different elements in the periodic table. But none of what all that information meant got worked out until a theory of the atom was developed, until Bohr and Schrödinger and those guys developed quantum theory. All of a sudden everybody said, "Aha, I can explain those lines because the atom has such and such a structure."

In much the same way, we're collecting the spectra, the sequences, of different genes, but the long-term goal of biology is to determine the functions of those sequences, that is, to understand as much as we can about the information encoded in the genome of the fertilized egg.

David Baltimore: A significant part of the biology community does not believe that sequencing the entire genome is the way to reach such an understanding. That's one of the reasons why the Genome Project is so controversial.

David Botstein: Perhaps I should explain why sequencing the entire genome is a controversial issue. As far as we know now, the informative part of the genome—the part that codes for proteins—is a small fraction of the total genome. Much of the DNA is junk, or of unknown and maybe unimportant function. The arguments that a large fraction of the DNA is relatively unimportant exist and are pretty convincing.

Most reasonable people estimate that the protein-coding regions compose on the order of 10 percent of the genome. The 10 percent I'm referring to are the bits of information in the information-theory sense—the exons. You can strip a human gene of its introns and insert only the exons into a bacterial cell, and the stripped gene functions, that is, makes a protein. That's been the result for all the human genes tried so far.

> *My favorite analogy with physics is spectroscopy. We're now cataloguing genes just like Fraunhofer catalogued atomic spectra. He had no idea what the lines meant in physical terms, but he knew they were important.*

Probably the great majority of biologists would initially say, "It makes obvious sense to sequence the informative bits first because sequencing with current technology is very expensive, laborious, and boring." But before the informative bits can be sequenced, they must be found. So the choice about the approach to sequencing the human genome is really not obvious. It depends on the answer to a technical question: Is it more expensive to figure out which are the informative bits and then sequence them, which is our current approach, or to sequence the entire genome and then find the informative bits? The first five-year plan of the Genome Project is agnostic on this issue. It says, "We want to develop the technology for faster and

cheaper sequencing as quickly as we can, and we are supporting pilot sequencing projects that lead in both directions." The compromise between the "let's go out and get every nucleotide" gang and the guys who thought that the idea was nuts was to say, "We're going to postpone most large-scale sequencing, and depending on how far we get in improving technology, we'll decide what approach to take on the human genome." Sequencing is the area that really needs some breakthroughs. If sequencing were about a hundred times cheaper or a hundred times faster, then it wouldn't make any sense not to sequence the whole genome.

Bob Moyzis: We'll return to the prospects for getting that hundredfold improvement in sequencing a bit later, but now I'd like to counter the notion that most of the genome is junk. Even if exons make up only 10 percent of the genome, that doesn't mean the other 90 percent of the genome is totally superfluous, that you can get rid of it without any effect. Remember that a few hundred years ago a lot of physiologists said the brain was useless because they had no idea what it did. The history of science is full of such statements.

I've spent several years identifying and cloning the human telomere, and we're now attempting similar work on human centromeres. Those regions don't code for proteins, but they're not junk. The telomeres ensure the stability of the chromosomes during DNA replication, and the centromeres are involved in the proper parceling out of the chromosomes during cell division. Unequal parceling out, or aneuploidy, is the major cause of both embryonic abnormalities and metastatic cancer. All other genetic defects added together do not add up to the human suffering caused by aneuploidy. Similarly, the regulatory regions necessary for controlling gene expression are not junk. They compose a significant fraction of the DNA and are often far removed from the genes they regulate.

I think the non-protein-coding regions are the most interesting regions of the genome because they are the regions that make it all work. There are many DNA codes other than the protein code, and determining the other codes is probably the most basic scientific justification for the Human Genome Project. It seems to me that when people say that 90 percent of the genome is junk, they really mean that those regions are uninteresting to their area of research. If you are interested in how proteins fold or how ions pass through cellular membranes, then the primary amino-acid sequences of the proteins encoded in DNA are probably the only aspect of the Genome Project that will interest you. Those are important and exciting areas of research, and the functioning of chromosomes is likely to shed *little* light on the answers. However, I believe that no molecular biologist interested in understanding how the genome works—how genes are differentially expressed in different tissues, for example, or how deletion of information causes genetic diseases—thinks the answers are only in the protein-coding regions. To quote Mary Lou Pardue, "One person's junk is another person's collector's item."

David Botstein: Okay, Bob, your point is well taken, but I think everybody is in agreement that no one's going to sequence from one end of the human genome to the other given current technology and the uncertainty about the function of most of the genome. The technology just isn't there to do it.

Right now, the Genome Project is funding a few large-scale sequencing

projects, that is, projects to sequence continuous stretches of DNA from one million to several million bases in length. Sequencing such long stretches has never before been attempted. But we are not sequencing any old stretch of DNA but rather are focusing on model-system DNA, which can be interpreted fairly easily, or on stretches that encompass well-studied families of genes such as the HLA complex, or on cDNAs.

Lee Hood: It's also necessary to support some biology along with the mapping and sequencing. Some of us at Caltech applied to both NIH and DOE for a grant for large-scale sequencing, and they both argued that we shouldn't do any biology as part of the Project. Well, the fact is that you're not going to get any good people to do the sequencing if you're not going to let them do any biology on the sequences they generate. It's insane to think that good laboratories are only going to sequence and not do anything else. They may take the money for sequencing, but they will end up spreading it around doing other kinds of things.

At Caltech we are sequencing the regions in the human and mouse genomes that code for the proteins of the immune system that recognize foreign antigens. Those proteins make up the receptors on the surfaces of T-cells. The T-cell receptor genes of the mouse and humans combined encompass between 6 million and 7 million base pairs of DNA. We've already sequenced close to 500,000 base pairs of that DNA.

We plan to set up a group whose primary purpose will be to push hard on sequencing as much DNA as possible. It will be a core of technicians managed by a senior postdoctoral fellow interacting with a group of more junior postdoctoral fellows interested both in sequencing

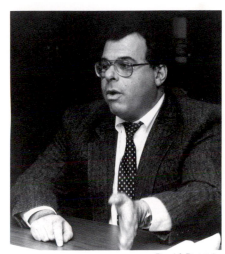

David Botstein

The approach to sequencing the human genome . . . depends on the answer to a technical question: Is it more expensive to figure out which are the informative bits [the protein-coding regions] and then sequence them . . . or to sequence the entire genome and then find the informative bits?

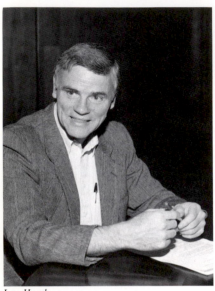

Lee Hood

The most widespread criticism is that the Project is taking away from other aspects of biological science and especially away from individual investigators . . . On the other hand, people don't seem to remember that the Genome Project is less than 1 percent of the total NIH research budget.

and biology. Also, as we do the large-scale sequencing itself, we will learn what new technologies need to be developed to get the job done efficiently. So the biology and the development of efficient sequencing technology will go hand in hand with the large-scale DNA sequencing.

David Cox: We have many different strategies for mapping and sequencing, and what the Genome Project is about right now is determining the most effective way to use them. The biological community has long been familiar with cloning DNA, making maps of restriction sites, and sequencing DNA, and those technologies are steadily being improved. So ultimately the entire human genome is going to be mapped and a large fraction of it sequenced. The issue is efficiency.

The money spent cloning and sequencing is a significant fraction of every laboratory's budget. If the maps and the cloned DNA were available, biologists could spend their time studying how the gene relates to the biology, and the science would move along much more efficiently and rapidly. So the rationale of the Genome Project is to put a lot of money up front into getting the maps of the human genome and thereby free up the rest of the scientific community to do biology. From a business point of view the Genome Project makes a lot of sense.

Norton Zinder: And the only way we're going to accomplish the goals in a reasonable time is through a targeted program. The goals are to develop the technology for mapping and sequencing the human genome and then to do the mapping and sequencing. It's as simple as that. It just takes work and money. The question is: How much work do we want to put in and how much money?

Bob Moyzis: Most reports, including that of the National Research Council's recommendation to Congress, indicated that $3 billion spread out over 15 years, which amounts to $200 million per year, was appropriate. If we reach that level of funding, it will be enough to generate the maps, but I question whether the necessary technology developments as well as the transfer of technology to industry can be accomplished within that budget.

The information from the Genome Project needs to be used for individualized medical diagnosis, and so we need to develop rapid, efficient ways to screen millions of people for hundreds of genes. Yet I see little current support for accomplishing that goal. Lee Hood is one of the few individuals thinking about and working on this problem. But still, by the standards of the biological community, the Project's current funding—$57 million from the DOE and $105 million from the NIH—makes it seem very much like big science, and as such it's been a target for criticism.

Lee Hood: The most widespread criticism is that the Project is taking money away from other aspects of biological science and especially away from individual investigators. That concern has not softened too much because the NIH isn't funding grants at very high levels and people feel the pinch. On the other hand, people don't seem to remember that the Genome Project is less than 1 percent of the total NIH research budget.

David Cox: From a psychological point of view the Project has led to a terrified scientific community. Researchers are saying, "Wait a minute. What am I going to do while you're making that map if I'm not getting any money to do my research?"

Bob Moyzis: There's also the fear that the Human Genome Project will stamp out the creativity of the individual researcher, that because it is a large project it will destroy the sociology that has produced so many dramatic advances in molecular biology over the last fifteen years. The Project requires a lot more coordination than biologists are accustomed to.

David Botstein: The goal is too big for standard cottage-industry science. We need to be able to think about the whole genome at once, and that requires more organization than we usually have. As Norton said, we need a targeted effort. The nice thing is that this large effort doesn't have to be on one piece of real estate. It can be, but it does not need to be.

David Galas: And in fact the effort is rather dispersed. The NIH probably will very soon have about ten genome centers located at universities, and the DOE currently has three centers at Los Alamos, Livermore, and Berkeley national labs. But we also have a lot of smaller projects at other national labs and a large number of individual research grants at universities. So, in a sense this project is certainly nothing like big science in any way it's ever been described before. The Genome Project is different from projects at any of the discipline-oriented NIH institutes in that it tends to be a bit more focused and a bit more integrated because the maps we're aiming for can't be made by just a couple of people. And all the people working on the Project have to coordinate their efforts. Ultimately, compiling, collating, and checking all the data will be the real problem.

Bob Moyzis: The size of this project is not totally outside the scale of what has been happening elsewhere in biology.

Individual lab efforts much larger than the physical-mapping effort at Los Alamos are not unusual. The Genome Project just makes more visible the movement toward larger, more coordinated research projects. The handwriting is on the wall, but many are reluctant to see it happen. As I mentioned earlier, there is a fear of losing control.

Lee Hood: Another concern of our critics is that this project won't produce anything useful for biology, that it is a misconceived project, and that it's boring science.

Bob Moyzis: Boring science is somebody taking for the 500th time yet another gene and sequencing the 200 nucleotides at the end to try to figure out whether there's another regulatory sequence out there that's going to somehow explain how the gene is turned on or off. That's molecular biology as it is currently done. My perception is that this project will revolutionize how people think about biology.

David Galas: Your comment reminds me of a poster, a satire on the state of molecular-biological research, that was displayed at a meeting on the Molecular Biology of Mammalian Gene Expression not too long ago. It was a generic poster outlining the formula for studying gene expression. This is what you do: You get a cDNA, you find the gene by hybridization, you look at expression in various tissues, you pull out the gene, you get the genomic clone, you sequence upstream, you sequence downstream, you do some gel-shift experiments, you do footprints, then you do direct mutagenesis, and then you show that this is the factor that binds this and that. Just plug in your favorite gene and it works! People learn something from that approach, but is it any less mindless than doing maps?

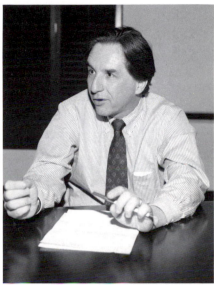

David Cox

From a psychological point of view the Project has let to a terrified scientific community. Researchers are saying, "Wait a minute. What am I going to do while you're making that map if I'm not getting any money to do my research?"

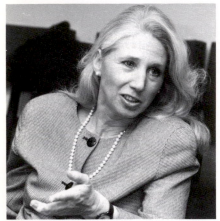

Nancy Wexler

The public thinks they have to wait fifteen years and then the human genome will be delivered on a platter, like the Hubble telescope, flaws and all. But as the genes spill out and the diseases are understood, the Project yields immediate benefits.

Nancy Wexler: To me the beauty of this project is that any new piece of information is immediately relevant. As soon as you obtain a sequence for a human gene, you can look at model organisms to find genes with similar sequences and perhaps identify the function of the gene. The public thinks that they have to wait fifteen years and then the human genome will be delivered on a platter, like the Hubble telescope, flaws and all. But as the genes spill out and the diseases are understood, the Project yields immediate benefits.

Bob Moyzis: That's an important difference between this so-called big science project and other projects, especially in the physical sciences. The infrastructure we are constructing—that's Norton's term—is useful long before it is finished. We should not, however, confuse this immediate usefulness with the ultimate goals. Multigenic traits, for example, will not be accessible until the linkage maps are complete. It's then that most of the fun begins.

David Cox: But I've heard many scientists ask, "How can I be sure that you will give me the tools from the Genome Project that I need to get on with my research?" Those not directly involved with the Genome Project feel they are being pushed out. A lot of thought currently taking place in the Genome Project is about how to get useful information out to the scientific community because that is the purpose of this project, and it has to start happening sooner than fifteen years, sooner than five years, and in fact sooner than two years.

The Genome Project must constantly assess what new tools can be made available to the scientific community and, at the same time, not jeopardize the whole reason for doing the project, which is to generate the maps in a cost-efficient and timely manner. Those two competing concerns must constantly be juggled.

There is a tool that the Genome Project will make available in the next year or so, a kit of 150 polymorphic DNA markers spaced evenly along the genome. That sparse version of the linkage maps we'll ultimately make will be the first product we give out to the community.

David Galas: As Nancy and Bob pointed out, the Genome Project is constantly generating not only new technologies and new data but also different ways of doing things in the molecular biology lab. As we go along, there's going to be a major increase in the usefulness of the Genome Project to the rest of biology with no decrease in the rate of the mapping.

Bob Moyzis: All the technology developed in the course of reaching the goals of the Genome Project becomes immediately useful for smaller projects. Even the large-scale physical-mapping projects have valuable spin-offs. Previously, students would spend their entire graduate career isolating, at best, one gene. Then they would pass it on to somebody else to do all the fun stuff of finding out what the gene does. Now that the physical-mapping projects make it possible to access large amounts of DNA quickly, a student can do some very interesting biology and do it a lot faster than he or she was able to do before.

David Botstein: This is the third or fourth field that I've watched grow. And what you see in a field that's really taking off is an exponential growth in the number of young people attending meetings. And that is what we're seeing in the genome business.

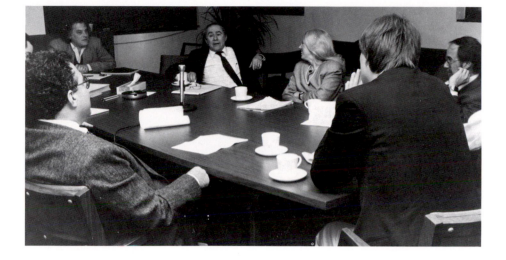

David Galas: Like it or not, the Genome Project is going to transform the science of biology in a major way. We will learn about so many things at a greater level of detail than ever before, and that detail will reveal principles that could not be approached up to now. The people who criticize the Genome Project on its scientific merit, who say it's boring, are largely lacking the vision to understand where this thing is going.

Lee Hood: The sound and fury from our critics has lessened slightly, but I suspect the volume will get turned up again as people go to Congress to try and squelch the genome initiative during the next budgetary hearings. Now that the Project is ongoing and the money is committed, I don't think the criticism will succeed in squelching it overtly. But, if our critics succeed in intimidating the NIH from spending money in ways that are consistent with the mission of the Genome Project, then they will have succeeded in squelching it by the back-door route. If most of the money gets spent on small projects that don't have much to do with the Genome Project itself, then the Project will flounder.

Right now the NIH is spending $8 billion a year on research, and the Genome Project is $105 million this year. So making the Genome Project into a more directed effort rather than spreading the money around is not going to change the character of American biological science in a fundamental way. That worry is unfounded.

The Genome Project is at the very beginning, and the NRC recommendation of $200 million per year is quite a bit more than we're now getting. So, quite apart from how well we're doing in managing the Project, if we've got a lot less money, the task will take longer. Frankly, the $200 million per year that the NRC suggested was really a guess. If anything, it'll cost more. So, we have to temper the suggested time line with the reality of the resources that we have available.

> *Like it or not, the Genome Project is going to transform the science of biology in a major way . . . The people who criticize the Genome Project on its scientific merit, who say it's boring, are largely lacking the vision to understand where this thing is going.*

Classical Linkage Mapping

Classical linkage analysis is used to determine the arrangement of genes on the chromosomes of an organism. By tracing how often different forms of two variable traits are co-inherited, we can infer whether the genes for the traits are on the same chromosome (such genes are said to be linked), and if so, we can calculate the genetic distance separating the loci of the linked genes. The order of and pairwise distances between the loci of three or more linked genes are displayed as a genetic-linkage map.

For simplicity, we will consider traits of the type that Mendel studied, namely, traits exhibiting two forms, or phenotypes, one dominant and one recessive. Each such Mendelian trait is determined by a single pair of genes, either *AA*, *Aa*, or *aa*, where *A* is the dominant allele (form) of the gene and *a* is the recessive allele. Many inherited human diseases fall into this category. The two phenotypes are the presence or absence of the disease, and they are determined by a single gene pair, either *DD*, *DN*, or *NN*, where *D* is the defective allele that causes disease and *N* is the normal allele. If *D* is dominant, as in Huntington's disease and retinoblastoma, a person who inherits only one copy of *D*, and therefore has the genotype *DN*, can manifest the disease. Alternatively, if *D* is recessive, as in neurofibromatosis, cystic fibrosis, and most other inheritable human diseases, a person must inherit a copy of *D* from each parent (genotype *DD*) to manifest the disease phenotype. The two members of a gene pair are located at corresponding positions on a pair of homologous chromosomes. The chromosomal position of the gene pair for trait "A" will be called locus A. In the figures the dominant phenotype will be referred to as dom "A" and the recessive phenotype as rec "a."

First let's consider the inheritance of two unlinked traits, "A" and "B." Here, unlinked means that the gene pairs for the two traits are on different chromosome pairs. Since the chromosomes on which the genes reside are inherited independently, the genes are also inherited independently. In other words each offspring of a parent with the genotype *AaBb* has an equal chance of inheriting *AB*, *Ab*, *aB*, or *ab* from that parent. The latter statement is the law of independent assortment discovered by Mendel. (See the discussion of Mendelian genetics in "Understanding Inheritance.")

Now let's suppose instead that traits "A" and "B" are linked and that a parent carries the dominant alleles *A* and *B* on one chromosome of a homologous pair and the alleles *a* and *b* on the other chromosome. The offspring usually co-inherit either *A* with *B* or *a* with *b*, and, in this case, the law of independent assortment is not valid. Thus to test for linkage between the genes for two traits, we examine certain types of matings and observe whether or not the pattern of the combinations of traits exhibited by the offspring follows the law of independent assortment. If not, the gene pairs for those traits must be linked, that is they must be on the same chromosome pair.

Question: What types of matings can reveal that the genes for two traits are linked?

Answer: Only matings involving an individual who is heterozygous for both traits (genotype *AaBb*) reveal deviations from independent assortment and thus reveal linkage. Moreover, the most obvious deviations occur in the test cross, a mating between a double heterozygote and a doubly recessive homozygote (genotype *aabb*). Recall that individuals with the genotype *AaBb* manifest both dominant phenotypes; those with the genotype *aabb* manifest both recessive phenotypes.

A Simplified Example: Consider a test cross between a double heterozygote (*AaBb*) and a double recessive homozygote (*aabb*). Without additional information, all we know is that the genes of the heterozygous parent could be arranged in any one of the three configurations shown in cases 1, 2a, or 2b. Recall, however, that a parent transmits only one member of each chromosome pair to each of its offspring, so each of the possible arrangements would yield a different result. In case 1, where the gene pairs for traits "A" and "B" are on different chromosome pairs, the offspring can exhibit all four possible two-trait phenotypes, each with a probability of 1/4, in agreement with the law of independent assortment. In cases 2a and 2b, where the gene pairs are linked (and we ignore the effects of crossing over, a phenomenon described below), the offspring exhibit only two of the four composite phenotypes, each with a probability of 1/2. Thus if the genes for traits "A" and "B" are linked, it would appear that the results of the test cross would depart significantly from predictions based on independent assortment.

The reader should note the difference in the arrangement of alleles in cases 2a and 2b and how each arrangement, or *linkage phase*, in the heterozygous parent leads to different two-trait phenotypes among the offspring. In case 2a, *A* and *B* are on one chromosome and *a* and *b* are on the other (a genotype denoted by *AB/ab*, where the slash separates the alleles on different chromosomes). Consequently, the offspring from this test cross exhibit either both dominant or both recessive phenotypes, each with a probability of 1/2. In case 2b, *A* and *b* are on one chromosome and *a* and *B* are on *different* members of the homologous pair (genotype *Ab/aB*), and so the offspring exhibit the other two composite phenotypes, each a combination of a dominant and a recessive trait and, again, each with a probability of 1/2. In this simplified example, it appears quite easy to distinguish linkage from independent assortment, provided the test cross results in a large number of progeny. However, in simplifying the example we have made a significant omission.

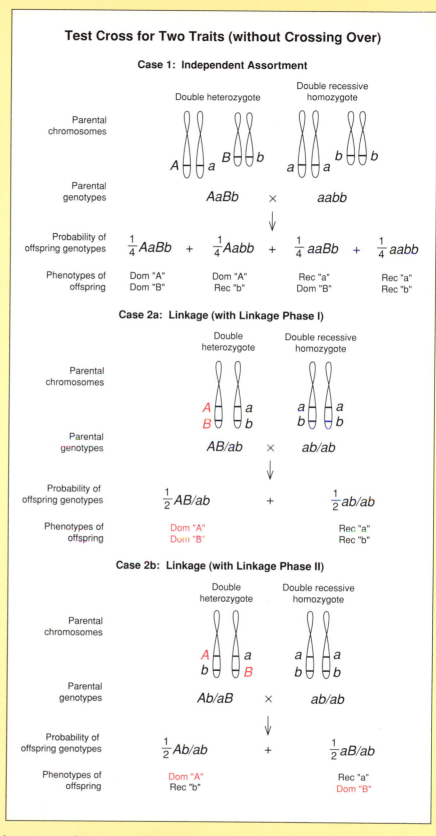

Test Cross for Two Traits (without Crossing Over)

Case 1: Independent Assortment

	Double heterozygote	Double recessive homozygote

Parental chromosomes

$A \quad a \quad B \quad b \qquad a \quad a \quad b \quad b$

Parental genotypes

$$AaBb \quad \times \quad aabb$$

$$\downarrow$$

Probability of offspring genotypes

$$\tfrac{1}{4}AaBb \quad + \quad \tfrac{1}{4}Aabb \quad + \quad \tfrac{1}{4}aaBb \quad + \quad \tfrac{1}{4}aabb$$

Phenotypes of offspring:

Dom "A" Dom "B"   Dom "A" Rec "b"   Rec "a" Dom "B"   Rec "a" Rec "b"

Case 2a: Linkage (with Linkage Phase I)

Double heterozygote   Double recessive homozygote

Parental chromosomes

$A \quad a \qquad a \quad a$
$B \quad b \qquad b \quad b$

Parental genotypes

$$AB/ab \quad \times \quad ab/ab$$

$$\downarrow$$

Probability of offspring genotypes

$$\tfrac{1}{2}AB/ab \qquad + \qquad \tfrac{1}{2}ab/ab$$

Phenotypes of offspring:

Dom "A" Dom "B"   Rec "a" Rec "b"

Case 2b: Linkage (with Linkage Phase II)

Double heterozygote   Double recessive homozygote

Parental chromosomes

$A \quad a \qquad a \quad a$
$b \quad B \qquad b \quad b$

Parental genotypes

$$Ab/aB \quad \times \quad ab/ab$$

$$\downarrow$$

Probability of offspring genotypes

$$\tfrac{1}{2}Ab/ab \qquad + \qquad \tfrac{1}{2}aB/ab$$

Phenotypes of offspring:

Dom "A" Rec "b"   Rec "a" Dom "B"

Question: Are two alleles on the same chromosome always inherited together?

Answer: No. During meiosis (the formation of eggs or sperms), two homologous chromosomes may exchange corresponding segments of DNA in a process called crossing over. Crossing over leads to formation of gametes that possess chromosomes containing new combinations of alleles, or recombinant chromosomes. Crossing over is not a rare phenomenon. In fact, each human chromosome pair within a germ-line cell undergoes, on average, about 1.5 crossovers during meiosis.

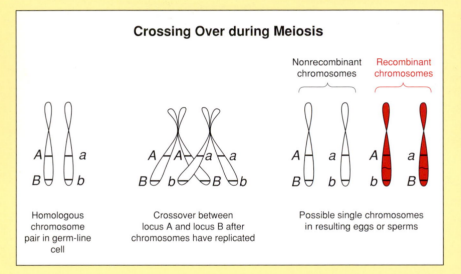

Crossing Over during Meiosis

Nonrecombinant chromosomes

Recombinant chromosomes

A *a*   *A* *A* *a* *a*   *A* *a* *A* *a*

B *b*   *B* *b* *B* *b*   *B* *b* *b* *B*

Homologous chromosome pair in germ-line cell

Crossover between locus A and locus B after chromosomes have replicated

Possible single chromosomes in resulting eggs or sperms

Example: Consider again a doubly heterozygous parent with the genotype *AB/ab*. That is, *A* and *B* are on one member of the homologous chromosome pair and *a* and *b* are on the other. During meiosis each chromosome is replicated and the resulting four chromosomes are parceled out so that only one enters each gamete. If crossing over does not occur between locus A and locus B (as assumed in case 2a above), each egg or sperm produced by the parent receives a chromosome containing either *A* and *B* or *a* and *b*. Those chromosomes are said to be nonrecombinant for traits "A" and "B." On the other hand, if crossing over happens to occur between locus A and locus B, as shown in the figure at left, then some gametes will receive a chromosome containing a new combination of alleles, either *A* and *b* or *a* and *B*. Those chromosomes (shaded red) are said to be recombinant for traits "A" and "B." (Note that only individuals who are doubly heterozygous for two traits can produce gametes containing chromosomes that are recombinant for those traits.) The appearance of a recombinant, an offspring containing a recombinant chromosome, is called a recombination event.

Question: How do recombination events complicate the determination of linkage between the genes for two traits?

Answer: When we include the possibility of recombinant offspring in cases 2a and 2b (above), the distinction between case 1 (independent assortment) and cases 2a and 2b (linkage) becomes less obvious.

A More Realistic Example: The figure on the page opposite shows the test crosses for cases 2a and 2b, this time including the possibility of recombinants among the offspring. The doubly heterozygous parent may produce recombinant chromosomes (shown in red), which can then be inherited to produce recombinant offspring. In each case the recombinants have the composite phenotypes that were absent when the possibility of crossing over was not included (see cases 2a and 2b above). In other words, both cases 2a and 2b can produce all four composite phenotypes, just as does case 1 (independent assortment). However, whereas in case 1 the probabilities of producing the phenotypes were equal, in case 2 the probability of producing recombinants is usually less than the probability of producing nonrecombinants. Thus linkage will be apparent from the results of a test cross provided three criteria are met: (1) the loci of the linked genes must be relatively close together; (2) a large number of progeny must be available to obtain good statistics (therefore we may have to examine a large number of matings); and (3) the test cross must involve only one possible linkage phase; that is, we must be able to infer which linkage phase is present in the heterozygous parent if indeed the genes are linked.

If these criteria are met, then we know which offspring are recombinants. Further, by comparing the number of recombinant offspring with the total number of offspring, we can arrive at an estimate of the probability of producing a recombinant. That probability is called the *recombination fraction* and, as we will see below, is related to the distance separating the loci of the linked genes.

We will also see that as the loci of two linked gene pairs get farther and farther apart, the recombination fraction for the two gene pairs approaches 0.5, so that the two recombinant phenotypes are produced with the same probability as the two nonrecombinant phenotypes. In other words, when the recombination fraction is 0.5, all four composite phenotypes are produced with equal probability, just as they are in case 1, and we infer that the gene pairs are unlinked even though they are on the same chromosome pair.

When we try to determine linkage among human traits, the problems we encounter are that human matings are not controlled (and therefore test-cross matings are rare), the data needed to infer the possible linkage phase in the heterozygous parent may not be available, and the number of offspring produced by two parents is typically much smaller than that produced by a pair of experimental organisms.

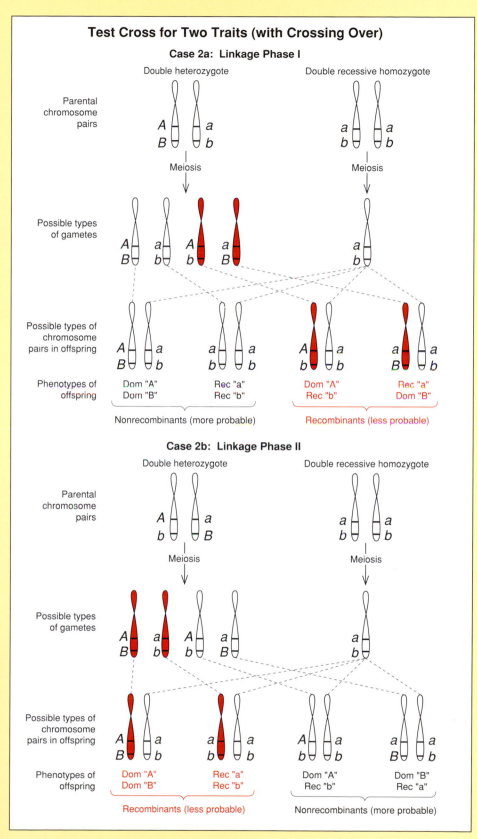

Test Cross for Two Traits (with Crossing Over)

Case 2a: Linkage Phase I

Double heterozygote · Double recessive homozygote

Parental chromosome pairs

Meiosis · Meiosis

Possible types of gametes

Possible types of chromosome pairs in offspring

Phenotypes of offspring

Dom "A" Dom "B" · Rec "a" Rec "b" · Dom "A" Rec "b" · Rec "a" Dom "B"

Nonrecombinants (more probable) · Recombinants (less probable)

Case 2b: Linkage Phase II

Double heterozygote · Double recessive homozygote

Parental chromosome pairs

Meiosis · Meiosis

Possible types of gametes

Possible types of chromosome pairs in offspring

Phenotypes of offspring

Dom "A" Dom "B" · Rec "a" Rec "b" · Dom "A" Rec "b" · Dom "B" Rec "a"

Recombinants (less probable) · Nonrecombinants (more probable)

Question: How do we estimate, from the offspring of a single family, the likelihood that two gene pairs are linked?

Answer: For simplicity, we consider a three-generation family for which we have enough information to infer the linkage phase in the heterozygous parent, if indeed the gene pairs for the two traits under study are linked. We can then identify which offspring are recombinants for the two traits, again under the hypothesis of linkage, and divide the number of recombinant offspring by the total number of offspring to obtain an estimate of the recombination fraction. Finally, we evaluate the likelihood of obtaining the data we have under two opposing hypotheses: that the gene pairs are linked, and that the gene pairs are unlinked. The ratio of the two likelihoods is a measure of how reliably the data distinguish linkage from independent assortment.

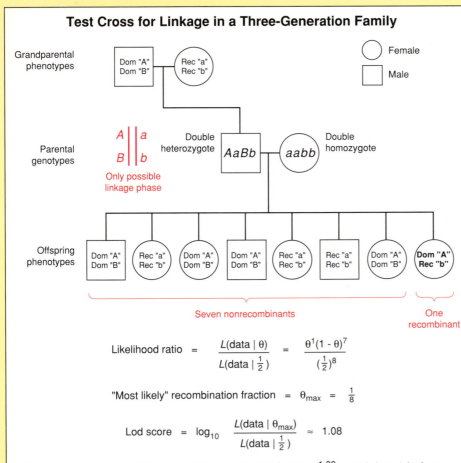

Test Cross for Linkage in a Three-Generation Family

Grandparental phenotypes

○ Female
□ Male

Dom "A" / Dom "B" — Rec "a" / Rec "b"

Parental genotypes

$A \parallel a$
$B \parallel b$
Only possible linkage phase

Double heterozygote *AaBb* — *aabb* Double homozygote

Offspring phenotypes

| Dom "A" Dom "B" | Rec "a" Rec "b" | Dom "A" Dom "B" | Dom "A" Dom "B" | Rec "a" Rec "b" | Rec "a" Rec "b" | Dom "A" Dom "B" | **Dom "A" Rec "b"** |

Seven nonrecombinants | One recombinant

Likelihood ratio $= \dfrac{L(\text{data} \mid \theta)}{L(\text{data} \mid \frac{1}{2})} = \dfrac{\theta^1 (1 - \theta)^7}{(\frac{1}{2})^8}$

"Most likely" recombination fraction $= \theta_{max} = \dfrac{1}{8}$

Lod score $= \log_{10} \dfrac{L(\text{data} \mid \theta_{max})}{L(\text{data} \mid \frac{1}{2})} \approx 1.08$

Data from this family indicate that the odds are about $10^{1.08}$, or 12.6 to 1 in favor of linkage between traits "A" and "B".

Example: Consider a test cross between a male double heterozygote (*AaBb*) and a female double recessive homozygote (*aabb*). The doubly heterozygous father inherited both dominant alleles from his father, and therefore, if the gene pairs for traits "A" and "B" are linked, the father must carry alleles *A* and *B* on the same chromosome. Thus, under the hypothesis of linkage, we know the linkage phase in the father, and therefore, we know that an offspring exhibiting one dominant and one recessive trait is a recombinant. Among the offspring shown here, one is a possible recombinant and seven are possible nonrecombinants. Thus the genes for traits "A" and "B" appear to be linked, with a recombination fraction of 1/8.

We need a method to evaluate the statistical significance of our results. The conventional approach is to apply maximum-likelihood analysis, which estimates the "most likely" value of the recombination fraction θ as well as the odds in favor of linkage versus non-linkage. We begin with the conditional probability $L(\text{data} \mid \theta)$, which is the likelihood of obtaining the data if the genes are linked and have a recombination fraction of θ. In particular, the likelihood of obtaining one recombinant and seven nonrecombinants when the recombination fraction is θ is proportional to $\theta^1 (1 - \theta)^7$, since θ is, by definition, the probability of obtaining a recombinant and $(1 - \theta)$ is the probability of obtaining a nonrecombinant.

We then determine θ_{max}, the value of θ at which L has its maximum value, or equivalently, at which $dL/d\theta = 0$. In this simple case, where we have only one linkage phase to consider, θ_{max} is identically equal to 1/8, the value we obtained by direct inspection of the data. (If both linkage phases are possible, both must be taken into account in the likelihood function.)

Next we compute the ratio of likelihoods $L(\text{data} \mid \theta = \theta_{max})/L(\text{data} \mid \theta = 1/2)$, where $L(\text{data} \mid \theta = 1/2)$ is the likelihood of obtaining the data when $\theta = 1/2$, or equivalently, when the gene pairs are unlinked. This ratio gives the odds in favor of linkage with a recombination fraction of θ_{max} versus nonlinkage. For this family we find that the odds are about 12.6 to 1 in favor of linkage with a recombination fraction of 1/8 versus independent assortment, or nonlinkage.

Geneticists usually report the results of linkage analysis in terms of a lod score, which is the logarithm (to the base 10) of $L(\text{data} \mid \theta = \theta_{max})/L(\text{data} \mid \theta = 1/2)$. For this family the lod score is about 1.1. A lod score of 3, which corresponds roughly to 1000-to-1 odds that two gene pairs are linked, is considered definitive evidence for linkage. The analysis of many families with large numbers of siblings is usually required to achieve lod scores of 3 or more.

Question: Why is the recombination fraction for linked gene pairs related to the distance separating the gene pairs?

Answer: If we assume that crossing over occurs with equal probability along the lengths of the participating chromosomes (an assumption first made by Thomas Hunt Morgan around 1910), then the distance between the loci of two gene pairs determines the probability that recombinant chromosomes will be formed during meiosis, which, by definition, is the recombination fraction. In particular, if two loci are far apart, a greater number of crossovers between the two will occur and recombinant chromosomes will be formed during a greater number of meioses than if the loci are close together. In other words, the value of the recombination fraction increases with the distance between the gene pairs, and thus it provides a measure of the physical distance separating the two pairs. Additionally, pairwise comparison of recombination fractions for several gene pairs on the same chromosome pair establishes the order of the loci along the chromosome pair.

Question: Once we have determined the recombination fractions for many pairs of genes, how do we construct linkage maps of the chromosomes?

Answer: First, we use the recombination fractions to separate the gene pairs into linkage groups. A linkage group is a set of gene pairs each of which has been linked to at least one other member in the set and all of which, therefore, must be on the same chromosome pair. Then, because the recombination fraction increases with the distance separating the loci of two gene pairs, we can use them to order the loci of the gene pairs. The ordering is carried out much as one would order a set of points on a line, given the lengths of the line segments joining the various pairs of points. Next each recombination fraction is converted to a genetic distance, a quantity defined below. Finally, the loci are plotted on a line in a manner such that the plotted distance between any two loci is proportional to the genetic distance between the two loci.

Construction of a Linkage Map

Linkage data

Interval between gene loci	Recombination fraction	Genetic distance (centimorgans)
AB	0.25	35
AC	0.16	20
AD	0.36	65
AE	0.44	110
BC	0.13	15
BD	0.22	30
BE	0.39	75
CD	0.30	45
CE	0.42	90
DE	0.30	45

Order of loci determined from recombination fractions

A   C   B   D   E

0.16   0.13   0.22   0.30

Linkage map

A   C   B   D   E

20   15   30   45

110 centimorgans

Example: The table shows the recombination fractions for a linkage group of five gene pairs, *Aa, Bb, Cc, Dd,* and *Ee.* The loci of these gene pairs are A, B, C, D, and E, respectively, and AB, for example, denotes the interval between locus A and locus B. The recombination fractions corresponding to the intervals AB, BC, and AC are 0.25, 0.13, and 0.16, respectively. Consequently, locus C is inferred to lie between locus A and locus B, as shown in the linkage map. All five loci can be ordered by this type of inference, as shown in the figure.

The next step is to convert the recombination fractions into genetic distances. The genetic distance between locus A and locus B is defined as the average number of crossovers occurring in the interval AB. When the interval is so small that the probability of multiple crossovers in the interval is negligible, the recombination fraction is about equal to the average number of crossovers, or to the genetic distance. However, as two loci get farther apart, the probability of multiple crossovers in the interval between them increases. Further, an even number of crossovers between two loci returns the alleles at those loci to their original positions and therefore does not result in the production of recombinant chromosomes. Consequently, the recombination fraction underestimates the average number of crossovers in the interval, or the genetic distance between the two loci. We therefore use what is called a mapping function to translate recombination fractions into genetic distances.

In 1919 the British geneticist J. B. S. Haldane proposed such a mapping function (see below). The table lists the genetic distance, according to Haldane's function, that corresponds to each recombination fraction, and those distances are displayed as a linkage map.

Question: What is Haldane's mapping function?

Answer: Haldane defined the genetic distance, *x*, between two loci as the average number of crossovers per meiosis in the interval between the two loci. He then assumed that crossovers occurred at random along the chromosome and that the probability of a crossover at one position along the chromosome was independent of the probability of a crossover at another position. (It follows from those assumptions that the distribution of crossovers is a Poisson distribution.) Using those assumptions, he derived the following relationship between θ, the recombination fraction and *x*, the genetic distance (in morgans): $\theta = \frac{1}{2}\left(1 - e^{-2x}\right)$, or, equivalently, $x = -\frac{1}{2}\ln(1 - 2\theta)$. Note that as the genetic distance between two loci increases, the recombination fraction approaches a limiting value of 0.5. Also, when the recombination fraction is small, *x* and θ are approximately equal. In practice geneticists treat them as equal for recombination fractions of 0.1 or less. As indicated, the unit of genetic distance is the morgan, or, more often used, the centimorgan, a distance between two loci such that on average 0.01 crossovers occur in that interval. Cytological observations of meiosis indicate that the average number of crossovers undergone by the chromosome pairs of a germ-line cell during meiosis is 33. Therefore, the average genetic length of a human chromosome is about 1.4 morgans, or about 140 centimorgans.

Question: How can we estimate the physical distance between the two gene loci from the genetic distance between them?

Answer: Since the average genetic length of a human chromosome is about 140 centimorgans and the average physical length of the DNA molecule in a human chromosome is about 130 million base pairs, 1 centimorgan corresponds to approximately 1 million base pairs of DNA. However, this correspondence is very rough because it is based on the assumption that the probability of crossing over is constant along the lengths of the chromosomes. In reality, however, the probability of crossing over varies dramatically from point to point, and a genetic distance of 1 centimorgan may correspond to a physical distance as large as 10,000,000 base pairs or as small as 100,000 base pairs. Also, because the probability of crossing over is higher in female humans than in male humans, genetic distances are greater in females than in males.

Example: Shown here are two genetic-linkage maps for chromosome 16, one derived from data for males and the other from data for females. The female linkage map is 70 centimorgans longer than the male linkage map. But we know from other data that the physical length of the DNA molecule in either a male or female chromosome 16 is the same (about 100 million base pairs). Note that the loci listed on the linkage map are those not of genes but rather of DNA markers (see "Modern Linkage Mapping").

CAVEAT: Classical linkage analysis can be applied only to genes for variable traits, and, most efficiently, to genes for single-gene variable traits such as many inherited human diseases. It can tell us whether the gene pairs for two or more variable traits are on the same homologous chromosome pair, but alone it cannot tell us on which chromosome pair the gene pairs reside. Furthermore, it can tell us the order of the gene pairs in a linkage group, but alone it cannot tell us where any one of the gene pairs is physically located. Finally, classical linkage analysis provides a genetic distance between two linked gene pairs, but that distance is not always proportional to the length of the DNA segment separating the gene pairs. Thus, classical linkage analysis alone does not help us to isolate the particular segment of DNA that contains a particular gene. However, when linkage analysis is applied to inherited variations in DNA itself, it does serve that function (see "Modern Linkage Mapping"). ∎

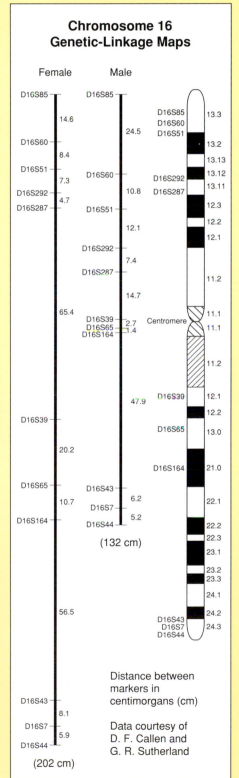

Chromosome 16 Genetic-Linkage Maps

Distance between markers in centimorgans (cm)

Data courtesy of D. F. Callen and G. R. Sutherland

Modern Linkage Mapping
with polymorphic DNA markers—a tool for finding genes

Problem: In "Classical Linkage Mapping" we showed how to construct maps that give the order of and genetic distances between gene pairs for variable, single-gene traits that are linked (lie on the same homologous chromosome pair). Prominent among the variable, single-gene traits of humans are inherited diseases. Several thousand such genetic disorders have been identified, and many of the genes for those disorders were mapped through classical linkage analysis. However, the maps included no reference to the physical reality of DNA, and therefore they did not provide the information necessary to isolate a segment of DNA containing a disease-causing gene. Then, in 1980, David Botstein, Raymond L. White, Mark Skolnick, and Ronald W. Davis transformed linkage mapping into a tool for finding genes.

The Botstein Idea: If we could compare the base sequences of corresponding regions of the DNA from several individuals, we would find many regions with identical sequences—but we would also find many regions where the base sequence varies slightly from one individual to another. Those variable regions are called DNA polymorphisms. Now suppose we have available DNA probes that can not only reveal the presence of variable regions but also distinguish one sequence variation from another. Suppose further that some of the variable regions are fairly stable, so that a given sequence within such a region is transmitted from one generation to the next. In other words, each variable region exhibits only a limited number of sequence variations among the population. Such a variable region, together with the DNA probe that detects the sequence variations within that region, is called a polymorphic DNA marker.

Polymorphic DNA markers are very useful for several reasons. First, because they are variable, we can construct a linkage map of DNA markers just as we construct a linkage map of the genes that determine variable phenotypic traits. That is, we trace the co-inheritance of pairs of DNA markers to determine the genetic distances between them. Second, we can trace the co-inheritance of a marker and a variable phenotypic trait to determine the genetic distance between the marker and the gene responsible for the variable phenotypic trait. Finally, we can use the DNA probe for a marker to find the physical location of the marker on a chromosome. The physical loci of the polymorphic DNA markers can then serve as landmarks in the search for a specific gene. For example, if we know from the linkage map that a gene for a particular phenotypic trait lies between two particular DNA markers, then the gene of interest can be found in the stretch of DNA connecting the physical loci of the two markers. In summary, DNA markers provide a way to connect loci on linkage maps with physical loci in the human genome, which in turn, provides a way to find genes of interest.

Question: What is an example of a base-sequence variation within a region that can turn the region into a DNA marker?

Answer: The base-sequence variation within a region must be easily detectable to make the region a candidate for a DNA marker. One type of detectable variation is a single base change that results in the creation or loss of a restriction-enzyme cutting site. Such sites are short sequences, four to eight base pairs in length, at which a restriction enzyme cuts a DNA molecule. For example, each cutting site for the restriction enzyme *Mbo*I has the base sequence 5′-GATC.

Example: Consider locus *a*, a variable region on a particular pair of of homologous chromosomes. The figure shows the DNA segments that compose locus *a* in the homologous chromosome pairs of two individuals. Also shown are the positions of the cutting, or restriction, sites for the restriction enzyme *Mbo*I within locus *a* and the distance between successive sites. Individual 1 carries two copies of a_1, a version, or allele, of locus *a* that has three restriction sites for *Mbo*I. Individual 2 carries one copy of a_1 and also a copy of another allele, a_2. Note that a_2 is missing the middle restriction site present in a_1. The absence of that restriction site is due to a change in a single base pair (shown in red). If *Mbo*I is allowed to cut the DNA from these two individuals, a_1 will be cut into two fragments of lengths 200 base pairs and 350 base pairs, whereas a_2 will be cut into one fragment of length 550 base pairs.

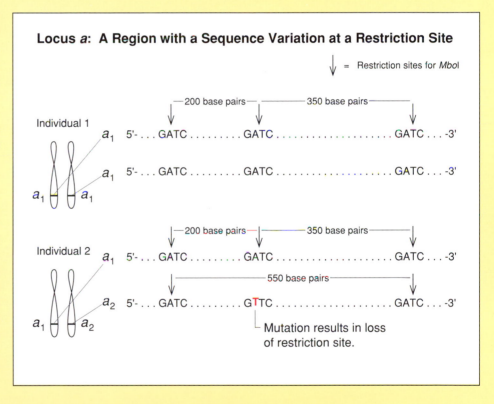

Locus *a*: A Region with a Sequence Variation at a Restriction Site

↓ = Restriction sites for *Mbo*I

Individual 1

a_1 5′-...GATC........GATC....................GATC...-3'
— 200 base pairs — — 350 base pairs —

a_1 5′-...GATC........GATC....................GATC...-3'

a_1 a_1

Individual 2

a_1 5′-...GATC........GATC....................GATC...-3'
— 200 base pairs — — 350 base pairs —

a_2 5′-...GATC........GTTC....................GATC...-3'
— 550 base pairs —

a_1 a_2

Mutation results in loss of restriction site.

Question: How do we detect which alleles of locus a *are present in the DNA molecules of two individuals?*

Answer: We measure the lengths of the fragments from locus *a* produced by cutting the DNA with *Mbo*I and note the differences between the lengths of the fragments from the two individuals. We do so by making a Southern blot (see "Hybridization" in "Understanding Inheritance"). We begin by extracting many copies of the DNA from the blood cells of each individual. We then chop up, or digest, the DNA in each sample with the restriction enzyme *Mbo*I. The next step is to separate the resulting fragments (called restriction fragments) according to length by gel electrophoresis (see "Gel Electrophoresis" in "Understanding Inheritance"). Because shorter fragments travel farther through the gel than longer fragments, the lengths of the fragments can be determined from their final positions on the gel. We then transfer (blot) the fragments onto a filter paper in a manner that preserves their final gel positions.

Next, we allow a radioactively labeled DNA probe from locus *a* to hybridize, or bind by complementary base pairing, to the restriction fragments. The probe hybridizes only to fragments from locus *a* and thereby reveals their positions and therefore their lengths. Finally, we make an autoradiogram of the filter paper in which the positions of the fragments that have hybridized to the probe are imaged as dark bands.

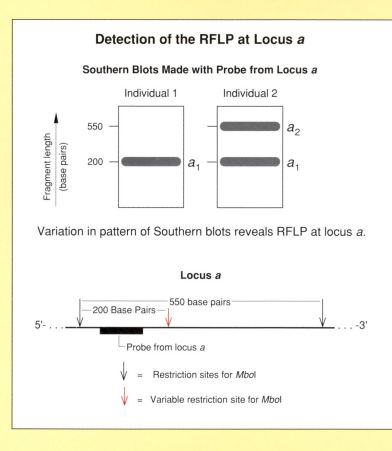

Detection of the RFLP at Locus *a*

Southern Blots Made with Probe from Locus *a*

Variation in pattern of Southern blots reveals RFLP at locus *a*.

Locus *a*

Example: The figure shows Southern blots for the DNA of individuals 1 and 2 made with the enzyme *Mbo*I and a probe for locus *a*. The position of the probe is shown in the diagram of locus *a*. That particular probe binds to the restriction fragments of length 200 base pairs from allele a_1 and to the restriction fragments of length 550 base pairs from allele a_2. Since individual 1 carries allele a_1 only, the Southern blot of individual 1 shows one band at a position corresponding to a length of 200 base pairs. Individual 2 carries alleles a_1 and a_2 and therefore has a Southern blot showing two bands, one at 200 base pairs and one at 550 base pairs. The variation within locus *a* that causes this difference between the two Southern blots (the presence or absence of a restriction site) is called a restriction fragment length polymorphism, or RFLP, which is one type of polymorphic DNA marker. (Another type of polymorphic DNA marker is described in "The Polymerase Chain Reaction and Sequence-tagged Sites.")

Question: How do we find polymorphic DNA markers?

Answer: Originally, this was done by a process involving patience and preferably luck. We randomly choose one clone from a collection of human DNA clones, use it as a probe in the making of Southern blots of the DNA of many individuals, and see whether the Southern blots vary from one individual to the next. A variation implies that the probe is part of a variable region of the genome and therefore defines that region as a polymorphic DNA marker. If the clone chosen does not reveal a difference, we continue choosing clones until a difference does show up. More recently, with the wide application of the polymerase chain reaction (PCR) and the discovery that there are a large number of highly variable, short di-, tri-, and tetranucleotide repeat sequences flanked by unique DNA sequences, it has become possible to select such regions of DNA and then develop them into highly polymorphic markers.

Question: How are polymorphic DNA markers used in linkage analysis?

Answer: In linkage analysis a polymorphic DNA marker is analogous to a gene that has two or more alleles. Each parent carries a pair of alleles of the marker, one on each member of a chromosome pair, so each parent may be either homozygous or heterozygous for the marker. Also, each parent transmits only one allele of the marker to each offspring.

Example: The figure at right shows an example of the inheritance of the RFLP at locus *a*. Beneath each parent and each of their six children is shown the Southern blot for the marker. The father is heterozygous for the marker, carrying alleles a_1 and a_2. Among the offspring three are heterozygous and three are homozygous for a_2. The heterozygous offspring have inherited the allele a_1 from their mother. Note that the alleles of a polymorphic DNA marker are inherently easier to trace than the alleles of a gene because the alleles of a polymorphic DNA marker are codominant. That is, none of them are recessive and each is directly observable.

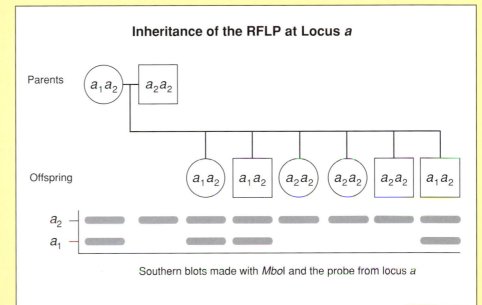

Inheritance of the RFLP at Locus *a*

Southern blots made with *Mbo*I and the probe from locus *a*

We can also trace the inheritance of two markers, find out whether they are linked (on the same chromosome), and determine the recombination fraction for the two markers and thus the genetic distance between their loci. The linkage analysis exactly parallels that described for phenotypic traits in "Classical Linkage Mapping." In particular, an informative mating, one that reveals linkage between a pair of markers, must involve a parent who is heterozygous for both markers.

Question: Why does the Genome Project have as one of its top priorities the construction of a high-density linkage map of polymorphic DNA markers?

Answer: By 1996 the Genome Project hopes to have produced a set of linkage maps, each containing polymorphic DNA markers spaced along each human chromosome at intervals of 2 to 5 centimorgans, genetic distances that roughly correspond to physical distances of 2 to 5 million base pairs of DNA. Such a set of maps will enable researchers to find any gene of interest relative to the loci of approximately 1500 markers. In other words, the markers will form a set of reference points along the genome.

Co-inheritance of Marker *c* and Disease Allele *D*

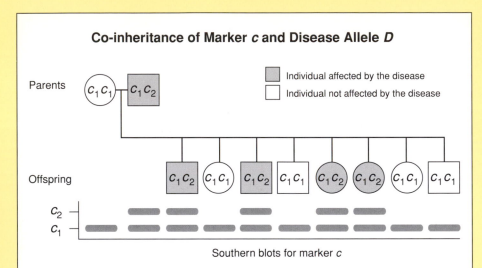

Since each offspring affected by the disease carries the c_2 allele of marker *c*, it appears that marker *c* and the disease gene are linked, and in this family allele c_2 is linked to the disease gene *D*.

Position of Disease Gene *D* on High-Density Linkage Map

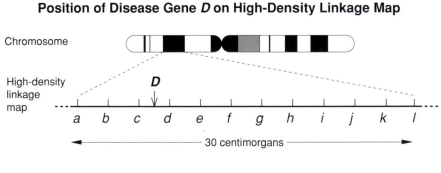

Linkage analysis shows that the disease gene *D* lies between markers *c* and *d*.

Example: Suppose we are interested in locating a mutant gene *D* that causes an inherited disease. We can find families affected by the disease and trace the co-inheritance of the disease with the reference markers on a linkage map. If we have a 2-centimorgan linkage map of highly informative markers (see "Informativeness and Polymorphic DNA Markers"), we can find markers flanking the gene that are less than 2 centimorgans away on either side. The pedigree in the figure shows the type of data needed to establish that the marker *c* and the disease gene *D* are tightly linked, that is, *c* and *D* are so close together that recombination events between them are rarely observed. Similar data between marker *d* and *D* would allow us to infer that *D* lies between *c* and *d*, as indicated in the lower part of the figure. This example shows the characteristic pattern of inheritance of an autosomal dominant disorder identified by allele c_2 of marker *c*.

Question: Once we have found DNA markers flanking a disease gene, how do we localize the disease gene on the DNA itself?

Answer: In addition to creating a linkage map of polymorphic DNA markers, the Genome Project is creating a physical map for each human chromosome. A physical map consists of an ordered set of overlapping cloned fragments that spans the entire length of the DNA molecule in the chromosome. As the physical maps and the linkage maps are constructed, the linkage map for each chromosome is being integrated with the physical map for that chromosome. That is, each locus on the linkage map will be associated with a locus on the physical map. Thus, if we find two markers that flank a disease gene, we will be able to ascertain how many base pairs of DNA separate the markers, and we will also have all that DNA available as cloned fragments. We therefore know that the disease gene is in one of those cloned fragments, and we can employ various methods to find the DNA segment that contains the gene. (Those methods are not necessarily straightforward, as explained on pages 111 and 142 of "Mapping the Genome.")

Example: The figure at right shows a schematic representation of a human metaphase chromosome (dark bands indicate A-T rich regions), a portion of a linkage map of polymorphic DNA markers, the position of a disease gene *D* on that map (as determined by linkage analysis), and the corresponding physical map of cloned fragments. Dotted lines connect the loci on the linkage map with the corresponding loci on the physical map and on the metaphase chromosome. Highlighted in red are the clones that must be searched to find the disease gene.

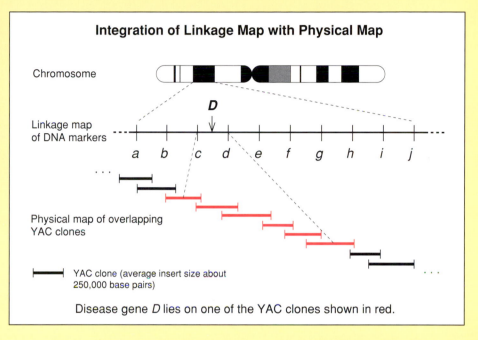

Integration of Linkage Map with Physical Map

Chromosome

D

Linkage map of DNA markers

a   b   c   d   e   f   g   h   i   j

Physical map of overlapping YAC clones

YAC clone (average insert size about 250,000 base pairs)

Disease gene *D* lies on one of the YAC clones shown in red.

CAVEAT: In practice we need flanking markers that are within 1 centimorgan of the gene on either side so that the search for the disease gene will involve no more than about 2 million base pairs of DNA. Consequently, the long-term goal of the Genome Project is to find enough highly polymorphic DNA markers so that they are spaced at intervals of 1 centimorgan on the linkage maps, or a total of about 3300 markers. If they are found by a random search, we will have to find about ten times that number to achieve the 1-centimorgan map. The search for markers has been accelerated in several ways. For example, new types of markers are being systematically sought (see pages 133–134 in "The Polymerase Chain Reaction and Sequence-tagged Sites"), and automated techniques are being developed to detect DNA markers in large numbers of individuals. ■

Informativeness of Polymorphic DNA Markers

Carl E. Hildebrand, David C. Torney, and Robert P. Wagner

As mentioned in "Modern Linkage Mapping," one of the five-year goals of the Human Genome Project is to find highly informative polymorphic DNA markers spaced at 2- to 5-centimorgan intervals along the genetic linkage map of each human chromosome. In this context, informative means useful for establishing through linkage analysis that the marker is near a gene or another marker of interest. Recall that linkage between two variable loci can only be determined from matings in which one parent is heterozygous (carries two different alleles) for the marker or gene at each locus (see "Classical Linkage Mapping"). Thus a marker is highly informative for linkage studies if any individual chosen at random is likely to be heterozygous for that marker. As shown below, markers with many alleles, or highly polymorphic markers, tend to be highly informative.

Informativeness can be quantitatively measured by a statistic called the polymorphism information content, or PIC. This statistic is defined relative to a particular type of pedigree: one parent is affected by a rare dominant disease and is heterozygous at the disease-gene locus (genotype *DN*, where *D* is the dominant, disease-causing allele of the gene and *N* is the normal allele of the gene). The other parent is unaffected by the disease (genotype *NN*). The polymorphic DNA marker in question has several alleles, a_i, which are codominant, that is, each one can be detected so that the genotype at the marker locus ($a_i a_j$) can always be determined for any individual. Moreover, the marker locus is linked to (on the same chromosome pair as) the disease-gene locus. The important property of this type of pedigree is that the genotypes of the parents and the offspring at both the marker locus and the disease-gene locus can always be inferred. In this context, an offspring is said to be *informative* if we can infer from his or her genotype which marker allele is linked to (on the same chromosome as) the disease allele and would therefore be co-inherited with the disease allele in subsequent generations.

The PIC value of the marker is defined as the expected fraction of informative offspring from this type of pedigree. The figure divides the possible matings from such a pedigree into three categories depending on the genotypes of the parents at the marker locus. Each category has a different fraction of informative offspring. Note that the marker locus is assumed to be near the gene locus, so recombination between the two is a rare event and is not taken into account. In (a) the disease-affected parent is homozygous at the marker locus (genotype $a_i a_i$) and therefore none of the offspring are informative. In (b) both parents have the same heterozygous genotype at the marker locus ($a_i a_j$). Then, if each possible type of offspring is produced with equal probability, half of the offspring are informative. For all other combinations of marker alleles in the parents, all offspring are informative. The fully informative matings are summarized in (c).

PIC is the expected fraction of informative offspring from the type of pedigree shown in the figure. Under the assumption of Hardy-Weinberg equilibrium (that in the general population the frequencies of the alleles at the marker locus are independent of the frequencies of the alleles at the disease

Mating Categories for Evaluation of PIC

PIC is the expected fraction of informative offspring from a mating between an affected individual carrying a single copy of a dominant disease allele D, and an unaffected individual. This mating is divided into three categories depending on which alleles a_i (i = 1, 2, ...) are present at the locus of a polymorphic marker with n alleles. Each category produces a different fraction of informative offspring. Recall that the genotypes of each offspring are known, but the arrangement of alleles on the chromosomes is not known. Thus an offspring is informative if his or her genotype allows us to infer that D and a_i are linked in the affected parent and will therefore be coinherited. Informative offspring are shown in red.

(a) k and l can take on any values

Affected parent

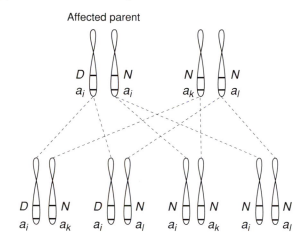

D = disease allele at disease locus
N = normal allele at disease locus
a_i = marker allele at marker locus
p_i = frequency of marker allele a_i

The affected parent is homozygous at the marker locus. Therefore, all offspring inherit a_i from the affected parent, and the inheritance of a_i cannot be used to predict the coinheritance of D.

Frequency of mating = p_i^2
Fraction of informative offspring = 0.

(b) $i \neq j$

Affected parent

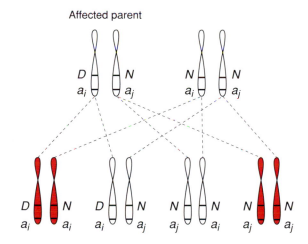

Both parents are heterozygous at the marker locus (genotype $a_i a_j$). In the absence of crossing over two types of offspring are informative (red), that is, we can deduce from the genotypes of those offspring that D and a_i are linked (or on the same chromosome) in the affected parent. Specifically, the offspring genotype $DNa_i a_i$ tells us directly that D and a_i were coinherited from the affected parent and therefore must be on the same chromosome. The offspring genotype $DNa_j a_j$, tells us that N and a_j were coinherited from the affected parent and by the process of elimination the D and a_i must be on the same chromosome in that parent.

Frequency of mating = $2 p_i p_j (2 p_i p_j)$
Fraction of informative offspring = 0.5

(c) $i \neq j$ and k, l can be any combination except i, j and j, i

Affected parent

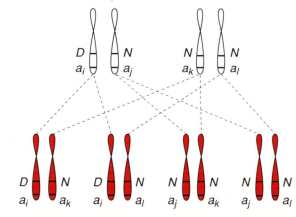
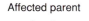

The affected parent is heterozygous at the marker locus, and the unaffected parent carries a different combination of marker alleles than that in the affected parent. Thus the genotypes of all offspring allow one to deduce that D and a_i are linked in the affected parent.

Frequency of mating = $2 p_i p_j (1 - 2 p_i p_j)$
Fraction of informative offspring = 1.0

locus) and the further assumption that a pair of alleles occurs with a frequency equal to the product of the two frequencies, we can determine the frequency of each mating category from the frequencies p_i of each marker allele a_i. Then (following Botstein et al., 1980 or Roychoudhury and Nei, 1988), to calculate PIC we multiply the frequency of each mating type by the expected fractions of informative offspring from that mating type and add the products:

$$\text{PIC} = 1 - \sum_{i=1}^{n} p_i^2 - 2 \sum_{i=1}^{n-1} \sum_{j=i+1}^{n} p_i^2 p_j^2 = 1 - \sum_{i=1}^{n} p_i^2 - \left(\sum_{i=1}^{n} p_i^2 \right)^2 + \sum_{i=1}^{n} p_i^4 \quad,$$

where $p_i =$ frequency of the marker allele, a_i and $n =$ number of different alleles. Thus to evaluate the PIC value of a marker, we must determine the frequencies of each marker allele. We present an example (from Weber et al., 1990) in which the polymorphic marker is on human chromosome 16 and has four alleles each containing the dinucleotide repeat $(GT)_n$, where n takes on the values 170, 168, 166, and 154. A population of 120 chromosomes indicated that the frequencies of those four alleles are 0.01, 0.12, 0.2, and 0.67, respectively. Using the equation for PIC, we find that the PIC value for this marker equals 0.44. Thus 44 percent of the offspring should be informative in the type of pedigree illustrated in the figure. Theoretically, PIC values can range from 0 to 1. At a PIC of 0, the marker has only one allele. At a PIC of 1, the marker would have an infinite number of alleles. A PIC value of greater than 0.7 is considered to be highly informative, whereas a value of 0.44 is considered to be moderately informative. A gene or marker with only two alleles has a maximum PIC of 0.375. Clearly markers with greater numbers of alleles tend to have higher PIC values and thus are more informative.

An alternative measure of the degree of polymorphism of a marker is the heterozygosity, the probability that any randomly chosen individual is heterozygous for any two alles at a marker locus having allele frequencies p_i. Thus, heterozygosity $= 1 - \sum_{n=1}^{n} p_i^2$, where $\sum_{n=1}^{n} p_i^2$ is the homozygosity. PIC, therefore, will always be lower than the heterozygosity and can be considered to be the heterozygosity corrected for partially informative matings. Polymorphic loci containing many tandem repeats of a short sequence two to six bases long tend to have many alleles and are thus good candidates for highly informative markers. Those markers can be detected using PCR (see "The Polymerase Chain Reaction and Sequence-tagged Sites"). ■

Further Reading

David Botstein, Raymond L. White, Mark Skolnick, and Ronald W. Davis. 1980. Construction of a genetic linkage map in man using restriction fragment length polymorphisms. *American Journal of Human Genetics* 32:314-331.

James L. Weber, Anne E. Kwitek, and Paula E. May. 1990. Dinucleotide repeat polymorphisms at the D16S260, D16S261, D16S265, D16S266, and D16S267 loci. *Nucleic Acids Research* 18:4034.

Jurg Ott. 1991. *Analysis of Human Genetic Linkage,*, revised edition. Baltimore: The Johns Hopkins University Press.

Arun K. Roychoudhury and Masatoshi Nei. 1988. *Human Polymorphic Genes.* New York/Oxford: Oxford University Press.

II: Maps, Markers, and the Five-Year Goals

Physical Mapping

Maynard Olson: The idea of the Genome Project is fundamentally a strong one, but when first broached, it was an idea whose time had *almost* come. Now, five years after the first serious proposals, we're actually beginning to do something. The early proponents could be called either visionaries or cranks, depending on how generous you are. Like Jules Verne and H. G. Wells, who had clear visions of space travel but no ideas of how to implement it, the early proponents of the Genome Project had the right instincts, but they were technically naive. Their predictions—that mapping the genome would take six months and that rough sequencing of a chromosome would take a similarly brief time—were simply nonsense. Mapping and sequencing the human genome is going to be expensive, and it's going to take a long time.

Bob Moyzis: In the last five years, however, we've had some technological breakthroughs that make the Genome Project feasible, especially the first step of constructing physical maps for the whole genome. When people first started talking about this project, most of them were unaware that Maynard was working on a method to clone very large pieces of DNA in YACs [yeast artificial chromosomes]. That new cloning method has now become the mainstay of a physical-mapping effort.

Without YACs, we would have been stuck with little pieces of the physical map and no way to put them together. To use an analogy, we would have had an interstate highway that was interrupted every mile or so by a stretch of dirt road or no road at all. That's better than nothing, but it's not as useful or efficient as a continuous highway.

David Cox: We should point out that the physical maps we're trying to construct are not just ordinary maps of landmarks and distances. Rather, each is a reconstruction of the DNA molecule in a chromosome as a set of cloned DNA fragments. The maps are made by isolating many copies of the whole genome, cutting the DNA molecules into relatively small pieces, and cloning the pieces. Then the challenge is to figure out how to hook those pieces together in the order in which they appear along each of the twenty-four different chromosomes in the human genome.

The mapping process is much like putting together the pieces of a one-dimensional jigsaw puzzle. In the case of a DNA puzzle, the pieces are cut so that they have overlaps with neighboring pieces, and the problem is to find the overlaps and thereby order the pieces. If you succeed in putting the puzzle together, you know the exact position of each fragment relative to all the other fragments, so you can pick out exactly those fragments that span a

region containing a gene of interest. Finally, you can then examine the fragments at the molecular level using all the standard techniques of molecular biology. [See "Physical Mapping—A One-Dimensional Jigsaw Puzzle."]

The difficulty in making a physical map is that often you get a few pieces hooked together to form a little island of the puzzle—that island is called a contig because it contains pieces of DNA that are contiguous in the genome—but then you get stuck because you can't find the overlapping pieces that would extend the island on each end. That's what Bob was referring to with his highway analogy. There are two reasons for getting stuck. First, the overlapping pieces you're looking for may have been lost in the cloning process, and second, your method for detecting overlaps may not be robust enough to find all of them. You end up with a whole bunch of little contigs, but you don't know how to put them together to form a whole DNA molecule. In other words, there are gaps in the puzzle.

Obviously, if you can start with larger pieces, larger cloned DNA fragments, you wind up with much longer contigs and many fewer gaps in the puzzle. That's why YACs were a breakthrough for mapping. YAC clones contain human DNA inserts that are, on average, about 300,000 base pairs in length, which is longer by a factor of 8 to 10 than the longest inserts in the clones used in earlier mapping projects. So we gained a factor of at least 10 in the speed of mapping.

Bob Moyzis: We gained speed, but more important, we gained the ability to build long contigs spanning several million base pairs of DNA. Contig maps had been constructed before in the search for disease genes, but only with great

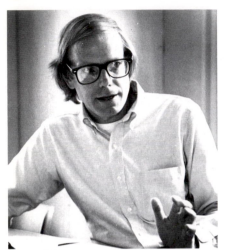

Maynard Olson

Like Jules Verne and H.G. Wells, who had clear visions of space travel but no ideas of how to implement it, the early proponents of the Genome Project had the right instincts, but they were technically naive. Their predictions that mapping the genome would take six months, and that rough sequencing would take a similarly brief time, were simply nonsense.

difficulty and only for relatively small stretches of a chromosome known to contain interesting genes. Those maps were built with lambda-phage or cosmid clones, which carry DNA inserts of 15,000 base pairs and 40,000 base pairs, respectively. Those numbers sound large, but to cover a whole chromosome 100 million base pairs in length would require about 7000 lambda-phage clones or 2500 cosmid clones. Furthermore, constructing a physical map of overlapping cloned segments requires at least five times those numbers to ensure adequate overlaps. So neither lambda-phage clones nor cosmid clones are ideal for mapping a whole chromosome.

But the real problem was already mentioned by David Cox. When we are constructing a contig, we often can't find the clones that extend the contig. In fact, a contig map made from cosmid clones typically consists of separate contigs whose average length is about 100,000 base pairs. Until YACs came along, that was the state of the art. We could construct a high-resolution physical map—a contig—for a region 100,000 base pairs in length, and if we wanted to, we could subclone the individual clones in the contig and apply standard sequencing techniques to go down to the highest-resolution map, which is the DNA sequence itself.

In addition we could make a low-resolution map of a chromosome using a technique called in-situ hybridization to map the DNA markers present on a linkage map of the chromosome onto the chromosome itself. The markers are separated, on average, by millions of base pairs. So knowing that a disease gene was flanked by two markers didn't necessarily lead to assigning the gene to a single contig because the available contigs were shorter—by a factor of 10 to 100—than the distance between

the markers. We needed a source of longer continuous pieces of DNA so that we could build contigs as long as the distance between the markers.

In the last few years the gap between a hundred thousand base pairs and several million base pairs has been filled in by two techniques. One, called pulsed-field gel electrophoresis, gives us fragments with an average length of about a million base pairs. That technique is useful but less so than first imagined because it does not always yield the same set of fragments, and further, it does not give us the DNA in a cloned form.

YAC cloning, in contrast, is a real breakthrough. It makes possible the construction of contigs a few million base pairs long. And such long continuous cloned regions bridge the gap between the high-resolution cosmid contigs and the low-resolution marker maps. We need *both* high connectivity, supplied by YACs, *and* high resolution, supplied by cosmids.

Maynard Olson: That's exactly why our five-year goal for physical mapping calls for the construction of contigs that span at least 2 million base pairs. Physical maps with such long-range continuity are essential. They are useful as navigational tools because once we find that a gene is flanked by two markers on a linkage map, we will be able to find a single contig containing both those markers and thus the gene that lies between them.

But maps are not merely navigational tools. They also provide a means of correlating many types of data. For example, we use maps to locate mountains, rivers, and city and state boundaries, but we also use maps to plot population density, average rainfall, climate changes, earthquake activity, and so on. And once we plot those data on a map, we start to see relationships.

Cytogeneticists, doctors, and molecular biologists are all making observations on the genomes of individuals on a daily basis, but without a map we have no way of correlating those data with other information about the genome. Once we have a continuous contig map, those data will become important. We'll be able to locate the exact site of, say, a chromosomal translocation, insertion, or deletion or a new DNA marker and to correlate that information with other facts about that region of the genome. A number of labs have already constructed YAC contigs spanning several million bases, and we can expect that kind of success to continue.

David Galas: The physical-mapping projects at Los Alamos and Livermore started early, and the people there began with the much smaller cosmid clones. Over the last few years they have built 100,000-base-pair contigs, which together compose a large fraction of chromosomes 16 and 19. And now they are using YACs to bridge the gaps between the short contigs and build the long contigs that we need. In fact, the whole community is learning to use YACs for physical mapping even though they do pose some problems. In particular, many YAC clones are chimeras. That is, they contain pieces of DNA from two or more locations in the human genome. Right now those chimeric clones are a tremendous headache for the mappers.

David Cox: It's like having a fifty-piece jigsaw puzzle in which ten of the pieces are from another puzzle but you don't know which ten.

David Galas: Presumably, chimeric clones are produced by recombination

between the human DNA inserts in two YACs that have entered the same yeast cell. The large amount of repetitive DNA in human DNA makes it a wonderful target for recombination in yeast. The best data about chimeric YACs come from Maynard's group at Washington University. Remember, YACs are relatively new, and chimeras were found among the clones propagated in *E. coli* too, until we came up with a strain of *E. coli* that was recombination-free. In the meantime it's very important that the mapping efforts continue despite the difficulties.

Bob Moyzis: In the last year our efforts at Los Alamos have effectively eliminated the YAC chimera problem. Starting with many copies of a single chromosome isolated by the specialized technique of flow sorting, Mary Kay McCormick has generated chromosome-specific YAC libraries of human chromosomes 16 and 21 that appear to be relatively free of chimeric clones.

The trick was to expose the yeast cells to extremely dilute YAC solutions so that the probability of two YACs entering a single yeast cell was greatly reduced and also to greatly reduce the number of recombinagenic broken DNA ends in the mixture. Clearly that's one approach to generating chimera-free YAC libraries. But other approaches need to be pursued as well, and our Russian collaborators, Vladimir Larionov and Natasha Kouprina, have had encouraging results using yeast mutants deficient in recombination.

Nancy Wexler: Perhaps we should discuss what motivates individuals to generate physical maps. It's an extremely difficult activity.

Bob Moyzis: I'm among those who are interested in the long-range order of the chromosome and therefore find the

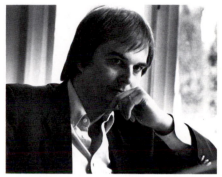

Bob Moyzis

The structural organization of human DNA holds the key to understanding function . . . . Those who are primarily interested in finding disease genes look upon physical mapping as spending time in the barrel. They are very impatient to get back to studying some interesting disease gene.

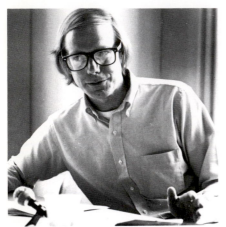

Maynard Olson

John Sulston, the originator of the nematode-mapping project . . . is famous for working out the complete embryonic lineage of the nematode. He literally spent several years in a closet looking through a microscope at those tiny, transparent worms and watching all the cell divisions that occur as the fertilized egg develops into the mature organism.

mapping effort intrinsically interesting. As I mentioned earlier, I firmly believe that the structural organization of human DNA holds the key to understanding function. I love solving structural problems. DNA is a beautiful molecule. I *see* the DNA in every living thing. I'm just amazed by nature and driven to understand how it works. But others, those who are primarily interested in finding disease genes, look upon physical mapping as spending time in the barrel. They are very impatient to get back to studying some interesting disease gene.

Maynard Olson: Those people are never going to get very much mapping done. Mapping is a complex activity, and only people obsessed with the task itself—those who don't sleep at night when they bump up against new obstacles—will see the job to completion.

Bob Moyzis: There's a not-so-subtle conflict between the mapping effort and the traditional interests of the human-genetics community. As I mentioned earlier, that community did not initiate the Human Genome Project, and I don't sense much interest on their part in global physical mapping.

Once we have mapped the regions containing known disease genes, there may be a strong push to focus in on those genes and abandon the mapping effort. For individuals like Nancy, who have dedicated most of their careers to isolating a single disease gene in the hope of finding a cure, such a focus is appropriate and commendable. But it is not the Human Genome Project.

Unfortunately, I don't see that there are very many Maynard Olsons out there who are interested in getting a complete physical map for its own sake. Maynard pioneered the physical

mapping of the baker's yeast genome [*Saccharomyces cerevisiae*], which is now just about complete. His work, as well as that of John Sulston on the nematode [*Caenorhabolitis elegans*], provided the models for how to go about making long-range physical maps. Maynard, perhaps you'd like to tell us a bit more about the motivations for making those maps.

Maynard Olson: In line with Norton's comments on his early work in bacterial genetics [see Part I of this discussion], the early efforts to map the genomes of yeast and the nematode illustrate the way in which science lurches forward. Both projects began roughly ten years ago and grew from entirely different motivations.

John Sulston, the originator of the nematode-mapping project, is a consummate biologist and, by his own characterization, a puzzle-solver. John is famous for working out the complete embryonic lineage of the nematode. He spent several years in a closet looking through a microscope at those tiny, transparent worms and watching all the cell divisions that occur as the fertilized egg develops into the mature organism. He documented the complete family tree leading from a single cell to a differentiated, multicellular organism with muscle and brain—or at least neurons—and so forth. A mature worm has a total of 959 somatic cells—cells that make up the body parts as opposed to those that produce eggs or sperm—and each worm produces those 959 cells by the same series of orderly cell divisions.

With that lineage in hand, people can, for example, use lasers to destroy a particular cell in a particular branch of the lineage and see whether other cells move in to take over the functions of the dead cell and its would-be progeny or whether the loss just causes a gap in the mature animal. John was very strong on the infrastructure development that we were talking about earlier. He recognized that the nematode would be a much more powerful experimental system if its cell lineage were sitting there making people think about nematode development in a different way.

John then went on to make a physical map of the nematode genome and that too was a pure infrastructure development. He had been around people like Fred Sanger, so, in a sense, he had grown up at the knees of the masters, but he had never done much work with DNA. Nonetheless, he understood that a physical map of the nematode genome would make that organism an even stronger experimental system, and he went after it.

Indeed, the physical map has made the nematode an immensely more powerful experimental system. Before the completion of that map, it was extremely difficult to isolate the DNA containing a nematode gene. Typically, a mutant worm was available that exhibited a specific functional defect, for example, a particular neuron might not develop or function properly in the mutant worm. Through controlled crosses, it was inferred that the defect was caused by a single mutant gene. Further, by tracing the co-inheritance of the defect with other variable nematode traits—again through controlled crosses designed to yield maximal information about linkage to other genes—the gene was located on a high-resolution genetic-linkage map [see "Classical Linkage Mapping."]

Clearly it's a lot easier to make linkage maps for experimental organisms than for humans because, first, crosses can be controlled, and second, huge numbers of progeny are available for analysis.

In the case of the nematode, a week or two of genetic-linkage mapping can often localize a gene to a region forty- to eighty thousand base pairs in length, but then that piece of DNA must somehow be isolated and cloned. Now that the nematode community has constructed a good physical map of overlapping cosmid clones and correlated it with the linkage map, the cosmids that are candidates for containing the gene of interest can be taken out of the freezer

When I first saw the basic pattern I thought, "The yeast genome has a definite physical structure, and if we could figure out the coordinates of the restriction-enzyme cleavage sites, it would be useful for genetics."

and the DNA from each cosmid can be injected into the gonads of a mutant animal. If that DNA contains the gene of interest, the defect is corrected in the resulting progeny. Then, since the DNA is in hand, the function of the gene can be pursued by the standard tools of molecular biology.

I took on the mapping of the yeast genome with a different motivation. My background is in physical chemistry, and I looked at mapping the yeast genome as a structural problem analogous, in spirit at least, to the first work on the atomic structure of proteins. I remember reading Max Perutz's description of his first good x-ray diffraction pattern from hemoglobin crystals. When he

saw all those spots on the film, he realized immediately that he was seeing the structure of those proteins at atomic resolution. He had not the slightest idea of how to interpret what he saw, and it took him twenty-five years to figure out how to do so, but he was very excited when he got those first data. He was sure, even then, that it would be useful for protein chemistry to know exactly where all the atoms were in a protein.

I had a similar experience when, for the first time, I saw the DNA fragments generated by digesting the yeast genome with a restriction enzyme all separated by length on an electrophoretic gel. At that time, 1974, restriction enzymes were not available commercially. Ben Hall, the yeast geneticist with whom I was working, obtained a little tube of the enzyme *Eco*RI from another laboratory. We wasted most of it by using the wrong buffer and so forth, but eventually we were able to cut some yeast DNA into fragments. We ran the fragments out on a gel, and we got the pattern of bands that made me think about the x-ray diffraction pattern of hemoglobin. The fragments were bunched together forming thousands of bands, more than you could count, but you could clearly see that the pattern comprised discrete bands. You could even see that the patterns for different yeast strains had subtle differences.

We eventually used those variations to do yeast genetics in a way that presaged the use of RFLPs as DNA markers in human genetics. When I first saw the basic pattern I thought, "The yeast genome has a definite physical structure, and if we could figure out the coordinates of the restriction-enzyme cleavage sites, it would be useful for genetics." My geneticist colleagues thought that I was crazy, but that is because—like most biologists—they were only interested

Most scientists with no experience in carrying out a large-scale mapping project—whether they are molecular biologists or not—assume that the six thousand DNA preparations and the one thousand gels represent most of the work. In fact, [for the yeast map] the ratio of time spent on specialized analysis to the time spent on routine fingerprinting and contig construction was 10 to 1.

in research that would directly address problems of biological function.

John's effort on the physical map of the nematode was more in tune with a preoccupation with immediate biological applications, whereas my efforts were motivated more by an innate belief in the importance of understanding structure. And like John I have a basic attraction to solving technical problems. My own motive for wanting to map the human genome is simply that human DNA has an exact structure, and there is a profound lesson in that.

Bob Moyzis: Maynard, perhaps you could describe how the yeast map was constructed, since it illustrates some of the difficulties of contig construction.

Maynard Olson: The basic challenge in constructing contigs of overlapping clones is to find the overlaps. One begins with a set, or a so-called library, of thousands of anonymous cloned fragments. I say anonymous because at the outset of mapping absolutely nothing is known about the fragments. The trick is to get just enough information about each fragment to be able to detect that one fragment overlaps another.

For the yeast project we picked clones at random, and then we created a fingerprint for each clone by cutting it up with a single restriction enzyme and separating the resulting fragments by length on a gel using electrophoresis. The lengths of the restriction fragments defined the fingerprint for the clone. If two clones have many restriction fragments of similar length in common, statistical arguments tell you that those two clones have a high probability of overlapping.

This procedure yielded not only contigs of overlapping clones but also a

restriction map for each yeast chromosome, a map that gives the distances between restriction-enzyme cutting sites along the chromosome. [See "Physical Mapping—A One-Dimensional Jigsaw Puzzle."] The average distance between the cutting sites on the yeast maps is approximately 2000 base pairs. The detailed physical maps are now providing a solid base for present efforts to sequence the entire yeast genome.

Bob Moyzis: That's a quick description, but you have estimated that the yeast map took 20 person-years to complete. How was that time spent?

Maynard Olson: Let's look at the routine work first. We analyzed roughly six thousand clones, obtaining a single-digest fingerprint for each. To produce most of the clones, we used lambda-phage vectors, which are derived from a widely used *E. coli* virus. The lambda clones each contained about 20,000 base pairs of yeast DNA. We also made a few hundred clones with cosmid vectors, and each of those clones contained about 40,000 base pairs of yeast DNA. Since the yeast genome contains about 15 million base pairs of DNA, our collection of clones provided nearly a tenfold sampling redundancy.

The clones were analyzed ten at a time on standard electrophoretic gels. Counting analyses that needed to be repeated and those that gave no useful data, nearly a thousand gels were run. Even though all that laboratory work was done by hand, it represents no more than 10 percent of the 20 person-years Bob mentioned. Moreover, that figure does not include one-time research and development activities such as software development and methodological research needed to come up with a workable strategy for finding overlaps and constructing contigs.

Most scientists with no experience in carrying out a large-scale mapping project—whether they are molecular biologists or not—assume that the six thousand DNA preparations and the one thousand gels represent most of the work. In fact, the ratio of time spent on specialized analysis to the time spent on routine fingerprinting and contig construction was 10 to 1.

What kinds of specialized analyses were needed? Significant effort went into tracking down errors and inconsistencies in the data. We had a data set of very high quality, but still we found that 5 percent of the fingerprints were problematic because the clones were biologically anomalous—they were unstable on propagation or were of arti-factual origin—and another 10 percent of the fingerprints were experimentally sus-pect—they were obtained from under- or over-digested DNA samples or involved mixed clones or incorrectly interpreted gel images.

Those special cases produced inconsis-tencies in the map, the most common being a branching contig. In other words, one contig would appear to branch into two when we attempted to accommodate all the fragments in the fingerprints of the clones in a linear order corresponding to a single contig. We used conservative criteria for recognizing overlaps, so very few of the inconsistencies resulted from placing clones in the wrong contigs. Most often, there was simply something wrong with the fingerprint data.

The key to building correct maps from reliable clone collections is to track down all the anomalies. Altogether we had about a thousand cases requiring special attention, and that attention had to come from skilled personnel and often required new experimental effort.

In addition, after the contigs were built, special experiments—none of them particularly satisfactory—were required to orient all the contigs in the same direction and align them with the chromosomes. Contigs built from lambda-phage and cosmid clones are rarely longer than 150,000 base pairs even when sensitive overlap-detection methods are employed. Therefore, the best-case scenario for a map the size of the yeast genome involves orienting and aligning one hundred contigs.

In reality, the yeast project dealt with several hundred contigs. For an average human chromosome the number would be closer to a thousand. Automation is not going to lessen the effort required to check and align large numbers of contigs, since it can only be applied to the routine activities that account for a small part of the total effort.

Bob Moyzis: Approaches similar to the one described by Maynard were used in the nematode mapping and the initial physical mapping of individual human chromosomes at Los Alamos and Livermore. At Los Alamos we realized that if more information could be rapidly obtained about each clone, then smaller overlaps could be detected, and hence, the initial mapping would progress faster. How could you obtain more information rapidly? That's where a low-resolution knowledge of the structural organization of human DNA proved useful.

Human DNA, unlike yeast and nematode DNA, is littered with multiple copies of various DNA sequences. The function of the repetitive DNA, if it has any, is unknown, leading some people to describe repetitive DNA as junk or parasitic DNA, as we mentioned ear-lier. Four particular sequences appear hundreds of thousands of times per

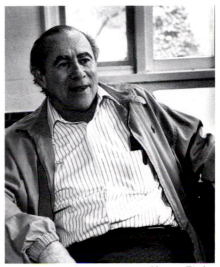

Norton Zinder

Though many people thought that the technical problems associated with large-scale mapping and sequencing would not be interesting to young people, the opposite seems to be true. Graduate students are tremendously enthusiastic about getting into this field.

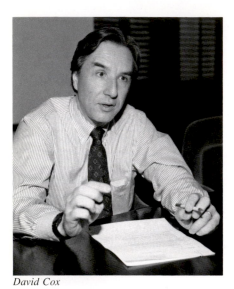

David Cox

People argue about which is the right technique for mapping the genome, and some are trying to push a given technique to its limit . . . when you search that hard, you end up making errors. Somebody is not the real father, or a tube is mislabeled, so . . . the new marker is not any closer to the gene than the markers you already have. Those mistakes happened in the search for the Huntington's gene.

genome and account for 5 to 10 percent of the DNA mass. Since our low-resolution studies indicated that those sequences were essentially randomly interspersed in human DNA, we realized that the locations of the four repetitive sequences in the restriction fragments of each clone would supply the needed extra information—and we could get that information rapidly.

One can show that for cosmid-sized fragments of a single chromosome, such repetitive-sequence fingerprints are essentially unique. David Torney at Los Alamos took this basic concept and developed a mathematically rigorous algorithm to identify pairs of overlapping clones. As predicted, our mapping initially progressed four to five times faster than the mapping of the nematode, which has about as much DNA as a single human chromosome. Our work has now progressed to the closure phase. The initial 550 cosmid contigs are being linked together with YAC clones to form between 50 and 100 contigs, each with an average length of 1 million to 2 million base pairs. [See "The Mapping of Chromosome 16."]

I'd like to point out that using fingerprints—even our repetitive-sequence fingerprints—to determine whether two clones overlap is a probabilistic approach to building contigs. A more powerful approach has recently been pioneered at Maynard's laboratory. The method involves first identifying a set of so-called sequence-tagged sites [STSs]—short segments of human DNA each with a unique base sequence—and then using the polymerase chain reaction to determine which STS is present in each clone. Any two clones that both contain the same STS by definition—and without question—overlap. STSs have become the main tool for map assembly as well as a universal map language.

Maynard Olson: It was obvious at the start of the Genome Project that we needed stronger overall strategies. YACs look like a promising way of keeping the analysis modular and reducing the number of modules—the number of clones and the number of contigs—to a more manageable number. However, even when YACs are used, the effort required to bring home a reliable, well-documented map is enormous.

Sequencing the human genome is going to be an even bigger job, but I doubt that it will prove to be as qualitatively difficult as mapping. And I am confident that it will be much more amenable to automation.

Norton Zinder: The beginning and end of any science—cosmology, anatomy, or molecular biology—is based on finding out where things are relative to each other. So the genome maps are fundamental. And though many people thought that the technical problems associated with large-scale mapping and sequencing would not be interesting to young people, the opposite seems to be true. Graduate students are tremendously enthusiastic about getting into this field. They find the rest of science crowded and in a way uninteresting.

A new generation of people will come into this field without the label of being molecular biologists and with a different mind-set. They see this field as wide open, as an opportunity to get lots of new information and data. And there's nothing more satisfying to a scientist than collecting lots of data.

In the days when I was doing almost nothing but making new bacterial mutants, I'd sit down at the end of the day and fill my notebook with the fifteen new mutants I had just knocked off, feeling very, very satisfied.

Bob Moyzis: The Genome Project is in essence a very large data-gathering effort—one that requires a lot more coordination than is normally found in biology. On the other hand, efforts to map the genome are divided among many laboratories. Los Alamos is mapping chromosome 16 and parts of chromosomes 5 and 21, Livermore is mapping 19, Washington University is mapping X and 7, and so on.

One reason for dividing the project by chromosome was to preserve the structure of the biological research community. No one wanted a large, monolithic organization dictating how the information would be gathered and disseminated. Each of the genome centers is using a different set of mapping strategies, depending on the talents and expertise of the scientists involved.

It's important to emphasize that there is no *right* way to generate a physical map and that many different techniques are needed to produce and confirm the map. As long as your map is translated into the STS language, how you obtained it is not relevant. Given the nature of molecular biologists, it will be obtained in any way that works. Under its present funding structure, the NIH may adopt the strategy of building a low-resolution, one-megabase, YAC map of the entire genome at one center. This map would be used as a framework for the construction of high-resolution maps at many different laboratories.

David Cox: Right now, in our work on chromosome 4 at UCSF, we're building contigs of overlapping YAC clones using a new type of linkage analysis called radiation-hybrid mapping to determine physical distances between unique DNA markers, and we're using in-situ hybridization to order the contigs and the DNA markers.

People argue about which is the right technique for mapping the genome, and some are trying to push a given technique to its limit. But no single technique will give us a reliable map of the genome. Each one is powerful only within a certain range of resolution, and at the limits of that resolution, it becomes inefficient and inaccurate.

The moral of the story is that we need to combine many different techniques if we're going to map the genome in a reasonable time.

Here's an example of what happens when you push linkage analysis to its limits. In searching for the Huntington's-disease gene, people were able to find DNA markers flanking the gene that were deduced from linkage analysis to be about 2.5 million base pairs apart. [See "Modern Linkage Mapping."] They went on to make a physical map of overlapping clones that spanned the region between the markers. But they wanted to narrow the search even further because finding a gene in 2 million base pairs of DNA is still a tough job. So they found new candidates for flanking markers and tried to find recombination events in afflicted families that would indicate the genetic distance between the new markers and the gene. [See "Classical Linkage Mapping" for a discussion of recombination events.]

Well, not very many recombination events take place within 2 million base pairs, so you have to scan the world for all the families afflicted with Huntington's disease in the search for

possible recombination events. The sad fact is that when you search that hard, you end up making errors. Somebody is not the real father, or a tube is mislabeled, so what you thought was a recombination event really is not, and the new marker is not any closer to the gene than the markers you already have. Those mistakes happened in the search for the Huntington's gene. All the workers in the field chased down a lot of garbage, and now the best we can do is to search through a region 2.5 million base pairs in length to find the gene. There's no additional recombination information at this time that allows us to find markers closer to the gene. Tomorrow there could be a new recombination event, but it's not very likely.

The moral of the story is that we need to combine many different techniques if we're going to map the genome in a reasonable time. Just as we need a series of microscope lenses with increasingly higher magnification to look not only at a whole cell but also at the small organelles within it, different mapping methods have different powers of resolution and we need all of them.

Bob Moyzis: Your point is well taken and it applies to contig building as well. For example, now that YACs are available, people argue that we should forget about cosmids because the contigs built from cosmid clones are relatively short. On the other hand, as soon as someone has a YAC contig, the first thing that person will do in order to find out more about what's in those YACs is to subclone them in cosmids or some other cloning vector. Smaller clones are much easier to work with, so cosmids will continue to play an important role in the mapping project. That is, of course, until we can directly sequence a 300,000-base-pair YAC.

Physical Mapping
a one-dimensional jigsaw puzzle

The human genome consists of forty-six double-stranded DNA molecules. Each molecule is made up, on average, of 130 million base pairs strung in a linear order between two sugar-phosphate backbones, and each is wound around proteins to form a chromosome. In order to study genes and other interesting regions of the genome at the molecular level, standard practice is to isolate the DNA and break up the long molecules into many fragments. We then make many identical copies of each fragment by cloning and pick out the clones of interest. Almost all methods for analyzing DNA at the molecular level require many copies of the fragment of interest. Therefore, cloning is essential for procedures such as finding the positions of restriction-enzyme cutting sites, determining the sequence of nucleotide bases in a particular DNA fragment, and identifying polymorphic DNA markers. However, in fragmenting the DNA molecules prior to cloning, we lose all information about the physical locations of fragments along the genome itself.

Problem: How do we find the chromosomal positions of known genes, polymorphic markers, and other cloned portions of the human genome?

Low-Resolution Physical Mapping by In-Situ Hybridization
In contrast to a linkage map, which specifies statistical distances between variable DNA markers and genes in terms of recombination fractions (see "Classical Linkage Mapping"), a physical map specifies physical distances between landmarks on the DNA molecule of each chromosome.

In-Situ Hybridization on Human Chromosome 21

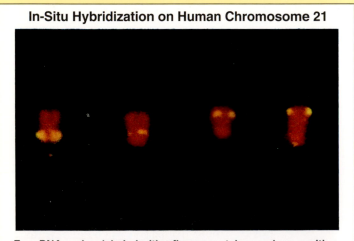

Four DNA probes labeled with a fluorescent dye produce positive hybridization signals at four locations along chromosome 21. Because metaphase chromosomes are made up of two nearly identical sister chromatids, each probe produces a pair of signals.

One standard low-resolution method for finding the physical position of a cloned fragment is in-situ hybridization on metaphase chromosomes. We first find a segment within the cloned region whose base sequence occurs nowhere else in the genome. We then synthesize many copies of a single strand of that unique segment and label each copy with a fluorescent tag to make it useful as a DNA probe. A solution containing the DNA probe is then applied to a spread of chromosomes that have been arrested at metaphase and fixed to a microscope slide. (Metaphase is the phase of cell division during which chromosomes have condensed to form the wormlike shapes easily visible under a light microscope.) Under appropriate conditions the probe binds, or hybridizes, only to the chromosomal DNA with a base sequence exactly complementary to that of the probe (see "Hybridization" in "Understanding Inheritance"). The position on a metaphase chromosome where the probe has hybridized is imaged with a fluorescence microscope as a bright spot. Because DNA molecules are wound very tightly during metaphase, the resolution achieved with in-situ hybridization is low, about 3 million base pairs. In other words, the hybridization signals from two probes less than 3 million base pairs apart will overlap one another and cannot be resolved into two distinct spots. In-situ hybridization using four cloned inserts as probes produced the bright spots on the metaphase chromosomes in the micrograph shown on the page opposite.

High-Resolution Physical Mapping by Construction of Contig Maps of Overlapping Clones

To determine the positions of genomic landmarks with much greater resolution, we can replace the chromosomes themselves with twenty-four contig maps, one for each of our twenty-two homologous chromosome pairs and one for each of our two sex chromosomes. A contig map is a set of contiguous overlapping cloned fragments that have been positioned relative to one another. In a complete contig map for a human chromosome, the cloned fragments would include all the DNA present in the chromosome and follow the same order found on the DNA molecule of the chromosome. As in any physical map, distances are measured in base pairs.

Using these contig maps, we can localize any cloned fragment or other DNA probe, again by hybridization, to a much smaller portion of the genome, namely to one of the cloned fragments in one of the maps. Moreover, we can determine the position of any DNA probe relative to all other landmarks that have been similarly localized. Once contig maps are constructed, the entire genome will be available as cloned fragments, and we will be able to use these clones to analyze any region down to the level of its base sequence.

Example: The figure at right is a schematic of a contig map for one chromosome. Right now, the top priority of the Human Genome Project is to construct a contig map for each of the twenty-four different chromosomes in the human genome. Those maps, when integrated with the corresponding genetic-linkage maps, will provide a means of finding the segments of DNA that contain disease genes (see "Modern Linkage Mapping"). The clones that make up the map also provide the material needed to sequence the human genome.

Many different strategies are being developed to make contig maps of human chromosomes. (Details of the Los Alamos effort to map a human chromosome are presented in "The Mapping of Chromosome 16.") Here we introduce the basic principles of contig-map construction.

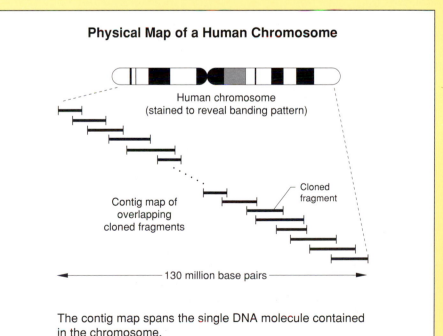

Physical Map of a Human Chromosome

Human chromosome
(stained to reveal banding pattern)

Contig map of
overlapping
cloned fragments

Cloned
fragment

←———— 130 million base pairs ————→

The contig map spans the single DNA molecule contained in the chromosome.

Question: How do we obtain the clones that compose the contig maps?

Answer: We prepare a collection, or library, of cloned human DNA fragments in a manner such that (1) essentially all parts of the genome are probably present in the library and (2) the human DNA fragments in the clones overlap one another. Overlaps among the cloned fragments are essential because they allow us to reconstruct the order in which the fragments appear along the genome.

Example: The figure illustrates the steps in preparing a library of cloned DNA fragments. We start by isolating the DNA from many human cells. Then we break up the DNA into a large set of overlapping fragments by partial digestion of the DNA with a restriction enzyme. A restriction enzyme digests a DNA molecule by recognizing and cleaving the molecule at every occurrence of a particular short sequence usually four to eight base pairs long. Such a site is called a restriction site and is marked on the figure by a dot. Since complete digestion would yield nonoverlapping fragments (every copy of a particular DNA molecule would be cleaved at the same places), we interrupt the digestion process before it reaches completion, thereby leaving many restriction sites intact at random locations along each molecule. (In the figure, cleavage is indicated by a vertical line through the restriction site.) Such partial digestion ensures that each resulting fragment will overlap other fragments in the set.

Next, each of these fragments is joined to a cloning vector to form a recombinant DNA molecule. A cloning vector is a small DNA molecule that, after entering a host organism (such as yeast or bacteria), is replicated by the cellular machinery of the host organism. The cloning vector shown here is a small circular DNA molecule that has been engineered to include a single cutting site for the restriction enzyme chosen to digest the sample of human DNA. Copies of the cloning vectors are cut at that site and are mixed with the human DNA fragments, and the enzyme DNA ligase is added to the mixture. The "sticky ends" of a cloning vector (which are formed by restriction-enzyme cleavage) bind to the "sticky ends" of a human DNA fragment, and the ligase catalyzes the chemical union of the sugar-phosphate backbones of the two DNAs into a recombinant DNA molecule. We then expose a population of the host organism to the recombinant DNA molecules, and, if we are lucky, each recombinant DNA molecule enters a host organism and is there replicated as the host replicates. Each host colony containing clones of a particular fragment is individually plucked and stored in a well of a 96-well microtiter dish where the cells can be grown up again and again. This library of clones provides a renewable supply of all the fragments that have survived the cloning process.

To create a contig map of a single human chromosome, many groups are starting with a chromosome-specific library of cloned fragments constructed by starting with many copies of a particular chromosome. Chromosome-specific libraries are being made by the National Laboratory Gene Library Project at Los Alamos and Livermore and are available to research groups throughout the world (see "Libraries from Flow-sorted Chromosomes").

The cloned fragments in a DNA library are "anonymous"; that is, we know nothing about them except their approximate length, which is determined by the length of the DNA insert that can be successfully incorporated into the cloning vector we have chosen. Until recently cosmids were the cloning vectors most often used for map construction. Cosmids reproduce in the bacterial host *E. coli*, and they accept DNA inserts ranging from about 25,000 to 45,000 base pairs in length. Therefore about 4000 cosmid clones could accommodate all the DNA in an average human chromosome. However, to achieve the overlaps among cloned fragments required in the construction of a contig map and to better assure that all the chromosomal DNA is represented in the clone library, the usual practice is to construct a library with up to ten times that number of cosmid clones.

Question: How do we position the cloned DNA fragments along the DNA molecules in the genome?

Answer: Positioning cloned DNA fragments is analogous to solving a one-dimensional jigsaw puzzle, but rather than looking for interlocking pieces, we look for detectable overlaps between clones, that is, for clones that have a unique stretch of human DNA in common. Because the number of pieces in the puzzle is so large, we need a rapid method for detecting overlaps between pairs of clones. If we could sequence each clone, we could identify overlaps unambiguously, provided the overlapping region is not a sequence that repeats elsewhere in the genome. However, given the current state of sequencing technology, that approach is totally impractical.

A practical and successful probabilistic method for detecting overlaps is to make a "fingerprint" of each clone (more precisely, of the human DNA insert within each clone) and compare the

Construction of a Library of Cloned DNA Fragments

Step 1: (a) Isolate many copies of the human DNA molecule to be mapped.

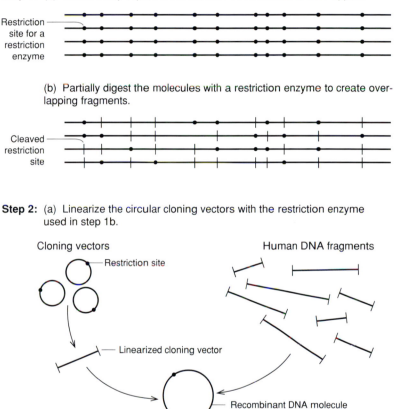

Restriction site for a restriction enzyme

(b) Partially digest the molecules with a restriction enzyme to create overlapping fragments.

Cleaved restriction site

Step 2: (a) Linearize the circular cloning vectors with the restriction enzyme used in step 1b.

Cloning vectors — Restriction site

Human DNA fragments

Linearized cloning vector

Recombinant DNA molecule

(b) Ligate cloning vectors and human DNA fragments to create recombinant DNA molecules.

Step 3: Facilitate the entry of recombinant DNA molecules into host cells, here the bacterium *E. coli*, and grow each host cell into an isolated colony, thereby producing many identical copies of that recombinant DNA molecule.

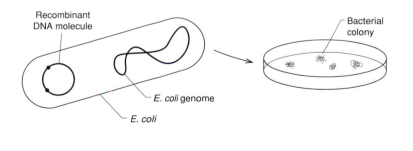

Recombinant DNA molecule

Bacterial colony

E. coli genome

E. coli

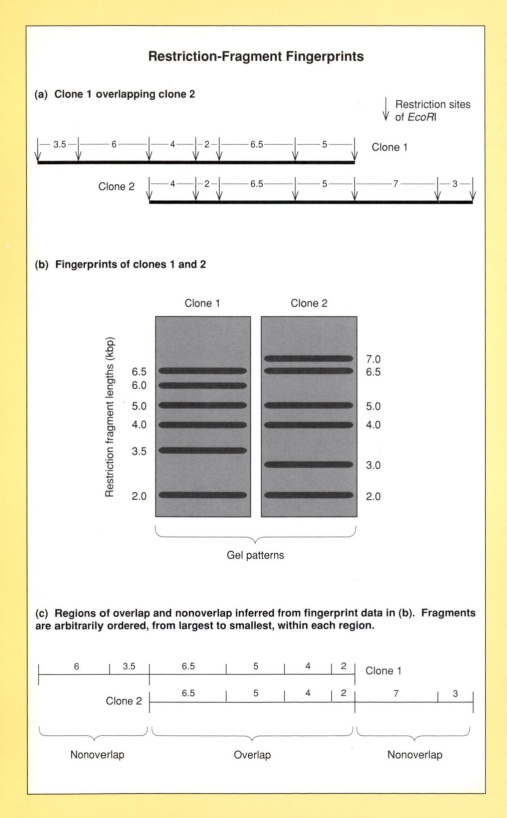

Restriction-Fragment Fingerprints

(a) Clone 1 overlapping clone 2

Restriction sites
of *Eco*RI

| 3.5 | 6 | 4 | 2 | 6.5 | 5 | Clone 1

Clone 2 | 4 | 2 | 6.5 | 5 | 7 | 3 |

(b) Fingerprints of clones 1 and 2

Clone 1   Clone 2

Restriction fragment lengths (kbp)

6.5
6.0

5.0

4.0

3.5

2.0

7.0
6.5

5.0

4.0

3.0

2.0

Gel patterns

(c) Regions of overlap and nonoverlap inferred from fingerprint data in (b). Fragments are arbitrarily ordered, from largest to smallest, within each region.

| 6 | 3.5 | 6.5 | 5 | 4 | 2 | Clone 1

Clone 2 | 6.5 | 5 | 4 | 2 | 7 | 3 |

Nonoverlap   Overlap   Nonoverlap

fingerprints. The simplest fingerprint of a cloned fragment is the one obtained by completely digesting about 10^{10} copies of the clone with a restriction enzyme and then determining the lengths of the resulting restriction fragments by gel electrophoresis. The restriction-fragment lengths determined from the gel constitute the restriction-fragment fingerprint of the clone.

Suppose we obtain restriction-fragment fingerprints of our clones by using the restriction enzyme *Eco*RI, which can cut DNA at every occurrence of the six-base-pair sequence GAATTC. Within a random sequence of the four DNA bases, any six-base-pair sequence occurs, on average, every 4^6, or about 4000, base pairs. Therefore the average length of the restriction fragments produced by *Eco*RI from a random sequence of the DNA bases is about 4000 base pairs. Now the sequence of bases in the human genome is not random, but nonetheless, the average length of the restriction fragments in the *Eco*RI fingerprints of a set of clones is about 4000 base pairs. Thus we expect that the human DNA inserts in two cosmid clones, each of which are, say, about 30,000 base pairs long, will have at least one restriction fragment in common if they overlap by more than about 15 percent.

Example: To illustrate the information content of fingerprints made by using the restriction enzyme *Eco*RI, consider two clones that are known to overlap as shown in part (a) of the figure. The cleavage sites for *Eco*RI are marked by arrows, and the distances between restriction sites are given in thousands of base pairs (kbp). Part (b) shows the restriction-fragment fingerprints obtained by completely digesting many copies of each clone with *Eco*RI. After several hours of electrophoresis, the restriction fragments of each clone have separated into distinct bands, each band consisting of all the restriction fragments with a particular length. (The bands are made visible by staining, and each gel is calibrated with fragments of known lengths.)

The region of overlap between the two clones shown in the figure yields four restriction fragments with lengths of 4, 2, 6.5, and 5 kbp. Thus the fingerprints of the two clones have four bands in common at the gel positions corresponding to those lengths. Suppose these two fingerprints were the only information we had about the two clones shown in the figure. We might suspect that the clones overlap one another and that the overlap region included four restriction fragments with lengths of 2, 4, 5, and 6.5 kbp. We might then partition the restriction fragments into a region of overlap and two regions of nonoverlap as shown in part (c) of the figure. Note that we would have no way to impose any further ordering on the restriction fragments present in the fingerprint.

Question: Can we infer that two clones overlap solely on the basis of their restriction-fragment fingerprints?

Answer: Since a restriction-fragment fingerprint is, in essence, just a list of restriction-fragment lengths, it gives us no information about the order of the fragments within each clone. Also, we can't tell whether the restriction fragments of the same length in two different fingerprints are copies of the same fragment. So the fact that the fingerprints of two clones have one or more restriction-fragment lengths in common does not provide unambiguous evidence that the two clones overlap. On the other hand, by taking into account statistical properties of restriction-fragment lengths, we can estimate the likelihood of overlap given the data. David Torney of Los Alamos has developed a rigorous formulation of the likelihood calculation that takes into account the distribution of the distances between cleavage sites in the genome (the distribution of *Eco*RI cleavage sites appears to be a Poisson distribution with an average spacing of 4000 base pairs), the errors in the measurement of restriction-fragment lengths (about 1 percent), and all possible ways in which the two clones might overlap. Since the declaration of a false overlap would lead to the merging of pieces of the map that are not contiguous on the genome and since such mistakes are very time-consuming to correct, a conservative approach is to declare an overlap only if the likelihood of overlap is 90 percent or greater. Given the simple restriction-fragment fingerprints shown on the page opposite, two clones must overlap by about 50 percent to yield such high likelihoods of overlap. Thus small overlaps are typically not detected with this conservative approach. As described in "The Mapping of Chromosome 16," the Los Alamos mapping group has devised a fingerprint that includes information about the presence of repetitive DNA sequences on the restriction fragments in each fingerprint. That additional information facilitates the detection of much smaller overlaps and therefore requires the fingerprinting of fewer clones to complete the contig map.

Question: How are pairs of clones with a high likelihood of overlap assembled into contigs, sets of contiguous overlapping clones?

Answer: Given the uncertainties in fingerprint data, assembling pairs of overlapping clones into contigs from those data alone is a difficult computational problem. The standard procedure is to find pairs of clones, link those pairs into groups, and then attempt to order all the restriction fragments within each group of clones in a self-consistent manner. The method is essentially an incremental approach. As each new clone is added to a contig, one tries to retain as much of the existing construction as possible even in the face of contradictory data.

A significant departure from the incremental procedure has recently been developed at Los Alamos. Map construction is treated as an optimization problem in which all available data are taken into account rather than only the data yielding high overlap probabilities. A description of this global approach to map construction is discussed in "Computation and the Human Genome Project." Here we illustrate the more standard procedure.

Example 1: Suppose that the fingerprints of clones A, B, and C reveal that clones A and B have five fragment lengths in common, A and C have six fragment lengths in common, and B and C have one fragment length in common. Furthermore, we have calculated from those data that the likelihood of A and B overlapping is 90 percent, of A and C overlapping is 95 percent, and of B and C overlapping is 10 percent. We would then assemble the three clones into a contig as shown in the figure, where some restriction fragments are placed in regions of overlap and the

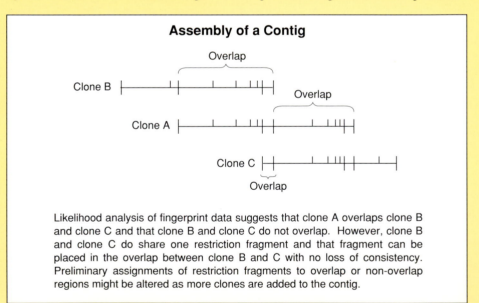

Assembly of a Contig

Likelihood analysis of fingerprint data suggests that clone A overlaps clone B and clone C and that clone B and clone C do not overlap. However, clone B and clone C do share one restriction fragment and that fragment can be placed in the overlap between clone B and C with no loss of consistency. Preliminary assignments of restriction fragments to overlap or non-overlap regions might be altered as more clones are added to the contig.

remaining ones are placed in the regions of nonoverlap. As we add other clones to the contig, we might have to revise the partitioning of the fragments into overlapping and nonoverlapping regions to construct a consistent ordering for the entire contig. Because of the uncertainties in fragment lengths and the possibility that fragments of equal length are not necessarily the *same* fragment, complicated computer algorithms are necessary to determine the most likely order of the clones in a contig. When the number of clones in a contig is much larger than the number required to span the region covered by the contig, we can order many of the restriction fragments that appear in each fingerprint and thereby help to avoid some false overlaps.

Example 2: Shown at right is a contig assembled on the basis of restriction-fragment fingerprints. The contig spans about 100,000 base pairs. Also shown is a restriction map deduced from the contig. The restriction map shows the order of and distances between restriction sites in thousands of base pairs or in kbp. The exact positions of some restriction sites (marked by the longer vertical lines that extend through the cloned fragments) have been determined by the fact that each lies at the end of one of the clones in the contig and therefore separates a region of overlap between two clones from a region of nonoverlap. Other restriction sites (marked by the shorter vertical lines) have been localized to a single overlap region but cannot be ordered further. Such sites have been arbitrarily located left to right on the contig in order of decreasing inter-site distance. This contig is representative of those used in constructing the recently completed physical map of the genome of baker's yeast (*Saccharomyces cerevisiae*). That map is, on average, eight clones deep. That is, any region is present in, on average, eight clones. Such

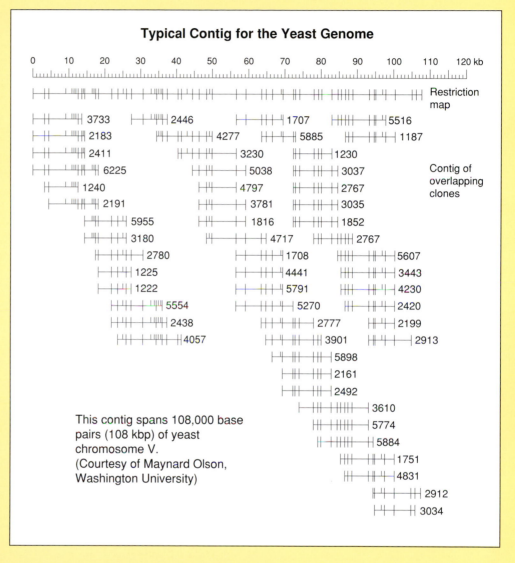

great redundancy provided information about the order of a large fraction of the restriction sites and greatly reduced the chance of a false overlap.

Question: *Do the disconnected contigs assembled by fingerprinting randomly selected clones steadily increase in length until they become connected?*

Answer: No. In a random fingerprinting strategy, both the numbers and sizes of the contigs grow fairly rapidly at first, but the rates of growth decrease after the existing contigs cover about two-thirds of the region to be mapped. The decrease in growth rate is due to the increasing probability that a randomly selected clone falls within a region for which a contig has already been assembled. Contig growth is also limited because small overlaps typically go undetected and some portions of the region being mapped may not have survived the cloning process. In fact, contigs assembled from cosmid clones typically stop growing after reaching lengths of 100 kbp.

Question: How do we order disconnected contigs along the chromosome and how do we check their accuracy?

Answer: Many types of lower-resolution maps can be used to position the contigs along a chromosome and to check that all the clones in a contig come from approximately the same region of the genome.

Example: The contigs constructed for yeast chromosomes, which had an average length of 100 kbp, were ordered relative to a high-density genetic-linkage map containing 400 markers spaced at an average physical distance of 30,000 base pairs. To check the integrity of each contig, the clones that form it were hybridized to very

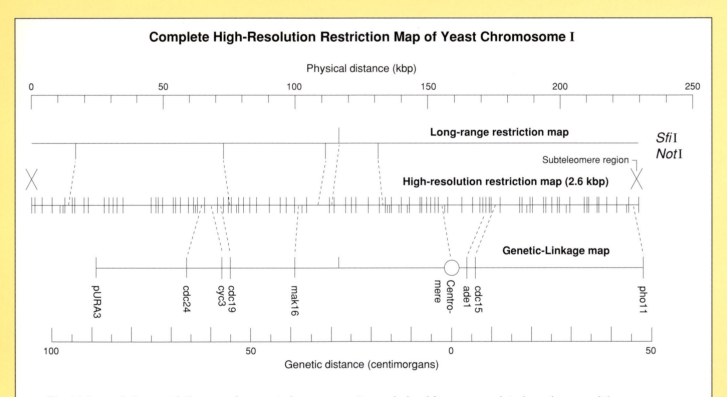

Complete High-Resolution Restriction Map of Yeast Chromosome I

The high-resolution restriction map for yeast chromosome I was derived from a completed contig map of the chromosome. The Xs mark the beginning of the subtelomeric regions which are known to lie a few thousand base pairs away from the telomeres (ends) of the chromosome. Restriction sites for the thirteen-base cutter *Sfi*I and the eight-base cutter *Not*I and markers on the linkage map of chromosome I are localized to particular restriction fragments on the high-resolution restriction map. (Courtesy of Maynard Olson, Washington University) long (over 100,000 base pairs) restriction fragments of DNA that had been separated by pulsed-field gel electrophoresis. If the clones assigned to a contig do in fact come from a single region of the genome, it is likely that all of them will hybridize to a single large fragment on the gel.

The figure shows the high-resolution restriction map deduced from the completed contig map of yeast chromosome I. Also shown is the alignment of the restriction map with two other maps: (1) the genetic-linkage map and (2) a long-range restriction map showing the distances between the eight-base restriction sites of the enzyme *Not*I and the thirteen-base restriction site of *Sfi*I. (The latter map was constructed using pulsed-field gel electrophoresis.) Markers on the genetic-linkage map and restriction sites on the long-range restriction map have been localized to particular restriction fragments on the contig map. Those correspondences are indicated by dotted lines.

The contigs being assembled for human chromosomes are being checked by a variety of techniques including in-situ hybridization and hybridization to the DNA from hybrid cells containing increasingly longer portions of the chromosome being mapped (see "The Mapping of Chromosome 16").

Question: After the contigs are ordered and checked for accuracy, how do we fill in the gaps between the contigs?

Answer: As mentioned earlier, the fingerprinting of randomly selected clones is not an efficient way to fill in the gaps between contigs after the existing contigs cover a large fraction of the region being mapped. Instead it is time to employ a directed strategy. One directed strategy involves identifying unique regions within the clones at the ends of a contig and using those regions as probes to pick out other clones that will extend the contig. If the contigs cover a very large fraction (95 percent) of the region being mapped, a single probe from the end of a clone may identify a new clone that spans the distance between two existing contigs and thus merges them into one. If not, then one must continue stepwise by creating an end probe from each added clone and screening the library of clones to find the next clone that extends the contig a bit farther. This procedure is called walking, and it is extremely time-consuming. Nevertheless, it has been used successfully to complete physical maps of the *E. coli* and yeast genomes. Those genomes are relatively small (containing 5 million base pairs and 13 million base pairs, respectively), and the gaps between contigs were small before walking was attempted.

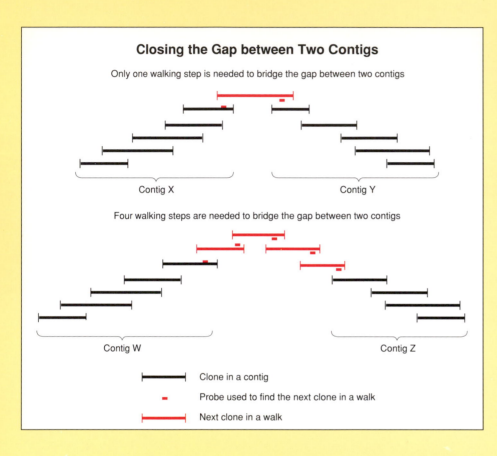

Closing the Gap between Two Contigs

Only one walking step is needed to bridge the gap between two contigs

Contig X   Contig Y

Four walking steps are needed to bridge the gap between two contigs

Contig W   Contig Z

— Clone in a contig

▬ Probe used to find the next clone in a walk

— Next clone in a walk

Example: The figure illustrates the merging of two contigs by either a single clone or several walking steps.

CAVEAT: A physical map is a very difficult puzzle to complete. As mentioned in the round table (see pages 108–109 in "Mapping the Genome"), the generic clone-to-fingerprint-to-contig cycle, which is amenable to automation and improved data-analysis algorithms, is only a small fraction of the work. The rest of the work required to close gaps between contigs and to track down inconsistencies such as the branching of one contig into two or more contigs involves many standard molecular-biology procedures, which, in the case of the human genome, must be carried out on an unprecedented scale. It is estimated that the completion of the yeast map took about 20 person-years of work, and the mapping of *each* human chromosome will take about 100 person-years. Further, mapping of human chromosomes presents some new challenges.

- An average human chromosome is ten times the size of the yeast genome, and the increased size calls for more efficient mapping strategies, such as working with larger clones.

- Unlike the genomes of yeast and *E. coli,* human DNA contains repetitive elements that require a new fingerprinting strategy to avoid inferring overlaps between clones containing long repetitive stretches of DNA near their ends.

- Experience has shown that regions containing repetitive sequences are often lost in the cloning process. Consequently, parts of the puzzle of each human chromosome may be missing, in which case completion of the map will require specialized techniques.

These challenges are being met in a variety of ways including the use of YAC cloning vectors, which accept DNA inserts eight to ten times larger than the inserts accepted by cosmids, and the use of STS markers, which, unlike restriction-fragment fingerprints, identify unique landmarks on the map and therefore eliminate the need for complicated probabilistic analyses to infer overlap between two clones. ■

STS Markers—
a common language for mapping

David Botstein: One new thing has come out of the Genome Project itself and the way it's organized, to wit, the STS idea, which was thought up by Maynard in response to a strategic problem. The strategic problem was how to connect all the physical maps together, how to get a universal language. There was no way to make sure that everybody uses the same name for the same region of the genome because everybody was using different methods.

Then Maynard came up with this brilliant idea of STSs, and what we did very well as a community was to get everybody to understand that here was a universal language that would benefit everyone. In absolutely record time a new idea was adopted by a whole group of people without any mandate from anybody. STSs are an enormous technical advance because the DNA is used to label itself. At least fifty labs are now using STSs.

Bob Moyzis: I've been quoted as saying that the STS idea was a conceptual breakthrough, and I believe that's true. Maynard, perhaps you would explain where the idea came from.

Maynard Olson: I saw large-scale physical mapping as a kind of Tower of Babel. People were subdividing the problem by chromosome and by chromosome region, and I saw us ending up with a bunch of contig maps expressed in completely incompatible languages. That is, each group was building a map from a different clone collection and

was using its own method for detecting clone overlaps. Consequently, we would have no convenient way to compare or crosscheck the maps. Eventually, the maps would have to be done again by whatever method proved to be the most generic.

The STS idea was to annotate each contig map with a series of unique landmarks. Each landmark, each STS, is just a short stretch of DNA—between 100 and 200 base pairs long—whose base sequence is found to be unique. Since the landmark is specified by a unique sequence of base pairs, it is called a sequence-tagged site, or an STS, and it can be unequivocally recognized and at the same time amplified by using the polymerase chain reaction [PCR].

The five-year plan includes the goal of generating a series of STSs for each chromosome separated by about 100,000 base pairs, but a series of more closely spaced STSs could eventually merge into the complete sequence.

I see the language of STSs playing a role similar to that of the ASCII code in the computer field. Once an early war between alternate standards was over, the ASCII code was adopted as the standard binary representation of a standard set of characters that are available on a standard typewriter keyboard.

The ASCII character set is woefully inadequate for today's word-processing needs because its roots are in a world view oriented toward typing. So when I try to read someone else's document on my computer, I may see a superscript where they had intended to have a Greek letter. Nonetheless, the fact that there was an ASCII code made a monumental difference to our ability to share information.

Similarly, the STS language enables us to share mapping information. In the late 1980s, when the feasibility of the Genome Project was being evaluated, the NRC committee struggled over the issue of generating incompatible maps, and we discussed the desirability of a common language for mapping. But at that time we had no experimentally practical technique to establish such a language. When the PCR was developed, it gave us an experimentally practical method for recognizing unique landmarks on the genome, and the sequences of those landmarks are the universal mapping language.

The crucial feature of STSs is that they have unique sequences. In other words, if we determine that two clones, one from each of two different clone collections, contain the same STS, we have no doubt that they come from the same region of the genome. Although the PCR is now the cheapest reliable method to recognize unique landmarks, one can imagine finding better recognition methods. However, I have no doubt that unique landmarks for the genome are going to remain short stretches of DNA with unique sequences, which is the essence of the STS concept.

The yeast map was constructed without STSs, and so the de facto landmarks on that map are the restriction sites at the ends of the particular clones that we used in its construction. We also made a restriction map specifying the distances between restriction sites. But restriction sites are repeated over and over in the genome, so they fail the most rudimentary test of an informative landmark. For example, if I give you a sample of yeast DNA and ask you whether it contains *Eco*RI site number 2708, you can't tell me whether it does or not. The restriction map does provide a back-up that would help to order a new set of clones, but a great deal of the original work would have to be done over to order a new set of clones.

In fact, almost all applications of the current yeast map are completely dependent on the clone collection used to make the map. Those clones are stored in a repository and have also been transferred to filters and sent out to laboratories where work on yeast is being done.

People use radioactively labeled DNA probes to pick out the clone on the filter that binds to the probe by complementary base pairing. Then they look at the database describing the map to see what part of the genome that clone comes from. That procedure works, but, say, ten years from now when we have the complete sequence of the yeast genome, our yeast clones will have become irrelevant.

It's going to be some decades before the human genome is sequenced completely. In this transitional period it would be a serious error to have the intermediate utility of the physical-mapping effort completely dependent on scores of clone collections, each created with one or the other of the different cloning systems now being used. The average lifetime of a cloning system is five years. By then we've generally found a better system. Not only would we have to store all those clones in vast repositories, but we'd have to create the clone collections over and over again because clones don't last forever. Every time you propagate a clone, you run the risk of losing some of the DNA insert and sometimes even gaining some DNA. So a map has to be based on something besides clones.

Norton Zinder: Biological entities don't last. Every time you handle them, it's trouble.

David Botstein: That point is worth amplifying. The original NRC report includes a whole set of references to a central storage place for DNA clones, what we used to call the Sears Roebuck of molecular biology. Those of us who are practical-minded were concerned that the Sears Roebuck could well have cost more than the research. It might have been our supercollider. But it became

I saw large-scale physical mapping as a kind of Tower of Babel. People were subdividing the problem by chromosome . . . and I saw us ending up with a bunch of contig maps expressed in completely incompatible languages.

clear very quickly that if an STS for some region of the genome has been identified, you can use the STS to pick out, from your own collection of clones, the clone containing that region. So the Sears Roebuck had become not only unnecessary but also undesirable.

Bob Moyzis: The idea that you can use an STS to pick out a clone of interest has already been tested experimentally in a number of labs. The base sequence of the STS can be transmitted electronically from one computer to another—no shipment of any material is involved. Along with the base sequence comes a protocol for a specific PCR that allows you to determine whether or not that STS is present in any given DNA sample.

In particular, the PCR can be used to screen a library of anonymous DNA clones to isolate the clone containing the STS. It is important to note that, although we all talk of *the* human genome, there are as many human genomes as there are humans. The region of the generic genome related to to some disease, for example, will have to be isolated from the DNA of many unaffected and disease-affected individuals in order to determine the DNA changes associated with the disease. STSs will be invaluable for that job.

Norton Zinder: The STS idea has another consequence: Anyone can play. Everyone thought you had to have a big lab to contribute to the Genome Project. But now anyone who provides an STS for a human DNA fragment with a reasonably well-defined location is contributing to the goals of the Genome Project.

Maynard Olson: When some of the large genome centers start producing long-range continuous maps, and by that I mean contigs that span millions of base pairs and that are separated by relatively small gaps, we're going to see a tremendous amount of detailed mapping in the smaller labs. People will hone in on particular regions of interest and add all kinds of annotations to the maps, not only new STSs, but also sites of translocations, mutations, genes, regulatory regions, and so forth.

We see that happening with the yeast map. People all over the place are annotating it in much the same way that road maps are annotated with information about the locations of parks, public buildings, and historic sites. Adding details to a map is easy compared with the initial construction of a map, but those details greatly increase the value of the map. In fact, to a large degree, they create the value of the map. Relatively large efforts are under way to create the initial contig maps for human chromosomes, but the little players will also get to contribute by straightening out the regions of the physical maps that they know a lot about. We've got to get some of the long-range physical maps out there, and then the community will do a superb job of annotating them.

When I suggested we could convert physical maps into pure information that could be stored in a computer, I didn't mean to imply that STSs do the whole job and that people outside the Genome Project would have to make their own contigs from earth, air, fire, and water. We'll still be sharing clones and other information about the contig maps. The purpose of STSs is to provide some bedrock to build on, some unique landmarks, that let you know where you are on the genome.

Bob Moyzis: The Genome Project's five-year goals for physical mapping are, in fact, to create a map for each human chromosome made up of contigs that are between 1 million and 2 million base pairs in length and that cover 95 percent of the chromosome, and second, to generate STSs spaced at intervals of 100,000 base pairs along each chromosome.

So we have to generate about 30,000 STSs. Some investigators initially thought that STS generation was an additional burden. However, now most laboratories consider STS generation to be a trivial part of physical mapping—a minor fraction of their total costs.

David Botstein: Generating an STS involves preparing a short DNA segment for sequencing, determining its base sequence, picking out unique primer sequences for the PCR, and then testing

the PCR for its ability to recognize and amplify that unique stretch of DNA.

We don't have a good estimate of how much it costs to generate each STS because people are generating STSs under different conditions and everybody's overhead is different. It's probably simpler to talk about the time required. I would say that if a person starts with a piece of cloned DNA, he can generate an STS from that clone in about two weeks.

The STS idea has another consequence: Anyone can play . . . anyone who provides an STS for a human DNA fragment with a reasonably well-defined location is contributing to the goals of the Genome Project.

Bob Moyzis: Yes, David, but one person can process many STSs in parallel. It's been our experience at Los Alamos that one person can generate approximately a hundred STSs per year. Therefore, generating each STS costs approximately a thousand dollars. And as I said, that is a small fraction of the total cost of physical mapping.

STSs are a means of annotating a contig map that's already constructed, but now that everybody's begun to accept the language of STSs, those markers are also being used as a primary means for building contigs, for detecting

whether two clones overlap. And unlike restriction-fragment fingerprints, which give only the probability of overlap, the presence of an STS in two clones is a guarantee of overlap.

So mapping can be carried out by first identifying a bunch of STSs and then finding pairs of clones containing the same STS. Clones that share an STS must overlap and thus belong in the same contig. This approach, called STS-content mapping, was pioneered at Washington University. It has become the approach used by most genome centers to construct the contig maps and to distribute the information in those maps.

David Botstein: That's been a major technological change in one year. We were looking at a lot of restriction-fragment fingerprint experiments a year ago, and now we're looking at a lot of STS-content experiments that are doing exactly the same thing, namely aligning one piece of DNA with another piece by detecting that the two overlap. There's no question that the STS-content paradigm is now the standard for physical mapping.

Bob Moyzis: That's the most efficient method for constructing a low-resolution map consisting of YAC-sized clones with unique landmarks spaced at intervals of 100,000 base pairs. But the most efficient method for creating a higher-resolution map with landmarks every few thousand base pairs is to fingerprint cosmid clones and create cosmid contigs covering the region within each YAC. We are geared to do that at Los Alamos and have found that it takes approximately two weeks to convert a YAC into a cosmid contig. Generating STSs at every few thousand base pairs would be much more work, at least by current methods.

125

STSs and Genetic Linkage Maps

Norton Zinder: Genetic-linkage maps can also be expressed in the language of STSs. All we have to do is generate an STS for each polymorphic DNA marker by sequencing each marker and developing a PCR to amplify a unique sequence within the marker.

Our five-year goal for the genetic-linkage maps is to find markers spaced evenly along the genome at genetic distances of 2 to 5 centimorgans, which translates into physical distances of 2 to 5 million base pairs. So we need about 600 polymorphic STSs—if they're equally spaced—to give us a pretty good genetic map of the genome, and we will need about ten times that number if we develop those markers from randomly chosen clones.

Nancy Wexler: People looking for disease genes probably haven't stopped to make an STS for each polymorphic DNA marker they are working with. We have discussed offering people some incentive either to do that themselves or to send their polymorphic DNA markers to some central place. In any case, the number of STSs is going to increase. The beauty of STSs is that they save real estate because you don't have to store clones.

Bob Moyzis: I expect that many of the polymorphic STSs will be generated around particular disease loci because PCRs can then be used to isolate the DNA of those variable sites directly from many patients. So we're going to have many more STSs than the number that is specified in the five-year plan. They may not, however, be generated with the desired spacing.

David Botstein: We need to remind people that there's no point in making a physical map if you don't have a high-density genetic-linkage map, that is, one on which the polymorphic markers are closely spaced.

Nancy Wexler: And only through the linkage map can we infer that a gene for a particular inherited trait is located near a particular marker. The folks working on genetic diseases are waiting avidly for the linkage maps.

> *Genetic-linkage maps can also be expressed in the language of STSs . . . We need about 600 polymorphic STSs—if they're equally spaced—to give us a pretty good genetic map of the genome, and we'll need ten times that number if we develop those markers from randomly chosen clones.*

Norton Zinder: At the moment most groups working on disease genes are retaining only those markers that turn out to be closely linked to the gene of interest, and they're discarding other markers that they come across. That's rather inefficient because the discarded marker might be relevant to genes in another region.

Nancy Wexler: People working on the same region often come up with different linkage maps, but they don't necessarily get around to resolving the differences. The managers of the Genome Project say the goal is to expedite getting the most accurate linkage map, and your funding is dependent on your sitting down with a committee and figuring out what experiments to do to resolve the discrepancies and connect the maps. That incentive seems to be working quite well.

Lee Hood: At Caltech we are developing automated techniques for genetic mapping. Present methods for identifying polymorphic DNA markers generally require gel electrophoresis and are therefore hard to automate. We are developing and automating an assay, the oligonucleotide ligase assay [OLA], which can readily identify known polymorphisms, in particular, those involving single-base changes.

The assay employs two DNA probes, about 20 bases long, that are complementary to adjacent regions in the genome. The polymorphism detected by the array includes the base at the 3' end of the 5' probe—the base directly adjacent to the 3' probe. The 5' probe has biotin attached to its 5' end; and the 3' probe has a reporter group at its 3' end. When the two probes are hybridized to the target DNA, DNA ligase will covalently join them if and only if there is perfect molecular complementariness between the probes and the target sequence. The sequences containing biotin are then pulled from the reaction mixture and assayed for the presence of the 3' reporter group.

If there is an exact match between the probes and the target sequence, then the 3' reporter group will be present on the biotin-labeled sequences that are pulled out of the mixture. If there is no match, then only the 5' probe will be pulled out from the mixture. Hence the assay is a simple plus or minus assay for the presence of a particular form [allele] of a polymorphism. A second 5′ probe can be synthesized complementary to the second allele of the polymorphism—and the same DNA can be assayed again. Thus we can determine whether an individual is homozygous or heterozygous for that polymorphism.

We are in the process of automating this entire procedure with a robotic work station. A single person can analyze 1200 assays in a day. This reaction can be carried out in the individual wells of a 96-well microtiterplate. We first amplify the target sequence in each well using PCR and then use the ligation assay. We're developing techniques for rapidly determining polymorphisms with two alleles so that OLA can be used to map entire chromosomes.

We're also working with Los Alamos to generate markers for chromosome 14 using a chromosome-specific library of clones. We're randomly sequencing cloned fragments from the library, picking out those regions from the DNA of six individuals and sequencing those regions again to identify frequent polymorphisms.

We have found that three or four polymorphisms often fall within a thousand base pairs and that these closely spaced markers are in partial linkage equilibrium, so that they provide highly informative markers for linkage analysis. In a relatively short period of time, we've generated seven such markers.

Now that a technique for identifying those markers in the DNA from any individual, namely, OLA, is semi-automated, if you want to use those markers to identify the relative position

of a particular trait on chromosome 14, you can readily do it.

Bob Moyzis: It's important to point out that if the genetic information obtained by this project is to be widely utilized, then automated techniques similar to those Lee just described must be developed.

Screening the whole genome for markers that are linked to a particular disease is still a very painful process for most laboratories, in part because those markers are not collected in any single place. That's why the Genome Project has decided to produce a kit of 150 reference markers spaced evenly over the genome at distances of about 20 million bases . . . the Project can create an appropriate infrastructure and deliver the goods to the scientific community.

David Cox: That's right, but in the meantime, screening the whole genome for markers that are linked to a particular disease is still a very painful process for

most laboratories, in part because those markers are not collected in any single place.

That's why the Genome Project has decided to produce a kit of 150 reference markers spaced evenly over the genome at distances of about 20 million bases. That effort involves identifying and collecting existing markers and supporting various individuals to search for probes in regions where no probes yet exist.

Those regions will be targeted by radiation-hybrid mapping or microdissection of chromosomes. Once the markers are collected, they will be put together in a package that will be sold at a reasonable price. Ray White and Helen Donis-Keller have each constructed a genetic-linkage map for the human genome. They say that they're happy to let other people have their markers. They just don't have the time and the money to distribute them.

Other available markers come with strings attached and rightly so because private companies have put a lot of money into generating them. The labs that have done the most work on the genetic map are often criticized for not sharing, but in many instances, they just don't have the infrastructure that allows them to share efficiently. On the other hand, the Genome Project can create an appropriate infrastructure and deliver the goods to the scientific community. The reference list is an immediate goal that can be fulfilled.

We must remember that the Genome Project is a product-oriented endeavor, and those who are funded are expected to come through with the product. In normal research, you can't always predict exactly what you're going to find, but here we have very specific goals.

The Polymerase Chain Reaction
and Sequence-tagged Sites *Norman A. Doggett*

Polymerase Chain Reaction

The polymerase chain reaction (PCR) is an in vitro method for selectively amplifying, or synthesizing millions of copies of, a short region of a DNA molecule. The reaction is carried out enzymatically in a test tube and has been successfully applied to regions as small as 100 base pairs and as large as 6000 base pairs. In contrast, DNA cloning is a nonselective in vivo method for replicating DNA fragments within bacterial or yeast cells. Cloned fragments range in length from several hundred to a million base pairs. (See "DNA Libraries" for further discussion of DNA cloning.)

PCR is particularly important to the Human Genome Project as a tool for identifying unique landmarks on the physical maps of chromosomes. The PCR can be used to detect the presence of a particular DNA segment in a much larger DNA sample and to synthesize many copies of that segment for further use as a probe or as the starting material for DNA sequencing.

Figure 1 illustrates the polymerase chain reaction. The reaction mixture contains:

- A DNA sample containing the target sequence.
- Two single-stranded DNA primers (short sequences about 20 nucleotides long) that anneal, or bind by complementary base pairing, to opposite strands of DNA at sites at either end of the target sequence. Such short DNA sequences are called oligonucleotides and can be synthesized in a commercially available instrument.
- A heat-stable DNA polymerase, an enzyme that catalyzes the synthesis of a DNA strand complementary to the target sequence and can withstand high temperatures.
- Free deoxyribonucleoside triphosphates (dATP, dGTP, dCTP, and dTTP), precursors of the four different nucleotides that will extend the primer strands.
- A reaction buffer to facilitate primer annealing and optimize enzymatic function.

The polymerase chain reaction proceeds by repeated cycling of three temperatures:

- Phase 1: Heating to 95°C to denature the double-stranded DNA, that is, to break the hydrogen bonds holding the two complementary strands together. The resulting single strands serve as templates for DNA synthesis.
- Phase 2: Cooling to a temperature between 55°C and 65°C to allow each of the primers to anneal (or hybridize) to its complementary sequence at the 3' end of one of the template strands.
- Phase 3: Heating to 72°C to facilitate optimal synthesis, or extension of the primer strand by the action of the DNA polymerase. The polymerase attaches at the 3' end of the primer and follows along in the 3'-to-5' direction of the template strand catalyzing the addition of nucleotides to the primer strand until it either falls off or reaches the end of the template strand (see "DNA Replication" in "Understanding Inheritance").

The figure shows the materials in the reaction mixture and the first three cycles of the reaction. The DNA synthesized in each cycle serves as a template in the next. Note that an exact duplicate of each strand of the target sequence is first created during cycle 2. Each subsequent cycle doubles the number of those strands so that after n cycles the reaction will contain approximately 2^n copies of each strand of the

128

Figure 1. The Polymerase Chain Reaction

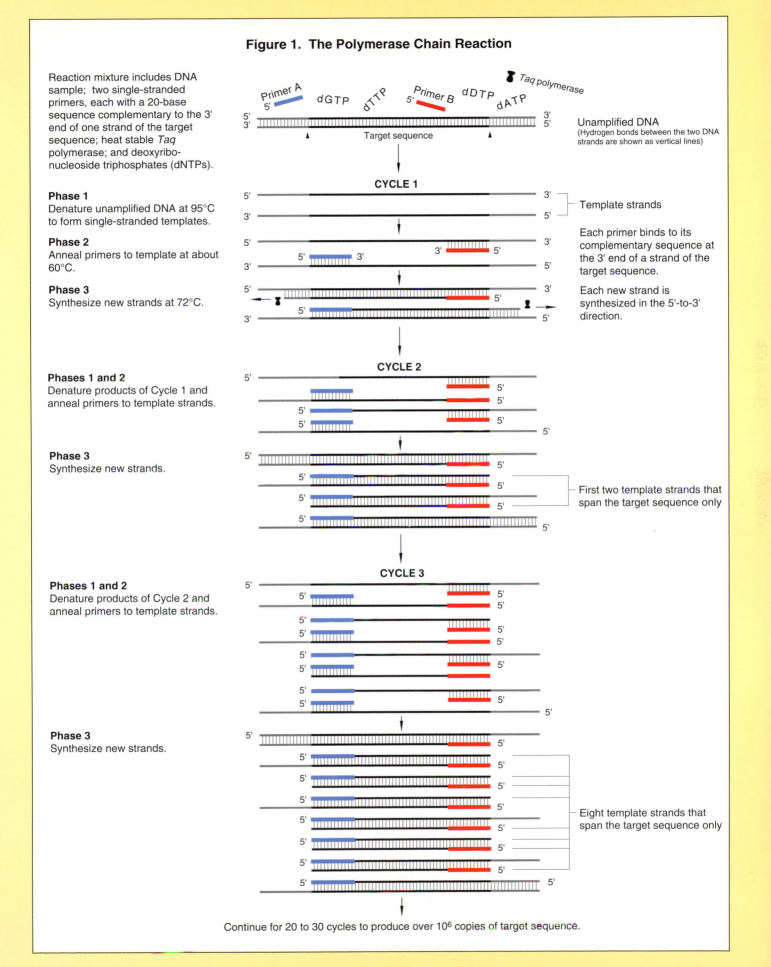

Reaction mixture includes DNA sample; two single-stranded primers, each with a 20-base sequence complementary to the 3' end of one strand of the target sequence; heat stable *Taq* polymerase; and deoxyribonucleoside triphosphates (dNTPs).

Phase 1
Denature unamplified DNA at 95°C to form single-stranded templates.

Phase 2
Anneal primers to template at about 60°C.

Phase 3
Synthesize new strands at 72°C.

Phases 1 and 2
Denature products of Cycle 1 and anneal primers to template strands.

Phase 3
Synthesize new strands.

Phases 1 and 2
Denature products of Cycle 2 and anneal primers to template strands.

Phase 3
Synthesize new strands.

Unamplified DNA
(Hydrogen bonds between the two DNA strands are shown as vertical lines)

CYCLE 1

Template strands

Each primer binds to its complementary sequence at the 3' end of a strand of the target sequence.

Each new strand is synthesized in the 5'-to-3' direction.

CYCLE 2

First two template strands that span the target sequence only

CYCLE 3

Eight template strands that span the target sequence only

Continue for 20 to 30 cycles to produce over 10^6 copies of target sequence.

target sequence. Typically the chain reaction is continued for 20 to 30 cycles in microprocessor-controlled temperature-cycling devices to create between roughly 1 million and 1 billion copies of the target sequence.

Taq polymerase, a heat-stable polymerase isolated from the bacterium *Thermus aquaticus* found in hot springs, is used in the reaction. The annealing temperature for the second phase of each cycle is chosen to be approximately 5°C below the temperature at which the primers no longer anneal to the target sequence. That so-called melting temperature varies depending upon the primer sequence. In particular because G-C base pairs (which have three hydrogen bonds) remain stable at higher temperatures than A-T base pairs (which have only two hydrogen bonds), primers containing mostly Gs and Cs have a higher melting temperature than those containing mostly As and Ts. The annealing temperature must be chosen carefully because if the temperature is too low, the primers will bind to sites whose sequence is not exactly complementary to the primer sequence resulting in the amplification of sequences other than and in addition to the target sequence. If the temperature is too high, the primers will not bind to the template strands and the reaction will fail.

Typically the initial DNA sample contains from 3,300 to 333,000 copies of the human genome (or 10 nanograms to 1 microgram of total genomic DNA). However, when working properly, the PCR will selectively amplify a unique target sequence contained in a diploid copy of the genome (6 picograms of DNA) isolated from a single cell. To evaluate the specificity of the reaction, that is, whether or not the reaction amplified a single target region, the reaction products are separated on a gel using electrophoresis. If a single region has been amplified, the gel will contain a single intense band containing the synthesized copies of the target sequence. The location of the band on the gel indicates the length of the amplified region. If more than one intense band appears on the gel, then more than one region of the genome was amplified by the reaction and the sequence of the primers appear more than once in the genome.

Sequence-tagged Sites

A sequence-tagged site (STS) is a short region along the genome (200 to 300 bases long) whose exact sequence is found nowhere else in the genome. The uniqueness of the sequence is established by demonstrating that it can be uniquely amplified by the PCR. The DNA sequence of an STS may contain repetitive elements, sequences that appear elsewhere in the genome, but as long as the sequences at both ends of the site are unique, we can synthesize unique DNA primers complementary to those ends, amplify the region using the PCR, and demonstrate the specificity of the reaction by gel electrophoresis of the amplified product (Figure 2).

Operationally, a sequence-tagged site is defined by the PCR used to perform the selective amplification of that site. The PCR is specified by the pair of DNA primers that bind to the ends of the site and the reaction conditions under which the PCR will amplify that particular site and no other in the genome.

STSs are useful because they define unique, detectable landmarks on the physical map of the human genome. One of the goals of the Human Genome Project is to find STS markers spaced roughly every 100,000 bases apart along the contig map of each human chromosome (see "Physical Mapping—A One-dimensional Jigsaw Puzzle" for a description of contig maps). The information defining each site will be stored in a computer database such as GenBank. That stored information will include the PCR primers, reaction conditions, and product sizes as well as the DNA sequence of the site. Anyone who wishes to make copies of the marker would simply look up the STS in the database, synthesize the specified primers, and run the PCR under the specified conditions to amplify the STS from genomic DNA. As described below, copies of the STS can be used to screen a library of uncharacterized clones and identify a clone containing the marker. Therefore, a database of such landmarks will eliminate the need to store and distribute a permanent set of DNA clones or probes for the physical maps.

Figure 3 outlines the procedure for finding an STS marker. One begins by sequencing a 200- to 400-base region of a cloned DNA fragment. The rough sequence can be obtained from a single run of a DNA sequencing gel (see "DNA Sequencing"). The sequence is then examined to find two twenty-base regions separated by 100 to 300 base pairs that might serve as unique primers for a PCR (see Figure 4). The primers are synthesized and then the PCR reaction is run on genomic DNA to see whether the reaction results in the selective amplification of the targeted region. If it does, then the amplified region becomes an STS. In our work at Los Alamos, we found that about half of the sequences we obtained from randomly selected clones yielded an STS.

STS Markers for Physical Mapping

STSs are being used to find pairs of overlapping clones for the construction of contig maps of human chromosomes. Since each STS is a unique site on the genome, two clones containing the same STS must overlap and the overlapping region must include the STS.

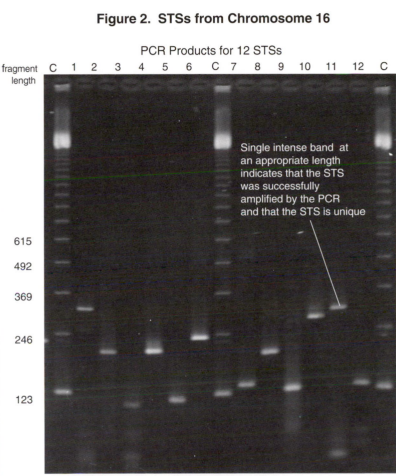

Figure 2. STSs from Chromosome 16

PCR Products for 12 STSs

Single intense band at an appropriate length indicates that the STS was successfully amplified by the PCR and that the STS is unique

Electrophoretic Gel

To check that a sequence-tagged site (STS) is a unique sequence on the genome, the polymerase chain reaction (PCR) defining that site is carried out on total genomic DNA and the products of the reaction are separated on a gel by electrophoresis. If the reaction amplifies that site and no other, all reaction products will have the same length (known from the sequence of that site) and will appear together as a single intense band on the gel.

At Los Alamos, twelve different STS markers are amplified in parallel by the PCR, and the products are separated on twelve separate lanes of a gel. The presence of only one intense band in each numbered lane of the gel shown above indicates that the STS is indeed a unique site. Fainter bands near the bottom of a lane are residual primers remaining after the PCR. The sizes of the amplified products are measured relative to a ladder of standard fragments (with known lengths that are multiples of 123 base pairs) that have been separated by length in the gel lanes marked C.

Before overlap can be detected, clones containing the same STS must be identified from among a collection of clones in a DNA library. If the individual cloned fragments have been permanently arrayed on nitrocellulose or nylon membranes,

Figure 3. Steps in Developing an STS Marker

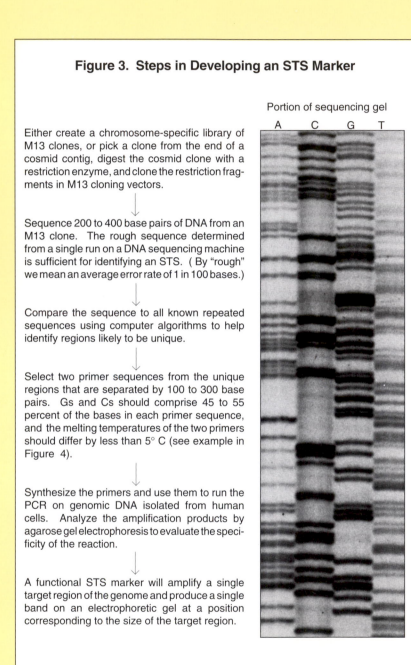

Portion of sequencing gel

A   C   G   T

Either create a chromosome-specific library of M13 clones, or pick a clone from the end of a cosmid contig, digest the cosmid clone with a restriction enzyme, and clone the restriction fragments in M13 cloning vectors.

↓

Sequence 200 to 400 base pairs of DNA from an M13 clone. The rough sequence determined from a single run on a DNA sequencing machine is sufficient for identifying an STS. (By "rough" we mean an average error rate of 1 in 100 bases.)

↓

Compare the sequence to all known repeated sequences using computer algorithms to help identify regions likely to be unique.

↓

Select two primer sequences from the unique regions that are separated by 100 to 300 base pairs. Gs and Cs should comprise 45 to 55 percent of the bases in each primer sequence, and the melting temperatures of the two primers should differ by less than 5° C (see example in Figure 4).

↓

Synthesize the primers and use them to run the PCR on genomic DNA isolated from human cells. Analyze the amplification products by agarose gel electrophoresis to evaluate the specificity of the reaction.

↓

A functional STS marker will amplify a single target region of the genome and produce a single band on an electrophoretic gel at a position corresponding to the size of the target region.

then clones containing a particular STS may be identified by hybridization to copies of an STS marker. First, copies of the STS are generated from genomic DNA by the PCR. The amplified copies are labeled with radioactive ^{32}P, denatured, and then applied to the membranes containing the arrayed collection of cloned fragments. The labeled markers will hybridize only to those clones containing DNA sequences complementary to those of the markers. Clones that are positive for the STS are imaged as dark spots on x-ray films that have been exposed to the membranes containing those clones.

A more rapid screening method involves dividing a library of clones into pools and using PCR to interrogate each pool for the presence of the STS. In the PCR-based screening method, primers are synthesized for each STS, and many pools are screened in parallel. If a particular pool of cloned fragments supports PCR amplification of the STS target sequence, then at least one particular clone in the pool must contain the target sequence. Using a clever pooling scheme described below, the identification of which pools support amplification will result in the identification of the particular clone or clones containing the STS.

STS Markers for the Chromosome-16 Physical Map

In line with the five-year goals of the Human Genome Project, the Los Alamos effort to construct a physical map of chromosome 16 includes developing STS markers spaced, on average, at 100,000-base-pair intervals along the chromosome. At present about 60 percent of chromosome 16 is covered by contigs made up of cosmid clones. On average each cosmid contig spans a distance of 100,000 base pairs. We are developing STSs by sequencing regions from the clones that lie at either end of each contig. Thus far a total of 325 sequences have been obtained from such clones and about 100 of these have been developed into STSs. The STS markers will be stored in GenBank so that anyone who wants to regenerate the markers and use them to identify clones containing those markers may do so.

The STS markers from the end clones of our cosmid contigs are serving several purposes. First, they are being used to screen a library of YAC clones for clones that may overlap two different cosmid contigs and therefore close the gap between them.

Our library of 550 YACs is specific for chromosome 16. That is, the YACs contain DNA inserts from human chromosome 16 only. Since those inserts have an average size of 215 kb, the total YAC library represents a one-time coverage of the DNA in chromosome 16. The construction of such chromosome-specific YAC libraries is an important breakthrough for physical mapping and is described in "Libraries from Flow-sorted Chromosomes."

We have partitioned the YACs into pools and are using a PCR-based screening strategy to identify YACs containing each STS. Our pooling scheme, devised by David Torney in the theoretical biology group at Los Alamos, has the advantage of detecting false positive and false negative results from the PCR (see "YAC Library Pooling Scheme"). Once a YAC clone containing an STS is identified, a PCR technique (known as inter-ALU PCR) is used to generate a set of probes from that YAC. The probes are hybridized to our arrayed library of cos-

---

Figure 4. Example of an STS

Rough Sequence—347 Bases (lower case letters indicate uncertainty in the base call)

```
                                              ┌ Primer A
5    5'-GAATTCCTGA  CCTCAGGTGA  TCTGCCCGCC │ TCGGCCTCCC  AAAGTGCTGG
51     GATTTACAGG  CATGAGGCAC  CACACCTGGC │ CAGTTGCTTA  GCTCTCTAAG
101    TCTTATTTGC  TTTACTTACA  AAATGGAGAT │ ACAACCTTAT  AGAACATTCG
151    ACATATACTA  GGTTTCCATG  AACAGCAGCC │ AGATCTCAAC  TATATAGGGA
201    CCAGTGAGAA  ACCAATGTCA  GGTAGCTGAT  GATGGGCAAa  GGgATGGGgA
251    CTGATATGCC  cNNNNNGACG  ATTCGAGTGA  CAAGCTACTA  TGTACCTCAG
301    CTTTtCATCT  tGATCTTCAC  CACCCATGGg  TAGGTGTCAC  TGAAaTT-3'
                   3'-CTAGAAGTG  GTGGGTACCC  AT-5'  ──────── Primer B
```

								Melting Temperature
Primer A	5'-GTT	TCC	ATG	AAC	AGC	AGI	CAG-3'	69.4°C
Primer B	5'-TAC	CCA	TGG	GTG	GTG	AAG	ATC-3'	68.7°C

The STS developed from the rough sequence shown above is 171 bases long. It starts at base 162 and runs through base 332. Primer A is 21 bases long and lies on the sequenced strand. Primer B is also 21 bases long and is complementary to the shaded sequence toward the 3' end of the sequenced strand. Note that the melting temperatures of the two primers are almost equal. A computer algorithm was used to pick out the two primer sequences and to calculate their melting temperatures.

---

mid clones. If clones from two different contigs yield positive hybridization signals, then the YAC must bridge the gap between the two contigs. So far we have identified 30 YACs containing the STSs from end clones of cosmids. These YACs and seventy-five others have been hybridized to the cosmid clones resulting in the closure of sixty-five gaps in the contig map of chromosome 16..

The same STSs are being used to localize each of our cosmid contigs to an interval on chromosome 16, defined by a series of mouse/human somatic-cell hybrids containing various portions of chromosome 16. Collaborators David Callen and Grant Sutherland of Adelaide Children's Hospital in Southern Australia have collected a panel of 50 hybrid cells that divide chromosome 16 into 50 intervals with an average size of 1.7 million bases. Using a hybridization-based method and, more recently, our STSs and a PCR-based strategy, they have screened the DNA in each hybrid cell and thereby localized each of 70 contigs to one of the 50 intervals defined by the hybrid-cell panel. Those 70 contigs represent about 10 percent of chromosome 16.

STS Markers for Genetic-linkage Mapping

So far we have suggested that an STS yields the same product size from any human DNA sample. However, STSs can also be developed for unique regions along the genome that vary in length from one individual to another. The PCR that amplifies

Figure 5. Polymorphic STSs—Highly Informative Markers for Linkage Analyis

(a) A Polymorphic STS

5'- unique sequence GTGTGT . . . . GT unique sequence -3'

$(GT)_n$

The number n of GT repeats varies among the population.

(b) Inheritance of the Polymorphic STS shown in (a)

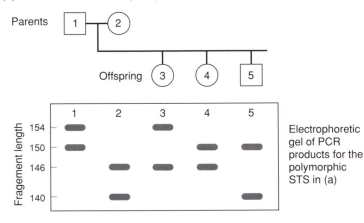

Electrophoretic gel of PCR products for the polymorphic STS in (a)

A variable locus containing a short repeated sequence, such as the dinucleo-tide repeat $(GT)_n$, flanked by two unique sequences can be developed into an STS. An example is shown in (a). The size of the amplified product for that STS will vary depending on the value of n at that locus, and therefore the STS is polymorphic. Each individual carries two copies of the STS marker, one on each chromosome of a homologous pair, and each copy may have a different value of n and thus be a different allele of the polymorphic STS.

The inheritance of the polymorphic STS in a five-member family is illustrated schematically in (b). The electrophoretic gel shows the PCR products for the STS from each family member. The two alleles carried by the father are different from the two alleles carried by the mother. The children inherit one allele of the STS from each parent.

Because markers developed around such repeat sequences have many alleles, the likelihood that a given individual is heterozygous for such a marker is high. As explained in "Classical Linkage Analysis," at least one parent must be heterozygous for two different markers (or genes) in order to establish linkage between the two. Thus markers that have many alleles are likely to be *highly informative* for linkage analysis. (See "Informativeness and Polymorphic DNA Markers.") Polymorphic STSs will help to attain the five-year goal to construct a genetic-linkage map of highly informative DNA markers spaced at genetic distances of 2 to 5 centimorgans along each chromosome of the human genome. Moreover, these STSs are easily located on the physical map and thus provide a convenient means for aligning the linkage map with the physical map of a chromosome.

the variable region will yield different product sizes depending on which variations of the region are present in the genome of a given individual. An STS from a variable region is, by definition, a polymorphic DNA marker, which can be traced through families along with other DNA markers and located on genetic-linkage maps (see "Modern Linkage Mapping").

Figure 5(a) shows an example of a unique region that has variable lengths and can be developed into a polymorphic STS. At either end of the region is a unique sequence about 20 nucleotides long that can serve as a primer sequence for the PCR. Between those two sequences is a simple tandem repeat, $(GT)_n$ (or GT repeated in tandem n times). Such dinucleotide repeats are scattered throughout the human genome as are tri-, tetra-, and penta-nucleotide repeats. Moreover, the number n of tandem repeats at a given locus along a chromosome is an inherited trait that tends to vary widely among the population. Thus each such variable locus has many different alleles (or forms), each one defined by the number n of tandem repeats between the unique sequences.

STSs are being developed for this abundant class of variable regions. Since the varying sizes of the PCR products from a polymorphic STS correspond to the alleles of that marker, PCR followed by gel electrophoresis of the amplified products is the method of detecting which alleles of the marker are carried by an individual [see Figure 5(b)].

Polymorphic STSs are particularly useful because they can serve as landmarks on both the physical map and the genetic-linkage map for each chromosome, and thus they provide points of alignment between the different distance scales on these two types of maps.

At Los Alamos we have identified the location of $(GT)_n$ repeats as part of our fingerprinting and mapping strategy (see "The Mapping of Chromosome 16"). We are now developing these regions into STSs for use in linkage mapping. ∎

YAC Library Pooling Scheme for PCR-Based Screening

David J. Balding and David C. Torney

The PCR is a rapid method for screening a library of clones for the presence of clones containing an STS. Usually the library is divided into pools of clones, and the PCR is run on each pool. The problem we address here is to design efficient and robust pooling schemes for such PCR-based screening. Two questions are relevant: (1) Given an arbitrary unique sequence, how should one pool a library of clones to find rare positive clones (those containing this unique sequence), using a reasonable number of pools and a minimum number of pools queried per positive? (2) How can the design of the pooling scheme be robust to experimental errors (false positives, false negatives) when querying pools with PCR? Clearly, we want to do group testing in a way that gives correct results even in the presence of experimental errors.

In answer to these questions, we designed a pooling scheme called a J-detector, capable of indicating either which j clones are positive for $j \leq J$, or whether more than J clones are positive. The scheme works in the presence of K experimental errors provided any one clone in the J-detector occupies at least $K+1$ pools that are not among the pools jointly occupied by any set of J other clones. For example, if $J = 1$, and $K = 0$, we require that, among the pools containing clone$_i$, there is at least one pool that does not contain clone$_j$ for all $i \neq j$. Thus we can distinguish one positive from two positives.

From information theory we know that the number of pools in a J-detector must be at least $J \log N$, where N is the number of clones in the library. We believe that t-designs (Beth et al., 1986) constitute optimal J-detectors, therefore we focused our efforts on improved methods for the construction of t-designs. A t-design has three parameters: v, the number of pools; k, the number of pools each clone occupies;

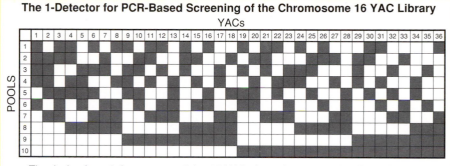

The 1-Detector for PCR-Based Screening of the Chromosome 16 YAC Library

The design for a 1-detector containing 36 YAC clones has ten pools. Each clone is in 5 pools and two clones occur jointly in no more than 3 pools.

and t, the maximum number of pools any two clones jointly occupy.

The chromosome 16-specific YAC library developed at Los Alamos contained 550 clones with an average insert size of approximately 215 kb, representing approximately a one-fold coverage of this chromosome. We chose to divide the library into 16 partitions each containing 36 clones and construct a 1-detector with $K = 1$ for the clones in each partition. In other words, the pooling scheme allows us to detect (1) which single clone among the 36 is positive for an STS or (2) whether there is more than one positive clone in the partition, even in the presence of an erroneous PCR reaction.

Assuming our YAC library represents uniform one-fold coverage of chromosome 16, the probability that more than one positive will occur in any of the 16 1-detectors is approximately 0.01. These 1-detectors (shown in the figure) are given by the t-design with parameters $v = 10$, $k = 5$, and $t = 3$. Note that the five pools containing one clone and the five pools containing another clone have at most three pools in common as $t = 3$.

Suppose only one clone in a 1-detector is positive for a given STS. Then even if one pool containing the positive clone yielded a false negative and only four pools containing that positive clone yielded positive results, one could use parsimony to tentatively iden-

tify the positive clone ($K = 1$). If the 1-detector contained two positive clones, at least seven pools would yield positive results (in the absence of experimental errors), a result readily distinguished from the five positive pools expected for a single positive clone. In fact, 4/7 of the time, only seven pools would be positive and all but three clones would be identified as negative. Thus, even when more than one clone in the 1-detector is positive for a given STS, the screening identifies a large number of negative clones, which can be eliminated from further consideration.

To identify which of the sixteen 1-detectors to screen, one could implement two levels of a four-way branching tree like that of Green and Olson (1990). Then, a maximum of 20 PCR reactions are required to identify each positive clone. Our pooling scheme has been successfully used to identify 30 YACs each containing a different STS. In almost all cases, PCR screening for each STS yielded five positive pools in a 1-detector, and the clone thereby identified as positive was always confirmed in subsequent analysis.

We plan to take advantage of the larger t-designs in future experiments. For example, the design with $v = 12$, $k = 6$, and $t = 4$ will accommodate 132 clones in its 12 pools. We found that the Biomek robot can create these pools given a bit-string representation. ∎

Sequencing cDNAs

Bob Moyzis: Since the Five-Year Plan was written, one of the new proposals that has surfaced is to sequence a large number of complementary DNAs, or cDNAs. Let's discuss the rationale behind this approach.

David Galas: Once it became clear that Maynard's idea about STSs was going to be a fruitful way to deal with physical mapping, the question arose: As long as we have to sequence short stretches of DNA to make STSs, why not choose those short stretches from cDNAs rather than from some random set of DNA fragments? cDNAs are interesting because they are copies of genes that actually get expressed as proteins in human cells.

We make cDNAs by isolating messenger RNAs, or mRNAs, from cells and using the enzyme reverse transcriptase to change those protein-synthesis templates back into the DNA message. But unlike the original DNA message, the cDNAs do not contain the noncoding regions, called introns, because RNA splicing has removed them [see "Gene Expression and cDNAs"]. Thus cDNA sequences are immediately useful for the identification of genes that are actually expressed as proteins, and they may even prove useful for studying protein structure and function if we get that far.

We think we can sequence a lot of cDNAs without slowing down the momentum of the mapping effort. This effort will probably catalyze a lot of activity in the community because it lends itself to independent participation by individuals in small labs. It's only when we try to collate, organize, and distribute the sequence data that we need a high level of coordination.

Bob Moyzis: Just as the genome mapping was divided by chromosome among various labs, the cDNA work can be distributed among different groups.

David Galas: Recently, people have found ways to make better libraries of cDNA clones, better in the sense that they more evenly represent the different mRNAs produced in the cell. These *normalized* cDNA libraries are trivial to produce in comparison with YAC

> *As long as we have to sequence short stretches of DNA to make STSs, why not choose those short stretches from cDNAs rather than from some random set of DNA fragments?*

libraries, and they're being generated in new cloning vectors designed to facilitate standard sequencing reactions. In six months to one year, we should have a bunch of good cDNA libraries being tested and sequenced.

We still don't know how easy it will be to map the cDNA sequences to specific chromosomes because not all cDNAs will be unique. On the other hand, preliminary data suggest that some STSs derived from human cDNAs will serve as STSs for other species, such as the mouse. Those cross-species STSs may help us enormously in comparing the mouse genome and the human genome.

Bob Moyzis: We should explain that different proteins and protein families share many similarities. Evolution

is conservative and did not re-invent the wheel every time a protein with a new function appeared. Rather, gene duplication and rearrangement was used to produce novel proteins. So, short stretches of a cDNA sequence may appear in many different human genes. Regions of this kind make poor STS markers because they tag multiple sites.

It is still uncertain what the overall efficiency of producing STSs from cDNAs will be. If the goal is to tag genes, genomic DNA sequencing may be just as efficient. For example, from our work on chromosomes 5 and 16, random STS generation appears to be uncovering a significant fraction of coding regions. This is not unexpected since with over 100,000 genes and a sequencing window of 400 nucleotides, approximately one third of the sequences should contain a piece of a coding region.

Therefore, as we make the 30,000 STSs for the physical map of the genome, we are likely to find pieces of approximately 10,000 genes. The advantage of sequencing cDNAs rather than random fragments of genomic DNA will depend on what other information—and how much—can be obtained by this alternative approach.

David Galas: The initial purpose of using cDNA sequences as STS markers is to find unique landmarks for mapping that also fall within expressed genes. As long as a cDNA is unique, it is useful for that purpose. Additionally, cDNAs may be useful for determining whether genes are distributed evenly across the whole genome or are clustered together in certain regions.

Bob Moyzis: Yes, we'll learn something about gene density from cDNAs as well as genomic sequencing. We may also have to revise our estimate of the number of genes in the genome. The present estimate of 50,000 to 100,000 genes is incredibly loose. It is based on theoretical arguments originally proposed by Haldane, which are now known to be based on false assumptions. The goal of the Human Genome Project is not only to map and sequence the genome, but ultimately to understand how it functions. At one extreme are people who believe that if we had the whole sequence of the human genome, we would be able to scan that sequence and find all of the protein coding regions, all the exons. But right now we don't know enough about the rules of the game to identify those regions unambiguously.

Neural-net programs like GRAIL, developed at Oak Ridge, are good, but not good enough. Some coding regions are very short, and these are hard to pick out directly from the sequence. Also, many genes have alternative sites for splicing out introns, so many messenger RNAs can be made from the same gene region. We can't yet predict from the DNA sequence which of those mRNAs are actually made. Consequently, at the opposite extreme are people who believe we must sequence every cDNA to unambiguously determine what protein is really being made from each particular gene. It seems clear that we'll need to sequence a lot of cDNAs in addition to sequencing the entire genome in order to learn the rules for finding genes.

Norton Zinder: I think the new emphasis on cDNAs may be very distracting to the goals of the Genome Project. cDNAs span about 10 percent of the genome, so if we sequence them with present technology, which is at least ten times more costly than what we are shooting for, then we will use up the whole genome budget on sequencing cDNAs.

David Galas: But the DOE is not proposing to sequence all the cDNAs but rather to sequence some cDNAs and use those sequences as a source of STS markers. We're putting a relatively small fraction of our resources, maybe a few percent, into finding out whether or not this approach will work. The cDNA effort will also mesh nicely with work on the mouse genome. The genetic-linkage map of the mouse is progressing very rapidly, in part because the mouse community is really behind the mapping effort. It is now apparent that genetic-linkage studies can be performed very efficiently in mice by crossing laboratory mice with wild mice from a different subspecies. Intraspecies crosses create offspring that are heterozygous for almost every genetic marker. In other words, each offspring carries two forms, or alleles, of almost every genetic marker. When those offspring are involved in controlled matings, a small number of successive generations of mice are sufficient to determine the genetic distances between many pairs of markers simultaneously.

The homology between the mouse genome and the human genome is very high. In fact, most of the cDNA sequences we find in humans will be present in mice with very little and sometimes no difference. People are often humbled at how closely we are related to mice. On the evolutionary scale, mice and humans have diverged a sufficiently short time ago that large stretches of mouse chromosomes can be matched up with corresponding stretches of human chromosomes. Therefore, the ordering of a bunch of cDNAs or a bunch of genetic markers will often be roughly the same on the mouse and on the human genomes. Consequently, studies of the mouse genome may provide some shortcuts for mapping certain regions of the human genome.

The NIH already has a program on mice, whereas the DOE genome program is largely focused on humans—and mostly on physical mapping. The coupling of the DOE genome program to the mouse project will most likely come through the cDNA work. We already have a huge mouse facility at the Oak Ridge Laboratory. It is the second largest such facility, the largest being at the Jackson Labs at Bar Harbor. We need to make those facilities available to the Genome Project, and we've recently funded a project at Oak Ridge.

Maynard Olson: The reason the cDNA sequencing proposals are worrisome is that they sound so good. We are all interested in discovering new human genes by any method that gives us solid information, and the sequencing of cDNAs appears to do that. But you have to ask yourself: Would I support a Human Genome Project whose principle goal was to make a catalog of cDNA sequences? For me, the answer is no. Such a catalog of cDNAs will be of exceedingly low quality. We have learned that the route from RNA to cDNA to protein is ragged around the edges. It involves RNA editing, errors in reverse transcription of RNA to cDNA, and so on.

Biology only gets more complicated as you get away from the genome. At the DNA level, the genome is analogous to a relatively simple kind of computer disk file. But RNA, as we've become increasingly aware, is an extremely complicated molecule. Because it is single-stranded, it can fold up in complex ways, which, in turn, affect its function.

By the time you reach the complicated structures of proteins, you've got the subtle complexity that makes biology possible. The Genome Project has to

cDNAs and Expressed Genes

Copy DNAs, or cDNAs, are being synthesized, cloned, and sequenced as a source of STSs, unique landmarks for the physical map of the human genome. A cDNA is a copy of the protein-coding regions (exons) of a gene. It is not made directly from DNA isolated from the genome but rather, as shown in the figure, from the messenger RNA, the template that is translated into a protein. These templates are valuable because, unlike genomic DNA, each mRNA is a continuous stretch of protein-coding nucleotides. Moreover, the existence of an mRNA is proof that the corresponding protein-coding gene is an active, or expressed, gene.

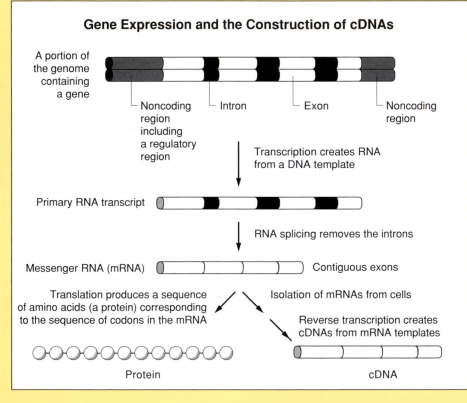

Gene Expression and the Construction of cDNAs

A portion of the genome containing a gene

Noncoding region including a regulatory region

Intron

Exon

Noncoding region

Transcription creates RNA from a DNA template

Primary RNA transcript

RNA splicing removes the introns

Messenger RNA (mRNA)

Contiguous exons

Translation produces a sequence of amino acids (a protein) corresponding to the sequence of codons in the mRNA

Isolation of mRNAs from cells

Reverse transcription creates cDNAs from mRNA templates

Protein

cDNA

cDNAs are synthesized in vitro. First, mRNAs are isolated from a population of tissue-specific cells. The isolated mRNAs represent only those genes that are being expressed in those particular cells. Each mRNA serves as a template in the synthesis of a complementary strand of DNA—the cDNA. The process of transcribing RNA into DNA, known as reverse transcription, is catalyzed by reverse transcriptase, an enzyme isolated from retroviruses, namely, RNA tumor viruses. The synthesized cDNAs are often shorter than the mRNA templates because of various processes that either degrade the mRNA or result in incomplete transcription. (Note that reverse transcriptase is not made by human cells. However, retroviruses, such as HIV, carry reverse transcriptase with them when they enter a host cell. The enzyme converts the viral RNA genome to DNA, which is then permanently incorporated into the genome of the host cell.)

After being synthesized in vitro, cDNAs are cloned. Cloned cDNAs have long been used for two purposes. First, cDNA libraries (random collections of cloned cDNAs) are used as sources of probes to identify the location of protein-coding regions in cloned fragments of genomic DNA. Second, particular mRNAs are isolated, converted to cDNAs, cloned, and then sequenced to determine the amino-acid sequence of the protein specified by the corresponding protein-coding gene.

The new emphasis is on sequencing short sections of cDNAs. If such a sequence is unique, it can be developed into a special kind of STS—one that is not only a unique, detectable landmark on the physical map of the genome but is also known to lie within an expressed gene. Furthermore, the cDNA sequence data provides some information about the protein encoded by the corresponding gene. ∎

be directed at the DNA because DNA is the Achilles heel of the cell. It's the one thing we have a chance of understanding. Higher-order phenomena of alternative RNA splicing, reverse-transcription artifacts, and complicated gene families will be invisible in the rough cDNA sequences, so a catalog of cDNA sequences would be a very frustrating thing to work with. The first thing you would want to do with such a catalogue would be to map all the cDNAs onto the physical map to determine their chromosomal location. If you had several seemingly different cDNAs all mapped to the same place, you would have to look again and decide whether or not they really were different.

Lee Hood: A number of U.S. groups are sequencing cDNAs. This method will allow one to readily identify interesting genes, but each cDNA library will allow one to identify only the small subset of genes that are abundantly expressed in a particular cell type.

Many important genes cannot be obtained by this approach because of the rarity of their mRNAs. Polymorphisms and multigene families may also be challenging to decipher. I believe there is merit in sequencing both genomic DNA and cDNAs. The issue of whether fragments of DNA sequence can be patented is obviously very controversial.

Bob Moyzis: The added value of most cDNAs comes once they are mapped. Obtaining the sequence of the cDNA is the most trivial part of the process. It's difficult to see the basis for patenting cDNA sequences.

Lee Hood: In contrast, the large-scale sequencing of interesting regions in the genome has a guaranteed payoff. At Caltech we're sequencing the immune receptor loci, which will very likely

lead to a much deeper understanding of autoimmune diseases and bring big biomedical and economic payoffs. If you focus sequencing efforts on DNA from the genome, you can direct those efforts to interesting regions. If you sequence cDNAs at random, it's the luck of the draw. Sequencing cDNAs is an inexpensive way of generating STSs to do physical maps. In the U.S., most scientists propose not to sequence the whole length of each cDNA but enough to generate unique genetic markers.

> *By the time you reach the complicated structures of proteins, you've got the subtle complexity that makes biology possible. The Genome Project has to be directed at the DNA because DNA is the Achilles heel of the cell. It's the one thing we have a chance of understanding.*

Norton Zinder: My own guess is that technological breakthroughs will make it easier to blindly sequence the entire genome than to pick out specific regions using cDNAs and then go back and sequence those regions.

Maynard Olson: We had a similar debate about whether to sequence 10 percent of the genome or the whole genome. These debates become meaningless when we think more ambitiously about

developing new technology. We're interested in seeing an order-of-magnitude reduction in sequencing costs. Now we are in a gray zone, and some people argue that the cost of sequencing is too high to justify sequencing the human genome but acceptably inexpensive to sequence all the cDNAs. If we are in this situation, we're unlikely to stay there.

Ultimately, we will want to sequence both the human genome and the cDNAs. In fact, I think that we're going to want to sequence both the human and the mouse genomes. Though we probably won't be able to find the exons by looking at the human DNA sequence alone, the way to find them is not to have some mishmash of cDNA sequences. We need to sequence the genomes of the human and the mouse, and maybe some other organisms, and then place them side by side and do comparisons. We should be putting more energy into the kind of technology development that would make that feasible.

If you want to study in detail the expression of a particular gene, you're going to have to do a lot of difficult experiments. We never claimed that lining up the mouse and human genome sequences would settle all the issues about which genes are expressed and which are not. But ask somebody who is trying to understand a particular gene whether he would like to compete in a situation where another lab had access to *both* the mouse and the human genomic sequence for the gene of interest while all he had was a bunch of cDNA clones. Then, you'd see more enthusiasm for mapping and a little less enthusiasm for cataloging cDNA sequences.

Bob Moyzis: If you want to understand how a gene works, when and where it gets expressed, and so on, you're never going to find that out from the cDNAs.

The Five-Year Goals

Bob Moyzis: I would guess that by the end of the Project's first five years, we will have some semblance of the high-resolution linkage maps, and, for some regions of some of the chromosomes, we will have reasonable physical maps. However, unless the effort on large-scale mapping increases, I don't think we will be able to complete the high-resolution physical maps on schedule—low-resolution contig maps, perhaps, but not the sets of closely spaced unique landmarks to go with the contig maps.

Maynard Olson: The prospect for meeting the Project's five-year goals doesn't look great at the moment, but that shouldn't be a matter of excessive concern. Right now we don't have enough mappers, in part because most molecular biologists are not trained in, nor are they necessarily good at, the analytical and technical skills required for the task. I think we will eventually recruit people who are not now working with DNA, and then momentum will build and the job will get done fairly quickly—although probably later than the famous five-year plan says. But remember, we asked for a $1-billion five-year plan—we're getting the half-price version. There will be a lag before new recruits enter the mapping effort, and we're in the lag phase now, but I predict that the maps will get done.

David Galas: At the moment physical mapping is perceived to be technology-limited. We are getting a lot of good mapping information, but the process is slow and tedious. However, it's foolish to think that the technology won't improve, and it may improve dramatically because a lot of innovation is still going on.

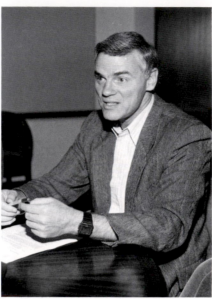

Lee Hood

So far the NIH leaders have been far too timid about making decisions that allow the money to be spent . . . appropriately. That has to change. If it doesn't . . . we're not going to come close to meeting the five-year goals.

Bob Moyzis: Our recent success at Los Alamos in producing chimera-free, chromosome-specific YAC libraries is an innovation that will have a significant impact on our own mapping effort as well as on the efforts of other genome centers. And we can expect to see other improvements in mapping technology. However, even now the technology is good enough, I feel, to complete the maps in five years.

The last ten years have seen major advances in technology development, such as YAC cloning. The major problem in achieving our goals is, as Maynard has mentioned, the lack of funding directed specifically at physical mapping and the lack of individuals who are truly interested in generating the maps.

Most of the people who would like to be funded by the Genome Project would rather try to improve mapping technology than make the maps. But if we can get the maps in five years with current technology, why spend the Project's money on technology improvements that will take five years to develop? It may be that in a hundred years we will be able to map a genome in a day, but I don't want to wait that long if the goal can be achieved in five years with current technology. I'd rather see technology-development money spent on the real bottlenecks, namely, sequencing and information management, analysis, and distribution.

Lee Hood: The Europeans seem more willing to give appropriate support to big projects. I'm not advocating creating a network of thirty-five laboratories to sequence one particular yeast chromosome, but that's what they did in Europe, and all 300,000 base pairs of the chromosome got sequenced. We haven't done a comparable project in the United States.

It's also obvious from the large investments in automation being made at CEPH [Centre d'Etude du Polymorphisme Humain] that the French government is willing to put a lot of money into carrying out very-large-scale linkage mapping. The CEPH scientists have built robots to make Southern blots of DNA from their repository of family cell lines. They will give those blots as well as probes for various DNA markers to about thirty labs and ask them to identify which forms of the markers are present in the blots.

The project is a big one, and it's attractive to the participating laboratories because they are going to get paid more than it's going to cost them to do the work. CEPH will then stand at least a chance of putting together a very good linkage map in a reasonably short time. You don't see that kind of commitment at any of the U.S. centers that are carrying out linkage mapping.

What the NIH is tending to do with its genome centers is to nickel-and-dime them to death. The centers put in reasonably ambitious proposals, and the proposals come back with cuts in equipment, in computers, in technicians, and so on. Most important, virtually all of the funding for technology development was cut. Much of the NIH budget is being spread over small projects that won't amount to much.

To turn this around, we need determined leaders in both the DOE and the NIH. They must make a commitment to spend money in ways that will get the objectives done. So far the NIH leaders have been far too timid about making decisions that allow the money to be spent programmatically and appropriately. That has to change. If it doesn't, I would agree with Bob: We're not going to come close to meeting the five-year goals.

Mapping a chromosome is an enormous task, and we in the United States are going to have to come to grips with that fact. If we're going to be stingy about supporting the people who have already taken on such big projects, we're not going to encourage other people to take them on.

The Five-Year Goals of the U.S. Human Genome Project

Genetic Map Complete a fully connected human genetic map with markers spaced an average of 2 to 5 centimorgans apart. Identify each marker by an STS.

Physical Map Assemble STS maps of all human chromosomes with the goal of having markers spaced at approximately 100,000 base pair intervals. Generate overlapping sets of cloned DNA or closely spaced, unambiguously ordered markers with continuity over lengths of 2 million base pairs for large parts of the human genome.

DNA Sequencing Improve current methods and/or develop new methods for DNA sequencing that will allow large-scale sequencing of DNA at a cost of 50 cents per base pair. Determine the sequence of an aggregate of 10 million base pairs of human DNA in large continuous stretches in the course of technology development and validation.

Model Organisms Prepare a genetic map of the mouse genome based on DNA markers. Start physical mapping on one or two chromosomes. Sequence an aggregate of about 20 million base pairs of DNA from a variety of model organisms, focusing on stretches that are 1 million base pairs long, in the course of the development and validation of new and/or improved DNA-sequencing technology.

Informatics: Data Collection and Analysis Develop effective software and database designs to support large-scale mapping and sequencing projects. Create database tools that provide easy access to up-to-date physical mapping, genetic mapping, chromosome mapping, and sequencing information and allow ready comparison of the data in these several data sets. Develop algorithms and analytical tools to interpret genomic information.

Ethical, Legal, and Social Considerations Develop programs addressed at understanding the ethical, legal, and social implications of the Human Genome Project. Identify and define the major issues and develop initial policy options to address them.

Research Training Support research training of pre- and post-doctoral fellows starting in FY 1990. Increase the numbers of trainees supported until a steady state of about 600 per year is reached by the fifth year. Examine the need for other types of research training in the next year.

Technology Development Support innovative and high-risk technological developments as well as improvements in current technology to meet the needs of the Genome Project as a whole.

Technology Transfer Enhance the already close working relationship with industry. Encourage and facilitate the transfer of technologies and of medically important information to the medical community.

(From *Understanding Our Genetic Inheritance. The U.S. Human Genome Project: The First Five Years, FY 1991–1995*. NIH Publication No. 90–1590, April 1990.)

III. Technological Challenges in the Genome Project

Improving Sequencing and Finding Genes

Bob Moyzis: Let's turn to the problem of improving sequencing technology. In order to carry out the vision Maynard gave—sequencing not only the human but also the mouse genome and all the human cDNAs and so forth—we need at least a hundredfold improvement in sequencing efficiency.

David Cox: There's another way to think about this problem. Suppose we focus not on sequencing the whole human genome, but on a more manageable goal—namely, finding out how to determine the sequence of 2 million base pairs of DNA accurately and rapidly. That achievement would have an absolutely revolutionary impact on human biology because it would provide an ideal tool for finding disease genes.

The search for the single dominant gene that causes Huntington's Disease illustrates my point. In 1983, a DNA marker that was very tightly linked to Huntington's Disease was identified by Jim Gusella and his colleagues. It's now 1992 and the Huntington's Disease gene has yet to be identified. The research has been narrowed down to a region of DNA 2.5 million base pairs long. Yeast artificial chromosomes and

other mapping techniques have allowed most of that region to be cloned, so we actually have the DNA in hand. A number of groups across the world are dedicated to the search, but we still don't have the Huntington's Disease gene. Why not? Well, in that 2.5 million base pairs of DNA, there are probably fifty different genes. And how do we find out which one is the Huntington's gene? There's just no easy solution.

> *The problem of finding a single base change in 2 million base pairs of DNA is going to be the standard problem in finding disease genes.*

Right now the approach is first to identify all of the genes in that region, say by hybridization to cDNAs, and then look for abnormalities in those genes. If the disease gene contains a DNA rearrangement, it's easy to identify. Or perhaps the messenger RNAs from the disease gene are different in size or amount from those of the normal gene. If we compare the messenger RNA of each of the fifty genes from a Huntington's patient and from a normal individual, we might be able to identify the disease gene.

But chances are that the Huntington's gene won't contain a DNA rearrange-

ment and won't change the size or the amount of the messenger RNA. So even if all fifty genes are identified, we will probably have to sequence all fifty genes from a Huntington's patient first, and then from unaffected individuals to identify changes present only in Huntington's patients but never in normal individuals. That will be the proof that you have found the Huntington's mutation. In fact, that exact strategy was used to prove that the cystic-fibrosis gene was indeed the disease-causing gene.

Suppose instead that you could sequence the whole region known to contain the Huntington's gene and find out what base changes are present only in Huntington's patients and never in normal patients. Then you could identify the disease gene immediately, and you wouldn't have to mess around finding all the genes in the region.

The problem of finding a single base change in 2 million base pairs of DNA is going to be the standard problem in finding disease genes. So if we had a way of sequencing 2 million base pairs accurately and rapidly, it would completely revolutionize how we went about finding human disease genes, and it would cut down the amount of work by at least a factor of ten. After sequencing the region, we could use PCR-based assays to examine very quickly the DNA from 100 normal individuals and thereby distinguish harmless polymorphisms from the disease-causing mutation. But we can't carry out this approach because present sequencing technology is simply too remedial.

Bob Moyzis: Whether we're searching for disease genes or wanting to sequence the whole genome, sequencing technology is currently not up to the job. However, incremental changes in current technology during the next few years are likely to increase the rate of sequencing to between a hundred thousand and a million nucleotides per day. Thin-gel technology, pioneered by Lloyd Smith and others, has been demonstrated to yield a tenfold improvement in through-put simply by increasing the voltage used to separate the DNA molecules. Further, parallel processing of samples using robotics or other more exotic techniques, such as flow cytometry, is being pursued. Advances in primer walking, such as those being developed at Brookhaven National Laboratory by Bill Studier, also look promising for the near term. We would need a major breakthrough to process a billion base pairs per day, but a million base pairs per day will be within reach at many laboratories in the next few years. As David Cox has said, at that rate most of the interesting goals of the Human Genome Project can be achieved.

David Galas: I agree that refinements in current technology will yield the tenfold to one hundredfold improvement that Bob is talking about. At that rate the bottleneck will not be sequencing but rather front-end preparation and back-end analysis. The back end, which includes entering short stretches of sequence, 300 to 800 bases long, that come off the sequencing machine into the database, assembling those sequences into long, contiguous se-quences, checking for errors, and so on, needs great improvement [see "DNA Sequencing"].

It's time for the DOE to do production-line or large-scale sequencing so we can find the hang-ups in those areas and address them. Sequencing technology itself should be seen as one module among many in this process, a module that can be changed as better technology comes along.

Lee Hood: I'm glad to hear you say that because a major output of the Genome Project is going to be DNA sequence data. Until now the DOE has done a super job of supporting the development of radically new sequencing technolo-gies, which may—or may not—lead to a hundredfold or a thousandfold increases in output, but we also need to do the systems integration required for large-scale sequencing projects with present technologies. That's the only way to learn the requirements for setting up production-line, large-scale, fully-automated technologies of the kind that will be needed to sequence the entire human genome.

Over the next ten years, we're hoping to get at least a hundredfold increase in sequencing throughput because that's what it will take to carry out the genome initiative. If we succeed, then I don't think academics will do the sequencing; it will be industry.

David Galas: The DOE is sponsoring some sequencing of model organisms now, and we're thinking seriously about setting up pilot sequencing projects, the principle goal of which would be to un-derstand the bottlenecks in production-line sequencing and to identify the places where new technology would really help.

So far we have only begun to scratch the surface of problems associated with sequence assembly and error checking.

We haven't had enough data to work on. Later, when sequencing costs and efficiencies, including front and back ends, improve by a factor of at least ten, it probably would be appropriate to start sequencing large, selected regions of the human genome.

Lee Hood: We should also encourage industry to get involved in such projects. Over the next ten years, we're hoping to get at least a hundredfold increase in sequencing throughput because that's what it will take to carry out the genome initiative. If we succeed, then I don't think academics will do the sequencing; it will be industry. Sequencing com-panies will get subcontracts from the government for large-scale sequencing. Industry needs to get involved now, so that when the technology is ready for high-throughput sequencing, they'll have skilled people to carry it out.

If we set up this large-scale sequencing effort now, I think we could produce a million base pairs of accurate, or finished, sequence per person, per year. We're still learning how to do this and various problems slow us down. The production of the DNA fragments for sequencing is not trivial. Each fragment must be sequenced five or six times to reduce sequencing errors. The assembly of long sequences from overlapping, short sequences is not fully automated, and the clones are not always faithful copies of the genome. To do large-scale sequencing we have to figure out how to make all these steps move faster in a reliable and integrated system.

Bob Moyzis: Determining the cor-rect sequence would seem to be very important, but we know that a single sequencing run can produce an error rate as high as 1 in 100. That means that the disease-gene hunts described by David Cox would be very inefficient. The sequencing of a 2-million-base region would produce 20,000 errors. That's an awful lot of data to check. Lee, how do you currently deal with errors?

Lee Hood: We deal with the errors in two ways. First we're doing the shotgun sequencing method, that is, we're picking many clones at random and sequencing them. Those clones overlap each other, so on average, we're sequencing each stretch of DNA between six and seven times. That gives us an error rate of perhaps 1 in 5000. Second, for each cloned fragment, we sequence about 15 percent of the cloning vector. Since the vector sequence is known, we determine the error rate for each run through the machine. Some runs have more errors because the chemical reactions used to prepare the DNA for the machines may have worked poorly and so forth. To my mind, the error rate in sequencing is not an insurmountable difficulty. It's true that an error rate of 1 in 100,000 is going to cost a lot of money, but if we can live with an error rate of 1 in 1000 or 1 in 5000, we'll be in good shape.

Many of the errors in sequencing are due to problems at the front end of the process. Cloning artifacts, such as deletions, for example, are not uncommon. Those artifacts are likely to be much more frequent in human DNA and mouse DNA because those genomes contain an abundance of repetitive sequences. Such sequences are probably a substrate for nonhomologous recombination, which, if it occurs during the cloning process, can create new sequences not present in the genomic DNA.

So any DNA that has lots of repetitive sequences is intrinsically less stable than DNA lacking repetitive sequences. We could use better cloning systems for minimizing those artifacts, but short of

that, we'll probably develop much better ways of checking clones to make sure they match their germ-line counterparts before we start analyzing them. Perhaps the hybridization-based technologies will be important both in mapping clones and in checking sequenced DNA for errors.

Ten years ago, if a good graduate student produced 12,000 base pairs of finished sequence in a year, that was considered very good. Today a machine can do 12,000 base pairs of rough sequence each day.

Bob Moyzis: Lee, what are you doing on the front and back ends of sequencing?

Lee Hood: At Caltech we haven't done much with the front-end problems because Applied Biosystems is developing a robot for doing the PCR and the standard sequencing reactions in a format that's consistent with placing the reaction products directly into a fluorescence sequencing machine. On the back end, we're working together with LOBE on two major projects. First, we're developing a laboratory management system to keep track of all the details that are a part of sequencing—where the fragments came from, how they've been treated, what time they were run on the machines, and so forth. Second, we're working on computer programs for assembling a long sequence from randomly generated short sequences. They still need a lot of work.

With the fluorescence sequencing machine, a computer program reads the order of the nucleotide bases directly from the sequencing gel and puts question marks in positions of ambiguity. Someone must look at the data and make decisions regarding those question marks. In the future, we should have better programs for *calling* the sequences. To do large-scale sequencing, we will have to automate this whole process in a way that requires a minimum of manual intervention.

Bob Moyzis: Earlier I voiced my optimism that these problems will be solved. I know you share that optimism.

Lee Hood: We need to remind ourselves of the progress we've made over the last ten years. Ten years ago, if a good graduate student produced 12,000 base pairs of finished sequence in a year, that was considered very good. Today, a machine can do 12,000 base pairs of rough sequence each day. Thus we've had an increase of several orders of magnitude in throughput. I think the front- and back-end problems are more straightforward and are going to be solved. The problem of getting good robots to prepare the reaction mixtures is technically less demanding than figuring out how to improve DNA sequencing throughput by two orders of magnitude.

David Galas: Given the uncertainty in meeting those demands, we have to plan on some large-scale sequencing using present-day, conventional technologies. But the new technologies are coming along, and there are two kinds. Those that push the present methods include multiplex sequencing, automated multiplex sequencing, capillary-gel electrophoresis, and automatic detection systems. And we can expect those developments to yield a tenfold improvement—maybe even more.

Then, there are three or four radically new technologies that could change things dramatically. One is the Los Alamos single-molecule-detection method [see "Rapid DNA Sequencing Based on Single-Molecule Detection"]. That's gotten to the point where they can actually detect single molecules.

A lot of progress is also being made on hybridization sequencing. Even if it doesn't work for precise sequencing, it'll work for gathering partial sequences of a lot of DNA extremely rapidly. The idea is to place huge numbers of short sequences, eight to ten bases long, on a little chip and determine which of those hybridize to the long fragment being sequenced. In its ultimate form, these hybridizations yield the full sequence, but even partial sequence information will be helpful for mapping and for finding homologous regions. Right now there's too much noise in the system, so the hybridization signals aren't clean. But those problems are being worked on, and I would say that the hybridization method is neck-and-neck with the Los Alamos single-molecule-detection scheme.

The other new sequencing method uses mass spectrometry. You start with the set of fragments produced by normal sequencing reactions. Remember, those are a set of nested fragments that increase in length stepwise, that is, one base at a time. You arrange to place a single charge on each of these, and then you use a laser to blast the stuff off a little plate into a vacuum. Because all the fragments are charged equally, you can use a device to separate them by mass and get the whole ladder of fragments laid out in a single measurement. It takes only a few milliseconds. If that method works with the required accuracy, you can read the sequence instantly. It requires measuring the mass of these

fragments to one part in a few thousand so that you can determine which base is at each place in the sequence. That's a radically new idea.

Lee Hood: The center at Caltech is focused on improving sequencing technologies, and there, we're taking two approaches. One is to implement a better design of the contemporary automated fluorescence sequencing machine by using better lasers, thin gels, pulse-field gel electrophoresis, and the like.

The second approach is to explore whether mass spectrometry can really be used for sequencing. As David Galas explained, the idea is to measure the mass of each of the fragments generated from the standard sequencing reactions. You can either measure the masses of the fragments from the four different dideoxy reaction mixtures, or if the resolution is higher, you can measure the masses of all the fragments from a combined mixture. For the latter, you have to have a resolution that can distinguish single-nucleotide additions.

David Galas: With three or four of these completely new ideas under development, my guess is that sooner or later one of them is going to work well enough for practical application and will revolutionize sequencing. My bet is that we're going to have some of these working within five to ten years, which is about when we were hoping to start doing some serious large-scale sequencing.

If one of these methods works, we'll be able to do what David Cox was talking about. We could sequence the chromosomes of an affected individual as well as the chromosomes of unaffected individuals, and we would be able to identify immediately what mutations were responsible for a given condition.

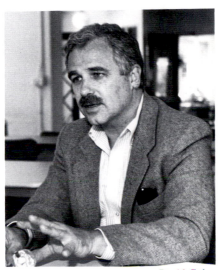

David Galas

With three or four of these completely new ideas under development, my guess is that sooner or later one of them is going to work well enough for practical application and will revolutionize sequencing. My bet is that we are going to have some of these working within five to ten years, which is about when we were hoping to start doing some serious large-scale sequencing.

Technology Development— an interdisciplinary challenge

Bob Moyzis: It's clear from the problems we're facing in mapping and sequencing that this project requires technological development in every area.

David Botstein: We're weak enough in technology that we really ought to invite people from other disciplines: chemistry, physics, robotics, and the like, to think about it. We hope that this issue of *Los Alamos Science* will reach people who can come out of the woodwork to help us. And I think it's really important to distinguish between what really helps and what doesn't help. We don't need a lot of physicists to turn themselves into biologists. But we do need physicists who have enough interest in the biology and enough patience to understand what the technical problems are.

I'll give you two examples from my own life. Around 1975 when I was at MIT, we were taking electron-microscope pictures of DNA. DNA looks like little worms with kinks in them. There's a lot of information in those little worms and we were using a map measurer to figure out how long the contour lengths were. We went to the computer group, which had a PDP-9, and we said, "Can you do this for us automatically?" And they said, "Get lost, kid, it's trivial." So finally, I got a Master's student and bribed him to look at this problem. He took it to his boss and they came back a month later and said, "Not only is it not trivial, but it's impossible. We can't do it." Of course what he really meant was that he didn't think he was going to get

anything out of solving the problem—it wouldn't get him tenure.

Today there is still no automatic equipment to make that measurement. It still can't be done. But we have to find a way to collaborate because I think that both sciences would benefit greatly.

Bob Moyzis: The cultural problem is very real. On the one hand biologists think of biological solutions to the problems. And one of the beauties of biology is that you can manipulate

> *Biologists think of biological solutions to the problems. And one of the beauties of biology is that you can manipulate a bug to do your work for you, so there's a resistance to tapping into the physical-science community.*

a bug to do your work for you, so there's a resistance to tapping into the physical-science community. It's only recently that low-key robotics has even entered biology. Maybe that's because molecular biologists think it's good for the soul to do these repetitive tasks.

On the other hand, if the physical scientists think they're being used to solve a trivial problem, they are never going to get interested. They have to feel that their contributions to the goals of this project are exciting and worth doing.

David Botstein: Steve Chu is a laser physicist who has been working with DNA at Stanford. He has invented a contraption that can stretch out an individual piece of DNA and measure its length by how far it stretches before it breaks. That's the kind of thing that would be fun to do. But Steve is unusual in that his brother is the biologist who invented the CHEF gel. So it's a special case because they talk to each other.

Every manipulation that we do in the Genome Project is suboptimal. For example, when people take pictures of in-situ hybridizations, they use cooled ccd-array cameras that are probably three generations old. Physicists wouldn't dream of using one of those. They're probably piling up as junk in the basement of the CERN accelerator.

Bob Moyzis: Certainly the general problem of image analysis or pattern recognition needs better solutions. We're using very antiquated technology, for example, in analyzing our gels. In many areas of biology, we're swamped and would love to find a way to automatically extract data, enhance images, and look for patterns, be they linear or three-dimensional.

David Botstein: Part of our five-year plan is technology development, but right now we don't know who are the right people to talk to. We think that we have employment for at least the next ten or fifteen years for these interdisciplinary guys. But they don't exist. They literally don't exist.

Nancy Wexler: We are trying to create a new kind of interdisciplinary science with a leg in not just physics and biology, but in other disciplines as well. We need to appeal to young people who are just beginning their training and who are willing to be a little experimental. We need meetings to define the issues and the problems and to bring people from different disciplines together. Then we need a specialized training program.

Maynard Olson: The Genome Project clearly needs a strong engineering component, and maybe that's another reason Wally Gilbert says the Project isn't science. Basic scientists often look down on engineering, but most don't know much about it. Some of the most creative things done in the 20th century have been engineering advances. When the dust settles on this century, we'll look back on two great technological revolutions: one in computers, the other in DNA technology.

Computers are largely an engineering advance. Early on new theoretical ideas about managing digital information and advances in solid-state physics were critical, but the real surge in computing power came when creative engineers took over and built better and better computers. We're not talking about building a slightly better mousetrap; we're talking about creating compositions of matter whose behavior differs qualitatively from anything people a few years before would have thought possible. Computers are an open-ended technology where a factor of ten improvement in memory or processing speed sets the stage for another factor of ten. At any given stage in the technology, it's always the imagination of the users that is limiting, but they catch up remarkably quickly.

There is a real analogy here between computers and DNA. I suspect that creative engineering on this basically monotonous chemical will open up applications in biology as important as those opened up by modern computers. The underlying idea behind computers was that if one got extremely good at processing digital information, one

could do an immense variety of things with it. Similarly, if we could analyze DNA—whether that means mapping, sequencing, or whatever—ten times better than we do now, it would yield tremendous opportunities for biological research and biomedical applications. When that happens, people won't be able to imagine working in the previous environment. What's more, the next factor of ten will have a similar impact.

Right now we're not working from this generic approach to DNA experimentation, but it will happen. I have my own ideas about how we might proceed, and I'm sure other ideas are out there. Such activities will not be a trivial mechanization of the present manual processes. It will mean taking a zero-based view of what we're trying to accomplish with DNA—and of the various physical tools that could be brought to bear on accomplishing those goals. That's the attitude we'll gradually grow into in DNA research. And I believe creative engineers will play a big role.

Lee Hood: We knew from the beginning that this project is about technology development, and to do that you need scientists who have interdisciplinary skills, who can talk to people, encourage new insights, and set up collaborations across different disciplines. These scientists are not easy to find. For the future, we need to establish training programs that cut across the different disciplines.

As far as getting things done now, we have to identify scientists who want to make a major commitment to the goals of the Project, either to produce highly informative genetic maps, or to make a physical map of a particular chromosome, or to do large-scale sequencing. Few scientists have

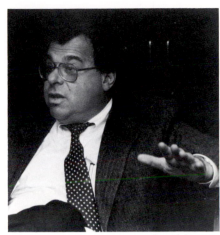

David Botstein

Part of our five-year plan is technology development, but right now we don't know who are the right people to talk to. We think that we have employment for at least the next ten or fifteen years for these interdisciplinary guys. But they don't exist. They literally don't exist.

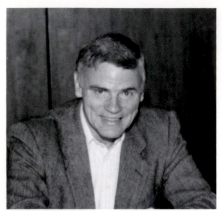

Lee Hood

The national labs are set up to do interdisciplinary projects, but until recently, they haven't been that strong in biology, and this project must be directed by scientists who really understand biology.

made this commitment. But if people who are now making the appropriate commitments were funded in an appropriate fashion, more people would be encouraged to take on these larger tasks.

At Caltech, we have a very strong interdisciplinary program by virtue of our NSF-funded Science and Technology Center. We have groups working on nucleic acid chemistry, computational problems, genetic mapping and DNA diagnostics, and large-scale sequencing. They are all housed together and are an incredibly interactive group. And it's the close interaction that really makes things happen.

Bob Moyzis: Lee, you were the prime mover behind development of automated sequencing machines. Tell us a bit about that development.

Lee Hood: I've been involved in technology development throughout my career. I got my Ph.D. training in protein chemistry and then switched over into molecular biology. Soon after Gilbert and Sanger came out with their groundbreaking sequencing techniques, we started trying to develop an automated sequencing machine.

For about three years, we went about it in the wrong way. We essentially tried to develop a very clever way of reading the standard four-lane radioactive gels. But each lane of a gel has its own artifacts, which may put the bands in one lane ahead of the bands in another, or create zig-zags in the mass scale from one lane to the next. Those artifacts are due to temperature anisotropies, and so forth.

My view now is that four-lane sequence analysis has intrinsic difficulties in accuracy, whereas putting all four reaction mixtures in one lane allows the fragments from each mixture to be

used as an internal standard against one another, so you get much more accurate sequence readings.

That is the approach we took in developing the automated fluorescent sequencing machine. Tim Hunkapillar first suggested the use of fluorescent tags on the DNA fragments produced by the enzymatic sequencing reactions. The tagged fragments are run down a single-lane gel past a laser, the laser causes the tags to fluoresce, and the color of the signal tells you which base was on the end of that fragment.

Lloyd Smith, a very good chemist from Stanford who joined our group in the early 1980s, developed those technologies. He'd had experience with lasers and was the right person at the right time. We also had a good organic chemist, Rob Kaiser, who could synthesize four different fluorescent compounds. So, putting together an interdisciplinary team of physical chemists, organic chemists, biologists, and then engineers, who could actually build the machine, was the key to making it work.

A lot of good universities are ideal places for interdisciplinary work because they have good departments in physics, computer science, engineering, and chemistry. Caltech is unusual because it is quite small, so it's easy for us to get to know people in different disciplines. That's much harder to do at the bigger universities.

On the other hand, the national labs are set up to do interdisciplinary projects, but until recently, they haven't been that strong in biology, and this project must be directed by scientists who really understand biology. For example, Bob Moyzis has contributed enormously to the genome center at Los Alamos.

Bob Moyzis: Thanks for the compliment. I have been somewhat frustrated by people from the physical sciences who seem interested in the mapping problem, in the physical reality of DNA, but who don't understand what the technical problems really are. A few years ago, mathematical types had a real obsession with modeling the best way to map the genome, and yet little of that theoretical work has had an impact on the experimental work.

Maynard Olson: That's because the modeling phase didn't pay adequate attention to experimental practicality. The mapping problem is dominated by the fact that the data aren't perfect, and a pristine model that assumes perfect data yields essentially no insight into the path that should be followed. So a purely theoretical approach to mapping problems won't help.

People in experimental physical chemistry, for example, have a better feel for the interplay between experiment and structure. The people who did the original molecular-beam experiments were very suspicious of pure theoreticians who wanted to take everything back to the wave equation. But they understood that there was quantization and that if they designed their detectors right, they could measure molecules in different quantum states, and they went on with the job. It also helped greatly that there were many investigators who were skilled in both theory and experiment. We do not have many people in biology with comparable breadth.

Norton Zinder: I've always had difficulty communicating with the theoretical physicists. Leo Szilard used to come to my lab suggesting experiments on DNA control and DNA synthesis that were meaningless because they were impossible to do. I spent four hours

talking to the *great god of physics*, Neils Bohr, who supposedly had great ideas about biology, but I never understood what he was talking about. He could not relate to the experimental system I was trying desperately to describe to him. So the theoretical physicists probably won't be of much help. But people working on materials science do appreciate the complexities of biology and know how to think about experimental systems.

Maynard Olson: I am also concerned about the present generation of molecular-biology graduate students. Too many of them don't know much about either molecules or biology. What they know is how to manipulate DNA, to do Northern blots and Southern blots, and site-directed mutagenesis and so forth. However, this problem may be a transitory response to two decades during which these protocols largely defined molecular biology.

The brighter young molecular biologists are beginning to study developmental biology and pathology, for example, and to work with transgenic mice. They're looking at livers again. They're starting to learn some biology, and some are starting to learn a lot about molecules. Biophysics is enjoying a renaissance with nice work on protein folding and recognition of macromolecules by other macromolecules.

Another new front will be people working on genome mapping. Those mappers—or whatever they're to be called—are going to be people with different backgrounds, and they'll be more specialized. Molecular biology has just been through a gold-rush phase, a phase when the techniques were crude and the participants were jacks-of-all-trades. They did the genetics, they did the sequencing, they did protein chemistry, and they made a start at getting out the

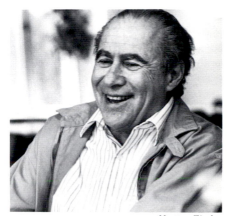

Norton Zinder

I've always had difficulty communicating with the theoretical physicists. Leo Szilard used to come to my lab suggesting experiments on DNA control and DNA synthesis that were meaningless because they were impossible to do.

information in DNA. But, just as serious mining operations require assayists, surveyors, lawyers, mining engineers, and the like, if we are going to get out all the information contained in the genome, we need specialists in all the techniques related to DNA analysis.

David Cox: This field is in its formative stages, and it's the obligation of the scientific community to identify areas where technology development can really help. Then it's up to the Genome Project to put money into those areas. The scientists who sit back and criticize the Project but don't know what they want or don't come forth with suggestions are missing a great opportunity.

We need requests that are posed carefully. If you want more rapid ways of sequencing the human genome, then the question remains: What's rapid enough? But if you say, "I want to sequence 2 million base pairs of DNA in the next eight months, can you do it or can't you?" then it's a concrete job and the question has a concrete answer.

The Genome Project is designed to solve concrete problems. We need new technology, but we also need to put it into action. This country is grappling on many fronts with the issue of getting technology out to the people who can use it. For example, the United States has invented a lot of the basic devices that are used in the electronics industry, but those devices are not being marketed or manufactured in the U.S. They're being manufactured in other countries. The goals of the Genome Project are not just to invent things but also to manufacture and come through with the goods. Inventing technology doesn't do the deed. It's delivering that technology that counts, and the Genome Project will be successful only if it does both.

David Galas: David Cox is right. We need to deliver good products to the biomedical community. But we should not forget that this is a fundamental science project as much as it is a medical

> *The Genome Project is forcing a bunch of researchers to cooperate and exchange information . . . that new way of working is going to change the sociology of how we do science. Rather than . . . working quietly in isolation and then giving a talk at a meeting maybe once or twice a year, many of us are learning a different way of doing projects, and I think it's all very healthy.*

one. At any time in this project, we're going to have some defined goals that we're working towards, but I don't think we should consider the present five-year goals as sacrosanct, or fixed. After all, they were made up by guys thinking about the way things were two or more years ago. We'll probably change the five-year goals, and those changes will depend on the changing technology.

Bob Moyzis: Watch it! Many of us drafted those five-year goals.

David Galas: Okay, let me give a really radical scenario. Let's suppose it turns out to be very easy to do the genetic and physical mapping for the mouse genome and extremely difficult to do it for the human genome. Then we ought to map everything on the mouse first and go back to humans later. The strategy we adopt will depend on how the technology works out.

This is an interesting time for biology. I think that most people don't realize how much the Human Genome Project is going to change the way we do biology. We're learning to take on huge tasks, and quite frankly, most of them are still above us. We are taking on tremendously broad goals, and we are realizing just how information-intensive this field is. We need new developments in automation, and we also need to interface with computers to the same extent that people in physics and chemistry do.

Five or ten years from now, I expect that the standard molecular-biology laboratory will be completely different from what it is today. There won't be any glassware. People will just have machines and computers. We will have automated the manipulations of DNA and animal cells, and we'll be able to go after fundamental biological problems with enormously powerful tools.

The Genome Project is forcing a bunch of researchers to cooperate and exchange information over computer networks, and that new way of working is going to change the sociology of how we do science. Rather than everyone going back to his or her lab, working quietly in isolation, and then giving a talk at a meeting maybe once or twice a year, many of us are learning a different way of doing projects, and I think it's all very healthy.

DNA Sequencing

An understanding of the structure, function, and evolutionary history of the human genome will require knowing its primary structure—the linear order of the 3 billion nucleotide base pairs composing the DNA molecules of the genome. Determining that sequence of base pairs is the long-term goal of the 15-year Human Genome Project. Both the merits and the technical feasibility of sequencing the entire human genome are discussed in Parts I and III of "Mapping the Genome." The bottom line is that sequencing technology is not yet up to the job.

In 1990, when the plans for the Genome Project were being made, the estimated cost of sequencing was $2 to $5 per base. That is, a single person could produce between 20,000 and 50,000 bases of "finished" sequence per year. The term "finished" sequence implies the error rate is very low (the conservatives say an error rate of 1 base in 10^5 is acceptable, and the less conservative say 1 in 10^3 or 10^4). A low rate is achieved, in part, by sequencing a given region many times over. The planners agreed that the costs of sequencing must be substantially reduced and that the rate of producing finished sequence must increase by a factor of 100 to 1000 for sequencing the entire human genome to become an affordable and practical goal.

On the other hand, sequencing technology has been improving steadily for the past two decades. In the early 1970s one person would struggle to complete 100 bases of sequence in one year. Then two very similar techniques were developed—one by Allan Maxam and Walter Gilbert in the United States and the other by Fredrick Sanger and his coworkers in England—that made it possible for one person to sequence thousands of base pairs in a year. Those techniques, for which the inventors were jointly awarded the Nobel Prize, still form the basis of all current sequencing technologies. Both methods are described in greater detail below.

Between 1975 and the present, the number of base pairs of published sequence data grew from roughly 25,000 to almost 100 million. During that time longer and longer contiguous stretches of DNA have been sequenced. In 1991 the longest sequence to be completed was that of the cytomegalovirus genome, which is 229,354 base pairs. By 1992 a cooperative effort in Europe had sequenced an entire chromosome of yeast, chromosome III, which is 315,357 base pairs. And now efforts are underway to sequence million-base stretches of DNA. Accomplishing such large-scale sequencing projects is among the goals for the first five years of the Genome Project.

In order to achieve this goal, each step in the multi-stage DNA sequencing process must be streamlined and smoothly integrated. Figure 1 outlines all the steps involved in the sequencing of long, contiguous stretches of genomic DNA, DNA isolated from the genome. The initial steps include cloning large fragments of genomic DNA in YACs or cosmids and using those clones to construct a contig map for the regions to be sequenced. The contig map arranges the cloned fragments in the order and relative positions in which they appear along the genome. The cloning and mapping steps are described elsewhere in this issue (see "DNA Libraries" and "Physical Mapping").

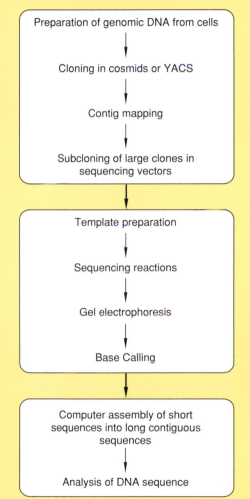

Figure 1. Steps in Large-Scale Sequencing

To determine the DNA sequence of the mapped region, the large DNA insert in each of the large clones must be broken into smaller pieces of a size suitable for sequencing, and those small pieces must be cloned. This subcloning is often done in the cloning vector M13, a bacteriophage whose genome is a single-stranded DNA molecule. M13 accepts DNA inserts from 500 to 2000 base pairs in length, propagates in the host cell *E. coli*, and is particularly convenient for the Sanger method of sequencing. Each of the small clones is then sequenced.

As mentioned above, all sequencing technologies currently in use are based on the Sanger or the Maxam-Gilbert method, which were developed in 1977. Both methods determine the sequence of only one strand of a DNA molecule at a time, and both methods involve three basic steps. Below we mix and match certain technical details of each method to simplify the description of these three steps. The real methods are described in Figures 4 and 5.

Figure 2. Nested Set of Labeled Fragments for Simplified Example

Original Strand	5'-^{32}P-ATGACCGATTTGC-3'
Labeled fragments ending in A	5'-^{32}P-A
	5'-^{32}P-ATGA
	5'-^{32}P-ATGACCGA
Labeled fragments ending in C	5'-^{32}P-ATGAC
	5'-^{32}P-ATGACC
	5'-^{32}P-ATGACCGATTTGC
Labeled fragments ending in G	5'-^{32}P-ATG
	5'-^{32}P-ATGACCG
	5'-^{32}P-ATGACCGATTTG
Labeled fragments ending in T	5'-^{32}P-AT
	5'-^{32}P-ATGACCGAT
	5'-^{32}P-ATGACCGATT
	5'-^{32}P-ATGACCGATTT

• Many copies of the strand to be sequenced are isolated and labeled with, say, the radioisotope ^{32}P, usually at the 5' end. The strands are chemically manipulated to create a nested set of radio-labeled fragments. By nested, we mean that each fragment in the set has a common starting point, typically at the labeled 5' end of the original strand, and the lengths of the labeled fragments increase stepwise, or one base at a time. In other words, the shortest fragment contains the radio label and the first base at the 5' end of the original strand. The next shortest fragment contains the label and the first two bases at the 5' end, and so on, up to the longest fragment, which is identical to the original strand.

• The fragments that make up the nested set are not prepared in one reaction mixture. Rather, copies of the original labeled strand are divided into four batches. Each batch is subjected to a different reaction, and each reaction produces labeled fragments that end in only one of the four bases A, C, T, or G. For example, if the sequence of the original labeled strand is 5'-^{32}PATGACCGATTTGC-3', the four reactions produce the four sets of labeled fragments shown in Figure 2. Together those fragments compose the complete set of nested fragments for the original strand. That is, the set includes all fragments that would be obtained by starting at the 5' end of the original strand and adding one base at a time.

• The fragments from the four reaction mixtures are separated by length using gel electrophoresis. A polyacrylamide gel is prepared with four parallel lanes, one for each reaction mixture. Thus each lane contains labeled fragments that end in only one of the four bases. Since polyacrylmide gels can resolve DNA molecules differing in length by just one nucleotide, the positions of all the labeled fragments can be distinguished. During electrophoresis, shorter fragments travel farther than longer fragments. Thus copies of the shortest fragment form a band farthest from the end at which the fragment batches were loaded into the gel. Successively longer fragments form bands at positions closer and closer to the loading end. Following electrophoresis, the radio-labeled fragments are visualized by exposing the gel to an x-ray filter to make an autoradiogram. Figure 3 shows the pattern of bands that would be created on the autoradiogram by the four sets of labeled fragments in Figure 2. Recall that each band contains many copies of one of those labeled fragments. The end base of those fragments is known by noting the lane in which the band appears, and the length of those fragments is determined from the vertical position of the band; fragment lengths increase from the bottom to the top of the autoradiogram. Therefore, the base sequence of the original long strand can be read directly from the autoradiogram. One starts at the bottom and looks across the four lanes to find the lane containing the band corresponding to the shortest fragments. Those fragments end at the base marked at the top of the lane. Then one continues up and across the autoradiogram, each time identifying the lane containing the band corresponding to the next longer fragments and thus identifying the end base of those fragments. The sequence of the original strand is thus read from its 5′ end, the common starting point, to its 3′ end.

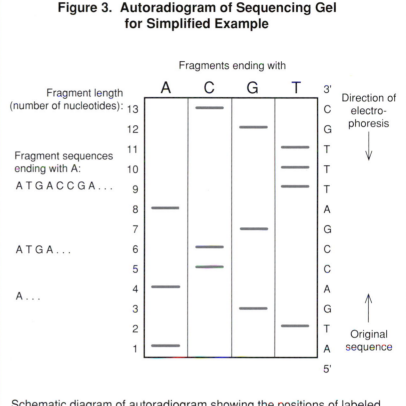

Figure 3. Autoradiogram of Sequencing Gel for Simplified Example

Schematic diagram of autoradiogram showing the positions of labeled fragments generated in four reaction mixtures from the sequence 5′-^{32}P-ATGACCGATTTGC-3′. The sequence in the 5′-to-3′ direction is read from the bottom to the top of the autoradiogram.

The Sanger and Maxam-Gilbert sequencing protocols differ in the reactions used to generate the four batches of labeled fragments making up the nested set. The Sanger method involves enzymatic synthesis of the radio-labeled fragments from unlabeled DNA strands. The Maxam-Gilbert method involves chemical cleavage of prelabeled DNA strands in four different ways to form the four different collections of labeled fragments. The details of the two procedures are described in Figures 4 and 5.

Figure 4. Maxam-Gilbert Sequencing Method

The Maxam-Gilbert sequencing protocol uses chemical cleavage at specific bases to generate, from pre-labeled copies of the DNA strand to be sequenced, a nested set of labeled fragments. Recall that the fragments in the set increase in length one base at a time from the 5' end of the original labeled strand. Four different cleavage reactions are used, and the reaction products are separated by length on four lanes of a gel to determine the order of the cleaved bases along the original labeled strand.

Two chemical cleavage reactions are employed; one cleaves a DNA strand at guanine (G) and adenine (A), the two purines, and the other cleaves the DNA at cytosine (C) and thymine (T), the two pyrimidines. The first reaction can be slightly modified to cleave at G only, and the second slightly modified to cleave at C only. In each reaction, cleavage of single-stranded DNA is accomplished by chemically modifying a specific base, removing the modified base from its sugar, and then breaking the bonds that hold the exposed sugar in the sugar-phosphate backbone of the DNA molecule.

(a) Cleavage Reaction for Guanine

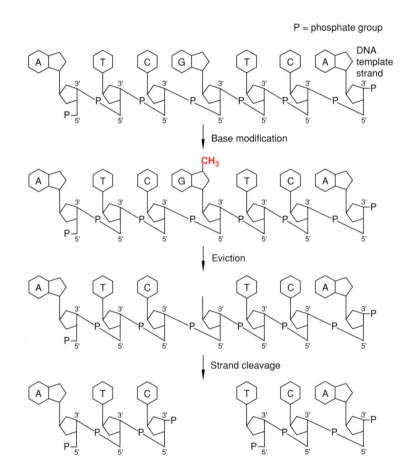

P = phosphate group

Dimethylsulfate is used to methylate guanine. After eviction of the modified base, the exposed sugar, deoxyribose, is then removed from the backbone. Thus the strand is cleaved in two.

The reaction that cleaves guanine is shown schematically in (a). A methyl group is added to guanine, the modified base is removed from its sugar by heating, and the exposed sugar is removed from the backbone by heating in alkali. To cleave at both A and G, the procedure is identical except that a dilute acid is added after the methylation step. The reactions that cleave at C, or at C and T, involve hydrazine to remove the bases and piperidine to cleave the backbone. The extent of the reaction shown in (a) can be carefully limited so that, on average, only one G is evicted from each strand, thus each strand is cleaved at only one of its guanine sites.

A radiolabeled strand to be sequenced and the fragments created from that strand by a single cleavage at the site of G are illustrated in (b). Each original strand is broken into a labeled fragment and an unlabeled fragment. All the labeled fragments start at the 5' end of the strand and terminate at the base that precedes the site of a G along the original strand. Only the labeled fragments will be recorded once all the fragments are separated on a gel and visualized by exposing the gel to an x-ray film to create an autoradiogram of the gel.

(b) Fragments from Single Cleavage at G

5'-^{32}P-ATGACCGATTTGC-3' ——— Labeled template strand

5'-^{32}P-AT-3'	5'-ACCGATTTGC-3'
5'-^{32}P-ATGACC-3'	5'-ATTTGC-3'
5'-^{32}P-ATGACCGATT-3'	5'-C-3'

Six different types of fragments are produced. Only three of those include the labeled 5' end of the original strand.

Given the four chemical cleavage reactions, we can outline the steps involved in Maxam-Gilbert sequencing.

Step 1: Preparation of Labeled Strands. Many copies of the DNA segment to be sequenced are labeled with radioisotope ^{32}P at the 5' end of the strand. If the DNA is cloned in double-stranded form, then the 5' ends of both strands are labeled. The DNA is then denatured, copies of one strand are isolated from copies of the other strand, and each strand is sequenced separately.

Step 2: Generating a Nested Set of Labeled Fragments. Copies of one labeled strand are divided into four batches, and each batch is subjected to one of four chemical cleavage reactions outlined above. The reactions cleave the template strands at G, G and A, C, or C and T, respectively. All labeled fragments in each batch begin at the 5' end of the original strand.

Step 3: Electrophoresis and Gel Reading. The fragments from the four reactions are separated in parallel on four lanes of a gel by electrophoresis. An autoradiogram of the gel shows the positions of the labeled fragments only. A schematic of the autoradiogram is shown in the figure. Each of the four lanes is labeled by the base or bases at which the original strand was cleaved. Fragments cleaved at C show up in two lanes, the one marked C and the one marked C and T. Fragments cleaved at T are identified by noting that they appear in the lane marked C and T, but do not appear in the lane marked C. Fragments ending in A or G can be similarly identified. Note that the fragment cleaved at the first base will not show up on the gel, so the first base at the 5' end of the original strand cannot be determined. As described in the main text, the band corresponding to the shortest fragments is at the bottom of the autoradiogram. The 5'-to-3' sequence of the original strand is read by noting the positions and lanes of the bands from the bottom to the top of the autoradiogram.

(c) Steps in Maxam-Gilbert Sequencing

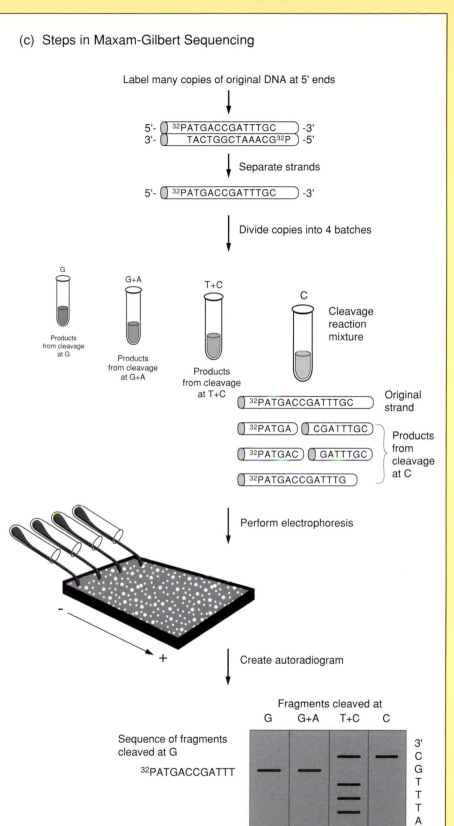

Figure 5. Sanger Sequencing Method

The Sanger method for sequencing, also known as the dideoxy chain termination method, generates the nested set of labeled fragments (see main text) from a template strand by replicating the template strand to be sequenced and interrupting the replication at one of the four bases. Four different replication reactions produce fragments that terminate in A, C, G, or T, respectively.

The replication reaction follows the path described in

"DNA Replication" (see box in "Understanding Inheritance"). A DNA primer is attached (by hybridization) to the template strand and deoxynucleoside triphosphates (dNTPs) are sequentially added to the primer strand by a DNA polymerase. However, dideoxynucleoside triphosphates, say, ddATPs, are present in the reaction mixture along with the usual dNTPs. If, during replication, ddATP rather than dATP is incorporated into the growing DNA strand, then replication stops at that nucleotide.

(a) Structure of dNTP and ddNTP

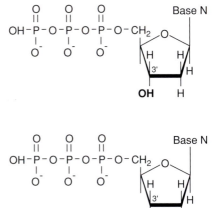

N = A, T, G, or C

Deoxynucleoside triphosphate (dNTP) (note hydroxyl group on 3' carbon of deoxyribosose).

Dideoxynucleoside triphosphate (ddNTP). Dideoxy analog lacks the hydroxyl group on the 3' carbon.

In (a) we show the difference between dNTP and ddNTP. The dideoxy analog lacks the hydroxyl group that is present on the 3' carbon of the sugar in dNTP and is needed to form an O-P-O bridge to the next nucleotide. Thus, the addition of a ddNTP to the growing strand prevents the polymerase from adding additional nucleotides, and the new synthesized strand terminates with the base N. Thus all the strands synthesized in the presence of ddATP have sequences that terminate at A. These strands are complementary to the template strand, and terminate opposite the site of a T on the template strand. Complementary strands terminating in either A, G, C, or T are produced by the inclusion in the reaction mixture of ddATP, ddGTp, ddCTP, or ddTTP, respectively.

(b) Dideoxy Chain Termination Reaction with ddATP

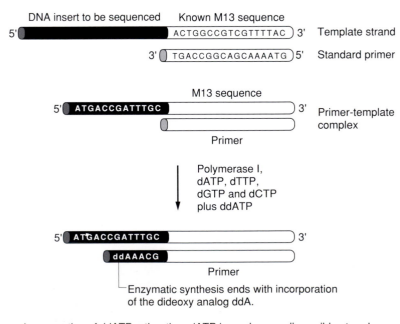

Incorporation of ddATP rather than dATP is random so all possible strands ending at ddATP are synthesized in the reaction.

As illustrated in (b), copies of the template strand to be sequenced must be prepared with a short known sequence at the 3' end of the strand. That short sequence will then hybridize to a DNA primer whose sequence is exactly complementary to that of the known sequence. The primer is essential to initiate replication of the templates by DNA polymerase. The most convenient method for adding a known sequence to the 3' end of the template strand is to clone the strand in the single-stranded cloning vector M13 so that a known M13 sequence will always flank the unknown DNA insert and can serve as the site for binding a standard primer. Also, the M13 cloning protocol automatically creates two types of clones, each type containing a DNA insert whose sequence is complementary to that of the other DNA insert. Thus, the two complementary strands may be sequenced and the two sequences cross-checked to ensure sequence accuracy.

(c) Steps in Sanger Sequencing

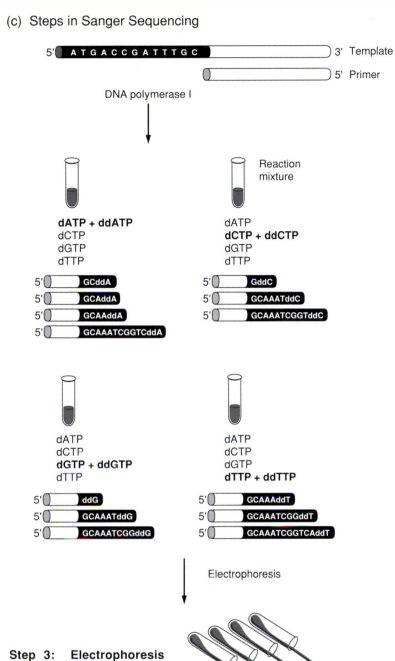

DNA polymerase I

Reaction mixture

dATP + ddATP
dCTP
dGTP
dTTP

5' GCddA
5' GCAddA
5' GCAAddA
5' GCAAATCGGTCddA

dATP
dCTP + ddCTP
dGTP
dTTP

5' GddC
5' GCAAATddC
5' GCAAATCGGTddC

dATP
dCTP
dGTP + ddGTP
dTTP

5' ddG
5' GCAAATddG
5' GCAAATCGGddG

dATP
dCTP
dGTP
dTTP + ddTTP

5' GCAAAddT
5' GCAAATCGGddT
5' GCAAATCGGTCAddT

Electrophoresis

In (c) we outline the three steps involved in the Sanger dideoxy sequencing method.

Step 1: Template Preparation. Copies of the template strand are cloned in M13. They are thus flanked at their 3' ends by a known sequence that will bind to a standard primer.

Step 2: Generating a Nested Set of Labeled Fragments. Copies of each template strand are divided into four batches, and each batch is used for a different replication reaction. Copies of the same standard primer and DNA polymerase I is used in all four reactions. To synthesize fragments, all of which terminate at A, the dideoxy analog ddATP is added to the reaction mixture along with dATP, dGTP, dCTP, dTTP the standard primer and DNA polymerase I. The ddATPs and one of the dNTPs are labeled with a radioactive isotope to produce radiolabeled strands. The figure shows a short template strand, the primer, the four reaction mixtures, and the labeled strands produced by each reaction. Note that the synthesized fragments from the four reaction mixtures compose the set of nested fragments needed to determine the order of the bases in the strand complementary to the template strand.

Step 3: Electrophoresis and Gel Reading. The fragments from the four reaction mixtures are loaded into four parallel lanes of a polyacrylamide gel and separated by length using electrophoresis.

An autoradiogram of the gel is read as described in the main text to determine the order of the bases in the strand complementary to that of the template strand. Again, since the bands corresponding to the shortest fragments are at the bottom of the autoradiogram, the 5'-to-3' sequence of the strand complementary to the template strand is read from the bottom to the top of the autoradiogram.

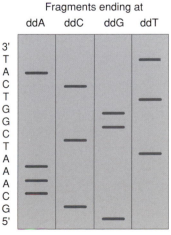

Autoradiogram of sequencing gel

Fragments ending at
ddA ddC ddG ddT

Sequence of strand
complementary to
template strand

3'
T
A
C
T
G
G
C
T
A
A
A
C
G
5'

The final step in both procedures is to separate the labeled fragments by length using gel electrophoresis (see "Gel Electrophoresis" in "Understanding Inheritance"). Since the fragment mobility in the gel varies as the reciprocal of the logarithm of the fragment length, shorter fragments are more widely separated from one another than longer fragments. That is, the resolution of fragment lengths decreases as the fragment length increases. Therefore, the range of fragment lengths that can be resolved in a single gel is limited to several hundred bases. Moreover, the separation of fragments in a standard gel (0.2 to 0.4 millimeters thick) is a relatively slow process. At least several hours are required to resolve fragment lengths from one to several hundred bases long. [More recently, very narrow gel-filled capillary tubes have been used to decrease the time needed for fragment separation. Several hundred bases can be resolved in tens of minutes and the resolution is high enough to read 1000 bases from a single gel.] The average error rate in a single sequencing run is about 1 base in 100. The errors are often due to inhomogeneities in the gel and various sequence-dependent conformational changes in the single-stranded fragments that affect their mobility in the gel.

Since only short stretches of DNA, several hundred to a thousand base pairs in length, can be obtained from a single sequencing gel, many short sequences must be generated separately and then combined to determine the sequence of a much longer DNA fragment. Various strategies have been developed to generate these short sequences from the larger fragment.

The "shotgun" approach is the most widely used in the larger sequencing projects. Copies of a long fragment to be sequenced are broken into much shorter fragments that overlap one another, and the short fragments are cloned. Those clones are then picked at random and sequenced. The sequence of the long fragment is determined by finding overlaps among the short sequences and assembling those sequences into the most likely order. Numerous computer algorithms have been developed to facilitate the assembly of long sequences.

Inevitably, gaps remain in the sequence of the long fragment, and they are filled by switching to a directed sequencing strategy. That is, the short clones are no longer sequenced at random, but rather, short sequences at the end of a continuous stretch of known sequence provide the information necessary to construct a probe to pick out a clone, or region of a clone, whose sequence will extend the known sequence. Most of the large sequencing projects to date have used a mixture of random and directed sequencing strategies to complete the sequence of long, contiguous stretches of DNA. The advantage of the random, or "shotgun," strategy is that in the course of picking clones at random and sequencing them, any given region is usually sequenced many times, thereby reducing the errors in the final sequence.

Almost all steps involved in sequencing are amenable to automation, and through automation many groups hope to increase both the throughput and the consistency of large-scale sequencing efforts. Several automatic sequencing machines have been

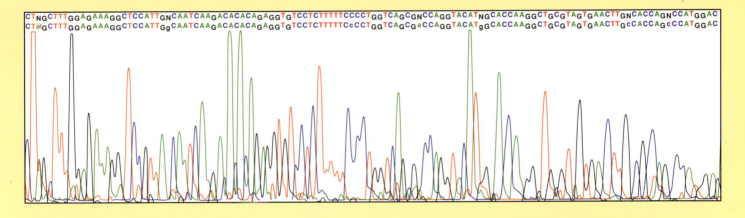

CTNGcTTTGGAGAAAGGCTCCATTGNCAATCAAGACACACAGAGGTGTCCTCTTTTTCCCCTGGTCAGCGNCCAGGTACATNGCACCAAGGCTGCGTAGTGAACTTGNCACCAGNCCATGGAC
CTalgCTTTGGAGAAAGGCTCCATTGgCAATCAAGACACACAGAGGTGTCCTCTTTTTCcCCTGGTCAGCGaCCAGGTACATggCACCAAGGCTGCGTAGTGAACTTGcCACCAGcCCATGGAC

on the market for a number of years. Those machines automate the steps of gel electrophoresis, gel reading, and the "calling" of the end bases of the successively longer fragments. The machines designed for high throughput require that the fragments produced by the four sequencing reactions be labeled with fluorescent dyes rather than radioisotopes, and they employ laser-induced fluorescence to detect the order of the labeled fragments as they migrate through the gel. Some machines use four parallel lanes for the fragments of the four reaction mixtures; others use a single gel lane for all the fragments. The output of a high-throughput sequencing machine includes a plot of the fluorescence signals versus time produced as the fragments migrate past the laser as well as the sequence of bases corresponding to the time sequence of the variously colored fluorescence peaks. Ambiguities in the data are also noted automatically (see Figure 6).

Under optimal conditions, the automatic sequencers are capable of producing 12,000 base pairs of raw data per day. However, much work remains to improve reliability and to organize the efficient use of those machines in large-scale sequencing projects. For example, problems associated with the preparation of clones for sequencing, the checking of the short sequences and assembling them into longer contiguous sequences, and the tracking of all procedures involved in sequencing need increased attention. So far, despite the availability of automatic sequencing machines, production of finished sequence remains a slow and expensive process. Those working on improving existing technologies and streamlining their use expect to achieve a tenfold increase in sequencing throughput within the next few years, and perhaps a hundredfold increase in ten years. Others are involved in developing radically new sequencing technologies that, if successful, might achieve the hundredfold to thousandfold increase needed to sequence the entire human genome. (See the discussion of new technologies in Part III of "Mapping the Genome" as well as "Rapid DNA Sequencing Based on Single Molecule Detection.") ■

Further Reading

T. Hunkapiller, R.J. Kaiser, B.F. Koop, L. Hood "Large-Scale and Automated DNA Sequence Determination." *Science*, October 4, 1991.

Figure 6. Output of Automatic Sequencing Machine

Each of four dideoxy sequencing reactions produces fragments labeled with a dye that fluoresces at a different wavelength. As the fragments from the four reactions migrate down a single lane of a polyacrylamide gel, they pass through a laser beam and produce a fluorescence signal. The machine automatically records the signal and calls the end base of the fragments based on the color (wavelength) of the fluorescence signal. The sequence of the strand complementary to the template strand is read from right to left corresponding to the 5′-to-3′ direction. The machine automatically generates the top sequence, recording any ambiguity in the base call as an N. A technician can resolve most such ambiguities by direct examination of the fluorescence signals. If the technician concludes with high certainty that a particular N is, for example, the base G, he or she replaces that N with a g in the bottom sequence.

Informatics— information handling and analysis

Bob Moyzis: We've been talking about improving technology to generate data much faster than we're now doing, and that brings up the problem of how to store, analyze, and distribute the data to the community. Even at the present rate, the genome centers have run smack into the issue of information handling.

David Galas: I want to emphasize that the principal resource to come from the Genome Project is an ongoing public database of information about chromosomes, segments of chromosomes, genes, and so on. So, even in this relatively early stage of the Project, we are focused on trying to envision that database and on organizing the information already available.

David Botstein: There are a lot of database types who are thinking about this problem, but at this point we don't have enough data to formulate the problem properly. Fully integrated databases for organisms don't really exist yet. In the long run, creating those databases is going to be a major problem. The Genome Project has established a joint informatics task force to address the problem, but it's a very contentious group. The one thing they agree on is that the database must be useful to biologists.

David Galas: In talking to biologists, computer scientists, and mathematicians, it's clear no one has a very good concept for the ultimate database. It is also clear that we must start with some kind of

database and then set up a process by which it can evolve to meet future need.

In a short term, the next couple of years, the genome database at Johns Hopkins is going to be our database, because it has no competitors. It has all the genetic data that people are willing to put into the public domain, and plans are now being laid for including physical-mapping data. That database is well

> The principal resource to come from the Genome Project is an ongoing public database of information about chromosomes, segments of chromosomes, genes, and so on. So, even in this relatively early stage of the Project, we are focused on trying to envision that database and on organizing the information already available.

conceived in present technology, and although it's clearly not at the cutting edge of database technologies, we have to do something now; we can't afford to wait. In the long term, either it will evolve into something quite different, or it will be replaced by something else.

Bob Moyzis: I think there is an incredible amount of data that is currently inaccessible in public databases, for example, the data sitting in DOE and

NIH genome centers. Just trying to get useful genetic-mapping data out of GDB, the Genome DataBase as Johns Hopkins, is a frustrating task. They're working hard at improving this resource, but it's still an enormous task. Until data flow from the genome centers to GDB is more efficient and until GDB becomes a more user-friendly database, I'm afraid much of the information will remain in local databases.

David Botstein: The more sophisticated computer-types think that major improvements in database structure are in the pipeline, so it's clear that we shouldn't lock ourselves in. Almost everybody believes that databases currently used by people who are not computer-science experts are going to have problems. And since the new methods put additional constraints and also additional liberties on how you do things, we must get everybody to preserve their data in such a way that they don't lose any essential parts.

Norton Zinder: We're trying very hard to put together a task force to look at this problem in a very serious way. We're also making minimal databases, so that people can get the data they want quickly and not get lost in the mountains of extraneous information that are presently being stored.

Nancy Wexler: We now have many collaborations organized around cells, parts of chromosomes, and disease genes, and they are forcing people to create databases. For example, seven different laboratories around the world collaborate on Huntington's disease. They're trying to figure out their own collaborative databases and communication systems, and people are getting locked into particular formats, so the database problem needs to be addressed before it becomes unmanageable.

David Galas: I think this worry of being locked into particular data structures and so forth is a red herring. There will always be a need to redo things, to turn over equipment, and so on. That is an ongoing cost of any database. But it is a misconception to think that choosing one format locks you in forever.

Software technology is now reaching the point where you can change from relational databases to the newer object-oriented databases. The change is not trivial, but you don't have to redo everything. Biologists are afraid, as David Botstein often says, of the Stalinism of setting standards, and they use that excuse to argue against doing anything. But we desperately need to do something now because people, particularly in the smaller labs, have to be able to have access to the data.

In some ways, David's argument that we need to wait cuts against the philosophy he espouses. That is, by not doing something now we cut out all the small labs. A small university is not going to have access to anything if there is no database. So it's a real problem. But the problem is not long for this world because the education of smart people like David and the biological community in general is going to come along rapidly.

We need a great deal more communication and coordination in the informatics area. The database issue is critical now. It is an administrative problem, a software problem, a networking problem, and a research problem. It's a mess and it needs to be addressed because data is our ultimate product.

Norton Zinder: Some informatics people want to completely restructure relational databases to apply, generically, to any world and to any problem. But

we have some finite problems that need immediate solutions.

David Galas: The handling of mapping data is one such problem, and the national labs recognized the need for sophisticated data handling a long time ago. Now, as Bob mentioned, the NIH centers are beginning to recognize the problem because they're having trouble dealing with all the data.

Bob Moyzis: They're beginning to realize they're all underfunded because the money they asked for is to do the biology and there's nothing left to do all of the other things.

David Galas: Before these centers really got started, the people involved were saying things quite antithetical to what they're now saying. So clearly there's a great deal of education in the community that needs to be done. We have a bit of a two-cultures problem. On one side you have those in mathematics and computational biology and on the other side are those with a classical biology background who are doing the good work in genome mapping. So we need informatics support for the mapping efforts.

Bob Moyzis: Other than STSs, for which it is easy to construct a database and share that information, management of mapping data is very difficult. At Los Alamos we have accumulated more information on chromosome 16 than we ourselves can access in an easy fashion. It has turned out to be a bottleneck for us. The problem of sending 4,000 clones someplace is easy compared with sending the information we've accumulated on chromosome 16 in some useful and intelligible format.

On the other hand, progress on map integration, analysis, and display under

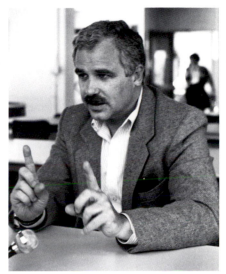

David Galas

Biologists are afraid . . . of the Stalinism of setting standards, and they often use that excuse to argue against doing anything. But we desperately need to do something now because people, particularly in the smaller labs, have to be able to have access to the data.

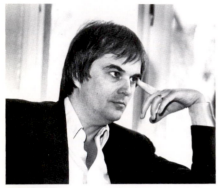

Bob Moyzis

If you have a bad fit between person and problem, it's frustrating all around. Certain aspects of this project are moving so fast that the informatics types need to come up with a quick and dirty solution to be of help.

the direction of Jim Fickett and others at Los Alamos have progressed to the point that I will make a prediction. Individual genome centers *must* consolidate their own data, or they will not produce a quality map. The idea that some central database, like GDB, can provide this function is nonsense. The central database should use the GenBank model. The *investigators* will produce the map. The central database will make it *available* in some consistent form.

David Galas: Another important area in informatics is research into future algorithms. We need new algorithms for doing pattern recognition in sequence data, for finding the genes among the sequence of bases, for finding similarities among sequences, and for assembling long stretches of sequence from short stretches.

Lee Hood: The information problems are tough. There are no programs that can search through a DNA sequence and unequivocally pick out the coding sequences. Scientists at Oak Ridge have made striking contributions to solving this problem. I think we're attracting good people into this field, people who know some biology. But there's really an enormous amount of work to be done. Scientists such as Chris Fields are incorporating various features of genes into their search algorithms, such as statistical asymmetries among groups of three bases or six bases in the protein-coding regions, properties of RNA splicing points and splicing boundaries, and so on. But we need to accumulate more sequence data and learn a lot more about those features before we'll have reliable algorithms for finding genes directly from the nucleotide sequence.

David Botstein: Another difficult problem is to figure out when one should be impressed with the similarity between

two sequences. A related problem is to find the similarities among sequences in a huge mass of data, which means lots of pairwise comparisons. Parallel computing is very appropriate for this task of making many comparisons of many sequences, and aligning them optimally. There are a few major mathematicians who work on this problem. The most prominent are probably Sam Karlen and Michael Waterman. The business is largely combinatorics.

David Galas: I understand from my mathematical colleagues that the mapping and sequencing data present some very important and interesting mathematical problems. And often those problems that the biologists think are trivial are really difficult for the mathematicians to solve rigorously and vice versa. For example, biologists have assembled physical maps from restriction fragment lengths, but to do it in a rigorous fashion turns out to be an NP-complete problem—which means that the number of computations required to do the problem increases exponentially with the number of fragments.

Bob Moyzis: Lander and Waterman took a rough cut at that problem, but to do it in a rigorous probabilistic sense is very tough indeed. David Torney at Los Alamos is working on this problem.

David Galas: Sequence-matching problems are also very difficult if the parameters are set in a sufficiently loose way, that is, if you allow gaps and insertions in the sequences to be matched. The difficulty of the comparison is dependent on the parameters in a way that's unexpected—at least to most biologists. The sequence-assembly problem is of the same kind—NP-complete, much like the traveling-salesman problem. An approximate solution is not too hard to get if you don't have too many short sequences to assemble into one. But when you're doing massive sequencing and trying to assemble the pieces in a rigorous and automated way, then you have to worry about the real nature of the problem. Other things, like quickly searching the database for particular sequences, sound difficult to a lot of biologists, but in fact database searches are not too hard. And many biologists can do it on their computers right now because the software is available.

We're really experiencing a blossoming of this interface between biology, mathematics, and computation. That interface holds a great deal of the future of biology, much like the automation problem in engineering.

We've talked about public databases, lab support, and research on algorithms, but you can't always distinguish one of them from the others. The lab biologist trying to do the mapping problem would say, "Give me some computer guys so I can do X." The computer guy will work on that for a while and say, "Okay, now you can do X." Then the lab guy says, "While you were fixing it so I could do X, I changed my mind. We've got this new technique, now I want to do Y." Developing software and techniques for ongoing, evolving technologies is a real problem.

Nonetheless, I want to make a distinction between developing software, showing people how to use it, and making it bulletproof, versus solving the much more abstract and esoteric problems. If done by the right people, the abstract problems are going to be extremely important. It's almost another two-cultures problem. Biologists say they want the mathematicians to be their computer programmers, but we also need to tackle the difficult mathematical problems.

Bob Moyzis: Very different kinds of people are interested in doing those very different types of problems. If you have a bad fit between person and problem, it's frustrating all around. Certain aspects of this project are moving so fast that the informatics types need to come up with a quick and dirty solution to be of help.

On the other hand, there are some major problems that aren't going to go away in two years and need more long-range kind of work. A few years ago many mathematical types were trying to develop models of the mapping problems, hoping to find the best strategy for mapping the genome. But molecular biologists, at least the more aggressive ones, aren't willing to wait around for anything. They want to get the job done on this project, and they'll switch midstream if a new technique comes on-line that looks better.

The *better* technique is very difficult to define because it depends on personal preference and skill at certain techniques not simply on some abstract measure of efficiency. Simulations of the mapping problems show only slight differences in the efficiency of different strategies and are really not that informative. So the mathematical problems have to be chosen with some care.

David Botstein: The recurrent dilemma that we haven't touched on at all is who will have access to the data. Most scientists want the data to be in a public database as soon as you read the sequences off your gel. But the sooner one releases the data, the less chance one has to check the data. It's a trade-off between speed and accuracy. There are also commercial and patent concerns because the sequences have many biotechnology spin-offs. That's a very difficult and touchy subject.

Most scientists want the data to be in a public database as soon as you read the sequences off your gel. But the sooner one releases the data, the less chance one has to check the data. It's a trade-off between speed and accuracy. There are also commercial and patent concerns because the sequences have many biotechnology spin-offs. That's a very difficult and touchy subject.

163

IV. Implications for Biology and Society

Biology and the Genome Project

Bob Moyzis: Everyone emphasizes the biotechnology and biomedical spin-offs from this project, but we're also creating an enormous resource for fundamental science, that is, for addressing some of the big open questions in biology.

Gene expression is one of those areas. For the information in the protein-coding sequence of a gene to be expressed as a protein, the DNA sequence is first transcribed into an RNA molecule and then the RNA sequence is translated into a protein. But genes are not actively making proteins all the time. What turns the gene on and off? Most of our models are based on experiments with organisms like *E. coli* where genes are either on or off. The rules of gene expression are much more complicated in humans. Some genes are expressed only in certain tissues and in varying amounts. Some are turned on at one point in development, then turned off again, and then re-expressed in another tissue.

The regulatory networks must be incredibly complicated, but at present we don't have the faintest idea how the expression of even a single human gene is regulated. We've identified some sequences near the gene that we know are important—promoter sequences, for example, that must bind to a special regulatory protein before the gene can

be turned on—but some regulatory signals may be very far from the genes themselves. When an individual human gene is put back into a cell in culture, it does not exhibit the exact kind of regulatory patterns as those observed in normal cells. Clearly we have a lot to learn.

> *In the future you'll be able to dial various sequences into a computer, and from those "area codes" and "molecular addresses" the computer will give you the 10,000 genes that are expressed in the kidney, for example, by virtue of those molecular addresses.*

Lee Hood: Once we have the sequences of the human genome, I expect we will find a lot of interesting patterns in the DNA that have to do with gene regulation. Indeed, those will constitute molecular addresses, which tell us in which cells and at what developmental stages the corresponding genes are expressed. We're going to have to figure out ways of deciphering those molecular addresses.

As another example, proteins have to bind to DNA to get it to coil and supercoil into a compact chromosome. I would guess that the DNA sequences that bind to these proteins will be made evident by a detailed analysis of the sequences in complete chromosomes. In the long term, I expect we'll be able to identify the regulatory sequences, that is, the binding sites of proteins, which turn genes on and off, and from those sequences we will deduce where that gene is expressed, when during development it's expressed, and the amplitude of its expression.

The regulatory site will be like a telephone area code, and in the future you'll be able to dial various sequences into a computer, and from those *area codes* and *molecular addresses*, the computer will give you the 10,000 genes that are expressed in the kidney, for example, by virtue of those molecular addresses.

Regulation is probably best understood in *E. coli*, which, of course, is a prokaryote, a cell with no nucleus. In the human, we know a lot about a few elements that regulate some genes, but not many. Extensive studies of gene regulation have been done on bacteria, the sea urchin, yeast, and *Drosophila*. But as far as understanding how a whole genome is put together so that the genes are expressed at the right time, in the right order, and in the right amounts, we have very little information.

David Galas: The global functioning on a whole chromosome won't be understood until we learn how the chromosome is organized not only in terms of the one-dimensional layout of the genes but also in terms of its three-dimensional structure. The basic structural unit of the chromosome is chromatin, which is a double loop of DNA wound around a protein center.

And many of us believe the structure of chromatin plays an important role in gene regulation.

The only things selected by natural selection are the protein products and whether they are turned on and off at the right time. That choreography must involve the detailed structure of the chromosome and how it winds and unwinds during the cell cycle. So if the Genome Project is really an effort to understand all the information encoded in the human genome, then as time goes on, the interests of the Genome Project will become closer and closer to those of structural biology, to the interplay between three-dimensional structures and biological functions.

The sequence information will be relevant not only to chromosome structure but also to protein structure. As we sequence cDNAs and thus determine more protein sequences, we hope to begin to understand how the primary sequences of proteins lead to the three-dimensional structures of the protein macromolecules themselves and therefore to their functions. I say *hope* because we don't know how a sequence of amino acids folds up into a stable protein structure. The protein-folding problem is indeed one of the great conundrums of modern biochemistry and biophysics. Nobody knows whether the problem has a real solution.

If, at the very least, we knew all the protein sequences and all the protein structures, we could figure out how they relate to each other. We don't know whether all the proteins are made up of a relatively small set of little structures, such as alpha helices and beta sheets, or whether each of the 100,000 different proteins is a distinct structure. Maybe there are only 500 elements or modules that are put together in different ways

and the various combinations give rise to all the existing proteins.

Bob Moyzis: Theoretically, you can show there hasn't been enough time since the universe began to create at random all the kinds of potential proteins that could be out there. Maybe all that evolution has done has been to mix and match a few hundred basic structural elements to make all the proteins we have. As we determine the sequence of more and more genes, that question will get answered.

David Galas: That idea of mixing and matching a few basic subunits proved relevant to the problem of how our immune system is able to generate a seemingly infinite variety of antibodies in response to foreign invaders. The antibody-diversity problem was solved by posing the existence of combinatorial rearrangements of a relatively small number of subunits with small variations added on here and there.

That explanation seems to have been borne out and provides a particularly elegant, almost mathematical solution to what seemed an almost unsolvable problem about fifteen years ago. The problem of gene regulation may have a similar solution. We may discover a small class of enhancers and promoter regions that form a hierarchy, a computer-program-like structure that governs regulation.

Bob Moyzis: At the risk of sounding like a broken record, I will point out again that this problem of regulation is relevant even to those primarily interested in human disease. Some types of thalassemia, which is the absence of a particular globin protein, are clearly caused by defects in the regulatory region that tells this gene whether or not to be expressed.

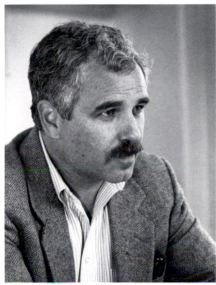
David Galas

What we're looking at in the human genome is a historical product of millions of years of evolution . . . . So evolutionary understanding is an inevitable consequence of the Genome Project. You could even characterize the Project as studying evolution.

A working hypothesis is that there are a limited number of *master* genes controlling regulation. The homeobox genes now being intensively studied in *Drosophila* development fall into that category. Their protein products are capable of binding to many different regions of DNA and regulating the expression of genes responsible for the structural development of an organism. And homeobox genes seem to have been conserved through evolution.

Of course the speculation that there are master genes just pushes the basic problem back one more level to how the master switches might be regulated. Again we have no answers, but this is an incredible time to be in biology because with the current explosion in biological knowledge, one has the feeling that we may solve many of these problems within our own lifetimes.

David Galas: What we're looking at in the human genome is a historical product of millions of years of evolution. The more detail we know about the human genome and the genomes of other species, the more we're going to understand about what processes were involved in getting us where we are. So evolutionary understanding is an inevitable consequence of the Genome Project. You could even characterize the Project as studying evolution.

We already know that molecular processes, the control of individual genes, and the structures of mammalian and bacterial viruses are Rube Goldberg-like arrangements. The reason for this seemingly ad hoc complexity is that these organisms and processes developed over time by natural selection and random variation.

At the heart of understanding evolution is understanding developmental

control—and that means gene control, turning on a battery of genes at one time versus another.

Bob Moyzis: It's astounding to realize that the tools we're developing to unravel the information content of the human genome will allow us to investigate the DNA from ancient tissues. We'll be able to choose specific STS markers and apply the PCR to very small DNA samples preserved in the

> *We'll be able to choose specific STS markers and apply the PCR to very small DNA samples preserved in the bones of our ancestors. It will be like going back in a time machine and finally pinning down some of the speculation about human origins.*

bones of our ancestors. It will be like going back in a time machine and finally pinning down some of the speculation about human origins. The more markers we get, the more we are going to be able to answer questions like, where did Cro-Magnon man really come from? People have now isolated DNA from ten-thousand-year-old human samples. This work is almost like science fiction.

David Galas: The plant record is much older. There's a lake in Minnesota where some leaves have been preserved in an anoxic sediment that dates back to 20 million years ago—they've gotten

DNA sequences from the rubisco genes of magnolias and sycamores. Those sequences are much the same as they are today. But there must be some other interesting DNA fossils in that sediment. This is a whole new area of exploration. In terms of evolutionary development, we're farthest along in understanding insect morphologies. Certain classes of Arthropoda have identical segments, like centipedes. Later in evolution came batteries of homeobox genes that caused differences to occur among those segments. Homeotic means changing, and homeotic mutations are those that change parts of the organism by changing individual segments—say, by making the second thoracic segment into an abdominal segment. In some cases you can take identical segments, lay on another level of genetic control, and produce a difference between the segments.

Clearly that's what has happened in the evolutionary branching among those various sorts of Arthropoda. We know that in the early embryonic development in *Drosophila* there are three or four genes, so-called segmentation genes, that lay down the initial segmented pattern of the organism. Then other genes turn on to produce changes among the segments. We're beginning to work out that circuitry now.

Bob Moyzis: Nobody on the Human Genome Project ever talks about development because the reality is that human development is particularly difficult to study.

David Galas: That's an important point. There are very important outstanding questions in development that can be answered in the nematode and in *Drosophila* and so forth. But nematode development, for example, is hardwired—you know where every cell goes. Every organism that develops properly through its time cycle with the same genome is identical. It's got the same cells in exactly the same position. That's not true for organisms even a little farther up the scale like *Drosophila*.

When you get to organisms with relatively complex brains, a large part of development is ultimately determined by the particular genome. It's completely stochastic relative to the kind of programming that appears in nematodes. For a decade or more people have been collecting genes in *Drosophila*, and it's only been very recently that they're starting to understand a little about how the genes are controlled relative to one another. That understanding is built up through controlled experiment.

Bob Moyzis: Obviously we're not going to be doing controlled experiments on human development, but we can work with mice, which are similar to humans in many ways. The mapping and sequencing of the mouse genome is part of the Genome Project. And once we have those tools, we can target genetic changes in mice that will give us clues about developmental questions.

The DOE has a history of being interested in agents that cause abnormalities in development, agents that alter the expression of a particular gene and thereby produce an abnormal embryo. The Oak Ridge people, for example, have a really nice set up for making transgenic mice, and they've been able to identify a number of interesting developmental genes in the mouse that have human homologues. And I believe that work will increase as a spin-off from the Human Genome Project. The Human Genome Project is focused on humans, but we need to study a lot of other organisms to understand human development and pathology.

Ethical, Legal, and Social Implications

Bob Moyzis: The Genome Project will have many practical consequences for society and maybe we should close this discussion by addressing some of them.

David Galas: Both the NIH and the DOE are devoting 3 percent of their total Genome Project budgets to the task of addressing the Ethical, Legal, and Social Implications [ELSI] of the public use of genetic information. [The NIH recently increased their allocation to 5 percent.] The ELSI working group was established by the NIH to identify the most pressing issues and to find ways to help make the new information a real benefit to society.

The basic problems . . . are not new—they will simply be exacerbated.

Nancy Wexler: ELSI is a very exciting aspect of the Genome Project. Traditionally, social issues and scientific work have been viewed as separate realms—scientists go into their labs, do their work, and when they finish, it's it up to society to take it as it comes. The Genome Project is different. Scientists like David Galas and Jim Watson recognized *up front* the need to pay attention to the social and ethical implications of their work, and by funding ELSI as an integral part of the Genome Project, they are taking responsibility for the initial examination of the effects it will have on our society.

David Galas: There are two important things to remember when we think about ethical and social issues in terms

of the Genome Project. First, there are no *new* problems. Issues concerning privacy, confidentiality, and discrimination will become much more pressing once the Genome Project generates the tools to diagnose genetic diseases presymptomatically. The *basic* problems, however, are not new—they will simply be exacerbated.

The second thing to keep in mind is that many ethicists, lawyers, and social scientists who speak out about the implications of the Genome Project are often somewhat ignorant of the fundamental science of genetics. We need everyone to learn and understand the difference between being a carrier of an abnormal gene and having a genetic disease, between the genetic markers for a disease and the disease gene itself, and between genetic probabilities and genetic certainties. Often, without the benefit of a solid background in genetics, people tend to adopt the attitude of naive genetic determinism, that there are good genes and bad genes or that genes alone control behavior. Those misunderstandings have been around a long time, and we have to start dealing with them.

Nancy Wexler: Education of both the general public and professional healthcare providers is among ELSI's high-priority goals. We are actively encouraging the leaders of voluntary health organizations and genetic-disease support groups to participate in public discussions geared toward creating a greater understanding of the nature of genetic disorders and the issues surrounding the Genome Project.

We are also encouraging the insurance industry to anticipate the challenges they will face as vast quantities of new genetic information become available to the public. In a way, the Project is quite a nuisance to the insurance providers.

UNRAVELING THE CHROMOSOME

E. Morton Bradbury

Central to biology is an understanding of the organization, structure, and functions of the chromosomes of higher organisms. Chromosomes contain the DNA molecules of the genome and are themselves contained within the cell nuclei of all eukaryotes, from single-celled yeast all the way up the evolutionary ladder to human beings. As pointed out by David Galas (pages 164–165 of "Mapping the Genome"), to understand the functions of the multitude of protein-coding and noncoding DNA sequences that will be determined by the Human Genome Project, we will need detailed knowledge of the three-dimensional structure of chromosomes and the structural changes that chromosomes undergo during the various phases of the cell cycle. Major advances in biology will be at the interfaces between the Human Genome Project, structural biology, and molecular biology of the cell.

The size of the human genome suggests the magnitude of the problem. The diploid human genome contains 6×10^9 base pairs or 204 centimeters of DNA molecules packaged into 46 chromosomes. It is generally believed that each chromosome contains a single DNA molecule several centimeters in length.

Studies of the yeast *S. cerevisiae*, a lower eukaryote that can be easily manipulated, have revealed three chromosomal elements that are essential to the faithful replication of each chromosome and to the subsequent separation of the two duplicate chromosomes into daughter cells during cell division. These are: (1) the very ends of chromosomes, called the telomeres; (2) a central region of constriction called the centromere that, after replication of a chromosome, is the last point of attachment between the resulting pair of sister chromatids; and (3) a DNA sequence required to initiate DNA replication, called an origin of replication.

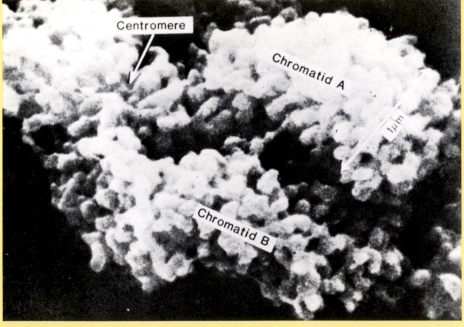

Figure 1. Human Metaphase Chromosome
A scanning transmission electron micrograph of a metaphase chromosome showing two sister chromatids attached at the centromeres. Each compact projection is thought to be a long loop of DNA (see Figure 2) packaged along with various proteins into a thick chromatin fiber. (Reprinted courtesy of U.K. Laemmli, Université de Genève.)

Figure 1 is a scanning transmission electron micrograph of a human metaphase chromosome, the highly condensed structure adopted by the chromosome during metaphase, one of the last phases of cell division. The chromosome has already replicated into two sister chromatids. The centromere connecting the sister chromatids (seen in the micrograph as a region of constriction) provides the point of attachment for the spindle apparatus that contracts and separates the replicated chromosomes into the daughter cells. The telomeres at the ends of each chromatid contain tandem repeated DNA sequences that cap, protect, and maintain the linear DNA ends of the chromosomes during replication.

Each of the 46 human chromosomes can be identified during metaphase by its length, the location of its centromere, and the particular banding pattern produced by staining the DNA of that chromosome. (Banding patterns can be seen in "Chromosomes: The Sites of Hereditary Information" in "Understanding Inheritance.") The origins of the distinctive banding patterns are not well understood but probably reflect a reproducible pattern of DNA folding induced by DNA-protein interactions specific to each chromosome. The DNA molecule is very tightly wound during metaphase. For example, human chromosome 16 is 2.5 micrometers long, whereas the DNA molecule in each sister chromatid is 3.7 centimeters long. In other words, the packing ratio of the linear DNA molecule in the metaphase chromosome is 15,000 to 1.

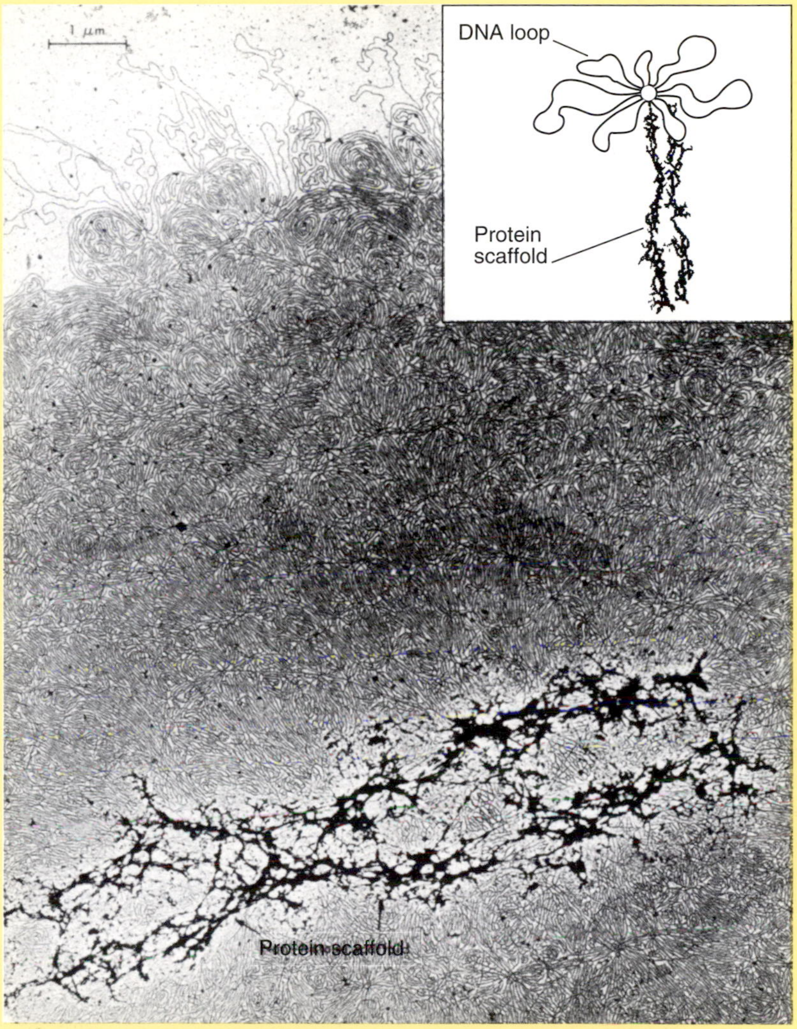

Chromosomal DNA Loops

When chromosomal material is isolated from the nucleus, the long DNA molecules are found to be associated with chromosomal proteins, whose weight is up to twice that of the DNA. The five histones, the many copies of which are equal in weight to that of DNA, are found in all eukaryotes and as explained below are involved in packaging the DNA in the chromosomes. The non-histone proteins are a heterogeneous group and many are associated with the various chromosome functions, such as replication, gene expression, and chromosome organization. Among the latter are a small group that bind most tightly to the DNA and form a scaffold for the chromosome. This protein scaffold has been made visible by gently treating metaphase chromosomes with detergents to remove the histones and most other nonhistone proteins. The remarkable structure that remains is shown in Figure 2. The residual protein scaffold, or "ghost," of the metaphase chromosome is surrounded by a halo of DNA. At higher

Figure 2. Chromosome Loops and Protein Scaffold
Above is a metaphase chromosome depleted of almost all chromosomal proteins. The remaining 2 to 3 percent of the proteins form a scaffold that retains the shape of the intact chromosome. Around the scaffold is a halo of loops of naked DNA. Each loop appears to begin and end at the same point along the protein scaffold (see insert). The number and sizes of these loops suggest that each may contain a single gene or a group of linked genes. (Reprinted courtesy of U.K. Laemmli, Université de Genève.)

resolution DNA loops can be observed to emerge from and return to the same point on the protein scaffold (see inset in Figure 2).

Two major scaffold proteins have been isolated, Sc1 and Sc2. Sc1 has been identified as topoisomerase II, an enzyme that relaxes supercoiled DNA by cutting through both strands of the DNA, thereby enabling the cut DNA ends to rotate, and then resealing the cut. The cuts made by topoisomerase II are essential for the separation of sister chromatids to the daughter cells.

The DNA loops in Figure 2 range in size from 5,000 to 120,000 base pairs and have an average size of about 50,000 base pairs. Thus the haploid human genome of 3×10^9 base pairs of DNA corresponds to 60,000 loops, which is close to the estimated numbers of genes, 50,000 to 100,000, in the human genome. Perhaps each DNA loop contains one or a small number of linked genes and therefore serves as both a genetic and a structural unit of eukaryotic chromosomes. This tantalizing conjecture was first made in 1978, and although it remains unproven, evidence in its favor has been accumulating.

Chromatin Contains a Repeating Subunit Structure

Having looked at some of the largest structural features of the chromosome, we now turn to what we know about the small, repeating substructures within a chromosome. DNA with its associated chromosomal proteins, histones, and nonhistone proteins, is called chromatin. In 1973 chromatin in isolated nuclei was first digested with micrococcal nuclease, an enzyme that cuts double-stranded DNA. The digestion yielded a ladder of DNA lengths in multiples of about 190 to 200 base pairs. Evidently DNA sequences spaced by 190 to 200 base pairs were more accessible to attack by micrococcal nuclease than the intervening DNA. This seminal observation showed that chromatin contained a simple, repeating subunit, known as the nucleosome.

For most somatic tissues, the nucleosome contains three elements, a stretch of DNA containing 195±5 base pairs, one copy of the histone octamer [(H3$_2$H4$_2$)(H2A,H2B)$_2$] and one copy of the histone H1. More prolonged micrococcal nuclease digestion reduces the length of the DNA in the nucleosome, thereby creating a slightly smaller unit, called the chromatosome, which contains 168±2 base pairs of DNA, the histone octamer, and H1. Such digestion often reduces the nucleosome to an even smaller unit contained within the chromatosome and called the nucleosome core particle. It contains 146±1 base pairs of DNA and the histone octamer (see Figure 3).

The nucleosome core particle has been obtained in large quantities and subjected to extensive structural studies. In 1974 neutron-scattering studies of the core particle in aqueous solution showed that it was a flat disc of diameter 100 angstroms and thickness 55 to 60 angstroms, with 1.7 turns of DNA coiled on the outside of a core of the histone octamer at a pitch of about 30 angstroms

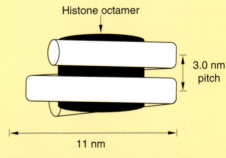

Figure 3. Nucleosome Core Particle
Structure of the nucleosome core particle determined from neutron scattering. The core particle is a flat disc, 100 angstroms in diameter and 55 to 60 angstroms thick.

(Figure 3). Subsequent x-ray-diffraction studies of crystallized core particles achieved a resolution of 6 to 7 angstroms. The crystal structure (Figure 4) not only confirmed the lower resolution solution structure achieved by neutron scattering but also showed that histones are in contact with the minor groove of DNA and leave the major groove available for interactions with the proteins that regulate gene expression and other DNA functions. The 7-angstrom-resolution crystal structure also revealed that DNA does not bend uniformly but rather bends gently and then more sharply around the histone octamer. Such a path implies that flexibility, or bendability, of DNA may be sequence-dependent and that the underlying DNA sequence along the molecule may determine the positions of some nucleosomes. The most recent work on nucleosome positioning shows that the bulk of nucleosome core particles are able to move along the DNA molecule between a cluster of positions separated by about 10 base pairs. This mobility is probably required during DNA replication and transcription to allow DNA polymerases and other enzymes access to specific DNA sequences.

Despite considerable effort to achieve higher resolution, the best data for the core particle structure is at a resolution of about 6 angstroms. However, the crystal structure of the isolated histone octamer has been solved to the higher resolution of 3.3 angstroms. This structure shows shapes of the individual histones and the nature of interhistone interaction of most but not all of the histone polypeptide chains. In particular, the basic N-terminal domains, comprising some 20 to 25 percent of the histone octamer, are not "seen" in the crystal structure, probably because they bind to DNA, and in the absence of DNA, they are disordered. These N-terminal domains contain all of the sites of the cell-cycle-dependent acetylation of lysines and phosphorylation of serines or threonines. Acetylation of lysine converts it from a positively charged residue, which can therefore bind to DNA, to a neutral acetylysine. It has been shown first that lysine acetylation is strictly correlated with transcription and DNA replication, and more recently, that histone acetylation drives the uncoiling of part of the DNA from the nucleosome to allow the initiation and progression of DNA replication and transcription.

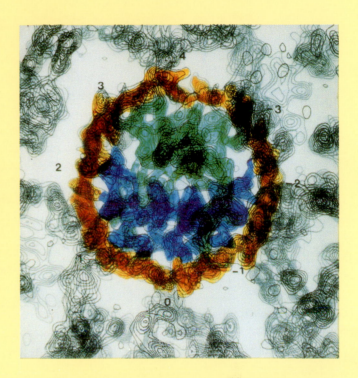

Figure 4. Crystal Structure of Core Particle
The structure of the nucleosome core particle as determined by x-ray diffraction is shown above. At a resolution of 6 to 7 angstroms, this top view of the core particle shows that the DNA (brown) does not follow a smooth path around the histone octamer (blue and turquoise) but rather bends sharply and then more gently. (Reprinted courtesy of Uberbacher and Bunick, Oak Ridge National Laboratory.)

Chromatosomes and Nucleosomes

A model of the structure of the chromatosome (Figure 5) has been inferred from the structures of the nucleosome core particle and the histone H1. The core particle has 1.7 turns of DNA at a pitch of 3.0 nanometers (30 angstroms) coiled around the histone octamer. Consequently, the chromatosome's 168 base pairs of DNA are long enough to complete two turns of DNA around the histone octamer. The chromatosome also includes the fifth histone H1. In the model structure shown in Figure 5, the histone H1 is bound to the outside of the coiled DNA where it might serve to modulate long-range interactions associated with reversible changes in chromosome structure during the cell cycle. During cell division chromosomes become more and more condensed until they reach metaphase. Then, when cell division is completed and the daughter cells enter interphase, the chromosomes assume a less-condensed configuration (see "Mitosis" in "Understanding Inheritance"). The long, flexible "arms" of H1 undergo a pattern of phosphorylations through this cycle, which may well modulate the long-range interactions required to coordinate these structural changes in the chromosomes. In support of this hypothesis is the fact that an increase in H1 phosphorylation has been correlated with the process of chromosome condensation to metaphase chromosomes. To describe the nucleosome beyond the model for the chromatosome requires a knowledge of the paths of the DNA that link one nucleosome to another. Our present lack of knowledge about those paths impedes our ability to pin down the higher-order chromatin structures that make up the chromosome.

Higher-Order Chromatin Structures

Although higher-order structures of chromatin cannot be resolved in the chromosome itself, they can be studied in solution. Chromatin, when placed in low ionic strength, 10-millimolar NaCl, forms a 10-nanometer-diameter fibril of nucleosomes, which is sometimes referred to as "beads on a string." This form is also observed when chromatin spills out of lysed nuclei. Neutron-scattering studies of the 10-nanometer chromatin fibril give a mass per unit length equivalent to one nucleosome per 10 ± 2 nanometers of fibril, or a DNA packing ratio of between 6 and 7 to 1. When ionic strength is increased to 150-millimolar NaCl, corresponding to normal physiological conditions, the 10-nanometer fibril undergoes a transition to the "30-nanometer" fibril. Neutron-scattering studies indicate that the diameter for this fibril in solution is 34 nanometers and the mass-per-unit length is equivalent to 6 to 7 nucleosomes per 11 nanometers of fibril, or a DNA packing ratio of between 40 and 50 to 1. Figure 6 shows the simplest model of the 34-nanometer fibril that is consistent with available structural data: it is a supercoil or solenoid of 6 to 7 radially arranged disc-shaped nucleosomes with a pitch of 11.0 nanometers and a diameter of 34 nanometers. Basic questions concerning the location of histone H1 and the linker DNA connecting the nucleosomes remain unanswered.

Packaging of Chromosome Loops

With these higher order chromatin structures in mind, we can imagine how the large transverse DNA loops present in the histone-depleted metaphase chromosome (see Figure 2) might be packaged in the normal chromosome. Since the average size of the

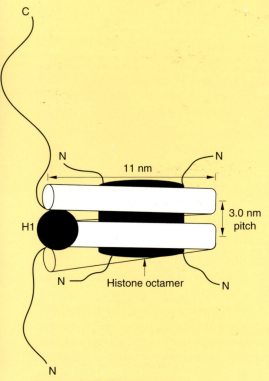

Figure 5. Model of the Chromatosome
The model includes the nucleosome core particle, an extra stretch of DNA, and the histone H1. The DNA makes two complete turns around the histone octamer, and H1 is bound to the outside of the coil at the place where the coil begins and ends. In this position H1 might server to modulate long-range interactions that modify chromosome structure during the cell cycle.

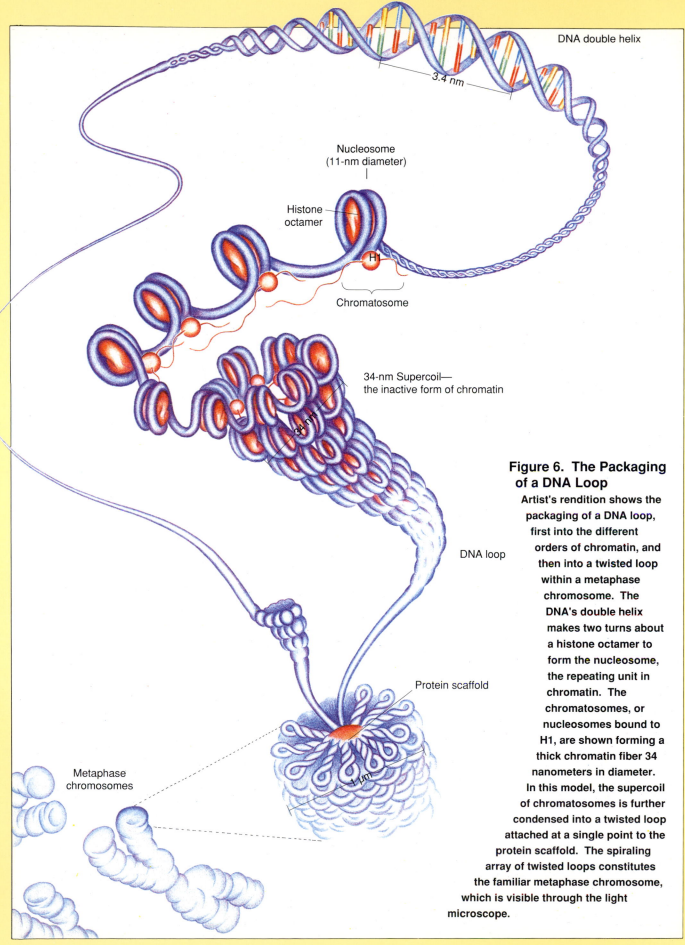

DNA double helix

3.4 nm

Nucleosome
(11-nm diameter)

Histone
octamer

H1

Chromatosome

34-nm Supercoil—
the inactive form of chromatin

34 nm

DNA loop

Protein scaffold

1 μm

Metaphase
chromosomes

**Figure 6. The Packaging
of a DNA Loop**

Artist's rendition shows the
packaging of a DNA loop,
first into the different
orders of chromatin, and
then into a twisted loop
within a metaphase
chromosome. The
DNA's double helix
makes two turns about
a histone octamer to
form the nucleosome,
the repeating unit in
chromatin. The
chromatosomes, or
nucleosomes bound to
H1, are shown forming a
thick chromatin fiber 34
nanometers in diameter.
In this model, the supercoil
of chromatosomes is further
condensed into a twisted loop
attached at a single point to the
protein scaffold. The spiraling
array of twisted loops constitutes
the familiar metaphase chromosome,
which is visible through the light
microscope.

DNA loops is 50,000 base pairs, or 17 micrometers in length, each loop of DNA can form a string of nucleosomes that are either coiled to form 2.6 micrometers of a 10 nanometer fiber, or supercoiled into 0.4 micrometers of a 34 nanometer fiber. Thus, to create the thickness of a sister chromatid (Figure 1), which is 1 micron in diameter, would require just one more order of chromatin folding above the 34 nanometer supercoil. Figure 6 shows a possible model of this final level of chromatin folding.

How is the packaging of DNA loops controlled in response to chromosome functions? Evidence suggests that the inactive form of chromatin is the 34-nanometer supercoil or solenoid of nucleosomes. For both DNA transcription and genome replication this supercoil of nucleosomes must first be uncoiled to the linear array of nucleosomes and then the DNA must uncoil even further to allow access of the transcriptional machinery or the replication machinery to the DNA sequences. Whenever DNA is constrained by proteins to form a loop, DNA supercoiling becomes an important consideration in understanding DNA structure-function relationships. DNA supercoiling has been subjected to extensive experimental and mathematical analysis.

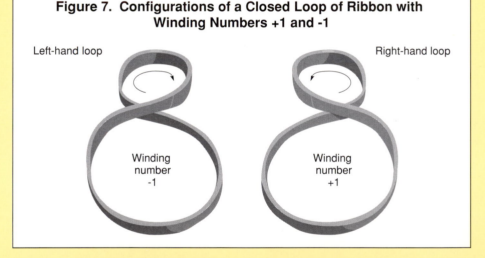

Figure 7. Configurations of a Closed Loop of Ribbon with Winding Numbers +1 and -1

Left-hand loop

Right-hand loop

Winding number -1

Winding number +1

Consider a model in which each DNA loop is firmly attached to the protein scaffold of a chromosome and is therefore somewhat analogous to a closed loop of ribbon. A closed loop of ribbon has a topologically invariant property known as the winding number, which is the number of twists in the ribbon plus the number of times the ribbon crosses itself, that is, coils about itself. The winding number is an integer or half-integer and remains constant unless the ribbon is cut. Each complete twist and each complete crossing adds $+1$ or -1 to the winding number depending on the direction of the twist or crossing. A right-handed twist (the same direction as the thread of a standard screw and the standard helical structure of a double-stranded DNA molecule) is positive, and a left-handed twist is negative. Similarly, a crossing that produces an extra right-handed loop in a loop of ribbon is positive, and a crossing that produces an extra left-handed loop in a loop of ribbon is negative (see Figure 7).

Now consider a loop of double-stranded DNA. Unconstrained DNA has 10.4 to 10.6 base pairs in each complete turn of the double helix. Taking the value 10.6 base pairs per helical turn, the twist (Tw) of a loop of unconstrained DNA consisting of N base pairs would be $N/10.6$. Because a double-stranded DNA molecule already has a helical structure, a loop of DNA further coiled about itself is said to be supercoiled. The linking number (Lk) of a closed loop of DNA is defined in terms of the twist and the number of supercoils, or writhe (Wr), through the equation $Lk = Tw + Wr$. Twists can be converted into supercoils, but Lk must remain constant in a DNA loop whose ends are fixed, in analogy with the constancy of the winding number of the loop of ribbon. If the loop is closed, the linking number must be an integer.

As an example, suppose three helical turns of a linear stretch of DNA are unwound and the ends are then joined. The linking-number change resulting from the unwinding is −3, and the loop can take on any of the three configurations shown in Figure 8. Moreover, the three configurations can be converted into one another without cutting the DNA. DNA configured as in (b) and (c) is said to be negatively supercoiled.

As shown in Figure 3, the DNA in the nucleosome core particle has 1.7 left-handed supercoils and in early studies it was expected that the linking-number change associated with the dissociation of a core particle would be −1.7. However, the experimentally determined linking-number change was −1.02. Although this difference was unexpected and initially controversial, it is easily explained by the change in twist between the DNA constrained in the core particle and free DNA in solution. The average DNA helical repeat on the core particle as measured from its crystal structure is 10.1 base pairs per turn. If we take the average helical repeat of free DNA as 10.6 base pairs per turn, the difference in twist between the DNA in the core particle and free DNA would be $146/10.1 - 146/10.6$ that is, 0.68. Thus the linking-number change associated with the core particle $\Delta Lk = -1.7 + 0.68 = -1.02$ as observed.

Now we can suggest how a DNA loop packaged as a 34-nanometer supercoil of nucleosomes (see Figure 6) could be unwound during interphase. If negative supercoils previously constrained by the nucleosomes are released, then negative supercoiling must be taken up by the linker DNA joining one nucleosome to another. This negative supercoiling would favor the unwinding of a 34-nanometer supercoil of nucleosomes. As suggested above, the acetylation of histones releases DNA that was negatively supercoiled about the histone octamer, presumably by unwinding DNA from the ends of the nucleosome.

The reverse process of chromosome condensation to the metaphase configuration (see Figure 1) requires that the 34-nanometer supercoil be further coiled into higher orders of coiling(s). Perhaps histone-H1 phosphorylation introduces additional supercoiling into a packaged DNA loop causing the higher order of coilings of metaphase chromosomes.

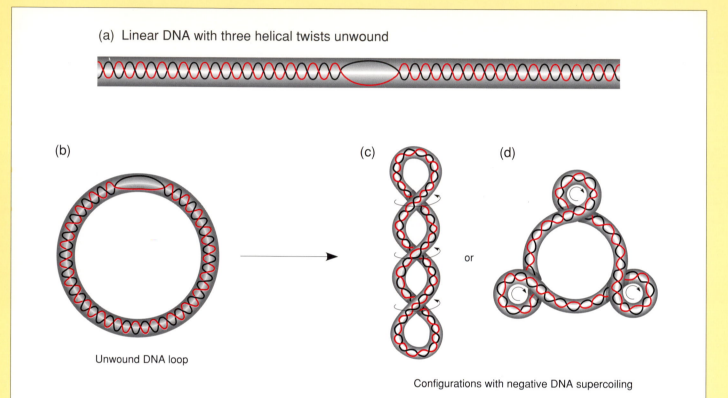

(a) Linear DNA with three helical twists unwound

(b)

Unwound DNA loop

(c)

or

(d)

Configurations with negative DNA supercoiling

Figure 8.   Negative Supercoiling of a Closed DNA Loop
If three helical twists of a linear, double-stranded DNA molecule are unwound as shown in (a) and the ends are then joined, the resulting DNA loop can take on the configurations shown in (b), (c), and (d). All three have the same linking number. In (b) the circular molecule is missing three helical twists that would be present in the normal structure. In (c) the three twists are restored and the loop forms a right-handed superhelix with three crossings in (d) the three twists are restored, but the loop forms three extra left-handed loops.   Configurations (c) and (d) are referred to as negative DNA supercoiling.

Figure 6 shows in outline the different orders of packaging of DNA loops into the different orders of chromatin structure and into metaphase chromosomes. It appears that the reversible chemical modifications of acetylation and phosphorylation of histones are involved in the structural transitions undergone by a chromosome during the cell cycle. These structural transitions are dictated by the functional requirements of chromosomes.

Conclusion

Despite recent advances in understanding centromeres and telomeres, we are still a long way from understanding the relationships between structure and function of eukaryotic chromosomes. Relevant to this understanding will be the sequence information from the Human Genome Project. Although much interest is now focused on the mapping and sequencing of genes, the noncoding DNA regions clearly contain information involved in the organization and functions of chromosomes. The constancy of the banding patterns of individual metaphase chromosomes reflects a highly reproducible pattern of long-range DNA folding, most probably directed by specific DNA-protein interactions and possibly by unusual DNA structures such as bent DNA segments. Superimposed on the very long-range order suggested by banding patterns is the packaging of the DNA loops by the histones together with other structural and regulatory proteins.

The existence of several subtypes of each histone raises the possibility that DNA loops containing different gene families could be packaged with different types of histones according to the requirements of the different cells. DNA control regions of active genes must be packaged in a fashion that makes them accessible to gene-regulating proteins, whereas regions containing permanently repressed genes of a particular cell type may be packaged so that they are inaccessible to such proteins. Such packaging may also determine the availability of DNA regions to chemical damage. Thus a knowledge of the organization of chromosomes is essential to an understanding of the central processes of cell differentiation and the orderly development of complex organisms as well as the processes of DNA damage in chromosomes. ∎

Further Reading

E. Morton Bradbury, "Reversible Histone Modifications and the Chromosome Cell Cycle." *BioEssays*, Volume 14, No. 1. January 1992.

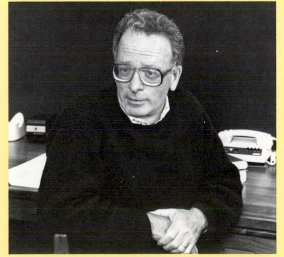

Morton Bradbury received a bachelor of science degree in physics and a Ph.D. in biophysics from King's College, University of London, in 1955 and 1958, respectively. After completing his postdoctoral research at Courtauld Research Laboratory, he was appointed head of the Department of Molecular Biology at Portsmouth (England) Polytechnic in 1962, where he remained until his appointment at UC Davis in 1979. He became leader of the Life Sciences Division at Los Alamos in 1988. Bradbury's research has been devoted to understanding whether chromosome organization and chromosome structure are involved in determining how a cell looks and behaves; the structure and function of active chromatin; and the process by which chromosomes condense prior to cell division. In pursuing his investigations, Bradbury has combined the results of measurements derived from the use of a wide range of techniques, including optical spectroscopy, nuclear magnetic resonance, x-ray diffraction, electron diffraction, and neutron diffraction. The recipient of numerous award and honors, Bradbury has also chaired a number of scientific organizations, including the British Biophysical Society, the International Council for Magnetic Resonance in Biology, and the Neutron/Biology Committee of the Institut Laue-Langevin. Bradbury is a member of HERAC and a member of the HERAC subcommittee on structural biology.

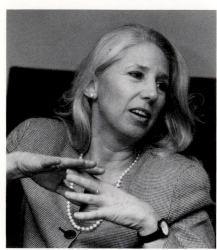

Nancy Wexler

Ultimately, the public will have to exert their democratic powers in order to implement the changes that meet their needs. The research and activities funded by ELSI are intended as a catalyst for public discussion of the problems and a foundation for their eventual solutions.

They have already worked out their actuarial tables, and they don't necessarily want to do that all over again. I don't believe that the insurance companies are welcoming future genetic-testing capabilities as a wonderful new tool that will enable them to better discriminate against people, but they need to figure out how the Genome Project will affect their business, what changes they can expect, and how they will handle these changes.

ELSI's Insurance Task Force includes representatives from the insurance industry, corporate benefit plans, and consumer and health groups who are all working together to come up with a plan of action for developing guidelines for insurance policy by 1993. It is significant that all these groups are working *together* in order to arrive at practical, realistic solutions to complex problems.

David Galas: In the past, society has largely ignored problems of genetic discrimination because too few people were affected. But a significant number of people have lost their health insurance or been discriminated against in employment because someone, in ignorance, decided they were at risk for some genetic disease. With the introduction of new genetic tests, more and more people will become vulnerable to such injustices.

Now, because the Genome Project has a very high visibility, we can stimulate society to come to grips with some fundamental problems. We need to address old problems like the confidentiality of medical records, what medical insurance really means in our society, and what it means to spread out risks. These problems are very difficult, and anyone who says they are going to be solved easily is just not thinking.

Nancy Wexler: Certainly, ELSI can't be counted on to *solve* all the problems. What ELSI *can* do is provide an infrastructure or framework for anticipating and describing the basic issues. We have begun to fund research grants, sponsor conferences, provide fellowships, and commission studies in order to stimulate positive changes.

We're trying to pave the way for practical responses to social challenges—old and new—through research, planning, and the development of public awareness. Ultimately, the public will have to exert their democratic powers in order to implement the changes that meet their needs. The research and activities funded by ELSI are intended as a catalyst for public discussion of the problems and a foundation for their eventual solutions.

David Galas: But we need to encourage people to submit proposals dealing with the hard issues that will impact the public directly. I've seen some of the proposals submitted to the DOE by the academic community, and in my view, many of them are unnecessary and rather off the mark. For example, I read one proposal aimed at studying the implications of the Human Genome Project for reductionism. Reductionism is a perfectly fine thing to study, but the Genome Project is not any more reductionist than the rest of biology.

We need studies and proposals that make specific suggestions about the legal agenda, educational programs, and pilot projects that will be really useful. A good example is the NIH-sponsored pilot project to study the problems associated with making a genetic test for cystic fibrosis available to the public. That study will focus on many significant issues such as confidentiality and methods of information delivery and genetic counseling.

David Cox: The pilot project on cystic-fibrosis testing was initially spearheaded by the Human Genome Project. Since the map of the human genome will allow for the isolation of many disease genes and the diagnostic testing of people at risk for those diseases, we believe that the cystic-fibrosis screening program will provide a valuable model for future genetic-screening programs.

Of course the NIH has for many years been involved with ensuring that the results of basic research on diseases are delivered to the public in the form of new medical services. After the cystic-fibrosis gene was cloned, we heard a lot of talk about a testing program, but at that time none of the NIH organizations were willing to put up the money to figure out in advance the best way to deliver screening and counseling to the general public. The community of scientists and healthcare professionals came forward and said, "This is a gap that is not being filled. If you guys say that the Genome Project is going to improve the quality of genetic services in our society, then you had better get on the stick!" And so we did. The Genome Project took the lead in initiating the pilot program, and as a result, the NIH called for applications for research grants to develop the best methods for delivering genetic services.

Nancy Wexler: The cystic-fibrosis pilot studies are being carried out by a group of seven research teams around the country. The research is supported by grants from three different NIH components—the National Center for Nursing Research [NCNR], the National Institute of Child Health and Human Development [NICHD], and of course, the National Center for Human Genome Research [NCHGR]. ELSI will be managing and coordinating the three-year study. All of the groups involved have a strong interest in the ways in which new genetic tests are integrated into clinical practice.

Rather than slow the science, we need to accelerate the creation of a social system that will be more hospitable to new information about our genes, our heritage, and our future. It's a big job, but it's very exciting.

David Cox: Developing methods of screening for cystic fibrosis is complicated by the fact that there are many different mutations of the gene that causes the disease, and at present the tests screen for most but not all of them. First, we have to decide what type of screening is and isn't possible, and then, what services should or should not be made available.

Eventually, the screening technology developed by the Project will be transferred to the commercial sector, but commercialization is a complicated issue. Many companies want to offer cystic-fibrosis screening because such a venture would be quite profitable. However, there are no regulatory systems in place that will ensure that the interests of the public are protected. We have no data that tell us exactly what problems to expect nor have we yet developed methods to address those that might arise.

The American Society of Human Genetics made a statement several years ago recommending against general population screening for cystic fibrosis until more information was available. Their recommendation made some companies very unhappy. Now there is increasing pressure to ignore that recommendation and to proceed with screening in answer to an inferred demand on the part of the community. That's why the pilot projects are so crucial. Without well thought-out regulations based on experience and sound data, every time a gene is cloned there will be a free market where new tests are offered without regard to the impact on the public.

It's clear that we need concrete and practical initiatives, involving both the public and the scientific community, that give suggestions as to how the Genome Project can be most beneficial to society. But suggestions that merely prohibit the main goal of the Project, which is to construct the tools for deciphering the human genome, will not be useful or beneficial. Balancing the long-term vision with more immediately practical concerns is very difficult, but it must be done if the Project is to use this country's resources to best advantage.

Nancy Wexler: The Genome Project is going to have a profound effect on people because it is so closely related to how we function, how we live, how we become ill, and how we heal ourselves. It would be foolish to try to slow down the advancing science—the advances promise better treatments for disease, better quality of life and health for society. Rather than slow the science, we need to accelerate the creation of a social system that will be more hospitable to new information about our genes, our heritage, and our future. It's a big job, but it's very exciting. ∎

[For further discussion of ELSI issues, see "ELSI: Ethical, Legal, and Social Implications" and "An Invitation to Genetics in the 21st Century."]

The Participants

David Baltimore received a B.A. in chemistry from Swarthmore College in 1960 and a Ph.D. in biology from Rockefeller University in 1964. In 1975 he shared the Nobel Prize in Physiology or Medicine with Howard Temin and Renato Dulbecco for "discoveries concerning the interaction between tumor viruses and the genetic material of the cell." In 1970, independently of but simultaneously with Temin, he discovered reverse transcriptase, making possible much of the innovative genetic research that followed. Baltimore has served in academic posts including postdoctoral fellow at MIT (1963–1964), postdoctoral fellow at Albert Einstein College of Medicine (1964–1965), research associate at the Salk Institute (1965-1968), associate professor at MIT (1968–1972), and Professor of Biology at MIT (1972–1990). He also served year-long appointments as American Cancer Society Research Professor and as Director of the Whitehead Institute. In July 1990 he became president of Rockefeller University; he resigned from that position in December 1991 but remains on the faculty. Baltimore has received numerous scientific awards and has been a leading spokesperson on many national and international issues related to science including genetic research, biological warfare, AIDS research, and the regulation of science.

David Botstein earned his A.B. from Harvard University in 1963 and his Ph.D. from the University of Michigan in 1967. He then joined the faculty of the Massachusetts Institute of Technology where he eventually became a Professor of Genetics. In 1990 he moved to his present position as Professor and Chairman of the Department of Genetics at Stanford University School of Medicine. Botstein's research has centered on genetics. The bacteriophage P22 was the focus of his earliest work, which included studies of DNA replication, recombination, assembly of the viral head, and DNA maturation. In the 1970s he studied the budding yeast *Saccharomyces cerevisiae* and developed novel genetic techniques to study the functions of the actin and tubulin cytoskeletons. In 1980 Botstein made a significant theoretical contribution to human genetics when he suggested, with collaborators, that restriction-fragment-length polymorphisms (RFLPs) could be used to produce a linkage map of the human genome and to map the genes that cause disease in humans. Botstein has won many scientific awards including the Genetics Society of America Medal (1985), the Allen Award of the American Society of Human Genetics (1989), and the 1992 Rosenstiel Award. He serves on the Advisory Council of the National Center for Human Genome Research and, along with R. W. Davis, is helping to organize the Stanford Yeast Genome Project.

David R. Cox earned his A.B. in biology from Brown University and his M.D. and Ph.D. in medicine and genetics from University of Washington in 1975. Since receiving his doctorate—except for a brief period of medical residency at Yale New Haven Hospital—Cox has been with the University of California at San Francisco. Currently, he is a professor in the Departments of Psychiatry, Biochemistry, and Pediatrics and is Director of the Medical Scientist Training Program at UCSF. Cox has served in several public advisory positions, has been a member of the Biomedical Sciences Study Section and the Mammalian Genetics Study Section at the NIH, and has served on the Scientific Advisory Board of the Genome Data Base at Johns Hopkins University.

David J. Galas earned his B.A. in physics at the University of California, Berkeley, and his M.S. and Ph.D. in physics at the University of California, Davis, and Lawrence Livermore National Laboratory. Before joining the faculty at University of Southern California in 1981, Galas spent four years at the Molecular Biology Department of the University of Geneva, Switzerland. His research interests have included the study of transposition of genetic elements and the study of DNA-protein interactions. He has developed several techniques used in molecular-biology research, including the widely used DNA "footprinting" method, a technique for determining specific DNA sites that interact with proteins and are involved in the regulation of gene transcription. In April 1990 Galas became the Department of Energy's Associate Director for Health and Environmental Research. Major DOE programs for which he is responsible include the Human Genome Project, the Structural Biology Program, the Global Change Research Program, and the Subsurface Science Program. Galas is a member of several federal advisory boards and scientific societies, and he chairs the Biotechnology Research Subcommittee for the Federal Coordinating Council on Science and Technology.

Leroy Hood received an M.D. from the Johns Hopkins Medical School and a Ph.D. in biochemistry from the California Institute of Technology. His research interests have been focused primarily on the study of molecular immunology and biotechnology. The Hood laboratory has played a major role in the development of automated microchemical instrumentation that permits the highly sensitive sequence analysis of proteins and DNA as well as the synthesis of peptides and gene fragments. More recently, Hood has applied his laboratory's expertise in large-scale DNA mapping and sequencing to the analysis of the human and mouse T-cell receptor loci—an important effort for the Human Genome Project. Hood is a member of the National Academy of Sciences and the American Association of Arts and Sciences. He has received numerous awards including the Louis Pasteur Award for Medical Innovation, the ARCS Foundation Man of Science Award for deciphering the message of DNA, and the Albert Lasker Basic Medical Research Award for studies of immune diversity. In 1990 he received the American College of Physicians Award of Distinguished Service for work in the development of instruments used to study modern biology and medicine. Currently, Hood is Bowles Professor of Biology and Director of the NSF Science and Technology Center for Molecular Biotechnology at the California Institute of Technology.

Robert K. Moyzis is Director of the Center for Human Genome Studies at

Los Alamos National Laboratory and is known for his work on human genome organization. His discovery of the human telomere is a landmark in the history of our understanding of chromosome structure and function. In the language of genetics, this sequence $(TTAGG)_n$, means "the end." Its isolation not only provided the necessary end-points of human chromosomes but also supplied the first evidence that unusual DNA structures can have biological importance as a second informational "code." Moyzis leads the physical-mapping effort at Los Alamos and continues to balance his research and administrative responsibilities in the genome center. He serves on numerous committees that oversee the DOE and NIH Human Genome Project, including the DOE Human Genome Coordinating Committee and the joint NIH-DOE Human Genome Advisory Committee. Moyzis received his B.A. in biology and chemistry from Northeastern Illinois University in 1971 and his Ph.D. in molecular biology from the Johns Hopkins University in 1978. Following postdoctoral and faculty appointments in the biophysics division at Johns Hopkins, he moved to Los Alamos in 1983. From 1984 to 1989 Moyzis led the Laboratory Genetics Group, taking his current position as center director in 1989.

Maynard V. Olson earned his B.S. in chemistry from the California Institute of Technology in 1965 and his Ph.D. in chemistry from Stanford University in 1970. His doctoral thesis concentrated on physical inorganic chemistry. Olson joined the faculty of Dartmouth College as an Assistant Professor of Chemistry in 1969. He spent one year on sabbatical leave at the University of Washington and returned in 1976 as a Research Associate in the genetics laboratory of Benjamin Hall. In 1979 he joined the Department of Genetics at Washington University, where he is now a Professor of Genetics. In 1989 Olson became an investigator at the Howard Hughes Medical Institute at Washington University. His research specialties are in yeast and human genetics with an emphasis on the long-range organization of eukaryotic genomes and the structure and function of eukaryotic chromosomes. Olson

has pioneered techniques for constructing physical maps, and in 1991 he completed a high-resolution physical map of the genome of the yeast *Saccharomyces cerevisiae*. He and his coworkers at Washington University developed the technology for cloning large DNA inserts in yeast artificial chromosomes (YACs). Olson is a member of the National Institutes of Health Program Advisory Committee on the Human Genome.

Nancy S. Wexler is an internationally respected authority on research into the genetic causes of human disease. In 1981 she began to study the world's largest known family with Huntington's disease, a family living along the shores of Lake Maracaibo in Venezuela. Over the years she and her colleagues have constructed a pedigree of over 12,000 people in the family and have collected blood samples from more than 3000 people. The samples led to the mapping of the Huntington's disease gene to the tip of human chromosome 4, which in turn led to the development of an effective presymptomatic test involving DNA markers that are tightly linked to the Huntington's disease gene. Wexler earned her A.B. from Radcliffe College in 1967 and her Ph.D. in Clinical Psychology from the University of Michigan in 1974. Wexler is President of the Hereditary Disease Foundation and Professor of Clinical Neuropsychology in the Departments of Neurology and Psychiatry of the College of Physicians and Surgeons at Columbia University. In addition to organizing and participating in many research collaborations, Wexler is a member of the Program Advisory Committee of NCHGR (National Center for Human Genome Research) and is chairperson of the Joint NIH/DOE ELSI (Ethical, Legal, and Social Implications of the Human Genome Project) Working Group.

Norton D. Zinder earned his A.B. from Columbia University in 1947 and his Ph.D. from University of Wisconsin in 1952. His first major discovery resulted from the attempt to induce matings between two strains of the bacterium *Salmonella typhimurium*. Zinder and Professor Joshua Lederberg found cell colonies that were the

product of a hitherto unknown process (now called transduction) in which bacteriophages act as carriers of genetic material from one bacterial strain to another. After receiving his doctorate Zinder joined the faculty of Rockefeller University as an assistant professor. In 1960 Zinder and a graduate student, Timothy Loeb, discovered seven new viruses that infected only "male" strains of *E. coli*. The viruses, f1 through f7, proved to be unusual. The genetic material of f1 was found to contain a single strand of DNA and f2 through f7 were the first known RNA bacteriophages (phages whose genetic material is RNA). Zinder and his group demonstrated in 1962 that replication of an RNA phage is not dependent on DNA and that its RNA acts both as genetic material and as a template for directing protein synthesis. Zinder was appointed a professor at Rockefeller University in 1964 and the John D. Rockefeller Jr. Professor in 1977. His recent research emphasizes genetic recombination of the bacteriophage f1 and the physical mapping of its genome by means of restriction enzymes. In addition, he has conducted extensive nucleotide sequence analyses of messenger RNA from both prokaryotes and eukaryotes. An active editor, author, and spokesman on the responsibilities of scientists, Zinder has chaired many scientific committees and advisory panels, including a committee that evaluated the Virus Cancer Program of the National Cancer Institute, the Section of Genetics, National Academy of Sciences (1979–1982), the NAS/NRC (BAST) Committee on the Disposal of Chemical Weapons (1982–1984), and the Committee of Industry-University Relationships (COGENE) of the International Council of Scientific Unions (1982–1984). He was one of the original members of the Committee on Recombinant DNA Molecules of the National Research Council of the National Academy of Sciences in 1974–1975. He received the Eli Lilly Award in Microbiology in 1962 and the National Academy of Sciences' United States Steel Foundation Award in molecular biology in 1966 "for the discovery of RNA phages and for the analysis of the mechanisms of their replication." In 1982 Zinder received the AAAS Award in Scientific Freedom and Responsibility. ∎

The Mapping of
Chromosome
16

Norman A. Doggett, Raymond L. Stallings,
Carl E. Hildebrand, and Robert K. Moyzis

Each human chromosome contains a single giant DNA molecule, ranging in size from 263 million base pairs (Chromosome 1) to less than 50 million base pairs (Chromosome 23). The chromosomes become visible at the time of cell division, when the proteins associated with the DNA undergo a series of protein–protein interactions that fold the chromosome into a shorter, thicker structure. At this stage, the chromosomes can be easily visualized if they are exposed to a fluorescent dye that binds specifically to DNA nucleotides; the dye imparts an overall red color to the chromosomes, as seen in the accompanying photomicrographs.

A further level of analysis allows the localization of individual genetic regions along the chromosome. Here one takes a segment of genomic DNA (for instance a restriction fragment derived from a recombinant DNA library) and allows it to search through the 46 human chromosomes immobilized on a glass slide to find its complementary (homologous) DNA sequence by forming Watson–Crick base pairs. For this analysis, both the "probe" DNA segment and the target chromosomal DNA are "denatured" into single strands of nucleic acid prior to the search-and-find annealing process. Furthermore, the probe DNA fragment is constructed to display its own fluorescent component so that when it finds its complementary DNA in the chromosome, the targeted region now glows with a second fluorescent color—here yellow.

The accompanying micrographs show the results of hybridizing human chromosomes with the full set of DNA fragments derived from purified chromosome 16. As a result, the two Chromosome 16s glow yellow all along their length (upper-right and lower-middle). When one or a few specific probe fragments are annealed, as shown in the inset, defined regions of the chromosome are highlighted, creating a preliminary genetic map that shows the location of the specific DNA segments within the chromosome. Finally, the base-pair sequence of the specific DNA segment can be determined, and its gene-coding regions identified at the nucleotide level.

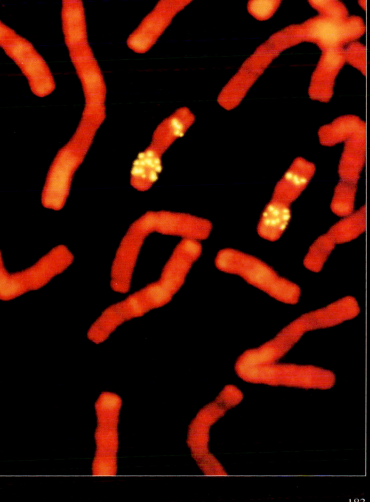

Setting the Stage

Both the molecular and the physical technology for constructing physical maps of complex genomes have developed at a blistering pace over the past five years, due largely to the initiation of the Human Genome Project. These technologies include the cloning of very large DNA fragments, electrophoretic separation of million-base-sized DNA fragments, and sequence-based mapping using the polymerase chain reaction (PCR) to identify unique sequences along the genome. The latter provides a language for interrelating various types of genome maps. The significance of these developments is discussed in Part II of "Mapping the Genome."

In 1988, when our laboratory initiated the physical mapping of chromosome 16, the cloning of very large DNA fragments in yeast artificial chromosomes (YACs) was just beginning in a handful of laboratories and only one library of YAC clones containing all the DNA in the human genome had been constructed worldwide. The total human-genomic YAC library was constructed at Washington University, where the technique of YAC cloning had originally been developed. The polymerase chain reaction had not yet become a standard tool of molecular biology, and the use of sequence-tagged sites (STSs) as unique DNA landmarks for physical mapping had not yet been conceived (see "The Polymerase Chain Reaction and Sequence-tagged Sites" in "Mapping the Genome"). Thus, in 1988 the most modern tools for large-scale physical mapping of human chromosomes were still waiting in the wings. On the other hand, a number of

[*Opening pages: large photomicrograph courtesy of Evelyn Campbell; inset image courtesy of David Ward, Yale University School of Medicine.*]

mapping techniques had been developed and were being applied to the genomes of some of the favorite organisms of molecular biologists.

Cassandra Smith and Charles Cantor had used pulsed-field gel electrophoresis to order the very large restriction fragments produced by cutting the *E. coli* genome with two rare-cutting restriction enzymes. The resulting long-range restriction map of *E. coli* demonstrated that pulsed-field gel electrophoresis is a way to study the long-range order of landmarks on the DNA of human chromosomes. Contig maps, or physical maps of ordered, overlapping cloned fragments, were near completion for the genomes of *E. coli* (about 5 million base pairs) and the yeast *S. cerevisiae* (about 13 million base pairs). Those maps were constructed using lambda-phage clones, which carry an average DNA insert size of 20,000 base pairs. Work had also begun on mapping the genome of the nematode (100 million base pairs) using cosmid clones. Cosmids carry the much longer average insert size of 35,000 base pairs.

The haploid human genome, which includes one copy of each human chromosome, has 3 billion base pairs and is therefore about 250 times the size of the yeast genome and 30 times the size of the nematode genome. When plans for the Human Genome Project were being discussed in the late 1980s, it was natural to consider dividing the human genome by chromosome and mapping one chromosome at a time.

Ongoing work at Los Alamos on human DNA and on adapting flow-sorting technology to separating individual human chromosomes set the stage for the Laboratory to play a key role in the Human Genome Project. In particular, as part of the National Gene Library Project, a group led by Larry Deaven had constructed twenty-four libraries, or unordered collections

of lambda-phage clones, each containing DNA from one of the twenty-four human chromosomes (see "Libraries from Flow-sorted Chromosomes"). Those chromosome-specific libraries were designed as a source of probes to find polymorphic DNA markers for constructing genetic-linkage maps (see "Modern Linkage Mapping") and as a source of clones for rapid isolation of genes using cDNAs, or coding-region probes, to pick out the appropriate clones from the libraries. Deaven and his group were also constructing larger-insert chromosome-specific libraries using cosmid vectors. The large DNA inserts were prepared by partially digesting sorted chromosomes with restriction enzymes, thereby creating overlapping fragments. The cloned fragments would therefore be useful in constructing physical maps of ordered, overlapping clones covering extended regions of human chromosomes. Among the first chromosome-specific cosmid libraries to be constructed at Los Alamos was one for human chromosome 16.

Human chromosomes range in size from 50 million base pairs for chromosome 21 to 263 million base pairs for chromosome 1. Chromosome 16, which is about 100 million base pairs in length, was chosen as our primary target for large-scale physical mapping. We selected chromosome 16 for a number of technical reasons including: (1) the availability of a hybrid-cell line containing a single copy of chromosome 16 in a mouse-chromosome background, which permitted accurate sorting of human chromosome 16 from the mouse chromosomes and thus the construction of a high-purity chromosome 16-specific library of cosmid clones for use in map construction; (2) identification of a chromosome 16-specific satellite repetitive-sequence probe permitting accurate purity assessments of sorted chromosomes; and (3) the availability,

Table 1. Disease Genes Localized to Human Chromosome 16

Location	Symbol	Cloned	Disease
16p13.3	HBA	Yes	Thalassemia
16p13.3	PKD1	No	Autosomal dominant polycystic kidney disease
16p13.3	MEF	No	Familial Mediterranean fever
16p13.3	RTS	No	Rubinstein-Taybi syndrome
16p12	CLN3	No	Batten's disease (juvenile-onset neuronal ceroid lipofuscionosis)
16q12	PHKB	No	Glycogen-storage disease, type VIIIb
16q13	CETP	Yes	Elevated high-density lipoprotein (HDL), (CETP deficiency)
16q22.1	LCAT	Yes	Corneal opacities, anemia, proteinuria with unesterified hypercholesterolemia (Norum disease)
16q22.1	TAT	Yes	Richner-Hanhort syndrome, oculocutaneous tyrosinemia II (TAT deficiency)
16q22.1	ALDOA	Yes	Hemolytic anemia (ALDOA deficiency)
16q24.3	APRT	Yes	Urolithiasis, 2,5 dihydroxyadenine (APRT) deficiency
16q24	CYBA	No	Autosomal chronic granulomatous disease
16q	CTM	No	Marner's cataract
16q	CMH2	No	Familial hypertrophic cardiomyopathy

through collaboration, of a panel of a large number of hybrid-cell lines containing portions of chromosome 16. This hybrid-cell panel enables probes from chromosome 16 to be localized into intervals along the chromosome having an average length of 1.6 million base pairs.

Chromosome 16 is also interesting to the biomedical community. It contains gene loci for several human diseases of both clinical and economic importance, including polycystic kidney disease, a class of hemoglobin disorders, and several types of cancer (including leukemia and breast cancer). Table 1 lists disease genes that have been localized to chromosome 16 through genetic-linkage analysis. A physical map of overlapping clones for chromosome 16 would facilitate rapid isolation of those genes not yet cloned.

It takes about 2500 cosmid clones laid end to end to represent all the DNA in chromosome 16 once, and so our chromosome 16-specific library of 25,000 cosmid clones represented a tenfold coverage of the chromosome. In 1988, with funds from the Department of Energy, we took on the physical mapping of chromosome 16.

Developing a Mapping Strategy

Our initial strategy for constructing an ordered-clone, or contig, map for chromosome 16 was to fingerprint cosmid clones chosen at random, determine the overlaps between pairs of clones from the similarities between fingerprints, and assemble the clone pairs into contigs, or islands of overlapping clones. This basic clone-to-fingerprint-to-contig strategy, which is described in "Physical Mapping—A One-Dimensional Jigsaw Puzzle" in "Mapping the Genome", had been applied successfully to the mapping of the *E. coli*, yeast, and nematode genomes. However, those maps of less complex genomes had taken many years of work. In addition, the human genome contains many classes of repetitive sequences that tend to complicate the process of building contigs. When faced with the mapping of human chromosome 16, which is about ten times larger than the yeast genome, we needed to develop a strategy that would increase the speed of contig building while retaining the required accuracy.

Lander and Waterman's 1988 analysis of random-clone fingerprinting suggested the key to increased mapping efficiency. That paper showed that the size of the smallest detectable clone overlap was an important parameter in determining the rate at which contigs would increase in length and therefore the rate at which contig maps would near completion. In particular, the calculated rate of progress increases significantly if the detectable clone overlap is reduced from 50 percent to 25 percent of the clone lengths.

In the mapping efforts for yeast and *E. coli*, the overlap between two clones was detected by preparing a restriction-fragment fingerprint of each clone and identifying restriction-fragment lengths that were common to the two fingerprints. With this method, two clones have to overlap by at least 50 percent in order for one to declare with a high degree of certainty that the two clones do indeed overlap. (See "Physical Mapping—A One-Dimensional Jigsaw Puzzle" for a description of restriction-fragment fingerprinting.) Clearly, increasing the information content in each clone fingerprint would make smaller overlaps detectable.

The Repetitive-Sequence Fingerprint

The unique feature of our initial mapping strategy was what we call the repetitive-sequence fingerprint. Repetitive sequences compose 25 to 35 percent of the human genome. The box at right shows the most abundant classes of repetitive sequences and the approximate locations of those sequences on human chromosome 16.

Various Classes of Human Repetitive DNA Sequences

Described below are the most abundant classes of repetitive DNA on human chromosomes. The figure shows the locations of these classes on chromosome 16. Numbers in parentheses indicate the size of continuous stretches of each repetitive DNA class.

Telomere Repeat: The tandemly repeating unit TTAGGG located at the very ends of the linear DNA molecules in human and vertebrate chromosomes. The telomere repeat $(TTAGGG)_n$ extends for 5000 to 12,000 base pairs and has a structure different from that of normal DNA. A special enzyme called telomerase replicates the ends of the chromosomes in an unusual fashion that prevents the chromosome from shortening during replication.

Subtelomeric repeats: Classes of repetitive sequences that are interspersed in the last 500,000 bases of nonrepetitive DNA located adjacent to the telomere. Some sequences are chromosome specific and others seem to be present near the ends of all human chromosomes.

Microsatellite repeats: A variety of simple di-, tri-, tetra-, and penta-nucleotide tandem repeats that are dispersed in the euchromatic arms of most chromosomes. The dinucleotide repeat $(GT)_n$ is the most common of these dispersed repeats, occurring on average every 30,000 bases in the human genome, for a total copy number of 100,000. The GT repeats range in size from about 20 to 60 base pairs and appear in most eukaryotic genomes.

Minisatellite repeats: A class of dispersed tandem repeats in which the repeating unit is 30 to 35 base pairs in length and has a variable sequence but contains a core sequence 10 to 15 base pairs in length. Minisatellite repeats range in size from 200 base pairs up to several thousand base pairs, have lower copy numbers than microsatellite repeats, and tend to occur in greater numbers toward the telomeric ends of chromosomes.

Alu repeats: The most abundant interspersed repeat in the human genome. The Alu sequence is 300 base pairs long and occurs on average once every 3300 base pairs in the human genome, for a total copy number of 1 million. Alus are more abundant in the light bands than in the dark bands of giemsa-stained metaphase chromosomes. They occur throughout the primate family and are homologous to and thought to be descended from a small, abundant RNA gene that codes for the 300-nucleotide-long RNA molecule known as 7SL. The 7SL RNA combines with six proteins to form a protein-RNA complex that recognizes the signal sequences of newly synthesized proteins and aids in their translocation through the membranes of the endoplasmic recticulum (where they are formed) to their ultimate destination in the cell.

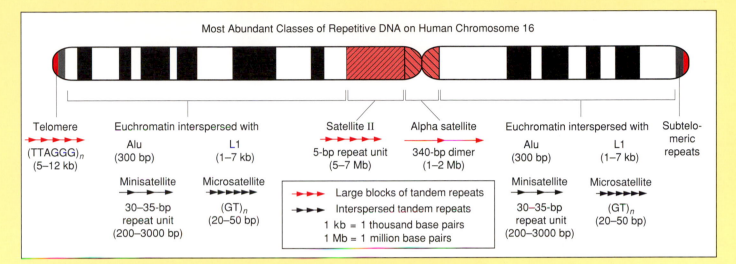

Most Abundant Classes of Repetitive DNA on Human Chromosome 16

| Telomere | Euchromatin interspersed with | | Satellite II | Alpha satellite | Euchromatin interspersed with | | Subtelomeric repeats |

Telomere
(TTAGGG)$_n$
(5–12 kb)

Euchromatin interspersed with
Alu (300 bp) | L1 (1–7 kb)

Satellite II
5-bp repeat unit
(5–7 Mb)

Alpha satellite
340-bp dimer
(1–2 Mb)

Euchromatin interspersed with
Alu (300 bp) | L1 (1–7 kb)

Subtelomeric repeats

Minisatellite
30–35-bp
repeat unit
(200–3000 bp)

Microsatellite
(GT)$_n$
(20–50 bp)

Large blocks of tandem repeats
Interspersed tandem repeats
1 kb = 1 thousand base pairs
1 Mb = 1 million base pairs

Minisatellite
30–35-bp
repeat unit
(200–3000 bp)

Microsatellite
(GT)$_n$
(20–50 bp)

L1 repeats: A long interspersed repeat whose sequence is 1000 to 7000 base pairs long. L1s have a common sequence at the 3′ end but are variably shortened at the 5′ end and thus have a large range of sizes. They occur on average every 28,000 base pairs in the human genome, for a total copy number of about 100,000, and are more abundant in Giemsa-stained dark bands. L1 repeats are also found in most other mammalian species. Full-length L1s (3.5 percent of the total) are a divergent group of class II retrotransposons—"jumping genes" that can move around the genome and are thought to be remnants of retroviruses. [Class II retrotransposons have at least one protein-coding gene and contain a poly A tail (or series of As at the 3′ end) as do messenger RNAs.] Recently, a full-length, functional L1 was discovered. It was found to code for a functional reverse transcriptase—an enzyme essential to the process by which the L1s are copied and re-inserted into the genome.

Alpha satellite DNA: A family of related repeats that occur as long tandem arrays at the centromeric region of all human chromosomes. The repeat unit is about 340 base pairs and is a dimer, that is, it consists of two subunits, each about 170 base pairs long. Alpha satellite DNA occurs on both sides of the centromeric constriction and extends over a region 1000 to 5000 base pairs long. Alpha satellite DNA in other primates is similar to that in humans.

Satellite I, II, and III repeats: Three classical human satellite DNAs, which can be isolated from the bulk of genomic DNA by centrifugation in buoyant density gradients because their densities differ from the densities of other DNA sequences. Satellite I is rich in As and Ts and is composed of alternating arrays of a 17- and 25-base-pair repeating unit. Satellites II and III are both derived from the simple five-base repeating unit ATTCC. Satellite II is more highly diverged from the basic repeating unit than Satellite III. Satellites I, II and III occur as long tandem arrays in the heterochromatic regions of chromosomes 1, 9, 16, 17, and Y and the satellite regions on the short (p) arms of chromosomes 13, 14, 15, 21, and 22.

Cot1 DNA: The fraction of repetitive DNA that is separable from other genomic DNA because of its faster re-annealing, or renaturation, kinetics. *Cot* 1 DNA contains sequences that have copy numbers of 10,000 or greater. ∎

Our work on the distribution of repetitive sequences had shown that the tandem-repeat sequence $(GT)_n$, where n is typically between 15 and 30, was scattered randomly across most regions of the human genome with an average spacing of 30,000 base pairs. The in-situ hybridization in Figure 1 shows that $(GT)_n$ is scattered throughout the arms of human chromosomes but is noticeably absent from the regions around the centromere. (The centromeric regions consists of large blocks of tandem-repeat sequences known as satellite DNA. Gene sequences are absent from these regions. Regions containing large blocks of tandem repeats are known as heterochromatin, and regions devoid of large tandem repeat blocks are known as euchromatin.)

We reasoned that the sequence $(GT)_n$ would appear, on average, about once in each cosmid clone containing a human DNA insert of 35,000 base pairs from the euchromatic arms of chromosome 16. Therefore, we could enrich the information content of the usual restriction-fragment fingerprint of each clone by determining, through hybridization of a radio-labeled $(GT)_{25}$ probe, which restriction fragments in each fingerprint contain the $(GT)_n$ sequence. As we will illustrate below, this information allowed us to detect overlaps between cosmid clones that were as small as 10 percent of their lengths.

To reduce the initial complexity of the mapping, we preselected from our chromosome 16-specific library of clones (through hybridization) those clones that were positive for the $(GT)_n$ sequence and negative for satellite DNA. In other words, we chose to build contigs around those sites in chromosome 16 that contain $(GT)_n$. Since those sites are widely scattered across the chromosome, we expected those contigs to cover the chromosome in a fairly uniform way except for

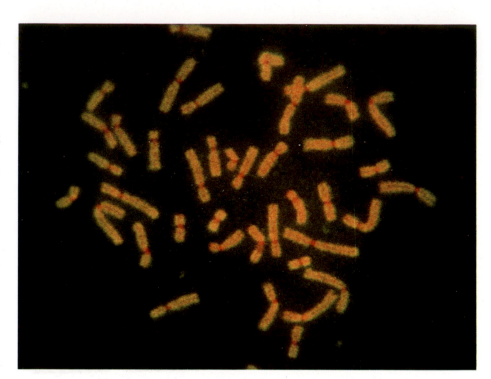

Figure 1. GT Hybridization on Human Chromosomes
The photomicrograph shows in-situ hybridization of human chromosomes using biotin-labeled $(AC)_{25}$ as a probe (yellow). $(AC)_{25}$ hybridizes to sites of the microsatellite repeat $(GT)_n$. Those sites are underrepresented at the centromeric regions of some chromosomes and at the distal half of Yq. However, $(GT)_n$ appears to be uniformly distributed on all euchromatic regions of the human genome.

the centromeric region, which can be mapped using an alternative approach. We identified about 3000 $(GT)_n$-positive clones from our library and made a repetitive-sequence fingerprint for each one.

The repetitive-sequence fingerprint was made by digesting each cosmid clone with restriction enzymes, sizing the resulting restriction fragments, and determining which of those fragments contain $(GT)_n$ as well as another type of repetitive DNA known as *Cot*1, which is also scattered throughout the arms of the chromosome (see box). *Cot*1 is the most abundant fraction of repeated DNA in the human genome, consisting predominantly of Alu and L1 repeated sequences.

The first step in fingerprinting was to isolate many copies of the DNA insert in each cosmid clone, divide those copies into three batches, and digest each batch with the restriction enzymes *Eco*RI, *Hin*dIII, and a mixture of both *Eco*RI and *Hin*dIII, respectively. The restriction fragments from each of the three digests were separated in parallel along three lanes of an agarose gel by electrophoresis. DNA fragments having known lengths were separated on adjacent lanes to determine the fragment lengths from each restriction-enzyme digest. The fragments in the gel were stained with ethidium bromide (a fluorescent dye that binds to DNA) and the gel was photographed under ultraviolet light to produce an image

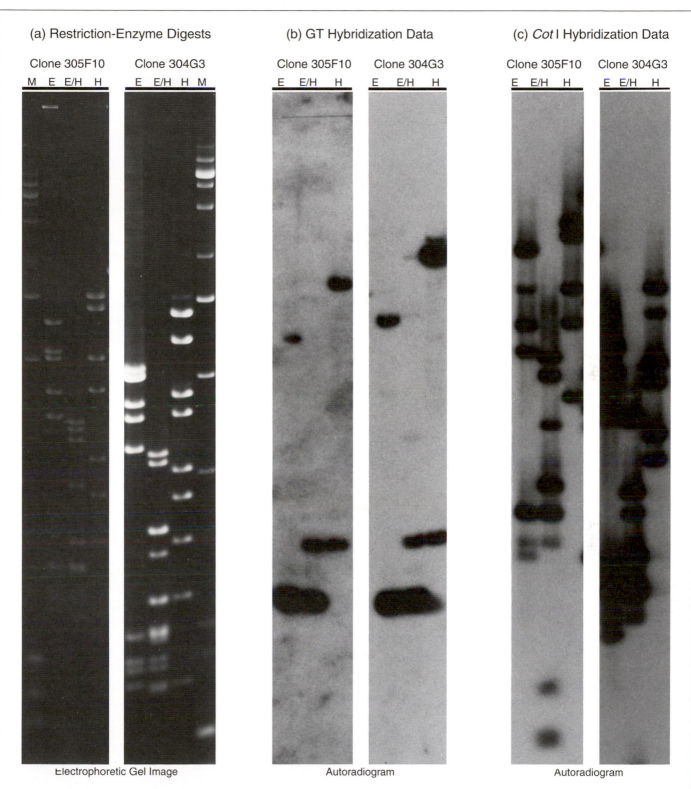

(a) Restriction-Enzyme Digests

Clone 305F10   Clone 304G3

M E E/H H   E E/H H M

Electrophoretic Gel Image

(b) GT Hybridization Data

Clone 305F10   Clone 304G3

E E/H H   E E/H H

Autoradiogram

(c) *Cot* I Hybridization Data

Clone 305F10   Clone 304G3

E E/H H   E E/H H

Autoradiogram

Figure 2. Repetitive Sequence Fingerprints of Two Overlapping Cosmid Clones
The repetitive-sequence fingerprint of a clone has three parts. The figure shows a comparison of those parts for two clones that have a high likelihood of overlap based on the similarities between their fingerprints. **(a)** Fluorescent images of DNA fragments separated by agarose gel electrophoresis. The three gel lanes for each clone contain the restriction fragments produced by completely digesting that clone with the restriction enzymes *Eco*RI (E), *Eco*RI and *Hind* III (E/H), and *Hind* III (H), respectively. The marker lanes (M) contain standard fragments of known lengths, which are used to calibrate the restriction-fragment lengths. **(b)** Autoradiographic images of the gels in (a) after hybridization with the GT probe. **(c)** Autoradiographic images of the gels in (a) after hybridization with the *Cot*1 probe. Clone 305F10 and clone 304G3 have identical GT-hybridization patterns, a strong indication of overlap.

showing the distinct bands of DNA fragments in the gel, each band made up of many copies of a particular restriction fragment. This gel image was then digitized with a CCD camera, the DNA fragments were assigned sizes according to their positions on the gel relative to the known fragment lengths using a commercial software package. These sizes were then stored in our mapping database. Figure 2 shows the gel images for two clones that were determined to overlap one another based on their complete repetitive-sequence fingerprints.

The second step in fingerprinting was to determine which restriction fragments contained $(GT)_n$ and $Cot1$ repetitive DNA. We accomplished this step using standard hybridization techniques. (See "Hybridization Techniques" in "Understanding Inheritance.") Specifically, DNA from each gel was transferred to two different nylon or nitrocellulose membranes using the blotting procedure developed by Edwin Southern in 1975. This blotting procedure preserves the relative positions that the DNA fragments have on the gel. Once the fragments are immobilized on the two membranes, radio-labeled copies of the $(GT)_n$ sequence are used as hybridization probes on one membrane and radio-labeled copies of the $Cot1$ sequences are used as probes on the second membrane. The bands of fragments that contain those sequences and therefore bind, or hybridize, to the radioactive probes can be visualized by exposing an x-ray film to the membrane, a process known as autoradiography. Alongside the gel images shown in Figure 2 are the corresponding autoradiographs, or blot images, produced by the $(GT)_n$ hybridization and $Cot1$ hybridization. Together, the gel image and the two blot images for each clone constitute the repetitive-sequence fingerprint of that clone.

The fingerprint data are scored by first noting the lengths of the restriction fragments on the gel image. Then the gel image and the two blot images for each clone are aligned to determine the hybridization score of each band of restriction fragments. To help us accomplish this task for thousands of clones in an efficient manner, Mike Cannon of the Computer Division at Los Alamos developed a computer program called SCORE. This program takes the fragment lengths determined from the gel image and creates a schematic of the gel image. The blot image is then scanned, and its image size is adjusted to match the schematic of the gel image. Each band is then scored for the presence or absence of a positive hybridization signal from the $(GT)_n$ probe and for the degree of hybridization of the $Cot1$ probe. $Cot1$ creates a low, medium, or high hybridization signal depending on whether the restriction fragment contains short, intermediate, or long stretches of $Cot1$ sequences. (Operation of the SCORE program is illustrated in "SCORE: A Program for Computer-assisted Scoring of Southern Blots" in "Computation and the Human Genome Project.")

Determining the Likelihood That Two Clones Overlap

Once the clones have been finger-printed and the fingerprint data scored and entered into the database, the next step is to determine from the similarities between fingerprints which pairs of clones overlap one another. The problem of determining clone overlap from such fingerprint data is probabilistic, as explained in "Physical Mapping—A One-Dimensional Jigsaw Puzzle." We have two types of information, the sizes of the restriction fragments and the hybridization scores for each fragment. The two questions we need to answer are: Given that the fingerprints of two clones share certain restriction-fragment lengths and hybridization scores, first, what is the probability that they overlap? and second, what is the extent of that overlap?

The first question was addressed by David Torney, a member of the Theoretical Biology and Biophysics Group at Los Alamos. He and his collaborator David Balding developed a complete statistical analysis of the problem, taking into account the known statistical properties of the restriction-fragment lengths, experimental errors in restriction-fragment lengths, hybridization errors, and the expected distribution of the repetitive sequences. They also developed a simplified computer algorithm based on their complete theoretical analysis and on extensive analysis of the actual fingerprint data generated at Los Alamos. That algorithm determines the likelihood that two cosmid clones overlap given the repetitive-sequence fingerprints of those clones.

Figure 3 illustrates how the information content in the repetitive-sequence fingerprint allows the detection of small overlaps. In particular, when $(GT)_n$ is present in the overlap region of two clones, the similarities between the repetitive-sequence fingerprints of those clones yield a nearly unambiguous signature of overlap, even if the region of overlap is small. In the example shown, clones A and B have only a 10 percent overlap, but the overlap region contains the single $(GT)_n$ sequence present on those clones along with two cutting sites for EcoRI and one cutting site for HindIII. Consequently the GT hybridization patterns on the blot images of the two clones are identical within experimental errors and contain one GT-positive band for each restriction-enzyme digest. The likelihood that two

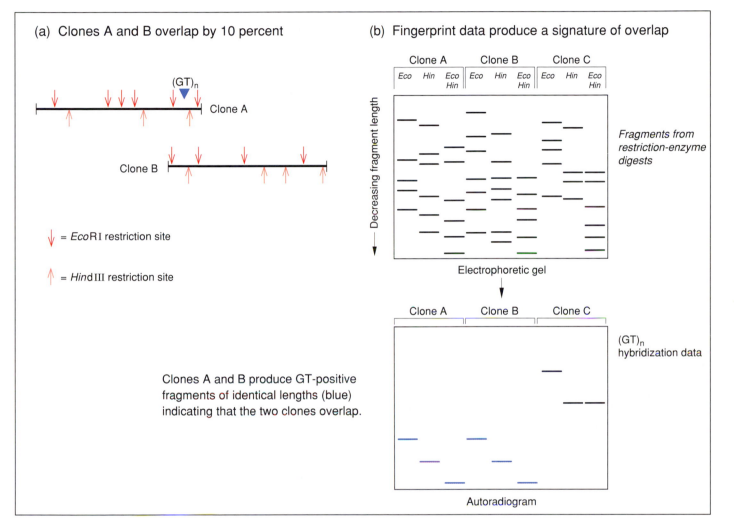

(a) Clones A and B overlap by 10 percent

(b) Fingerprint data produce a signature of overlap

(GT)$_n$

Clone A

Clone B

↓ = *Eco*RI restriction site

↑ = *Hin*dIII restriction site

Clone A   Clone B   Clone C

| Eco | Hin | Eco Hin | Eco | Hin | Eco Hin | Eco | Hin | Eco Hin |

Decreasing fragment length

Fragments from restriction-enzyme digests

Electrophoretic gel

Clones A and B produce GT-positive fragments of identical lengths (blue) indicating that the two clones overlap.

Clone A   Clone B   Clone C

(GT)$_n$ hybridization data

Autoradiogram

Figure 3. Detection of Small Clone Overlaps Using Repetitive-Sequence Fingerprints

Shown in (a) is a diagram of two clones, A and B, that overlap by 10 percent of their lengths. Arrows indicate restriction (cutting) sites for the restriction enzymes *Eco*RI and *Hin*dIII. Clones A and B each contain a single (GT)$_n$ site, which happens to occur in the short overlapping region. Shown in (b) is a diagram of the restriction-fragment fingerprints and corresponding (GT)$_{25}$ hybridization data produced from clones A and B as well as a third clone C. The identical (GT)$_n$ hybridization pattern from clones A and B is sufficient information to infer that the two clones have a very high likelihood of overlap.

such identical patterns would arise from non-overlapping clones is extremely low. In general, if two cosmid clones from our chromosome-specific library produce the same GT-hybridization pattern, they have an extremely high probability of overlapping, even if they share only one GT-positive region.

The detailed computer algorithms used to estimate the probability of clone

overlap from the fingerprint data will not be presented here. Suffice it to say those algorithms are based on Bayes' theorem for conditional probabilities and use parameters for estimating errors in restriction-fragment sizes and hybridization results that were determined through detailed statistical analysis of the experimental conditions. The computer algorithms were used to examine all

possible pairs of fingerprinted clones and determine the probability of overlap for each clone pair.

Assembling the Contig Map

As illustrated in "Physical Mapping—A One-Dimensional Jigsaw Puzzle," restriction-fragment fingerprint

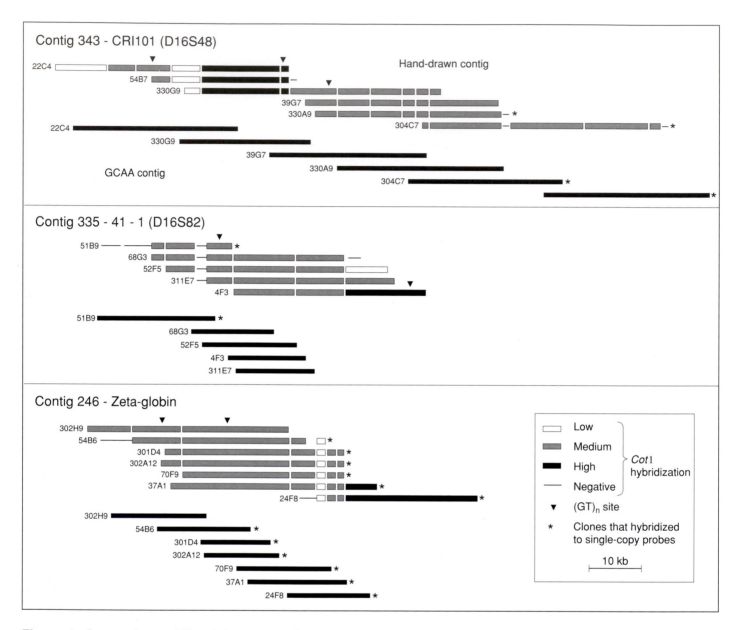

Figure 4. Comparison of Hand-drawn and Computer-generated Cosmid Contigs from Chromosome 16.
Groups of overlapping clones are arranged into contigs showing the linear arrangement and extents of clone overlap deduced from repetitive-sequence fingerprint data. The hand-drawn representations show which restriction fragments were positive for GT and *Cot* 1 hybridization probes and provides a partial ordering of the restriction fragments. The corresponding GCAA-generated contig shows the extent of overlap between clones and the contig length. Additions to GCAA are planned that will enable the algorithm to generate contigs similar to the hand-drawn contigs. As shown, the GCAA contigs sometimes differ in length from the hand-drawn contigs.

data can be used to assemble islands of contiguous, overlapping clones showing the position of each clone relative to the others and the extent of overlap between each pair of overlapping clones.

Initially we assembled contigs by sorting the output of the pairwise overlaps into sets of multiply overlapping clones. More recently Jim Fickett and Michael Cinkosky of the Laboratory's Theoretical Biology and Biophysics Group developed a "genetic algorithm" for contig assembly called GCAA, which has sped up this process considerably. The algorithm is based on optimization theory. Figure 4 compares hand-drawn cosmid contigs for chromosome 16 with versions generated by the genetic algorithm. The hand-drawn contigs are sometimes more accurate, but each one takes many hours to construct. In contrast, the computer algorithm can handle data from thousands of clones and construct hundreds of contigs automatically in a short time. It also allows manual changes to be made through interactive software. The genetic algorithm has been invaluable to our mapping efforts, as has the whole suite of informatics tools developed at Los Alamos for managing, analyzing, utilizing, and sharing mapping data. Some of those tools are described in

"Computation and the Genome Project."

About 3145 GT-positive cosmid clones and an additional 800 GT-negative cosmid clones were fingerprinted and then assembled into contigs in the manner described above. The clones formed 576 contigs with an average size of 100,000 base pairs and containing, on average, four or five clones. The largest cosmid contig spanned approximately 300,000 base pairs. These contigs cover about 58 million base pairs, or 58 percent of chromosome 16. There were also 1171 singletons (single fingerprinted clones not contained within a contig). Experiments discussed below suggest that the singletons cover 26 percent of the chromosome. Together the 4000 fingerprinted clones cover about 84 percent of chromosome 16.

If the minimum detectable overlap between clones is 50 percent of the clone lengths, the equations of Lander and Waterman suggest that one would have to fingerprint about 16,000 clones of an average length of 35,000 base pairs to reach an average contig size of 100,000 base pairs for a chromosome the length of chromosome 16. We reached an average contig size of 100,000 base pairs after fingerprinting only 4000 clones. That reduction was due to two factors. First, the repetitive-sequence fingerprints enabled the detection of clone overlaps composing between 10 and 25 percent of the clone lengths depending on the positions of the $(GT)_n$ sites. In fact, the average length of each detected overlap region was 20 percent of the clone lengths. Second, we did not fingerprint clones at random but rather preselected clones containing $(GT)_n$. By focusing our mapping efforts around regions of $(GT)_n$ sites, we effectively reduced the size of the region that was being mapped during the initial phases of mapping. These two factors resulted in the rapid construction of relatively large cosmid contigs.

Several other features are distinctive about our cosmid-fingerprinting approach. By sizing the restriction fragments from each clone, we know the extent of overlap between clones in a contig, and therefore we can estimate the length of each contig. In contrast, mapping methods that determine clone overlap from hybridization-based or STS data alone cannot determine the extent of the overlap or the length of the contigs without further analysis. Restriction-fragment lengths also provide us with information to generate partially ordered restriction maps for each contig. Finally, as a result of the GT and $Cot1$ hybridizations, we know which fragments contain GT repeats and which fragments contain $Cot1$ DNA. A GT repeat at a given site in the genome varies in length among the population and therefore provides a source of polymorphic markers for genetic-linkage mapping. Our contig map thus provides the positions of fragments containing those potential markers. The $Cot1$ hybridization is useful because fragments that do not hybridize to the $Cot1$ probe are free of the most abundant classes of repetitive DNA and are therefore likely to contain single-copy sequences, which may be candidates for genes. Finally, as the map is further developed and the repetitive-sequence distribution more accurately determined, it may reveal new insights into genome organization and the molecular evolution of mammalian chromosomes.

Evaluation of the Cosmid Contig Map

After constructing the 576 cosmid contigs, we first wanted to ascertain their distribution on chromosome 16. David Callen and Grant Sutherland in Australia located 140 of our cosmid contigs on their panel of mouse/human hybrid cells. The 50 different hybrid cells in their panel contain, in addition to the full complement of mouse chromosomes, increasingly longer portions of human chromosome 16, starting from the far end of the long arm of the chromosome (see Figure 5). In effect, the panel divides the chromosome into bins, or intervals, 1.6 million base pairs in length. They found the 140 cosmid contigs to be distributed evenly over the intervals defined by the hybrid-cell panel.

Second, to evaluate the accuracy of the contigs, we picked 19 pairs of clones from 11 different contigs and checked whether each pair that had been assigned to the same contig hybridized to the same large restriction fragment and therefore came from the same region of chromosome 16. The DNA for these experiments was isolated from a mouse/human hybrid-cell line containing human chromosome 16 only. Eight rare-cutting restriction enzymes were used to make eight different complete digests of the DNA, and the resulting large restriction fragments were separated in parallel by pulsed-field gel electrophoresis. The fragments were then blotted onto filters, and each filter was probed with one clone from each pair. This analysis confirmed that the two members of each of the 19 clone pairs came from the same region of the genome.

A second check on contig accuracy involved hybridization of 43 single-copy probes (probes containing sequences that appear only once in the human genome) to membranes containing a gridded array of our 4000 fingerprinted clones. The single-copy probes were graciously provided by a large number of collaborators and associates. Ideally, if a single-copy probe hybridizes to more than one clone, those clones should be contained within a single contig and

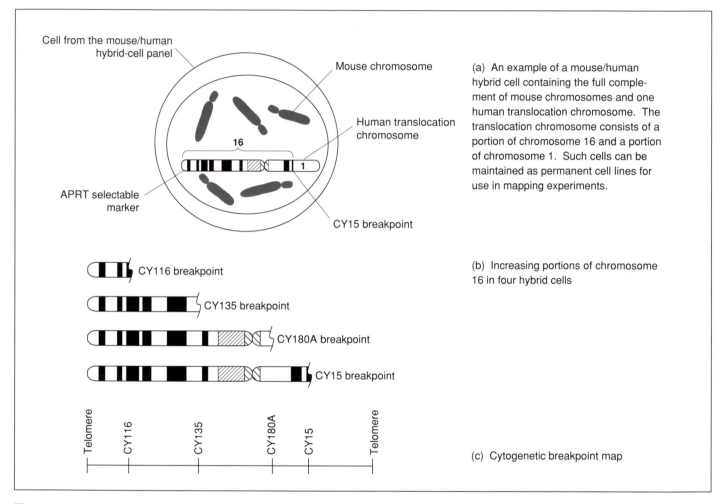

Cell from the mouse/human hybrid-cell panel

Mouse chromosome

Human translocation chromosome

16

APRT selectable marker

CY15 breakpoint

(a) An example of a mouse/human hybrid cell containing the full complement of mouse chromosomes and one human translocation chromosome. The translocation chromosome consists of a portion of chromosome 16 and a portion of chromosome 1. Such cells can be maintained as permanent cell lines for use in mapping experiments.

CY116 breakpoint

CY135 breakpoint

CY180A breakpoint

CY15 breakpoint

(b) Increasing portions of chromosome 16 in four hybrid cells

Telomere — CY116 — CY135 — CY180A — CY15 — Telomere

(c) Cytogenetic breakpoint map

Figure 5. Hybrid-Cell Panel and the Cytogenetic Breakpoint Map for Chromosome 16
A panel of 50 different mouse/human hybrid cells, each containing an increasingly longer portion of chromosome 16 starting from the tip of the long arm of the chromosome, is a convenient tool for constructing a low-resolution physical map of the chromosome. The hybrid cells are formed by fusing mouse cells with human cells and growing them in a medium in which only those cells containing a particular gene (APRT) can survive. Thus APRT is called a selectable marker. It is near the end of the long, or q, arm of chromosome 16. During the fusion process and subsequent growth, human chromosomes that lack the selectable marker are lost, resulting in a mouse/human hybrid containing a single human chromosome 16. The 50 different hybrids were derived from a collection of patients' cells that had each undergone translocations (breakage and rejoining) of chromosome 16 with another human chromosome. (a) The type of hybrid cell produced by the fusion process and selectively grown for inclusion in the panel is shown. The hybrid cell contains the full complement of mouse chromosomes and one chromosome produced by a translocation between human chromosomes 16 and 1. Because this chromosome includes the portion of the q arm of chromosomes 16 containing APRT, it survived the fusion and selective growth process. (b) Increasing portions of chromosome 16 contained in some of the hybrid cells of the panel are shown. The panel contains 50 hybrid cells and, in effect, divides the chromosome into intervals with an average length of 1.6 million bases. Each portion ends at a so-called breakpoint of the chromosome, a natural site of chromosomal translocation. (c) A cytogenic map of chromosome 16 indicating the locations of the breakpoints in (b). The complete cytogenetic breakpoint map derived from the hybrid cell panel contains 50 breakpoints separated by intervals with an average length of 1.6 million base pairs. A human DNA probe or clone from chromosome 16 can be localized to a region between two breakpoints by showing that it hybridizes to the DNA from all hybrid cells containing that region and *does not* hybridize to the DNA from the hybrid cell in which that region is absent.

should overlap one another because they contain the same unique sequence. Our analysis showed no unequivocal false-positive overlaps in our contigs, and it also enabled us to detect overlaps between some singleton clones and our existing contigs.

The hybridizations of single-copy probes to the gridded arrays of fingerprinted clones also allowed us to estimate how much of chromosome 16 is covered by our fingerprinted clones. Out of 43 probes, 25 hybridized to clones within contigs, 11 hybridized to singletons, and 7 did not hybridize to any of the fingerprinted clones. These results suggest that our cosmid contigs cover 58 percent of chromosome 16, and the singleton cosmids cover 26 percent of the chromosome for a total coverage of 84 percent.

Our goal was to construct a map composed of at most 100 contigs, each having an average size of about a million base pairs. Having already achieved substantial coverage, we were at a point where continued random fingerprinting of cosmid clones was no longer the most efficient way to achieve this goal. At that point the likelihood of fingerprinting a new clone that was not yet represented in contigs was diminishing, while the likelihood that the new clone would fall within pre-existing contigs was increasing. The gaps between cosmid contigs could be closed by a directed approach called chromosome walking (see Figure 9 in "DNA Libraries") but to "walk" from one cosmid clone to the next would be a very slow and labor-intensive process.

Fortunately, by that time YAC technology had matured. In 1991 Mary Kay McCormick at Los Alamos successfully constructed chromosome 21-specific YAC libraries from flow-sorted chromosomes using a modified cloning technique. Eric Green and Maynard Olson at Washington University, in collaboration with Bob Moyzis and coworkers at Los Alamos, had developed a substantial number of STS markers for chromosome 7 from our chromosome 7-specific library of M13 clones (a library of cloned single-stranded DNA fragments for sequencing). They thereby demonstrated the feasibility of generating large numbers of STS markers for use in physical mapping.

Green and Olson had already used STS-content mapping to construct a contig of YAC clones covering the region surrounding the cystic-fibrosis gene. In particular, they had developed a set of STS markers from pre-existing genetic-linkage markers, which had been used to find the gene, and from cDNAs for sequences within the cystic-fibrosis gene. Then they used those STSs to screen a YAC library made from total-genomic human DNA and pick out the YAC clones containing each marker. Two YACs that contain the same STS marker must overlap because each STS is a unique sequence that has been shown to appear only once on the genome. Thus, based on the STSs contained in each YAC, they were able to construct a contig of overlapping YAC clones spanning about 1.5 million base pairs and containing the cystic-fibrosis gene.

These advances made it feasible for us to consider closing the gaps in our cosmid contig map with YAC clones from chromosome 16. We decided that the most efficient strategy would be to work with a chromosome 16-specific YAC library.

Improving YAC Cloning Techniques

YACs are cloning vectors that replicate as chromosomes in yeast cells and can accommodate human DNA inserts as large as 1 million base pairs. These large inserts are extremely useful for attaining long-range continuity in contig maps, and therefore the use of YAC clones in large-scale mapping of the human genome was becoming widely adopted by 1990.

From our point of view, however, prior to McCormick's work at Los Alamos on improving YAC cloning techniques, YAC cloning had some serious drawbacks. First, large amounts of human DNA were required to construct YAC clone libraries because the efficiency of transforming yeast cells by the addition of a YAC clone was relatively low. Consequently, creating a chromosome 16-specific library of YAC clones from the small DNA samples obtained by sorting chromosomes would be difficult if not impossible.

Second, we knew that 30 to 50 percent of the clones in most YAC libraries were chimeric, that is, they contained DNA from two or more nonadjacent regions of the genome. Such clones can be produced when more than one YAC or partial YAC recombinant molecule enters a yeast cell, and, during the transforming process, the human DNA inserts in these recombinant molecules recombine with each other to produce a YAC containing two different human inserts instead of only one. Chimeras are also produced when two DNA fragments are accidentally ligated prior to their ligation with the vector arms of the yeast artificial chromosome.

Chimeric YACs can be identified during the construction of contig maps, but when a large percentage of clones in a YAC clone library are chimeric, the difficulty of map construction increases considerably and the process is error-prone.

These two major difficulties were overcome in 1991 when McCormick succeeded in constructing a chromosome 21-specific YAC library from sorted chromosomes. Not only was she able to work with small amounts of DNA but also only a few percent of the resulting clones are chimeric. The modified cloning techniques she developed to accomplish this technical tour de force are described in "Libraries from Flow-sorted Chromosomes." Following this breakthrough, McCormick applied the new YAC-cloning techniques to the construction of a chromosome 16-specific YAC library for specific use in our mapping effort.

Closing Gaps in the Contig Map with YACs

The YAC library for chromosome 16 contains about 550 clones, and the clones contain inserts with an average size of 215,000 base pairs. Assuming that our 576 cosmid contigs are randomly distributed over chromosome 16, we estimate that the average gap between cosmid contigs is 65,000 base pairs. Thus each gap should be closed with a single YAC clone. Figure 6 outlines our procedure for incorporating YAC clones into the cosmid contig map. We first develop STS markers from the end clones of our cosmid contigs. We then use PCR-based screening to pick out YAC clones that contain each STS and therefore overlap with the cosmid contig from which the STS was derived. Details of this work are presented in "The Polymerase Chain Reaction and Sequence-Tagged Sites" in "Mapping the Genome," and the design of the pooling scheme used to screen the YAC library is described in an accompanying sidebar "YAC Library Pooling Scheme for PCR-based Screening."

Figure 7 presents the results of screening the library for one STS. To date, we have made 89 STS markers from end clones of cosmid contigs and have incorporated 30 YAC clones into the contig map by showing that they contain STSs derived from those end clones.

Figure 6. YAC Closure of Gaps in the Cosmid Contig Map

Both STS markers and YAC inter-Alu PCR products are being used to identify overlaps between chromosome 16 YAC clones and our cosmid contigs. The procedure is outlined below.

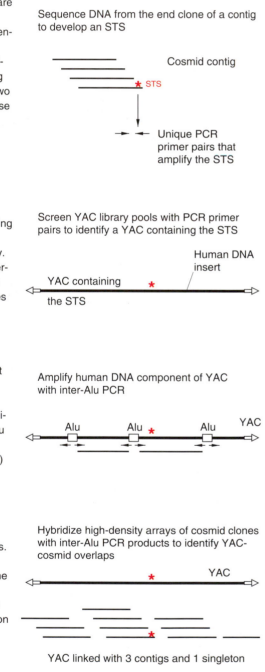

(a) Sequence-tagged sties (STSs) are generated from the end clones of cosmid contigs. This involves sequencing about 300 base pairs from the end clone, identifying a pair of candidate primer sequences, synthesizing the primers, and checking that the two primers, when used in the polymerase chain reaction, will amplify a single region of the genome. If so, the amplified region is an STS.

Sequence DNA from the end clone of a contig to develop an STS

(b) YAC clones containing the STS are identified by PCR-based screening of pools of YAC clones from our chromosome 16-specific YAC library. A YAC containing the STS must overlap the cosmid clone from which the STS was derived. Figure 7 illustrates the steps in the screening process.

Screen YAC library pools with PCR primer pairs to identify a YAC containing the STS

(c) To identify all cosmid clones that overlap with a YAC, inter-Alu PCR products are generated from each YAC and labeled for use as a hybridization probe. (Note that the inter-Alu products represent only a portion of the human insert in the YAC clones.)

Amplify human DNA component of YAC with inter-Alu PCR

(d) The probe is then hybridized to membranes containing high-density arrays of fingerprinted cosmid clones. Cosmid clones that yield positive hybridization signals must overlap the YAC. A single YAC often overlaps several cosmid contigs, as shown in the figure. However, the hybridization data do not determine the relative positions of the cosmid contigs.

Hybridize high-density arrays of cosmid clones with inter-Alu PCR products to identify YAC-cosmid overlaps

YAC linked with 3 contigs and 1 singleton

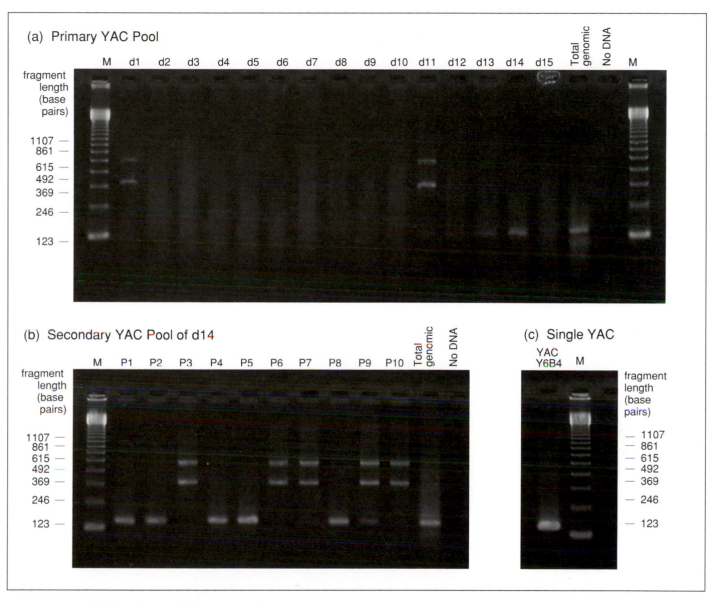

Figure 7. PCR-based Screening of YAC Library Pools for Clones Containing an STS

Our library of 540 YACs was divided into 15 sets of 36 YACs each. These 15 sets are called the primary pools, or detectors, and are numbered d1 through d15. The 36 YACs in each primary pool are then divided into 10 secondary pools (p1 through p10) according to David Torney's design for the 1-detector (see "YAC Library Pooling Scheme for PCR-based Screening" in "Mapping the Genome"). Each of the 36 YACs occur in 5 pools of the 1-detector. (a) An electrophoretic gel in which the PCR products produced by screening the primary pools for STS 25H11 have been separated by length. The lane third from the right, marked "total genomic DNA," contains the STS 25H11, which was amplified from total-genomic human DNA. In this experiment only detector 14 produced a PCR product that has the same length as STS 25H11. Multiple bands at different lengths in lanes d1 and d11 indicate PCR amplification of regions other than STS 25H11 and can therefore be ignored. (b) To determine which YAC was responsible for the positive signal from primary pool d14, we screen the 10 secondary pools composing the 1-detector for d14. Five of these pools, p1, p2, p4, p5, and p8, were identified as positive for STS 25H11. YAC clone Y6B4 was the only YAC that occurred in each of these five pools. (Multiple bands in p3, p6, p7, p9, and p10 were again the result of spurious PCR amplification and did not match the length of STS 25H11.) (c) Finally, the PCR was run on YAC Y6B4 only. The results confirm that this YAC contains STS 25H11. This pooling strategy allows error correction of false negatives in the secondary pools. If less than five positives were identified, this would increase the number of likely candidate YACs that could then be individually checked to find the correct YAC. In other pooling strategies, false negatives lead to the loss of YAC candidates.

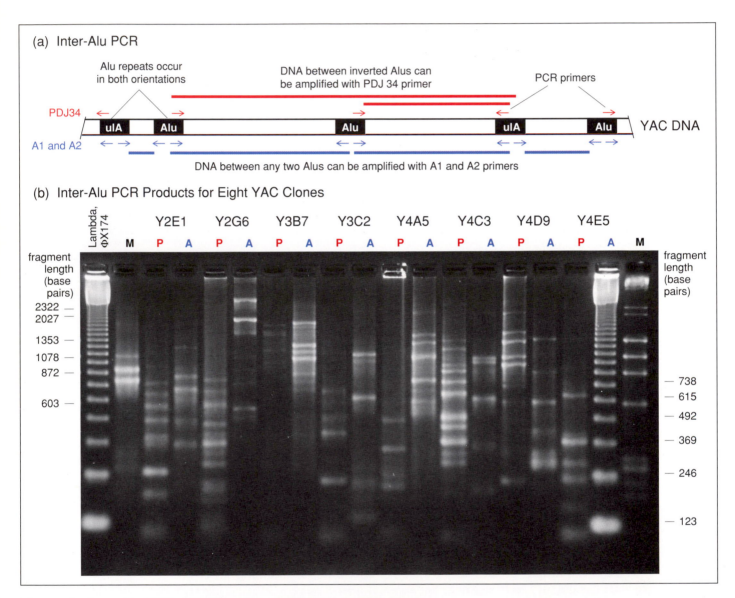

Figure 8. Inter-Alu PCR Amplification of DNA from YAC Clones

(a) Primers whose sequences match the ends of the Alu repetitive sequence can be used in the polymerase chain reaction to amplify the DNA occurring between of Alu sequences in the human DNA insert of a YAC clone. Alu sequences are 300 base pairs long, occur on average at intervals of 3300 base pairs in the human genome and are absent from the yeast genome. As shown in the figure, Alu sequences can be oriented in opposite directions along the DNA in the genome. The figure shows two sets of Alu primers. Those marked PDJ34 match only one end of the Alu sequence and therefore can amplify DNA between Alu sequences of opposite orientation. Primers A1 and A2 match either end of the Alu sequence and therefore can amplify DNA between any two Alu sequences. The polymerase chain reaction can be used to amplify regions up to several thousand base pairs in length. (b) Agarose gel containing inter-Alu PCR products of YAC clones. Alu primers PDJ34 (from Pieter de Jong, LLNL) or A1 and A2 (from Michael Scicillano, M.D., Anderson Hospital) were used in the PCR to amplify human DNA from eight different YAC clones and the amplified products were separated by electrophoresis on eight lanes of the gel shown in the figure. The first two and last lanes contain fragments of known lengths and are used to calibrate the lengths of the PCR products. Inter-Alu PCR products range in size from 100 base pairs to greater than 2500 base pairs. Each of the YACs shown yielded from 5 to 15 such PCR products.

Table 2. Results of Hybridization of Inter-Alu PCR Products to YACs

Number of cosmid contigs overlapped by a single YAC	0	1	2	3	4	5	6	>6
Number of YACs	105	133	84	41	24	12	6	6

Each YAC clone has an average insert size of 215,000 base pairs, so we expect many of them will bridge the gaps between two or more cosmid contigs. To find those contigs, we adopted a hybridization strategy which is less time-consuming than the STS approach. YAC clones are not good hybridization probes for detecting overlaps between human DNA inserts because the yeast DNA in those clones contains sequences that are homologous to human DNA and can produce false-positive hybridization signals. We need, instead, to generate DNA probes from each YAC clone that we know are derived from the human DNA insert in that clone. An efficient procedure, known as inter-Alu PCR, is outlined in Figure 8(a). The procedure uses the polymerase chain reaction to amplify DNA that lies between Alu sequences within the human DNA insert of the YAC. Alu sequences are found in human DNA but not in yeast DNA. Therefore, if primers from the ends of the Alu sequence are used in the polymerase chain reaction, the reaction will amplify regions of the human DNA insert only. Figure 8(b) shows a gel containing the amplified products derived by applying inter-Alu PCR to each of eight YAC clones. Each lane of the gel contains PCR products from one YAC clone. The average number of PCR products was about six.

The inter-Alu PCR products from each YAC clone were then radiolabeled with ^{32}P nucleotides and annealed with Cot1 DNA, a process that covers any Cot1 repetitive sequences that might be present. The PCR products were then ready to be used as a hybridization probe to screen the 4000 fingerprinted cosmid clones. To facilitate screening, the 4000 fingerprinted clones were fixed on membranes in a high-density, gridded array. Each membrane accommodates 1536 clones, so the entire set of fingerprinted cosmid clones was arrayed on three membranes (see Figure 9). Cosmids that yield positive hybridization signals must contain a DNA sequence present in the YAC clone from which the hybridization

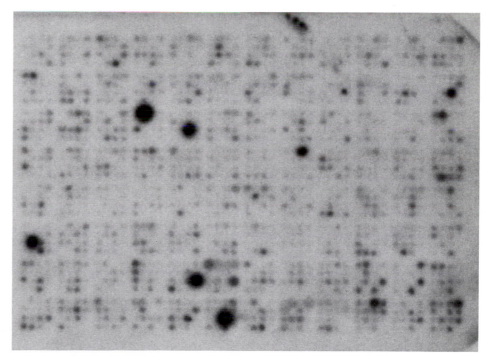

Figure 9. Hybridization of Inter-Alu PCR Products to Cosmid Clones

The figure shows an autoradiogram of a membrane containing 1536 cosmid clones. The clones from the wells of 16 different microtiter plates (8 rows and 12 columns for 96 clones per plate) were stamped onto a membrane the size of the microtiter plate by a high-precision robotic device. The resulting gridded array of clones provides a convenient tool for hybridization experiments. The darker and larger dots are the result of hybridization of YAC inter-Alu PCR products to specific cosmid clones. Here the PCR products from YAC clone Y3A12 hybridized to cosmid clones from 2 different contigs. The results suggest that the YAC clone overlaps those cosmid contigs. The automated robotic gridding device that makes the hybridization grids was designed and built by Pat Medvick, Tony Beugelsdijk, and Bob Hollen in the MEE-3 group. A photograph of the device appears on the opening pages of "DNA Libraries" and is discussed in "Libraries from Flow-sorted Chromosomes."

(a) Subcloning of YAC 16.3

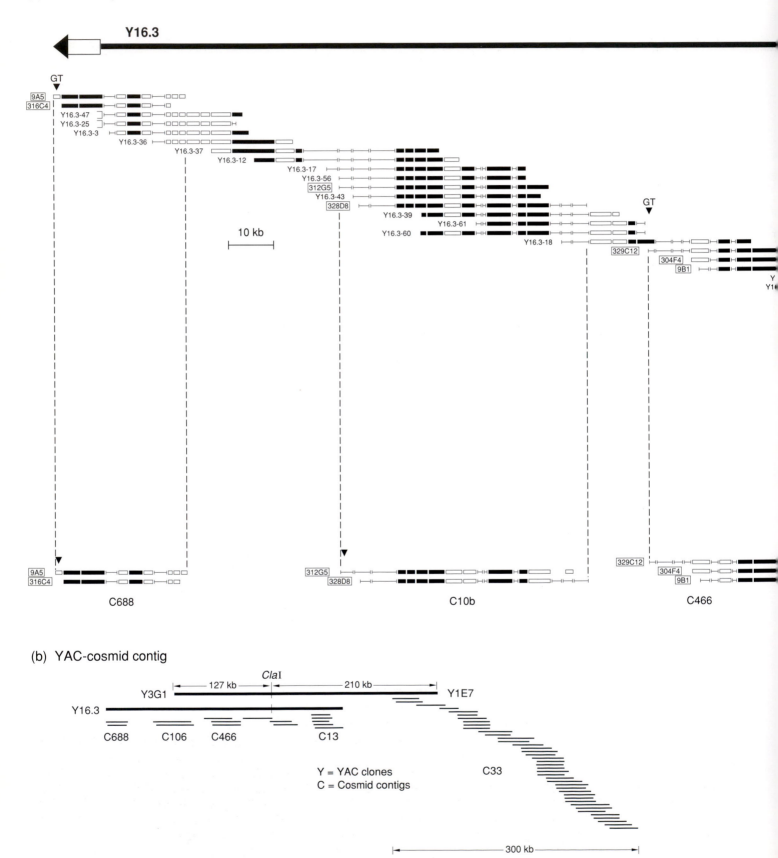

(b) YAC-cosmid contig

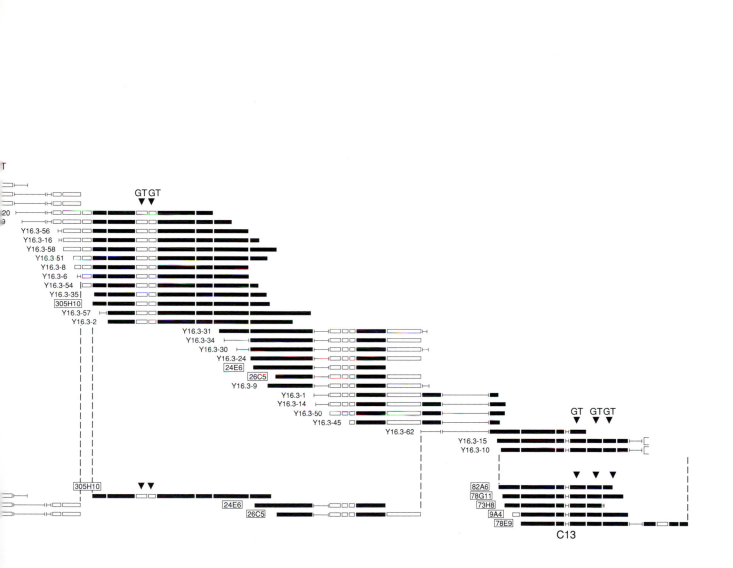

Figure 10. Confirmation of YAC-Cosmid Overlaps by YAC Subcloning

Hybridization experiments using inter-Alu PCR products from YAC clone Y16.3 suggested that this clone bridges the gaps between four cosmid contigs. To confirm that result, Y16.3 was subcloned into cosmid vectors and, as shown in (a), the resulting cosmid subclones were fingerprinted and assembled into a contig spanning the YAC. Five cosmid contigs from our chromosome 16 map were then aligned with the YAC subclone contig, based on their repetitive-sequence fingerprints. These results confirm the overlaps deduced from the hybridization experiments. Overlap of Y16.3 with an additional contig, C688, was detected by repetitive-sequence fingerprinting of the cosmid subclones of Y16.3. Thus, four out of five cosmid contigs that overlap this YAC were detected by the hybridization of inter-Alu PCR products to the high-density arrays of fingerprinted cosmid clones. (b) Other hybridization experiments have indicated overlaps with two other YACs and a sixth cosmid contig. Together these three YACs and six cosmids cover over 600,000 base pairs in chromosome 16.

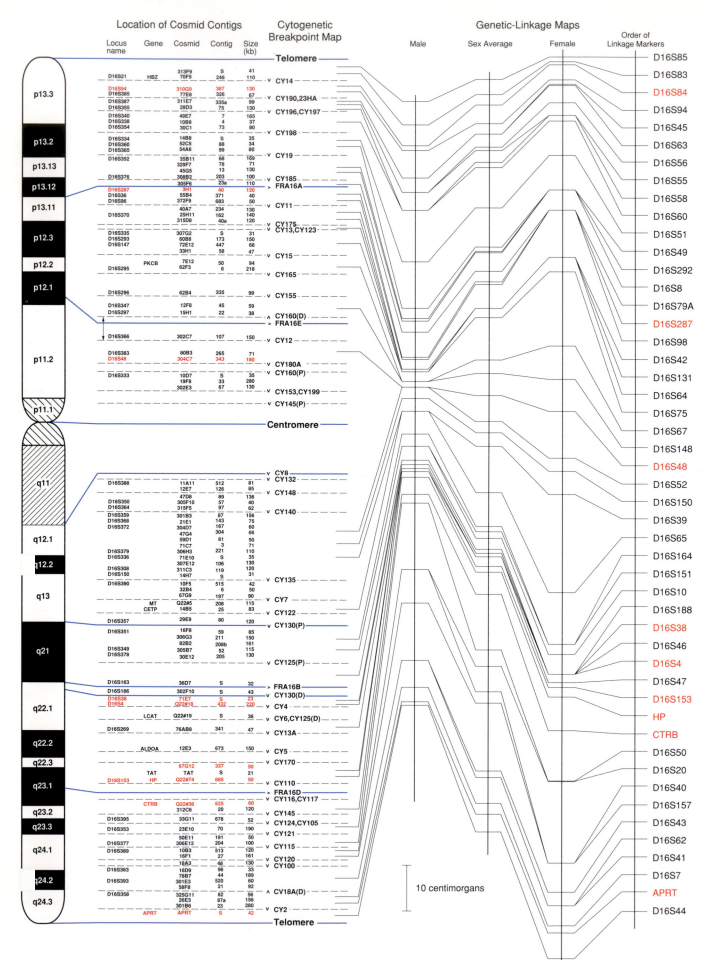

probe was derived. Consequently, the cosmid clone is highly likely to overlap the YAC clone.

To date we have generated inter-Alu PCR products from 411 YAC clones and hybridized those products to the arrays of fingerprinted cosmid clones. As shown in Figure 9, the inter-Alu products yield intense hybridization signals. The hybridization results enabled us to incorporate 334 YAC clones into our cosmid contig map. The PCR products from 133 YAC clones showed overlap with only a single cosmid contig and therefore extended those contigs but did not close any gaps in the map. Other YACs were shown to overlap as many as six separate cosmid contigs. Table 2 (page 199) lists the number of YACs whose PCR products hybridized to clones in one, two, three, four, five, or more than five cosmid contigs. The hybridization results also enabled us to join 203 singletons into the YAC-cosmid contigs. The number of YAC cosmid contigs in our map is now 462, and the average contig size has grown from 100,000 base pairs to 218,000 base pairs. The total number of "islands" in the map (462 YAC-cosmid contigs plus 54 YAC singletons) cover 94 percent of chromosome 16. Overlaps between YAC and cosmid clones were detected by hybridization of YAC inter-Alu PCR products to cosmid clones.

Verification of YAC-Cosmid Contigs

Our implicit assumption in the discussion above was that if the inter-Alu PCR products from a YAC hybridize to a cosmid clone, the human DNA insert in the YAC clone overlaps the human insert in the cosmid clone, and thus the two are from the same region of chromosome 16. However, we have discovered that chromosome 16 contains a number of low-abundance repetitive sequences (see "What's Different about Chromosome 16?"). Those repetitive sequences would not have been masked by annealing the PCR products with $Cot1$ repetitive DNA prior to hybridization. Therefore, if the inter-Alu PCR products from a YAC clone contain those low-abundance repeats, they would hybridize to cosmid clones that did not necessarily overlap the YAC clone. Consequently, we used an independent method to confirm the inferred overlaps between YACs and cosmid contigs.

Our procedure involved subcloning the DNA insert in each of seven YAC clones into cosmid vectors, generating a repetitive-sequence fingerprint for each of the resulting cosmid subclones, and comparing the fingerprints of the subclones to each other and to the fingerprints of the original set of fingerprinted cosmid clones to detect overlaps. Figure 10(a) shows how the cosmid subclones of YAC 16.3 overlapped among themselves and linked up with members of our original set of fingerprinted cosmid clones. Hybridization of inter-Alu PCR products had indicated that the YAC 16.3 clone overlapped four cosmid contigs. The results of subcloning the YAC confirmed the hybridization results. Two more YAC clones were found to overlap this region based on hybridization of their inter-Alu PCR products. This YAC-cosmid contig currently contains two of these YACs and six cosmid contigs, and

Figure 11. The Integration of Physical and Genetic-Linkage Maps of Chromosome 16

Physical and genetic-linkage mapping data presently available for chromosome 16 are summarized in the figure on this spread. Together they provide a resource for isolating a variety of genes on the chromosome. At right are three genetic-linkage maps showing genetic distances (in centimorgans) of 49 polymorphic DNA markers derived from male, female, and sex-averaged linkage data. These data were compiled by the Second International Workshop on Human Chromosome 16 and are based on analysis of pedigrees in CEPH (Centre d'Etude du Polymorphisme Humain). The coordinates of the physical mapping data are defined by (1) the cytogenetic map showing the dark and light Giemsa-stained bands of chromosome 16; and (2) the cytogenetic breakpoint map, the set of fifty horizontal lines that are positioned along the chromosome bands at the fifty breakpoints of chromosome 16 determined from the mouse/human hybrid-cell panel (see Figure 6). A cosmid clone from our contig map can be localized to a region or interval between two breakpoints by showing that it is present in the DNA of hybrid cells containing the chromosomal region corresponding to that interval but absent in the DNA of hybrid cells lacking that region. Each of 140 cosmids, and thus the contigs in which they reside, have now been placed into one of the 50 intervals. The YACs that overlap those 140 contigs are thereby regionally localized as well. The DNA in the cosmid contigs and YACs that have been located on the breakpoint map covers 21 million base pairs, or about 21 percent of the chromosome. In a separate effort, polymorphic DNA markers from the linkage map have been located onto the breakpoint map thereby integrating the linkage map with the cytogenetic breakpoint map and with the cosmid contigs located on the breakpoint map. We have also integrated the linkage map directly with our cosmid contigs by hybridizing 50 gene and polymorphic DNA markers to our high-density arrays of fingerprinted clones and identifying which clones contain those genes and markers. Shown in red are cosmids that have been both regionally localized and shown to contain a marker from the linkage map.

it spans a region over 600,000 base pairs long [see Figure 10(b)]. In most instances the overlaps inferred from the hybridization of YAC inter-Alu PCR products were confirmed by the analysis of YAC subclones. In one instance, the inter-Alu PCR products contained a low-abundance repeat and produced a false YAC-cosmid overlap. Such false overlaps can be avoided by mapping the locations of these low-abundance repeats. Additional experiments showed that 85 to 90 percent of the cosmids that overlap a YAC are identified by the hybridization of YAC inter-Alu PCR products. In general, our verification experiments suggest that YAC inter-Alu PCR products provide convenient and reliable probes for integrating YACs into cosmid contig maps.

Integration of the Physical Map with the Genetic-Linkage Map

As discussed in Part I of "Mapping the Genome," genetic-linkage analysis with polymorphic DNA markers is often the only way to find the approximate location of genes that cause inherited disorders. The polymorphic DNA markers that are tightly linked to, or usually co-inherited with, certain diseases are located close to the causative gene (see "Modern Linkage Mapping"). To find the gene, those markers must be located on a contig map and the cloned DNA in the neighborhood of the markers can then be searched for the causative gene. In other words, the genetic-linkage map must be integrated with the physical map.

Although our contig map is not yet complete, we have been locating previously cloned genes and polymorphic DNA markers on our cosmid contigs. Here, again, the high-density arrays of fingerprinted cosmid clones are an invaluable resource. Gene and DNA-marker probes are radioactively labeled and hybridized to these arrays to determine which cosmids contain those genes or markers. Alternatively, if a gene or marker exists in a cosmid from another library, we can fingerprint that clone to integrate it with our existing contigs. Using both of these approaches, we have now located more than 50 genes and DNA markers on cosmid contigs, thereby integrating our cosmid contigs with genetic-linkage maps.

Earlier we mentioned that 140 contigs have also been localized to intervals between breakpoints on the cytogenetic breakpoint map of chromosome 16 derived from the panel of 50 mouse/human hybrid cells (see Figure 5). In addition, hybridization experiments show that inter-Alu products from 82 YAC clones overlap those localized contigs. The YAC clones and cosmid contigs now localized to intervals on chromosome 16 cover 21.4 million base pairs. Figure 11 summarizes the integration achieved so far between the linkage maps, the cytogenetic breakpoint map, and our cosmid contig map.

Application of the Map toward the Isolation of Disease Genes. The integrated maps provide potent resources to identify, isolate, and sequence regions

Figure 12. Chromosome-16 Maps at Different Levels of Resolution

Maps of chromosome 16 are being made by several different techniques and at a wide range of resolutions. The figure shows only a few of the landmarks on each map and also indicates the level of resolution presently available for each. The three low-resolution maps include a cytogenetic map, the hybrid-cell, or cytogenetic-breakpoint map, and the genetic-linkage map. At higher resolution is the cosmid contig map, which presently consists of separate contigs that are being connected by YAC clones. At the highest level of resolution, which is the sequences of bases in the genome, STSs are being generated to serve as unique physical landmarks. These landmarks can be located on all physical maps at all levels of resolution. The position of STS N16Y1-10 is traced from one level of resolution to another. It can be amplified, or duplicated millions of times, by the polymerase chain reaction using the two unique primers shown at the bottom of figure. At the top of the figure is shown the position of the STS (red) determined by in-situ hybridization to cosmid clones from which the STS was derived. In-situ hybridization localizes the STS to a region 3 to 4 million bases in length in bands 16q12.1 and 16q12.2. The STS is also shown regionally localized to the interval between breakpoints CY7 and CY8 on the hybrid-cell cytogenetic map. The intervals on this map have an average size of 1.6 million bases. The particular STS shown is not polymorphic, and therefore it cannot be located on the genetic-linkage map through linkage analysis. However, the DNA markers on the linkage map have been regionally localized on the hybrid-cell map. The alignment between the two maps allows us to infer that the STS lies between markers 16AC6.5 and D16S150 on the genetic-linkage map. The next higher level of resolution is provided by contig maps of overlapping cloned fragments. The figure shows a YAC clone containing the STS as well as a cosmid contig from which the STS was derived. The YAC clone must overlap the cosmid contig because they both contain the same STS. The position of the YAC relative to the cosmid contig is known because all inter-Alu PCR products from the YAC clone hybridized to all clones in the cosmid contig. The STS was derived from the right end clone of the cosmid contig. The information at the highest level of resolution is the base sequence of the STS determined in the process of developing the PCR protocol that recognizes and amplifies this sequence whenever it appears in a DNA sample.

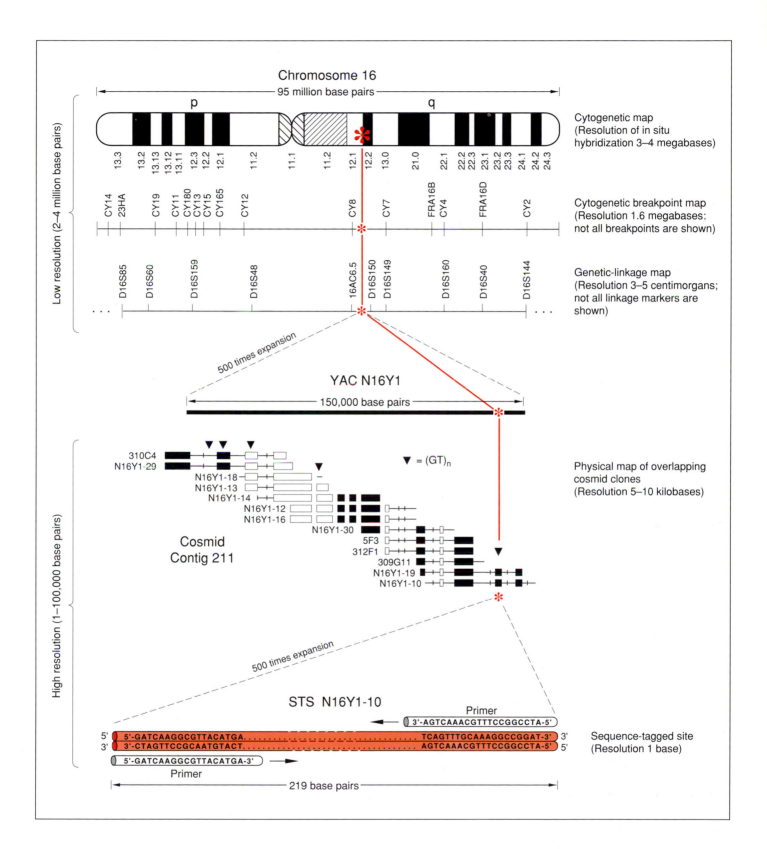

Chromosome 16

← 95 million base pairs →

p   q

Low resolution (2–4 million base pairs)

Cytogenetic map
(Resolution of in situ hybridization 3–4 megabases)

13.3 13.2 13.13 13.12 13.11 12.3 12.2 12.1 11.2 11.1 | 11.1 11.2 12.1 12.2 13.0 21.0 22.1 22.2 22.3 23.1 23.2 23.3 24.1 24.2 24.3

CY14 23HA CY19 CY11 CY180 CY13 CY15 CY165 CY12 CY8 CY7 FRA16B CY4 FRA16D CY2

Cytogenetic breakpoint map
(Resolution 1.6 megabases; not all breakpoints are shown)

D16S85 D16S60 D16S159 D16S48 16AC6.5 D16S150 D16S149 D16S160 D16S40 D16S144

Genetic-linkage map
(Resolution 3–5 centimorgans; not all linkage markers are shown)

500 times expansion

YAC N16Y1

← 150,000 base pairs →

High resolution (1–100,000 base pairs)

310C4
N16Y1-29
N16Y1-18
N16Y1-13
N16Y1-14
N16Y1-12
N16Y1-16
N16Y1-30
5F3
312F1
309G11
N16Y1-19
N16Y1-10

▼ = (GT)$_n$

Cosmid Contig 211

Physical map of overlapping cosmid clones
(Resolution 5–10 kilobases)

500 times expansion

STS N16Y1-10

Primer
3'-AGTCAAACGTTTCCGGCCTA-5'

5'-GATCAAGGCGTTACATGA.....................TCAGTTTGCAAAGGCCGGAT-3' 3'
3'-CTAGTTCCGCAATGTACT.....................AGTCAAACGTTTCCGGCCTA-5' 5'

5'-GATCAAGGCGTTACATGA-3'
Primer

← 219 base pairs →

Sequence-tagged site
(Resolution 1 base)

associated with genetic diseases and other inherited variations.

These maps include the overlap relationships between cosmid contigs and YACs, the regional localization of contigs, YACs, and STSs, and the integration of the genetic-linkage map with the physical contig map.

Figure 12 illustrates the levels of resolution at which information about chromosome 16 is available and also illustrates how STSs serve to integrate the various types of information and levels of resolution. These mapping data, in combination with the resources used to generate the data (the high-density arrays of cosmid clones, the pooled YAC library, the STSs, and the hybrid-cell panel), are already proving useful for the isolation of disease genes and other important regions on chromosome 16. For example, these resources were used to complete the map for the metallothionein gene family, to isolate the chromosome 16 microdeletion region associated with Rubinstein-Taybi syndrome, and to identify chromosome 16-specific repetitive DNA sequences associated with rearrangements of this chromosome that accompany a type of acute nonlymphocytic leukemia.

Several national and international collaborative efforts (described in the accompanying box) are now underway to isolate a variety of disease genes on chromosome 16. Each of these efforts takes advantage of the physical mapping progress on chromosome 16, and collectively they illustrate how the physical mapping of the human genome already has far-reaching significance in the field of medicine.

Completing the Map and Looking toward the Future

In line with the mapping goals stated in the Human Genome Project's Five-Year Plan, the completed map of chromosome 16 will have at most 100 contigs with lengths of between 1 and 2 million base pairs. The contigs will be ordered along the chromosome and represent at least 99 percent of the DNA within it. Moreover the map will be dotted with STS markers at intervals of 100,000 to 200,000 base pairs. Every region of the chromosome will then be rapidly accessible by STS screening of a genomic YAC library.

To complete this final map, we will be making a second YAC library of chromosome 16 by using a restriction enzyme whose restriction sites have a distribution pattern different from those of Cla1 (which was the restriction enzyme used in the construction of the first YAC library). A directed approach will then be used to screen this library (and a total genomic library if necessary) for YACs that extend the current YAC-cosmid contigs. We expect that most of the remaining gaps can be closed in this manner. The ongoing development of STSs from the original 576 cosmid contigs will provide the framework for an STS map at a resolution between 100,000 and 200,000 base pairs.

The approach we used to map chromosome 16 is resulting in a high-resolution map of this chromosome. The repetitive-sequence fingerprinting of cosmid clones, the subsequent assembly of contigs, and the evaluation of contig accuracy and chromosome coverage through hybridization experiments have produced a robust map with information on sizes, ordering, and sequence complexity of DNA restriction fragments. Mapping data of this type are invaluable for interrelating chromosome structure with function. Already the chromosomal distribution of $(GT)_n$ repeats has been determined from those data.

With the advent of YAC and PCR technologies, it is now possible to rapidly produce a lower-resolution map of an entire chromosome. YAC clones are 10 to 20 times larger than cosmid clones, so far fewer are needed to create a complete contig map. The assembly of contigs by STS-content mapping is relatively efficient and straightforward. Although physical maps constructed from YAC clones and STS markers will not be as useful for elucidating the structure-function relationships of chromosomes as those made from cosmid clones, the YAC maps still permit immediate access to genes or regions of medical and scientific importance. Consequently, in developing a strategy to map a second chromosome, chromosome 5, we chose to exploit the new technologies. Deborah Grady at our Laboratory and John Wasmuth at the University of California, Irvine, have begun a collaborative effort using chromosome-specific STSs and YAC libraries to rapidly generate a relatively low-resolution map of chromosome 5. Their strategy and some early data are presented in "Mapping Chromosome 5." ∎

Collaborations on the Isolation of Disease Genes on Chromosome 16

Polycystic Kidney Disease (PKD1). Polycystic kidney disease is a common dominant single-gene disorder (affecting at least 1 in 1000 Caucasians) that is responsible for cystic kidneys, accompanied by hypertension and renal failure. The principal locus for the genetic defect, PKD1, has been assigned to chromosome band 16p13.3 by genetic linkage with polymorphic DNA markers shown to reside in that band.

Steve Reeders (Yale University School of Medicine), Anna-Maria Frischauf (Imperial Cancer Research Fund), and collaborators have constructed both a long-range restriction map (covering 1 million base pairs) and an ordered contig map (covering 75,000 base pairs) that span the entire PKD1 region. Construction of the contig map by cosmid walking from multiple start sites within the region was greatly aided by the use of two chromosome 16-specific cosmid libraries constructed at Los Alamos. A gene-by-gene search is now being carried out in the region to identify candidate disease genes (genes that are expressed in the kidney and that have alleles that are specific to affected individuals). This effort will probably soon lead to the identification of the gene that is responsible for the disease.

Batten's Disease (CLN3). Batten's disease is a juvenile-onset neurodegenerative disease with incidence rates of up to 1 in 25,000 live births. It is characterized by the accumulation of autofluorescent fatty pigments in neurons. The responsible locus (CLN3) is inherited in an autosomal recessive pattern. That is, the defective allele must be present on both chromosomes in order for the disease to be manifested. The gene responsible for this disease has been mapped to the region between two polymorphic markers in the chromosomal band 16p12.

We have found thirteen cosmid contigs and one YAC clone from our physical map that lie in this same interval, and in collaboration with groups in London (Mark Gardiner), the Netherlands (Martijn Breuning), and Australia (David Callen), we are developing new polymorphic DNA markers from these contigs in an attempt to find markers that are closer to the disease locus. We have used prior knowledge of the repetitive-sequence fingerprint of four of these cosmid clones to develop STSs containing GT-repeat sequences present on these clones. Since GT repeats tend to be variable in length, we expect these STSs to be polymorphic and therefore useful for linkage analysis. We are now evaluating their informativeness in linkage studies. (Genetic-linkage markers for the remaining cosmids are being developed by the other laboratories with the aid of the fingerprint data.) The development of these new genetic-linkage markers in the Batten's-disease region will allow the disease gene to be localized to a manageable region (approximately 1 million bases). Then construction of a detailed physical map starting from the existing contigs and YACs in the region can be completed. The availability of the Los Alamos clones in the Batten's region has substantially reduced the extensive work that would have been required to find genetic-linkage markers from this region and to construct a complete map of the region.

Familial Mediterranean Fever (FMF). FMF is an autosomal recessive form of arthritis that is characterized by acute attacks of fever with inflammation of the lining of the abdominal cavity (peritonitis), pleural cavity (pleurisy), and joints (synovia). The gene frequency among non-Ashkenazic Jews, Armenians, Turks, and Middle Eastern Arabs is comparable to the gene frequency for cystic-fibrosis defects among Caucasians (1 in 25). As with Batten's disease, genetic-linkage markers flanking the disease locus have been identified by researchers led by Dan Kastner at the National Institutes of Health. We are working with that group to identify contigs and YACs that lie within this region so that additional genetic-linkage markers can be developed.

Rubinstein-Taybi Syndrome (RTS). RTS is characterized by abnormal facial features, broad thumbs and big toes, and mental retardation. RTS is a rare disorder that accounts for an estimated 1 in 500 institutionalized cases of mental retardation. Almost all cases seem to arise from spontaneous mutations. Three patients with RTS have been found to have translocations involving the short arm of chromosome 16. Using fluoresence in-situ hybridization, Martijn Breuning (Leiden University) was able to pinpoint the location of breakpoints in two of these patients relative to cosmids that he had ordered in the region in his group's effort to map breakpoints associated with ANLL M4. One of these cosmids, RT1, appeared to be very close to the breakpoints and was found to be deleted in 6 out of 24 patients. By screening our gridded arrays of chromosome 16 cosmids with RT1, Breuning identified one cosmid, 316H7, that overlapped RT1 by 10 kilobases. This overlapping cosmid was also hybridized to metaphase chromosomes from the two patients with RTS. In both cases, Breuning found three signals, one on the normal chromosome 16, a second signal on the aberrant chromosome 16, and a third on the chromosome that the p arm of 16 had translocated to. These results indicated that cosmid 316H7 spanned both translocation breakpoints in these RTS patients. Since the gene(s) responsible for RTS is likely to be disrupted by these breakpoints, the identification of cosmid 316H7, which spans the breakpoints, opens the door for identification of the gene(s) that causes this syndrome.

Acute Nonlymphocytic Leukemia (ANLL). In contrast to PKD1, CLN3, and FMF, which follow a Mendelian pattern of inheritance, acute nonlymphocytic leukemia is a polygenic trait, that is, it involves the interaction of several genes. A high frequency of rearrangements (inversions and translocations involving both the p and q arms) of chromosome 16 is associated with a specific subtype of acute nonlymphocytic leukemia known as ANLL subtype M4 (see "What's Different about Chromosome 16?"). This association suggests that chromosome 16 may contain at least one of the genes involved in the progression of the disease state and that the chromosomal rearrangements disrupt the functioning of that gene. We are collaborating with groups in the United States, Australia, and the Netherlands to isolate the chromosomal breakpoint regions associated with ANLL. Our prior identification of chromosome 16-specific repeats that map near these regions is aiding the search for the breakpoint regions. Genes that are disrupted as a result of the chromosomal rearrangements will be candidates for having a role in ANLL.

Breast Cancer. Like ANLL, breast cancer appears to be a polygenic trait involving specific alterations of chromosome 16 in addition to alterations in other genes. Deletions in the q22 region of chromosome 16 that are not always detectable at the gross microscopic level occur at a relatively high frequency in the malignant cells of breast tumors. These deletions are readily detectable using fluorescence in-situ hybridization by noting the absence of a positive hybridization signal from a probe that usually hybridizes to the deleted region and the presence of a signal from a second probe that hybridizes to the centromere. We have sent cosmid clones from the q arm of chromosome 16 to Joe Gray (UCSF), who is attempting to pinpoint the region of deletion associated with breast cancers. A gene-by-gene search through the deleted region will presumably lead to the identification of a gene whose function suppresses the development of cancer (tumor-suppressor gene). ∎

Further Reading

D. T. Burke, G. F. Carle, and M. V. Olson. 1987. Cloning of large segments of exogenous DNA into yeast by means of artificial chromosome vectors. *Science* 236:806–812.

D. C. Schwartz and C. R. Cantor. 1984. Separation of yeast chromosome-sized DNAs by pulsed field gradient gel electrophoresis. *Cell* 37:67–75.

R. Saiki, S. Scharf, F. Faloona, K. Mullis, G. Horn, H. Erlich, and N. Arnheim. 1985. Enzymatic amplification of beta-globin genomic sequences and restriction site analysis for diagnosis of sickle cell anemia. *Science* 230:1350–1354.

R. Saiki, D. H. Gelfand, S. Stoffel, S. Scharf, R. Higuchi, G. T. Horn, K. B. Mullis, and H. Erlich. 1988. Primer directed amplification of DNA with a thermostable DNA polymerase. *Science* 239:487–491.

M. Olson, L. Hood, and D. Botstein. 1989. A common language for physical linkage mapping of the human genome. *Science* 245:1434–1435.

C. L. Smith, J. G. Econome, A. Schutt, S. Klco, and C. R. Cantor. 1987. A physical map of the *Escherichia coli* K12 genome. *Science* 236:1448–1453.

D. L. Daniels and F. R. Blattner. 1987. Mapping using gene encyclopaedias. *Nature* 325:831–832.

Y. Kohara, K. Akiyama, and K. Isono. 1987. The physical map of the whole E. coli chromosome: Application of a new strategy for rapid analysis and sorting of a large genomic library. *Cell* 50:495–508.

M. V. Olson, J. E. Dutchik, M. V. Graham, G. M. Brodeur, M. Frank, M. MacColin, R. Scheinman, and T. Frank. 1986. Random-clone strategy for genomic restriction mapping yeast. *Proceedings of the National Academy of Sciences of the United States of America* 83:7826–7830.

A. Coulson, J. Sulston, S. Brenner, and J. Karn. 1986. Toward a physical map of the genome of the nematode *Caenorhabditis elegans. Proceedings of the National Academy of Sciences of the United States of America* 83:7821–7825.

A. V. Carrano, J. Lamerdin, L. K. Ashworth, B. Watkins, E. Branscomb, T. Slezak, M. Raff, P. J. De Jong, D. Keith, L. McBride, S. Meister, and M. Kronick. 1989. A high-resolution, fluorescence-based, semiautomated method for DNA fingerprinting. *Genomics* 4:129–136.

S. Brenner and K. J. Livak. 1989. DNA fingerprinting by sampled sequencing. *Proceedings of the National Academy of Sciences of the United States of America* 86:8902–8906.

G. A. Evans and K. A. Lewis. 1989. Physical mapping of complex genomes by cosmid multiplex analysis. *Proceedings of the National Academy of Sciences of the United States of America* 86:5030–5034.

A. G. Craig, D. Nizetic, J. Hoheisel, G. Zehetner, and H. Lehrach. 1990. Ordering of cosmid clones covering the Herpes simplex virus type I (HSV-I) genome: A test case for fingerprinting by hybridization. *Nucleic Acids Research* 18:2653–2660.

L. L. Deaven, M. A. Van Dilla, M. R. Bartholdi, A. V. Carrano, L. S. Cram, J. C. Fuscoe, J. W. Gray, C. E. Hildebrand, R. K. Moyzis, and J. Perlman. 1986. Construction of human chromosome-specific DNA libraries from flow-sorted chromosomes. *Cold Spring Harbor Symposia on Quantitative Biology* 51:159–167.

N. E. Morton. 1991. Parameters of the human genome. *Proceedings of the National Academy of Sciences of the United States of America* 88:7474–7476.

R. K. Moyzis, K. L. Albright, M. F. Bartholdi, L. S. Cram, L. L. Deaven, C. E. Hildebrand, N. E. Joste, J. L. Longmire, J. Meyne, and T. Schwarzacher-Robinson. 1987. Human chromosome-specific repetitive DNA sequences: Novel markers for genetic analysis. *Chromosome* 95: 375–386.

D. F. Callen, E. Baker, H. J. Eyre, and S. A. Lane. 1990. An expanded mouse-human hybrid cell panel for mapping human chromosome 16. *Annals of Genetics* 33:190–195.

C. F. Callen, C. E. Hildebrand, and S. Reeders. Report of the second international wokshop on human chromosome 16. Submitted for publication.

E. S. Lander and M. S. Waterman. 1988. Genomic mapping by fingerprinting random clones: A mathematical analysis. *Genomics* 2:231–239.

R. K. Moyzis, J. M. Buckingham, L. S. Cram, M. Dani, L. L. Deaven, M. D. Jones, J. Meyne, R. L. Ratliff, and J.-R. Wu. 1988. A highly conserved repetitive DNA sequence, (TTAGGG)$_n$, present at the telomeres of human chromosomes. *Proceedings of the National Academy of Sciences of the United States of America* 85:6622–6626.

J. Meyne, R. L. Ratliff, and R. K. Moyzis. 1989. Conservation of the human telomere sequence (TTAGGG)$_n$ among vertebrates. *Proceedings of the National Academy of Sciences of the United States of America* 86:7049–7053.

F. Rouyer, A. de la Chapelle, M. Andersson, and J. Weissenbach. 1990. An interspersed repeated sequence specific for human subtelomeric regions. *The EMBO Journal* 9:505–514.

R. L. Stallings, A. F. Ford, D. Nelson, D. C. Torney, C. E. Hildebrand, and R. K. Moyzis. 1991. Evolution and distribution of (GT)$_n$ repetitive sequences in mammalian genomes. *Genomics* 10:807–815.

J. L. Weber and P. E. May. 1989. Abundant class of human polymorphisms which can be typed using the polymerase chain reaction. *American Journal of Human Genetics* 44:388–396.

A. J. Jeffreys, V. Wilson, and S. L. Thein. 1985. Hypervariable 'minisatellite' regions in human DNA. *Nature* 314-:67–73.

M. F. Singer. 1982. Highly repeated sequences in mammalian genomes. *International Review of Cytology* 76:67–112.

B. A. Dombroski, S. L. Mathias, E. Nanthakumar, A. F. Scott, and H. H. Kazazian, Jr.. 1991. Isolation of an active human transposable element. *Science* 254:1805–1808.

H. F. Willard. 1989. The genomics of long tandem arrays of satellite DNA in the human genome. *Genome* 31-737–744.

R. J. Britten and D. E. Kohne. 1968. Repeated sequences in DNA. *Science* 161:529–540.

R. K. Moyzis, D. C. Torney, J. Meyne, J. Buckingham, J. M. Meyne, J.-R. Wu, C. Burks, K. M. Sirotkin, and W. B. Goad. 1989. The distribution of interspersed repetitive DNA sequences in the human genome. *Genomics* 4:273–289.

R. L. Stallings, D. C. Torney, C. E. Hildebrand, J. L. Longmire, L. L. Deaven, J. H. Jett, N. A. Doggett, and R. K. Moyzis. 1990. Physical mapping of human chromosomes by repetitive sequence fingerprinting. *Proceedings of the National Academy of Sciences of the United States of America* 87:6218–6222

E. M. Southern. 1975. Detection of specific sequences among DNA fragments separated by gel electrophoresis. *Journal of Molecular Biology* 98:503–517.

A. P. Feinberg and B. Vogelstein. 1983. A technique for radio-labeling DNA restriction endonuclease fragments to high specific activity. *Analytical Biochemistry* 132:6–13.

T. M. Cannon, R. J. Koskela, C. Burks, R. L. Stallings, A. A. Ford, P. E. Hempfner, H. T. Brown, and J. W. Fickett. 1991. A program for computer-assisted scoring of southern blots. *Biotechniques* 10:764–767.

D. J. Balding and D. C. Torney. 1991. Statistical analysis of DNA fingerprint data for ordered clone physical mapping of human chromosomes. *Bulletin of Mathematical Biology* 53:853–879.

J. W. Fickett and M. J. Cinkosky. A genetic algorithm for assembling chromosome physical maps. Submitted for publication.

D. F. Callen, N. A. Doggett, R. L. Stallings, L. Z. Chen, S. A. Whitmore, S. A. Lane, J. K. Nancarrow, S. Apostolou, A. D. Thompson, N. M. Lapsys, H. J. Eyre, E. G. Baker, Y. Shen, R. I. Richards, K. Holman, H. Phillips, and G. R. Sutherland. High resolution cytogenetic-based physical map of human chromosome 16. Accepted for publication in *Genomics*.

R. L. Stallings, N. A. Doggett, C. Callen, S. Apostolou, P. Harris, H. Michison, H. Breuning, J. Sarich, C. E. Hildebrand, and R. K. Moyzis. Evaluation of a cosmid contig physical map of human chromosome 16. Accepted for publication in *Genomics*.

M. K. McCormick, J. H. Shero, M. C. Cheung, Y. W. Kan, P. A. Hieter, and S. E. Antonarakis. 1989. Construction of human chromosome 21-specific yeast artificial chromosomes. *Proceedings of the National Academy of Sciences of the United States of America* 86:9991–9995.

E. D. Green, R. M. Mohr, J. R. Jones, J. M. Buckingham, L. L. Deaven, R. K. Moyzis, and M. V. Olson. 1991. Systematic generation of sequence-tagged sites for physical mapping of human chromosomes: Application to the mapping of human chromosome 7 using yeast artificial chromosomes. *Genomics* 11:548–564.

E. D. Green and M. V. Olson. 1990. Chromosomal region of the cystic fibrosis gene in yeast artificial chromosomes: A model for human genome mapping. *Science* 250:94–98.

M. K. McCormick, E. Campbell, L. Deaven, and R. Moyzis. Non-chimeric yeast artificial chromosome libraries from flow sorted human chromosomes 16 and 21. Submitted for publication.

E. D. Green and M. V. Olson. 1990. Systematic screening of yeast artificial-chromosome libraries by use of the polymerase chain reaction. *Proceedings of the National Academy of Sciences of the United States of America* 87:1213–1217.

D. L. Nelson, S. A. Ledbetter, L. Corbo, M. F. Victoria, R. Ramirez-Solis, T. D. Webster, D. H. Ledbetter, and C. T. Caskey. 1989. Alu polymerase chain reacgtion: A method for rapdi isolation of human-specific sequences from complex DNA sources. *Proceedings of the*

T. Beth, D. Yungnickel, and H. Lenz. 1985. *Design Theory*. Zurich: Bibliographisches Institut.

National Academy of Sciences of the United States of America 86:6686–6690.

P. A. Medvick, R. M. Hollen, R. S. Roberts, D. Trimmer, and T. J. Beugelsdijk. 1992. Automated DNA hybridization array construction and database design for robotic control and for source determination of hybridization responses. *International Journal of Genome Research* 1:17–23.

R. L. Stallings, N. A. Doggett, D. Bruce, M. K. McCormick, A. Ford, D. C. Torney, J. Dietz-Band, C. E. Hildebrand, and R. K. Moyzis. Approaching closure of a human chromosome 16 contig physical map using inter-Alu PCR products from a chromosome specific YAC library. Submitted for publication.

G. G. Germino, D. Weinstat-Saslow, H. Himmelbauer, G. A. J. Gillespie, S. Somlo, B. Wirth, N. Barton, K. L. Harris, A.-M. Frischauf, and S. T. Reeders. 1992. The gene for autosomal dominant polycystic kidney disease lies in a 750-kb CpG-rich region. *Genomics* 13:144–151.

M. Gardiner, A. Sandford, M. Deadman, J. Poulton, W. Cookson, S. Reeders, I. Jokiaho, L. Peltonen, H. Eiberg and C. Julier. 1990. Batten Disease (Spielmeyer-Vogt disease, juvenile onset neuronal ceroidlipofuscinosis) gene (CLN3) maps to human chromosome 16. *Genomics* 8:387–390.

E. Pras, I. Aksentijevich, L. Gruberg, J. E. Balow, L. Prosen, M. Dean, A. D. Steinberg, M. Pras, and D. L. Kastner. 1992. Mapping of a gene causing familial mediterranean fever to the short arm of chromosome 16. *New England Journal of Mediciane* 326:1509–1513.

M. H. Breuning, H. G. Dauwerse, G. Fugazza, J. J. Saris, L. Spruit, H. Wijnen, M. Tommerup, C. B. van der Hagen, K. Imaizumi, Y. Kuroki, M.-J. van den Boogaard, J. M. de Pater, E. Mariman, B. Hamel, H. Himmelbauer, A.-M. Frischauf, R. L. Stallings, G.-J. B. van Ommen, and R. C. M. Hennekam. 1992. Submicroscopic deletions of chromosome 16 in patients with Rubenstein-Taybi syndrome. Submitted for publication.

R. L. Stallings, N. A. Doggett, K. Okumura, and D. Ward. 1992. Chromosome 16 specific repetitive DNA sequences that map to chromosome regions known to undergo breakage/rearrangement in leukemia cells. *Genomics* 13:332–338.

T. Sato, F. Akiyama, G. Sakamoto, F. Kasumi, and Y. Nakamura. 1991. Accumulation of genetic alteration and progression of primary breast cancer. *Cancer Research* 51:5794–5799.

WHAT'S DIFFERENT ABOUT CHROMOSOME 16?   *Raymond L. Stallings and Norman A. Doggett*

Human chromosome 16 is different from most other human chromosomes in that it contains a larger-than-average fraction of repetitive sequences. As we will describe below, during the course of constructing a contig map for chromosome 16, we discovered several new low-abundance repetitive sequences that are present only on chromosome 16 and that may be implicated in the etiology of certain genetic diseases.

Repetitive sequences are frequently referred to as junk DNA because it has been difficult to determine whether these sequences have any role in the organization and functioning of eukaryotic genomes. Repetitive sequences are also referred to as selfish DNA because they represent such a large fraction of these genomes. For example, the fraction of repetitive DNA in the human genome is estimated to be between 25 and 35 percent. The fact that some classes of repetitive sequences, such as the alpha satellite DNA found in primates, have mutated rapidly over evolutionary time scales lends credence to the notion that at least some repetitive sequences represent mere clutter and play no functional role.

In contrast, work led by Bob Moyzis here at the Laboratory has shown that the repeat sequences that make up the functional centromeres and telomeres of human chromosomes have been highly conserved throughout evolution and serve very important functions. The centromeric repeat sequences are essential to the proper replication and parceling out of chromosomes to daughter cells during cell division. The telomeric tandem repeats maintain the ends of the chromosomes during replication. Some simple microsatellite repeat sequences, such as $(GT)_n$, are so widely distributed throughout all eukaryotic genomes that it is difficult to believe they don't have some functional significance. (See "Various Classes of Human Repetitive DNA Sequences.")

Regardless of whether different classes of repetitive sequences have specific functions or, as Orgel and Crick suggest, are "the ultimate parasite," many of these sequences are of medical interest. Recent findings demonstrate that some human repetitive sequences undergo rapid mutations or facilitate chromosomal rearrangements and that both types of changes can lead to human genetic diseases. The fragile site on the human X chromosome is an example. Like other fragile sites, the fragile X site is so named because the X chromosome at that site appears to have a non-staining gap or break under certain experimental conditions. The fragile X site is located on the X chromosome within the region Xq27.3. Fragile X is inherited in a Mendelian fashion. Recent cloning of the fragile X region and subsequent analysis showed, first, that it contains the trinucleotide tandem repeat sequence $(CCG)_n$, and second, that the tandem repeat can undergo significant amplification (that is, n can increase significantly) between one generation and the next. Moreover, amplification of $(CCG)_n$ seems to be the cause of a very common form of mental retardation that has long been associated with the presence of the fragile X site.

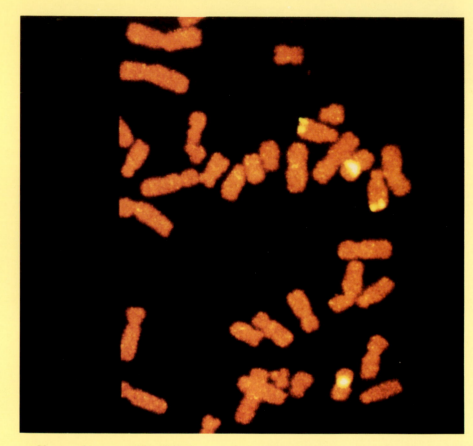

Photograph courtesy of David Ward,
Yale University School of Medicine

Shortly after the dramatic discovery of the fragile X site came reports that amplification of another trinucleotide repeat on chromosome X, $(CTG)_n$, is responsible for spinal and bulbar muscular atrophy and that amplification of the $(CTG)_n$ repeat on chromosome 19 is responsible for myotonic dystrophy. Evidently, when those tandem repeats undergo spontaneous amplification within germ-line cells, they disrupt the functioning of a gene or of the regulatory region for a gene in an offspring derived from a gamete containing the amplified sequence. The increasing level of amplification from one generation to the next is accompanied by an increase in the symptoms of the disease, a genetic process that has been termed anticipation. For example, amplification of $(CTG)_n$ that occurs in one generation may cause cataracts, and its further amplification in a subsequent generation will cause full-blown myotonic dystrophy.

Repetitive sequences other than trinucleotide tandem repeats have also been implicated in genetic disease. For example, it was recently discovered that the insertion of a truncated L1 sequence in the gene for blood-clotting factor VIII was responsible for a spontaneous case of hemophilia A. Similarly, de novo insertion of Alu repeats into the cholinesterase gene led to inactivation of the gene, and a comparable insertion in the NF1 gene caused the common dominant disorder known as neurofibromatosis type 1.

Our group and a group at Leiden University have recently determined that there is extensive sequence homology between two widely separated regions of chromosome 16, band 16p13 on its short arm and band 16q22 on its long arm. The homology could explain why rearrangements occur between those chromosomal regions in acute nonlymphocytic leukemia (ANLL). The sequence homology between the two bands is due to the presence of low-abundance repetitive sequences at multiple loci in bands 16p13, 16p12, 16p11, and 16q22.

We discovered those repetitive sequences on chromosome 16 in the course of developing the contig map of chromosome 16. As we grouped pairs of overlapping clones into contigs, we encountered an anomaly—a set of 78 clones, all of which seemed to overlap other clones in the set. Thus the clones appeared to form a single contig, or island of overlapping clones, much larger than the average contig, which contained only four or five clones. However, when we tried to position the clones to form a single contig, we found that they could not be placed in a linear order, but rather the contig branched in many directions and included many clones that seemed to be piled on top of one another. Our inability to construct a linear contig indicated that many false overlaps had been deduced from the fingerprint data because of the presence of some unknown repetitive sequence in the clones.

We went on to analyze the 78 clones using a variety of techniques. Fluorescence in-situ hybridization of five of the clones revealed that each one hybridized to as many as three locations on chromosome 16, and those locations occurred in four bands of chromosome 16: 16p13, 16p12, 16p11, and 16q22 (see page 214). The hybridization results and further analysis indicated that the four bands contain low-abundance repetitive sequences that are found only on chromosome 16. Characterization of one of those sequences revealed that it was a minisatellite-type sequence that did not possess homology to any of the known minisatellites. The concensus repeat unit of the sequence is

TCCT X TCCT CTTCCACCCT CAGTGGATGA TAATCTGAAG GA,

where X is any sequence containing between 2 and 9 nucleotides. The results of in-situ hybridization of this consensus repeat to chromosome 16 is shown in the opening pages of "The Mapping of Chromosome 16." High-stringency hybridization of the consensus sequence to Southern blots containing DNA from humans, the rhesus monkey, rat, mouse, dog, cow, rabbit, chicken, and yeast produced positive hybridization signals only from human and monkey DNA. Apparently, the sequence is present only in primates and therefore could be relatively recent in origin.

We estimate that the low-abundance repetitive sequences specific to chromosome 16 together occupy between 2 million and 6 million base pairs of the chromosome. Moreover, those sequences appear to overlap the breakpoint regions involved in the rearrangements of chromosome 16 commonly observed to accompany the particular subtype of acute nonlymphocytic leukemia referred to as ANLL subtype M4. Those chromosomal rearrangements include an inversion around the centromere between breakpoints in bands 16p13 and 16q22, a translocation between the homologs of chromosome 16 involving bands 16p13 and 16q22, and deletions in 16q22. Recom-bination between the low-abundance repetitive sequences in bands 16p13 and 16q22 could lead to the observed inversions and translocations. Therefore it is not unreason-able to consider that the repetitive sequences may be causally related to the inversions and translocations that occur in the chromosomes of leukemia cells. The isolation of repetitive sequences common to bands 16p13 and 16q22 is facilitating the isolation of the breakpoint regions and any gene(s) that may reside at those breakpoints.

We have discovered not only low-abundance repetitive sequences in the euchromatic arms of chromosome 16 but also novel repetitive sequences at the pericentromeric regions (regions near the centromere) of human chromosome 16 and at locations on other human chromosomes. The latter repetitive sequences are distinct from

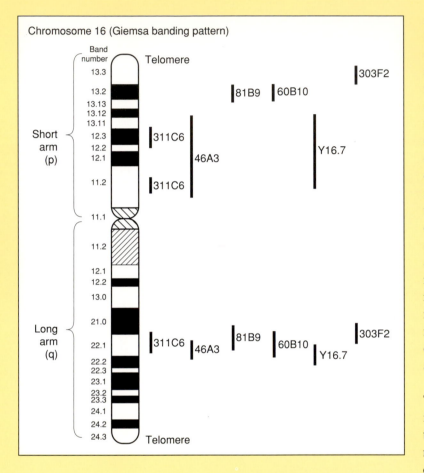

Chromosome 16 (Giemsa banding pattern)

any of the five satellite sequences (α, β, I, II, III) that are commonly found in the centromeric region of all human chromosomes. Previous work at the Laboratory had revealed that a large block of chromosome-specific, satellite-II-variant DNA occurs at the pericentromeric region of the long arm of chromosome 16 (at 16q11.1) and that a chromosome-specific α-satellite variant occurs in the centromeric region of chromosome 16. We have identified a new repetitive sequence that appears as a large block on the pericentromeric region of the short arm of chromosome 16 (at 16p11.1) and is also found in the telomeric regions of chromosome 14 (see page 212). This block of repetitive sequence at 16p11.1 composes almost 2 percent (or 2 million base pairs) of chromosome 16. In addition, we have found another repetitive sequence that maps to 16p11.1 and 15q11.1.

The region 16p11.1 appears to be quite rich in novel repetitive DNA sequences that map to a few other human chromosomes. Another minisatellite, MS29, maps to 16p11.1 and to chromosome 6. The MS29 locus at 16p11.1 is polymorphic in that it is absent from some human chromosomes 16. Several other unusual chromosome-16 variants have also been reported that appear to have extra material added in band 16p11.1 The extra material is C-band negative; that is, it does not darken when stained by the special techniques that usually darken only the centromeric regions. Also, the extra material is not composed of α-satellite DNA.

With the extensive amount of repetitive DNA found at 16p11.1, one might expect to find occasional amplification of this region. The amplification of this DNA does not appear to have any phenotypic effect, although the possibility of increased risk of aneuploidy cannot be ruled out. Also, the possibility that further amplification in successive generations could have detrimental effects cannot be ruled out. ■

Further Reading

C. R. Bryke, W. R. Breg, R. P. Venkateswara, and T. L. Yang-Feng. 1990. Duplication of euchromatin without phenotypic effects: A variant of chromosome 16. *American Journal of Medical Genetics* 36:43–44.

J. Buxton, P. Shelbourne, J. Davies, C. Jones, T. Van Tongeren, C. Aslanidis, P. de Jong, G. Jansen, M. Anvret, B. Riley, R. Williamson, and K. Johnson. 1992. Detection of an unstable fragment of DNA specific to individuals with myotonic dystrophy. *Nature* 355:547–548.

J. G. Dauwerse, E. A. Jumelet, J. W. Wessels, J. J. Saris, A. Hagemeijer, G. C. Beverstock, G. J. B. Van Ommen, and M. H. Breuning. 1992. Extensive cross-homology between the long and short arm of chromosome 16 may explain leukemic inversions and translocations. *Blood* 79:1299–1304.

B. A. Dombroski, S. L. Mathias, E. Nanthakumar, A. F. Scott, and H. H. Kazazian. 1991. Isolation of an active human transposable element. *Science* 254:1805–1810.

D. L. Grady, R. L. Ratliff, D. L. Robinson, E. C. McCanlies, J. Meyne, and R. K. Moyzis. 1992. Highly conserved repetitive DNA sequences are present at human centromeres. *Proceedings of the National Academy of Sciences of the United States of America* 89:1695–1699.

G. M. Greig, S. B. England, H. M. Bedford, and H. F. Willard. 1989. Chromosome-specific alpha satellite DNA from the centromere of human chromosome 16. *American Journal of Human Genetics* 45:862–872.

E. J. Kremer, M. Pritchard, M. Lynch, S. Yu, K. Holman, E. Baker, S. T. Warren, D. Schlessinger, G. R. Sutherland, and R. I. Richards. 1991. Mapping of DNA instability at the fragile X to a trinucleotide repeat sequence p(CCG)$_n$. *Science* 252:1711–1714.

A. R. La Spada, E. M. Wilson, D. B. Lubahn, A. E. Harding, and K. H. Fischbeck 1991. Androgen receptor gene mutations in X-linked spinal and bulbar muscular atrophy. *Nature* 352:77–79.

M. M. LeBeau, R. A. Larson, M. A. Bitter, J. W. Vardiman, H. M. Golomb, and J. D. Rowley. 1983. Association of an inversion of chromosome 16 with abnormal marrow eosinophils in acute myelomonocytic leukemia: A unique cytogenic-clinicopathologic association. *New England Journal of Medicine* 309:630–636.

R. K. Moyzis, K. L. Albright, M. F. Bartholdi, L. S. Cram, L. L. Deaven, C. E. Hildebrand, N. E. Joste, J. L. Longmire, J. Meyne, and T. Schwarzacher-Robinson. 1987. Human chromosome-specific repetitive DNA sequences: Novel markers for genetic analysis. *Chromosoma* 95:375–386.

K. Muratani, T. Hada, Y. Yamamoto, T. Kaneko, Y. Shigeto, T. Ohue, J. Furuyama, and K. Higashino. 1991. Inactivation of the cholinesterase gene by Alu insertion: Possible mechanism for human gene transposition. *Proceedings of the National Academy of Sciences of the United States of America* 88:11315–11319.

S. Ohno. 1972. So much "junk" DNA in our genomes. In *Evolution of Genetic Systems*, edited by H. H. Smith. New York: Gordon and Breach.

L. E. Orgel and F. H. C. Crick. 1980. Selfish DNA: The ultimate parasite. *Nature* 284:604–607.

R. L. Stallings, A. F. Ford, D. Nelson, D. C. Torney, C. E. Hildebrand, R. K. Moyzis. 1991. Evolution and distribution of (GT)$_n$ repetitive sequences in mammalian genomes. *Genomics* 10:807–815.

R. L. Stallings, N. A. Doggett, K. Okumura, and D. C. Ward. 1992. Chromosome 16 specific repetitive DNA sequences that map to chromosomal regions known to undergo breakage/rearrangement in leukemia cells. *Genomics* 13:332–338.

M. R. Wallace, L. B. Anderson, A. M. Saulino, P. E. Gregory, T. W. Glover, and F. S. Collins. 1991. A de novo Alu insertion results in neurofibromatosis type 1. *Nature* 353:864–866.

Z. Wong, N. J. Royle, and A. J. Jeffreys. 1990. A novel human DNA polymorphism resulting from transfer of DNA from chromosome 6 to chromosome 16. *Genomics* 7:222–234.

Mapping Chromosome 5 *Deborah Grady*

Constructing physical maps of complex genomes relies on the ability to isolate DNA segments for detailed analysis and to position those segments along the genome by identifying physical landmarks within them. The chromosome-16 physical map, now nearing completion, is a high-resolution map of DNA segments that have been isolated through cloning in cosmid and YAC vectors. The cloned fragments have been assembled into contigs and positioned along the chromosome based on detailed information about the positions of restriction sites, repetitive sequences, and the unique physical landmarks called STSs, or sequence-tagged sites. The chromosome-16 contig map provides information at a resolution of about 10,000 base pairs and will prove useful in studying chromosomal structure and organization.

In view of the need to complete physical maps of other chromosomes both rapidly and efficiently, we are adopting a different approach in mapping a second chromosome, chromosome 5. The goal is to construct a lower-resolution map consisting of (1) a series of STSs spaced evenly across the chromosome; and (2) YAC contigs assembled and ordered along the chromosome on the basis of their STS content. The project is being carried out in collaboration with John Wasmuth of the University of California at Irvine.

Our starting strategy utilizes the Los Alamos technologies for constructing chromosome-specific libraries to rapidly build a map covering 60 percent of the chromosome. The first step is to create a "framework" map of STS markers spaced at intervals of 0.5 to 1 million bases along chromosome 5. Given the statistics associated with generating STS markers at random and the fact that chromosome 5 is 194 million bases long, we will have to generate at least 400 STS markers to produce an STS map with a resolution of 1 million base pairs. We are developing the STS markers from a chromosome 5-specific library of M13 clones constructed at Los Alamos specifically for this purpose. Generating an STS involves sequencing a short cloned fragment of genomic DNA and identifying unique primer pairs from that sequence, which, when used in the polymerase chain reaction (PCR), will amplify a unique site in the genome. (See "The Polymerase Chain Reaction and Sequence-tagged Sites.")

Wasmuth is localizing the position of each STS to one of the intervals along human chromosome 5 defined by a panel of 30 hamster/human hybrid cells each containing various portions of chromosome 5. This localization is accomplished by determining through PCR screening which hybrid cells contain the STS and which do not. This method allows regional localization at a resolution of between 5 and 10 million base pairs. Plans are being made to refine the localization to a resolution of 200,000 base pairs using radiation-hybrid mapping. This mapping technique is analogous to genetic-linkage mapping in that distances are measured by how often two markers on the same chromosome become separated from one another. In linkage studies the separation is due to crossing over during meiosis, and the frequency of crossing over, the so-called genetic distance, is not necessarily proportional to the physical distance. In radiation-hybrid mapping the separation occurs through radiation-induced chromosome breakage, and the frequency of the radiation-induced breakage between two markers is linearly proportional to the physical distance separating the markers. Moreover, the technique is readily applied to any unique markers, in particular, to STSs.

Once generated and regionally localized on the chromosome, each STS will be "anchored," or located, on a non-chimeric YAC clone from a chromosome 5-specific YAC library, which has been constructed at Los Alamos. The cloning technique used to construct non-chimeric clones from flow-sorted chromosomes is discussed in "Libraries from Flow-sorted Chromosomes."

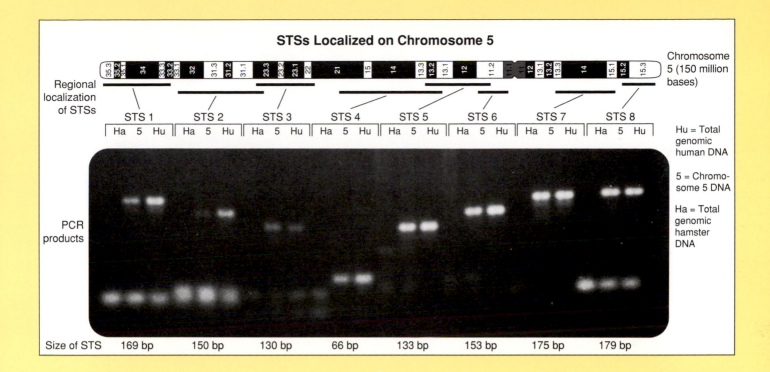

The non-chimeric YACs, localized along chromosome 5 by their STS content, will provide a solid base on which to build YAC contigs covering the chromosome. At Los Alamos, we will concentrate on mapping the short arm of chromosome 5 (52 million base pairs). Special emphasis will be placed on the region of chromosome 5 involved in the Cri du chat syndrome, one of the most common terminal-deletion syndromes in humans.

The figure (above) illustrates our early work on STS generation and regional localization. The upper portion shows the regional localization along chromosome 5 of eight STSs generated from our chromosome 5-specific M13 library. The regional localization (indicated with bars) will be reduced to intervals of 5 to 10 million bases once all available hybrid cells are screened for the presence of each STS.

The photograph in the lower portion of the figure shows the results of testing for the existence and uniqueness of each STS. The three gel lanes for each STS show the PCR products generated from total-genomic human DNA (right lane), chromosome-5 DNA (middle lane), and total-genomic hamster DNA (left lane) using the primer pairs that operationally define each STS. The PCR products from the three reactions were separated in parallel in a 3 percent agarose gel and stained with ethidium bromide to visualize the DNA. In all cases a single PCR amplification product of the same size resulted from the total-genomic human DNA and the chromosome-5 DNA. The hamster DNA served as a control to ensure that a positive signal from the chromosome-5 DNA did not represent a spurious signal arising from hamster DNA. In all cases, the hamster DNA yielded no PCR product. The test also shows that human/hamster hybrid cells can be screened for an STS without concern that false positive signals will arise from the hamster DNA in the hybrid cell. The PCR results demonstrate the existence of each STS as a unique landmark on chromosome 5 and the specificity of the PCR protocol defining each STS. The size of each STS is given at the bottom of the figure. ■

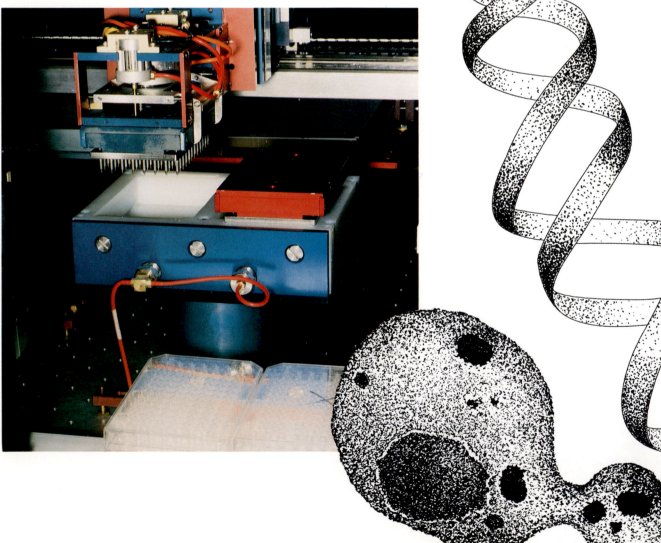

recombinant clones for mapping and sequencing DNA

LIBRARIES

Larry L. Deaven

Until the 1970s it was nearly impossible to isolate and purify single genes in sufficient quantity for biochemical analysis and DNA-sequence determination. The difficulty was largely due to the small size of many genes (2000 to 10,000 base pairs, or 2 to 10 kbp) and the large size of complex genomes such as the human genome (3 billion base pairs). In order to obtain 1 milligram of a 2-kbp human gene, such as the β-globin gene, all of the DNA in all of the cells of twenty-four people would have to be used as the starting material. Even if it were practical to obtain that much DNA, the problem of separating the DNA sequences that encode β-globin from the rest of the DNA would be very difficult. A solution to this problem was found during the recombinant-DNA revolution through the development of a technique called molecular cloning. By using molecular-cloning techniques, a small fragment of DNA can be duplicated, or amplified, into an unlimited number of copies.

Shown on these pages are the two common host cells for molecular cloning, the bacterium E. coli *and the yeast* S. cerevisiae; *a popular cloning vector, the λ phage, with its icosahedral head and long tail; a membrane containing a gridded array of recombinant clones to which DNA probes have been hybridized; and a robotic device developed at the Laboratory that creates those gridded arrays.*

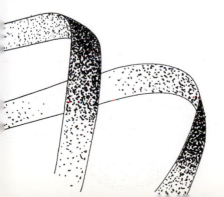

Molecular cloning of a gene requires three ingredients: one copy or a few copies of the gene to be cloned, a biological cloning vector, and a host cell. Cloning vectors are small molecules of DNA, often circular, that can be replicated within a host cell. Host cells are usually single-celled organisms such as bacteria and yeast. The first step of the cloning process is to combine the DNA fragment containing the gene sequence with the DNA of the cloning vector. If the vector DNA is circular, the circle is cut and the gene to be cloned is joined to each end of the opened circle. The new, somewhat larger circle of DNA is called a recombinant molecule, as is any molecule formed from a cloning vector and an inserted DNA fragment. The recombinant molecule can now be allowed to enter a host cell, where it is duplicated by the replication machinery of the host cell. Each time the recombinant molecule is replicated a new copy of the gene it contains is produced. Furthermore, each of the two daughter cells formed by the division of the original host cell receives copies of the recombinant molecule. When the host cell has grown into a colony, it is referred to as a recombinant clone, and the DNA fragment contained within each cell of the colony is said to have been cloned.

If we apply the cloning process to the production of 1 milligram of the human β-globin gene, a few copies of the gene would be inserted into plasmid cloning vectors. (Plasmids are small circular DNA molecules found in bacteria.) The recombinant plasmids would then be added to *E. coli* bacterial cells. Some of the cells would be entered, or "transformed," by a recombinant plasmid and would begin to produce copies of the cloned β-globin gene. Using this approach, just 2 liters of nutrient solution would produce enough *E. coli* cells to yield 1 milligram, or many

trillions of copies, of the β-globin gene. Molecular cloning removed the barriers that had prevented the biochemical and molecular analysis of individual genes in complex genomes.

During the recombinant-DNA revolution of the 1970s molecular cloning was also applied to the study of entire genomes with even more dramatic results. In that application, instead of cloning one gene at a time, all of the DNA in a genome is cut into small fragments and each of those fragments is cloned. The resulting collection of cloned fragments is called a DNA library. The word "library" was chosen because collectively, those cloned fragments contain all of the genetic information in an organism. Like a library of reference books, a library of cloned human DNA, for example, represents a collection of reference material for studying the genetic information in human beings. However, whereas conventional libraries are ordered collections of information, DNA libraries are unordered and uncharacterized collections of recombinant clones. Those collections provide the starting materials for almost all the current techniques used to decipher the instructions contained in DNA.

Two general features of libraries make them a remarkable resource. First, individual clones from a library can easily be isolated from the other clones. If the host cells are bacteria, a small portion of the library can be placed on a culture dish where each bacterium will form a colony of identical cells. Each colony can then be transferred to an individual culture dish and grown into a large population. Since each population contains a different cloned DNA insert, any region of the genome can be made accessible for analysis and sequencing. Second, a DNA library is a renewable resource. The clones can be grown individually or collectively

to replace any portions of the library that have been consumed. Therefore, a library is, in a sense, permanent. It can be repeatedly used or shared with other laboratories with little or no depletion of the original recombinant clones.

Just as there are legal libraries and medical libraries and scientific libraries, there are various types of DNA libraries. Each type is classified according to the vector used in library construction and the source of insert DNA. For example, DNA libraries constructed from the DNA in human cells are called human-genomic libraries. Ideally they contain all of the DNA sequences present in the human genome. Human cDNA libraries contain only those sequences utilized in protein coding. They are constructed by isolating messenger RNA (mRNA) molecules from human tissue and converting them into complementary DNA (cDNA) by the action of the enzyme reverse transcriptase. The cDNA fragments are then cloned. Because mRNA molecules are derived from the protein-coding portions of genes (see "Protein Synthesis" in "Understanding Inheritance"), cDNA libraries contain the sequences within genes that are expressed as proteins. Thus a brain cDNA library would be made from the mRNAs in brain cells and would contain only those DNA sequences expressed as brain proteins. Similarly, a liver cDNA library would contain those DNA sequences whose expression as protein is necessary to the proper functioning of liver cells.

A library is further classified according to the vector used in its construction. Since different vectors tend to carry DNA inserts with a limited range of lengths, classification by cloning vector, in effect, specifies the average length of the inserts within the recombinant clones of the library. Each type of library offers particular advantages for particular applications.

A primary goal of the Human Genome Project is to construct a physical map of each human chromosome. A physical map of a chromosome is an ordered collection of clones selected from one or more DNA libraries. Collectively, those clones carry inserts that include all of the DNA in the chromosome, and through the mapping process each cloned insert is ordered according to its position along the length of the chromosome (see "Physical Mapping" in "Mapping the Genome"). Thus the construction of a physical map is somewhat analogous to the cataloging of documents in a conventional library. Many of the recent improvements in cloning technology have been due to the initiation of the Human Genome Project and specifically to the need for physical maps of each human chromosome. Libraries with large DNA inserts make the mapping process both faster and easier, so considerable attention has been given to the development of cloning systems that can faithfully maintain and propagate large DNA inserts.

Although much effort is directed to ordering, or physical mapping, of the clones in a library, unorganized libraries are also useful tools. Through a process called library screening, cloned fragments of DNA that contain a sequence of interest can be retrieved from a library. The sequence of interest might be a region of a chromosome that contains a gene or some other genetic landmark. To find a particular clone, the library is screened with a DNA probe whose sequence is identical to a small portion of the region of interest. The probes may be synthesized, but often they are obtained from small-insert genomic-DNA libraries or from cDNA libraries. For example, a labeled probe containing a unique DNA sequence from the hemoglobin gene can be used to identify the clones in a DNA library whose inserts contain all or a portion of that gene.

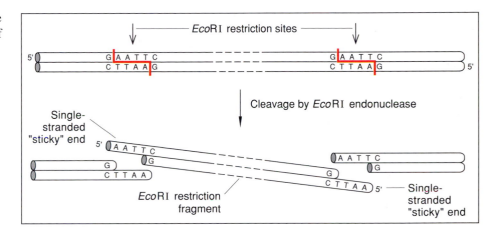

Figure 1. Restriction-Enzyme Cleavage
A restriction enzyme cleaves DNA at each recognition site on the DNA molecule. In this illustration the restriction enzyme is *Eco*RI, which cleaves DNA having the sequence 5′-GAATTC. Both strands of the DNA are cleaved between the G and A bases, leaving a tail with the sequence TTAA on each cut end. The tails are complementary to each other, so two pieces of DNA that have both been cleaved with *Eco*RI can be joined end-to-end to make a recombinant molecule. If a DNA molecule has tails that facilitate joining, it is said to have sticky ends.

DNA libraries are vital to much of the research in molecular genetics and to most of the activities sponsored by the Human Genome Project, including the construction of physical maps, the sequencing of DNA fragments, the isolation of genes, and the search for polymorphic genetic-linkage markers. Details of those activities are discussed elsewhere in this issue.

This article points out applications of DNA libraries but focuses primarily on the libraries themselves. It includes a brief history of the discoveries that led to the first DNA libraries and descriptions of the various types of libraries, their construction and manipulation, and the pioneering work here at Los Alamos National Laboratory on the construction of human-chromosome-specific DNA libraries.

Historical Background

The ability to construct libraries of recombinant clones depends on a very long series of discoveries and technological developments in DNA biochemistry. These include the discovery that DNA is the carrier of genetic information in 1944, the determination that DNA has a double-helical structure in 1953, and the unraveling of the genetic code in the 1960s. However, the first essential step in the origin of recombinant-DNA technology was the discovery in 1970 of a group of bacterial enzymes now called class-II restriction endonucleases, or simply restriction enzymes. Those enzymes help to protect the bacterium from the DNA of invading viruses by recognizing certain specific sequences in DNA and cleaving the viral genome within or near those recognition sites. (The bacteria produce other enzymes, called methyltransferases, that prevent the restriction enzymes from cutting the bacteria's own DNA.)

Figure 1 shows how the restriction enzyme *Eco*RI cuts double-stranded DNA into fragments. *Eco*RI is called a six-base cutter because it recognizes

Figure 2. Construction and Propagation of Recombinant Molecules

A circular DNA molecule containing an origin of replication, which allows the replication machinery of *E. coli* to reproduce the molecule, is used as a vector to carry foreign DNA into a host cell. The DNA of the circular vector and linear molecules of target DNA are digested or cut with the same restriction enzyme (*Eco*RI). The result is linear vector molecules and fragments of target DNA, which all have complementary "sticky" ends that permit the molecules to be joined by DNA ligase. When the vector and insert are joined, the resulting recombinant DNA molecule is inserted into an *E. coli* cell. Billions of copies of the recombinant molecule are made as the transformed cell replicates through many generations to form a bacterial colony. Each copy contains the short fragment of human DNA that was inserted into the original recombinant molecule.

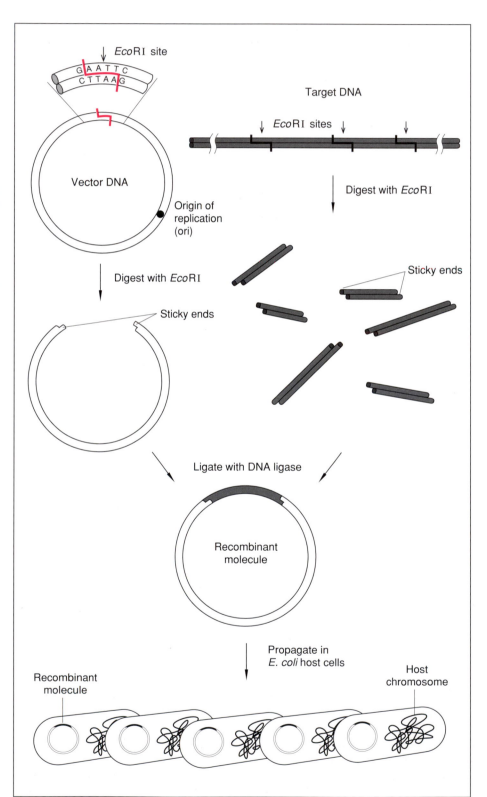

the six-base DNA sequence 5′-GAATTC and can cut DNA molecules at every site where that sequence occurs.

Like the recognition sequences of most restriction enzymes, that of *Eco*RI is a "palindrome," meaning that the sequence on one strand is identical to the complementary sequence on the other strand when both are read in the 5′-to-3′ direction. *Eco*RI cuts the phosphodiester bond between the G and the A nucleotides on both strands. Thus the enzyme produces a staggered cut so that the two cut ends have single-stranded tails, or so-called sticky ends. Those ends are useful for making recombinant molecules because any two fragments generated by the same restriction enzyme have identical sticky ends and therefore can be held together by hydrogen bonding. The two fragments can then be permanently joined, or recombined, by enzymes called DNA ligases.

Restriction enzymes provide a tool for cutting DNA in a reproducible way and they produce fragments that can easily be joined to other similarly cut fragments. Moreover, the many different restriction enzymes make it possible to cut large molecules of DNA into fragments of a controlled average size. In addition to six-base cutters, there are four-base and eight-base cutters. If the four bases A, T, G, and C were distributed randomly in DNA molecules, on average a given four-base sequence would occur every 256 base pairs, a given six-base sequence approximately every 4 kbp, and a given eight-base sequence approximately every 66 kbp. In actual practice, restriction-enzyme cleavage sites, or restriction sites, do not occur at random. For example, since the enzyme *Not*I recognizes the eight-base sequence 5′-GCGGCCGC, it would be expected to produce fragments averaging 66 kbp in length after all available sites are cut. But when *Not*I

is allowed to completely digest human DNA, that is, to cut all its restriction sites in a sample from the human genome, it produces fragments that have an average length of 1 million nucleotides because its recognition sequence is rarer than expected (in particular the sequence 5′-CG is rare in mammalian genomes). Nevertheless, by selecting the proper restriction enzyme, it is possible to repeatedly cut DNA molecules into fragments of different average lengths. Fragment size may also be adjusted by allowing the enzyme to cut only a portion of the available restriction sites. For example, if *Eco*RI is permitted to cut only one 5′-GAATTC sequence in five, the resulting average fragment size will be 20 kbp rather than 4 kbp. This "partial digestion" is accomplished by using a shorter incubation period or a lower concentration of enzyme than a complete digest would require. The ability to reduce large molecules of DNA to smaller fragments of controlled average size is a critical step in the construction of libraries because most cloning vectors accept only DNA inserts whose lengths fall within a limited range.

Just two years after the discovery of restriction enzymes, the first experiments were performed that created recombinant DNA molecules. DNA containing genes from a bacterium and from a bacterial virus was inserted into the genome of simian virus 40, a virus that infects mammalian cells. The two types of DNA were initially in the form of closed loops. The restriction enzyme *Eco*RI was used to cut the loops and the resulting linearized molecules were joined to form recombinant molecules. The ultimate objective of that work was to use the simian virus as a biological vector to carry foreign genes into mammalian cells and to see if the foreign genes would be expressed in their new environment. Concerns over the potential hazards of recombinant

molecules halted research on gene transfer into mammalian cells for several years; nevertheless, the experiment clearly demonstrated that a restriction enzyme would cut DNA in a predictable manner and that restriction fragments from two different organisms could be joined.

Shortly after that experiment, molecular cloning techniques were extended and improved. In one set of experiments, a plasmid containing a single *Eco*RI restriction site as well as a gene for resistance to the antibiotic tetracycline was purified from *E. coli* and a method was devised for introducing the plasmid into other *E. coli* cells that were not resistant to tetracycline. The transformed cells were then grown on agar (a culture medium) mixed with tetracycline. Some of the bacteria grew into colonies, demonstrating that they had taken up the plasmid and that it was functioning. Following that experiment, the plasmid was recombined with a second plasmid containing a gene for resistance to the antibiotic kanamycin. The recombinant plasmids also transformed host cells and conferred antibiotic resistance. Finally, experiments demonstrated that DNA from two different species could be recombined and propagated as a recombinant plasmid. A gene encoding a ribosomal RNA in the toad *Xenopus laevis* was recombined with *E. coli* plasmid DNA and propagated in *E. coli* host cells. The general approach for those experiments is shown in Figure 2.

As more experience was gained in recombinant-DNA technology, new cloning vectors were developed and methods for growing and handling recombinant molecules were further improved. The possibility of cloning fragments of DNA that represented all of the genetic information in the human genome began to look achievable. An intermediate step in this direction was the construction of a recombinant-DNA library from the DNA in fruit flies (*Drosophila melanogaster*) in 1974. Several recombinant plasmids containing either unique-sequence or repetitive-sequence inserts were isolated from the library and localized or mapped to specific regions of the *Drosophila* chromosomes. That work suggested the potential value of constructing libraries from the total DNA in a complex organism, selecting clones from the library that contain genes of interest, and then using those clones to find the chromosomal location of the cloned gene sequences. Further progress led to the construction of a library of DNA from human embryonic liver tissue in 1978 and the selection of clones from the library that contained human α- and β-globin genes. That experiment clearly demonstrated that DNA libraries could provide a starting point for mapping the human genome and for studying gene structure and expression.

Library Construction

Continued progress since 1978 has made it possible to construct many kinds of recombinant-DNA libraries. Libraries differ in the preparation of the target DNA, the choice of the host strain, and the design of the cloning vector. Each variation produces a library that has advantages for specific applications. The most significant characteristics of a library are usually determined by the choice of the cloning vector, so a description of the vectors currently in use provides a convenient way of defining the variety of libraries.

This article focuses primarily on the four types of vectors currently used in constructing libraries for the physical mapping of complex genomes. In common use today are plasmids, bacteriophage (phage) genomes, cosmids, and yeast artificial chromosomes (YACs).

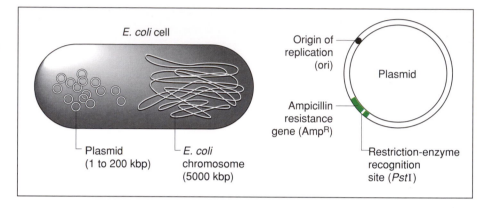

Figure 3. Plasmids

Plasmids are small, circular DNA molecules that occur naturally in *E. coli* and other bacteria. They all contain a replicon, a DNA sequence that enables the host bacterium to replicate them. The replicon includes an origin of replication (ori). Many contain restriction-enzyme cleavage sites and DNA sequences that encode antibiotic-resistance genes. For instance, the plasmid shown here contains an ampicillin-resistance gene and a single cleavage site for the restriction enzyme *Pst* I. These natural properties were exploited to adapt plasmids for use as the first vector systems.

The first three vectors are all referred to as *E. coli*-based systems because they are propagated within the common intestinal bacterium *Escherichia coli*. The fourth is called a yeast-based system because propagation occurs within the baker's yeast *Saccharomyces cerevisiae*.

Whereas the original versions of some of these vectors were similar to wild-type organisms, the modern vectors are highly engineered for a variety of uses. For example, DNA sequences not essential for replication have been removed from some wild-type vectors to provide space for large DNA inserts. Molecular biologists have also inserted sequences into the vectors that help in incorporating and manipulating DNA inserts and in recovering the inserts from recombinant clones.

E. coli-based Cloning

Plasmids. As mentioned above, plasmids were the first vectors to be used in constructing recombinant clones.

These small chromosomes are often found in *E. coli* cells along with the main bacterial chromosome. Plasmids are circular, double-stranded DNA molecules that range in length from 1 to 200 kbp and are thus considerably smaller than the main chromosome, which is about 5 million base pairs long (see Figure 3).

Plasmids frequently contain genes that are advantageous to the bacterial host. Among these are genes that confer resistance to antibiotics and genes that produce restriction enzymes. Every plasmid also includes DNA sequences called replicons, each of which contains an origin of replication and the other elements the plasmid needs in order to be replicated by bacteria. Although some types of plasmids replicate only when the main chromosome replicates and tend to exist as a single copy within the host cell, most plasmids commonly used as cloning vectors replicate independently of the main chromosome and exist in multiple copies, from ten to five hundred, within the host. The entry of a plasmid, whether engineered or natural, into a

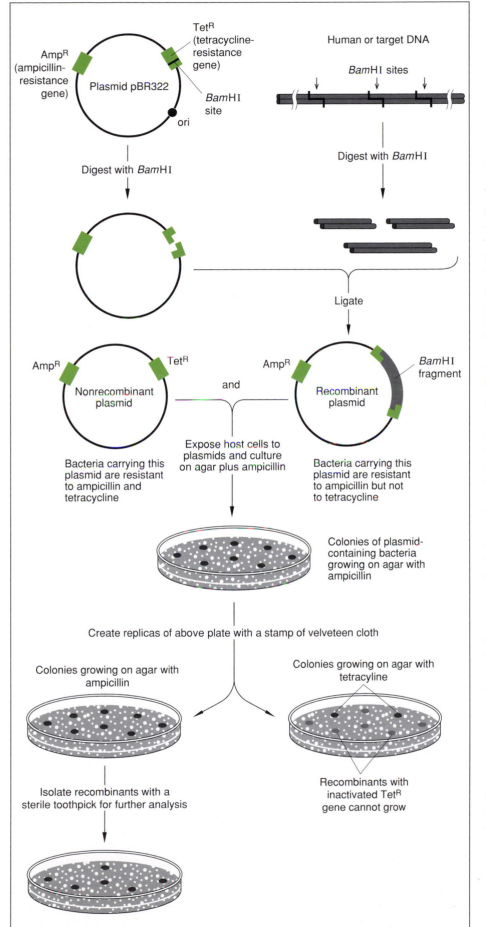

Figure 4. Selection of Recombinant Clones

The plasmid vector pBR322, containing genes for ampicillin resistance and tetracycline resistance, allows clones containing foreign-DNA inserts to be distinguished from clones lacking inserts. Digestion with *Bam*HI opens the circular molecule at a point within the tetracycline resistance gene. A target DNA fragment produced by *Bam*HI digestion can then be inserted to make a circular recombinant plasmid. The presence of the insert inside the tetracycline gene inactivates the gene. Thus nonrecombinant plasmids provide resistance to both ampicillin and tetracycline, whereas recombinant plasmids provide resistance only to ampicillin. A population of plasmid-free host cells is exposed to the plasmids and then spread on culture dishes containing agar mixed with ampicillin. Only host cells that were transformed by either recombinant or nonrecombinant plasmids multiply and form clones in the presence of ampicillin. A portion of each clone is transferred to each of two other dishes in a way that preserves the relative positions of the clones. One dish has ampicillin in the agar; the other has tetracycline. The recombinant clones are those that grow in ampicillin and do not grow in tetracycline. This selection technique, called insertional inactivation, was used in the early plasmid vectors. Now it is more common to use a single antibiotic resistance gene as a selectable marker and select transformed cells directly on the basis of response to the appropriate antibiotic. The formation of nonrecombinant plasmids is suppressed by chemical techniques (such as removing the phosphate groups from the ends of the vector so that the ends can not bind to each other).

bacterial cell is called transformation. The exact mechanism of entry is unknown, but all the methods for increasing the frequency of transformation involve increasing the permeability of the pores in the bacterial membrane, which presumably allows the plasmid to pass through. Even when those methods are employed, only a small fraction (1 in 10,000) of the cells in a bacterial population are stably transformed when exposed to a solution containing plasmids.

The naturally occurring plasmids used as cloning vectors in the 1970s contained features that could be exploited both in the cloning process and in the process of selecting or identifying clones containing recombinant plasmids. Figure 4 illustrates such a plasmid. It contains a single cutting site for the restriction enzyme *Bam*HI. The restriction site is located in the middle of a gene conferring resistance to the antibiotic tetracycline. To form a recombinant plasmid, the vector is cut at that site with *Bam*HI and then ligated with a fragment of target DNA that was also produced by digestion with *Bam*HI. The DNA insert thus separates the antibiotic-resistance gene into two pieces and inactivates the gene. If a bacterial cell is transformed by that recombinant plasmid, that host cell will be sensitive to tetracycline. A bacterial cell transformed by a plasmid with no insert will be resistant to tetracycline. Thus the tetracycline-resistance gene not only contains a cloning site, or site for insertion of a foreign DNA fragment, but also acts as a selectable marker to differentiate recombinant clones containing DNA inserts from clones containing plasmid vectors but no foreign DNA insert.

The plasmid vectors developed in the early 1970s were useful, but they had many limitations. They replicated poorly, had a limited number of selectable markers, and contained restriction sites for at best two restriction enzymes. The plasmids used today have been engineered to overcome these limitations. Some plasmids even contain regulatory regions that facilitate the expression of foreign genes contained within the DNA insert and genes that can change the color of a bacterial colony and thus allow visual identification of clones containing recombinant plasmids.

However, plasmids have two limitations that cannot be overcome. First, plasmids are inefficient at transforming bacteria. Second, plasmids containing long DNA inserts are particularly inefficient at transformation, and tend to lose portions of the inserts as they are replicated. Therefore, plasmids are usually used to carry short inserts on the order of 4 kbp in length. To clone all the DNA in the haploid human genome (3 billion base pairs) would require 750,000 plasmids each containing a different DNA insert. To find a particular gene in such a library, all of those clones would have to be screened. Those limitations spurred the development of new cloning vectors with higher transformation efficiencies and the ability to accommodate larger inserts. The first of the new vectors was the genome of a bacterial virus, bacteriophage λ.

Bacteriophage λ. Bacteriophage, or phage, are viruses that infect bacteria. Being extremely simple biological systems, they had been extensively studied since the 1930s. In the 1970s they were seen as promising cloning vectors because their DNA genomes are readily replicated by the cellular machinery of the host bacterium and because, unlike plasmids, they have a natural and efficient mechanism of entry into a bacterial host.

An intact λ phage has a protein coat consisting of an icosahedral head and a rod-like tail. The head contains the phage genome, a double-stranded linear DNA molecule about 48 kbp in length, with short, complementary single-stranded ends of 12 nucleotides each. Those cohesive ends are called *cos* sites. During replication, the phage tail attaches to a bacterial host cell, and the phage genome enters the host's interior. There the DNA molecule may incorporate itself into the bacterial chromosome. Alternatively, in the "lytic" life cycle used in cloning, the DNA cyclizes by base pairing of the *cos* sites and begins to express genes involved in the replication of phage DNA. Initially, the replication process forms a long strand of DNA that consists of hundreds of copies of the λ-phage genome. Such a strand is called a concatamer. Then the phage DNA directs the synthesis of proteins for the head and tail as well as enzymes that cut the concatamer into individual λ genomes and package each one into a phage head. When the cell contains between 100 and 200 new phage particles (about 20 minutes after infection), λ proteins cause it to rupture, or "lyse," and the released phage particles infect surrounding cells (see Figure 5).

A phage particle added to a monolayer, or "lawn," of bacterial cells growing on an agar plate produces through that infection cycle a clear area called a plaque containing lysed bacterial cells and replicated phage. A visible plaque contains a population of from 1 to 10 million identical phage particles.

A section in the middle of the λ-phage genome contains a cluster of genes that are unnecessary for its replication in *E. coli* cells. To make the λ-phage genome into a vector, either the DNA is cut or that middle section of DNA is removed, leaving the left and right end fragments (called arms) that are essential for λ replication. The arms are then attached to an insert. If the insert is not too different in size from the DNA that it

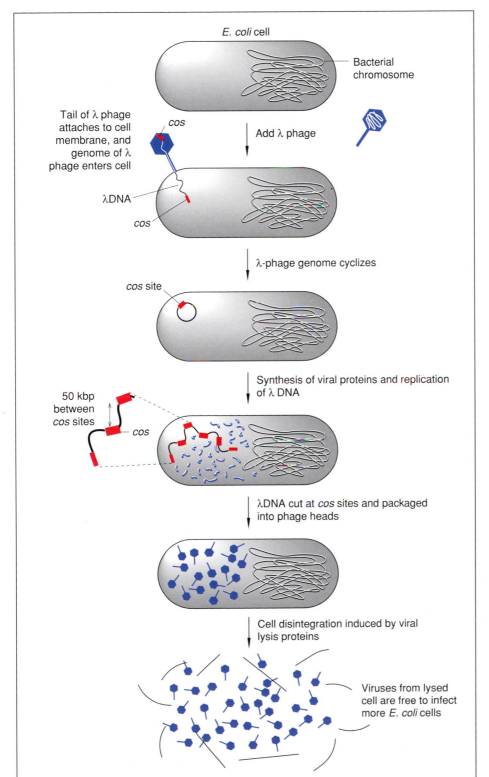

E. coli cell

Bacterial chromosome

Tail of λ phage attaches to cell membrane, and genome of λ phage enters cell

Add λ phage

cos

λDNA

cos

λ-phage genome cyclizes

cos site

Synthesis of viral proteins and replication of λ DNA

50 kbp between cos sites

cos

λDNA cut at cos sites and packaged into phage heads

Cell disintegration induced by viral lysis proteins

Viruses from lysed cell are free to infect more E. coli cells

Figure 5. Lambda-Phage Lytic Life Cycle

The tail of a phage particle attaches to the surface of a host *E. coli* cell and the phage genome enters the cell. The genome cyclizes by base pairing of the complementary, single-stranded "terminus" on each end (the cohesive ends or *cos* sites). The viral DNA then directs the synthesis of proteins necessary for its replication and enzymes and structural proteins necessary for the assembly of phage particles. The product of genome replication is a long chain, or "concatamer," of many copies of the viral chromosome joined end to end at the *cos* sites. When 100–200 copies of the viral DNA have been made, the concatamer of DNA is cleaved at the *cos* sites into individual phage chromosomes by phage enzymes that recognize and cut them. Phage enzymes then package these genomes into phage particles that are released by cell lysis and can infect new bacterial cells.

replaces, the resulting recombinant DNA molecule can be packaged to make an infective λ particle.

Packaging is performed in vitro using "packaging extracts" that include the enzymes and structural proteins needed for head and tail assembly. Packaging extracts are isolated from two strains of E. coli engineered from natural strains whose chromosomes contain λ DNA (as a result of the phage's nonlytic life cycle). Under appropriate growth conditions each of the engineered strains makes some of the proteins necessary to package λ-phage particles. If a single strain produced all the packaging proteins, phage coats would form inside the cell and the cells could not be used as a source of packaging extracts. Therefore in each strain the λ DNA has a mutation that prevents the bacterium from producing one protein essential for assembly of λ-phage particles. The strains differ in which protein is missing. The unassembled phage proteins are extracted from cells of each strain and combined in vitro with each other and the recombinant DNA so that the DNA can be packaged into phage particles. Once the phage particles have been produced in a test tube, the phage infection cycle described above will, in a very short time, generate recombinant phage clones containing millions of copies of the insert DNA.

As suggested above, for the packaging to work the size of the insert must be similar to the size of the phage DNA it replaces (or if no phage DNA was removed, the insert must be small). In practice, inserts usually range from 12 to 22 kbp in length. With inserts of 20 kbp the DNA in the human genome could be fragmented and included in a library made up of 150,000 recombinant λ-phage particles, a considerable improvement over the 750,000 plasmids that would be required. Phage also have the advantage of transforming hosts

far more efficiently than plasmids do; typically one phage particle in ten infects a host bacterium.

A cloning vector based on λ phage was first used in 1974. Since that time many versatile and sophisticated vectors have been derived from the wild-type phage (see Figure 6). This progress is due in large part to the extensive studies of the genetics and physiology of bacteriophage beginning in the late 1930s and continuing today. Without that accumulation of detailed knowledge, the use of λ phage as a central tool of molecular biology would have been delayed and might well not have been developed at all.

Cosmids. Bacteriophage-λ vectors made it possible to construct libraries with inserts of up to 22 kbp. However, many genes contain on the order of 35 to 40 kbp. In order to clone those genes as single inserts, a vector with greater capacity was needed. In 1979 the first account was published of a successful library based on a more capacious vector called a cosmid.

Cosmids were engineered to combine desirable features of plasmids and λ phage (including the cos site, whence the word "cosmid"). Phage can transform hosts efficiently and maintain long inserts without deletions. Nevertheless, the size of their inserts is limited because a λ-phage head can hold no more than 52 kbp of DNA, and the phage requires 30 to 40 kbp for replication and packaging. On the other hand, plasmid vectors need only a replicon for reproduction in host cells, a drug-resistance gene for use as a selectable marker, and restriction sites for inserting foreign DNA. A cosmid is designed to reproduce as a plasmid and be packaged as a λ phage. It contains all the necessary ingredients for reproduction in E. coli and for other cloning functions and is only 5 to 6 kbp long. Cosmids can therefore accept

inserts as large as 47 kbp and still be packaged in a phage protein coat to facilitate entry into host cells.

This synthetic vector is grown as a plasmid in E. coli and then isolated. To prepare the circular vector for cloning, it is cleaved by a restriction enzyme to produce a linear molecule containing a cos site. Next a DNA insert is ligated with the vector. The ligation produces long concatamers in which inserts alternate with vectors. When phage packaging extracts are added to the concatamers, the cos site in each vector is cleaved, producing individual phage chromosomes. Chromosomes in the appropriate size range are packaged into phage particles that can infect bacteria. Once inside the host cell, the recombinant DNA cyclizes and reproduces as a plasmid. Because inserts in cosmids have an average size of about 40 kbp, a cosmid library containing all of the DNA in the human genome would require approximately 75,000 clones, about half as many as a λ-phage library would require. Unfortunately, some cosmids, if not maintained under optimal conditions, may lose portions of their inserts during replication.

Yeast-based Cloning

Yeast Artificial Chromosomes. Cosmid vectors fulfilled some of the needs for longer cloned inserts. However, during the 1980s new genes were discovered that are too large to be cloned as single fragments in cosmids, and attempts to map large segments of the human genome were hindered by the small size of the inserts in λ and cosmid libraries. A new cloning system that accommodates longer inserts was first reported in 1987. The recombinant molecules are called yeast artificial chromosomes (YACs) because they are maintained and reproduced as chromosomes in yeast

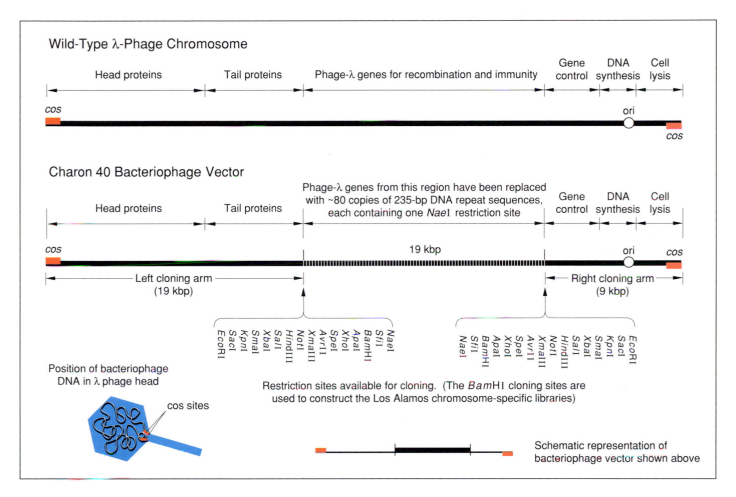

Figure 6. Engineering the Genome of Wild-Type λ Phage into a λ-Phage Vector

The genome of the wild-type lambda phage is divided into six regions according to the locations of genes that encode various functions. In the vector Charon 40, a region that is not necessary for replication is replaced with 80 copies of a 235-base-pair sequence that contains a cleavage site for the restriction enzyme *Nae*I. When Charon 40 is cut with *Nae*I, the repeat-sequence region is reduced to small fragments that can be separated from the cloning arms of the vector by gel electrophoresis. The section of Charon 40 on each side of the repeat-sequence region (enlarged) contains a single restriction site for each of a number of restriction enzymes. These sites have been added to Charon 40 to increase its versatility as a cloning vector.

host cells. The vector arms contain a yeast centromere, two yeast telomeres, and a yeast origin of replication, the elements necessary for yeast cells to replicate the recombinant molecules in the same way they replicate yeast chromosomes.

YAC vectors, like cosmid vectors, are highly engineered and are produced as plasmids in *E. coli*. The first YAC vectors were single plasmids containing all the yeast sequences listed above as well as a plasmid replicon, one or more markers to use in selecting *E. coli* cells containing YAC vectors, and two restriction sites for the same enzyme: one between the sequences that give rise to the telomeres and one at which to insert target DNA. Cloning with these YAC vectors is similar in approach to λ-phage and cosmid cloning. The vector is cleaved at the insertion site and between the telomere sequences. The cleavage produces two vector arms that are ligated with the insert to produce a YAC. The YAC is then allowed to transform a yeast cell; once inside the host cell, it behaves as a stable chromosome.

The YAC vector carries a gene that suppresses the host strain's production of a red pigment. The commonly used cloning site is within that suppressor gene. If nonrecombinant YAC vectors

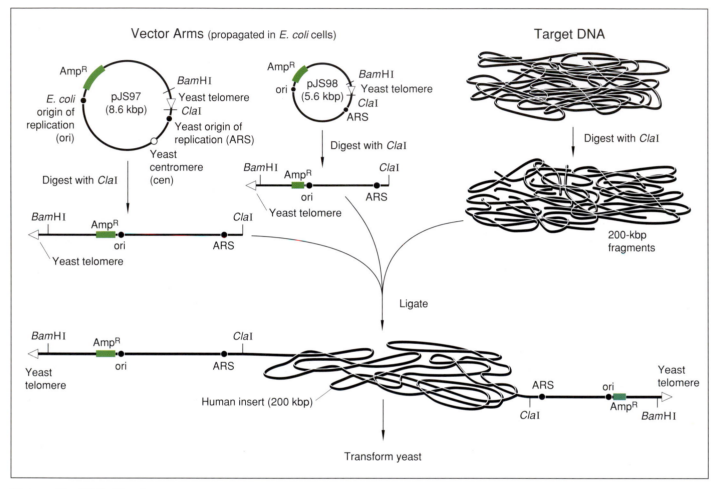

Figure 7. YAC Cloning

The two arms of the YAC shown are manufactured separately in *E. coli* as plasmids pJS97 and pJS98. Each contains an ampi-cillin-resistance gene, an *E. coli* replicon (including an origin of replication) so that it can propagate as a plasmid, a yeast origin of replication (labeled ARS), a yeast telomere, and several restriction sites, including one for *Cla*I located at the end of the telomere. Only pJS97 contains a yeast centromere and a pigment-suppressor gene that changes the color of yeast colonies. The plasmids are linearized and the target DNA is fragmented, both by cutting with *Cla*I. The vector arms thus produced each have a yeast telomere sequence at one end (arrow) and a *Cla*I tail at the other end. The fragments of target (human) DNA are then ligated to the vector arms to form a YAC that can transform yeast cells. Promoters for T7 RNA polymerase (not shown) are located near the *Cla*I restriction site. These sequences are used in generating RNA probes from the ends of the insert.

transform yeast cells, the resulting yeast colonies are white. Insertion of target DNA inactivates that gene, causing the formation of red rather than white yeast colonies and providing a rapid means of identifying the colonies that contain the target DNA.

In 1991 a new type of YAC vector was reported that has additional advantages (see Figure 7). This vector is produced as two separate plasmids: one carries the centromere and serves as one arm of the YAC, and the other serves as the second YAC arm. Each arm has a selectable marker to identify transformed hosts, and the arm containing the centromere also contains a pigment-suppressor gene used to monitor the number of YACs

in each host cell and their stability against deletions. Again the host strain produces red pigment. When one YAC is present in each cell, the colony is pink; the presence of two YACs in each cell causes the colony to be white; and an unstable colony (one in which some cells are losing the YAC as they divide) has red and pink sectors.

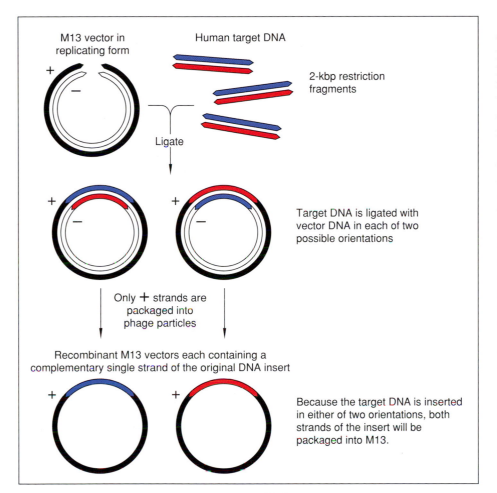

The YAC cloning system has the advantage of being able to maintain and propagate inserts up to a million base pairs long. The average insert size in many YAC libraries is 200 to 400 kbp, five to ten times the average size in a cosmid library, and the human genome may be covered in 7500 YAC clones.

A major disadvantage of the YAC cloning system is that it often produces chimeras. Chimeras are YACs whose inserts are composed of more than one piece of target DNA. For example, a chimeric YAC with a 400-kbp human insert may contain 300 kbp from human chromosome 3 and 100 kbp from human chromosome 10. Chimeras complicate the construction of physical maps of overlapping clones, and they must be identified to avoid mapping errors. Unfortunately, identifying chimeras is laborious. Moreover, since 40 to 60 percent of the clones in most YAC libraries are chimeric, chimeras add a significant amount of work to the mapping process. Techniques developed at the Laboratory for producing nonchimeric YACs are described in "Libraries from Flow-sorted Chromosomes."

Figure 8. Cloning in Bacteriophage M13

The double-stranded circular replicating form of the phage genome is recovered from infected *E. coli* cells and then cut with a restriction enzyme. The resulting vector is ligated to target DNA cut with the same enzyme. The recombinant molecules are allowed to enter bacteria as plasmids do. Inside the bacterium, they replicate themselves and produce phage proteins. Only the + strands of the phage genome are packaged as viral progeny. Nevertheless, roughly equal amounts of both strands of the insert are obtained because some inserts enter phage DNA molecules oriented so that one strand of the insert is incorporated into the phage's + strand, and some inserts enter so that the complementary strand is incorporated into the + strand. Finally the + strands are packaged into phage particles and leave the host cell (without damaging it).

To allow the generation of probes from the ends of the DNA inserts, each arm contains a promoter sequence from the T7 phage that is located near the sites of attachment to the insert. RNA polymerase from phage T7 can bind to the promoters and transcribe the ends of a DNA insert into RNA. These RNA "end probes" are useful in characterizing the YAC inserts. For example, one can try to hybridize either end probe from one YAC to all of the other YACs in a library and thus locate overlapping YACs for chromosome walking.

Bacteriophage M13. Another vector used to construct libraries is derived from the filamentous *E. coli* phage M13. M13 clones are particularly convenient for DNA sequencing. An M13 phage particle consists of single-stranded DNA packaged into a narrow cylindrical protein coat. The strand of DNA in the phage particle is designated as the + strand. When the phage infects *E. coli* cells, the DNA replicates to form about 300 double-stranded (+/-) copies, but only the + strands from those copies are packaged into progeny virus particles. Figure 8 shows the method of cloning with M13. The double-stranded form is used as the cloning vector. Small fragments (about 2 kbp) are inserted into any of several restriction sites engineered into the M13 phage vector. The recombinant molecules enter the host cells as plasmids and replicate as phage. The + strands produced by the replication are used as a template for Sanger dideoxy sequencing (see "DNA Sequencing" in "Mapping the Genome"). Because the sequence at the M13 insertion site has been determined, an oligonucleotide (short DNA sequence) can be synthesized to serve as a universal primer for the dideoxy sequencing of any DNA fragment that is cloned into M13.

Host Cells

Host cells are as important in cloning as vectors. To work well in cloning, host cells should be as accessible as possible to the introduction of the vector, they should facilitate library screening, and they should alter inserts as rarely as possible. In addition, while host organisms should provide conditions for robust growth of recombinant molecules, they must also be sufficiently disabled to have no significant probability of surviving outside of laboratories. The need for safe cloning systems was a major concern for scientists in the early years of recombinant-DNA research, and progress was delayed until host bacterial strains were developed that had many features to prevent the escape of transformed cells from laboratories. For example, the weakened strains require chemicals not likely to be found in nature and have cell walls that burst in the presence of low salt concentrations or a trace of detergent. In hindsight many of the concerns about unexpected, hazardous properties of recombinant organisms have turned out to be unwarranted. Nevertheless, the early guidelines and regulations helped reassure the public that recombinant-DNA procedures would not result in

new diseases or the spread of bacterial antibiotic resistance.

Once the issue of safety was appropriately addressed, the development of host-vector systems accelerated, in large part because of the wealth of information available on the genetics and biochemistry of *E. coli* cells. Some vectors are so specialized that they can be propagated only in a single host strain. Others can grow in a wide variety of strains so that a host strain can be selected according to the requirements of a specific cloning application. In general, strains of bacteria that produce restriction enzymes are avoided because those strains do not propagate inserts that contain a susceptible cleavage site. Some strains of bacteria produce enzymes called methyltransferases that add methyl groups to certain bases in DNA. Those enzymes protect bacteria from their own restriction enzymes by altering the structure of recognition sites. Strains with active methyltransferase genes are also unsuitable for cloning because they would produce recombinant DNA molecules that could not be cleaved by certain restriction enzymes and therefore could not be used in experiments involving those enzymes. For bacteriophage-λ vectors, host strains must be susceptible to λ infection. For plasmid cloning, strains free of nonvector plasmids must be used in order to recover the recombinant molecules without contamination by other plasmids. Other interactions between vectors and host cells can serve to identify and isolate cells that contain vectors. For example, a host strain that requires a particular amino acid can be used with a vector that contains a gene for the production of the amino acid. When grown on a medium lacking the amino acid, only bacteria that have incorporated the vector will survive.

Wild-type *E. coli* produce enzymes that recombine DNA strands containing

homologous sequences. Because human DNA contains many sequences that are repeated in various places in the genome, there was considerable concern that recombinant inserts would be rearranged and deleted when propagated in *E. coli*. From the beginning strains of *E. coli* deficient in recombination enzymes were used in cloning. Now many such strains have been engineered, and reports of DNA rearrangements are far outnumbered by studies that find no rearrangements after extensive propagation of recombinant molecules. There are, unfortunately, a few types of sequences that are known to replicate poorly or not at all in the *E. coli* environment, primarily repetitive sequences such as the DNA in the centromeric region of a chromosome.

As might be expected of the relatively new YAC-*S. cerevisiae* system, the choice of host strains is limited; in fact, only two are available. The desired features are similar to those for *E. coli* strains: ease of transformation, stable maintenance of artificial chromosomes, and compatibility with various selection and recovery systems. The two yeast host strains in widespread use differ primarily in the selectable markers they contain, and because YACs can be readily transferred from one strain to the other, the features of the two host strains are complementary. A useful addition to the available yeast host strains would be a strain deficient in recombination pathways, which would reduce the incidence of chimeric inserts in YACs.

Genomic Libraries Constructed from Cellular DNA

As mentioned previously, the first libraries to contain DNA inserts from total cellular DNA were constructed using phage vectors. Those early

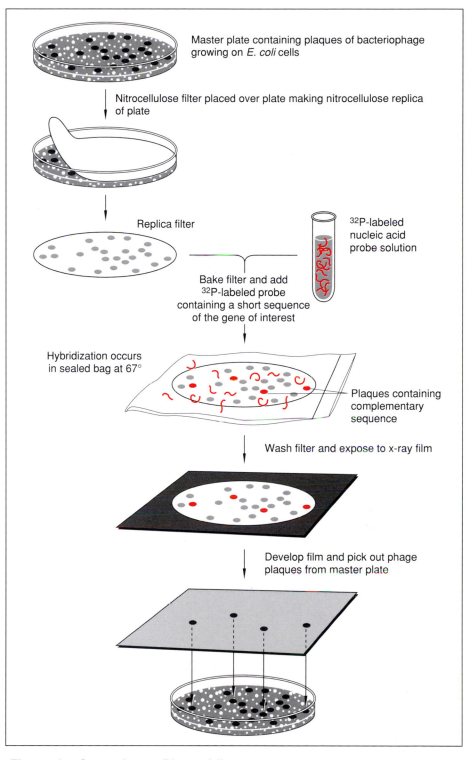

libraries, like many used today, were designed to facilitate the isolation of genes and nearby regulatory sequences for studies of gene structure and function. Because a single gene might span several fragments in the library, a library designed to be searched for genes should consist of overlapping cloned fragments. Then a series of cloned fragments that overlap each other and span the entire gene can be identified. Overlapping fragments are made by partially digesting with a restriction enzyme the DNA extracted from many cells. In partial digestion of target DNA, the restriction enzyme cleaves a random subset of the restriction sites in each of the many copies of the target molecules and thereby produces a population of overlapping fragments, which can be used in constructing a library of overlapping clones.

To identify clones in the library that duplicate all or part of a gene of interest, the library must be screened with a gene probe, a single-stranded short segment of DNA or RNA composed of a sequence complementary to the sequence of the gene. The first probes were cDNAs constructed from specialized cells that produce large amounts of specific mRNAs. Later, it became possible to construct cDNA libraries that contained sequences complementary to most of the mRNAs found in specific tissues, such as brain tissue.

As illustrated in Figure 9, the first step in screening a bacteriophage library with a gene probe is to grow a lawn of *E. coli* host cells in a set of agar-coated Petri dishes. About 150 to 200 recombinant phage particles from the library are added to each plate. When plaques have formed, a filter membrane is placed on each agar surface. Some phage particles from each plaque adhere to the membrane, so a pattern of invisible spots identical to the pattern of plaques on the Petri plate is formed on

Figure 9. Screening a Phage Library

Recombinant phage from the library are allowed to form plaques on a set of master plates. A nitrocellulose filter membrane is placed on the surface of the agar. Some phage adhere to the membrane, providing a copy of the plaque arrangement. The filter is first treated with sodium hydroxide to lyse the phage particles and denature the DNA they contain. The filter is then baked to prevent the DNA from renaturing and to fix it in position. The membrane is exposed to a radioactively labeled probe, which hybridizes only to those spots containing a DNA sequence complementary to the probe sequence. Then the radioactive spots are detected by making a sandwich consisting of a sheet of x-ray film and the filter enclosed in a plastic wrap. When the x-ray film is developed, spots appear at the same positions as the positions of the plaques in the Petri dish that hybridized to the probe.

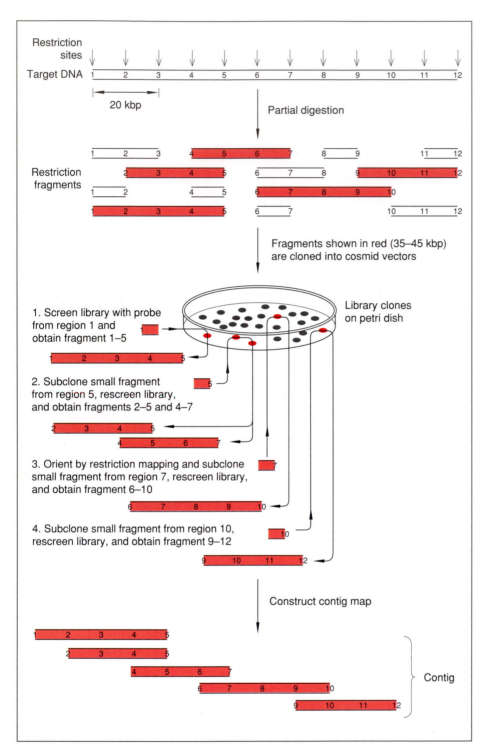

Figure 10. Chromosome Walking

The aim of this technique is to recover fragments of cloned DNA that span a gene or any DNA region of interest. A DNA library constructed from partially digested DNA provides a source of overlapping cloned fragments of the entire genome. A DNA probe known to be close to the gene of interest is used to screen the library for fragments that contain sequences complementary to that of the probe. In the illustration, the probe comes from region 1 and the screening shows that fragment 1–5 contains that region. Now a small single-copy portion of the DNA in region 5 is used as a probe to identify other clones in the library that contain DNA from region 5. In our example, this second screening identifies two fragments: 2–5 and 4–7. A third screening using a probe from region 7 identifies the fragment 6–10. The process is repeated until clones containing the entire region of interest have been identified.

the filter membrane. Each spot is composed of phage particles from a single plaque. A radioactively labeled probe is then allowed to hybridize to the DNA on the membrane. Any spots on the membrane that contain DNA complementary to the probe become radioactively labeled. When a labeled spot is identified, the plaque corresponding to that spot can be located in the Petri dish. Each such plaque contains all or part of the gene (or of a member of the gene family) of interest. The phage in those plaques can then be isolated and regrown to provide more DNA for further study of the gene.

If no single clone in the library of overlapping clones includes the entire gene, a process called chromosome walking is used to identify a series of overlapping clones whose inserts span the gene sequence (see Figure 10). In this technique, the clone identified by the initial gene probe is cut into smaller fragments with one or more restriction enzymes. A short segment of single-copy DNA from one end of the clone insert is then used as a probe to re-screen the library and identify an overlapping clone. A probe from the endmost fragment of the second clone is then generated and used to find a third clone that overlaps the second. The process continues until the set of overlapping clones spans the entire gene. Chromosome walking thus produces a contig map of the region containing the gene (see "Physical Mapping" in "Mapping the Genome"). Sometimes a segment of DNA within the gene is not present in the library, in which case several libraries must be used to complete the walk. Each step in chromosome walking takes a few weeks to a month. If a phage library is used, as many as several hundred thousand phage plaques must be screened with each probe, and the distance covered with each step in the walking process may be only 1 to 1.5 kbp. Obviously the use of libriaries with large inserts is advantageous. The workload is reduced by a factor of about two if a cosmid library is used, and by a further factor of five to ten if a YAC library is available. Here again cloning systems capable of carrying larger and larger inserts are desirable.

Another kind of library made from total cellular DNA is a library of the DNA in a "monochromosomal" hybrid-cell line. Hybrid-cell lines are constructed by inducing cells from two different species to fuse together to become one cell. Hybrids are commonly made by fusing human cells with mouse or Chinese hamster cells. Initially, the hybrid cell contains two complete sets of chromosomes, one from the human cell and one from the rodent cell. However, each time the hybrid cell divides, it tends to lose some of its human chromosomes. Some of the hybrid cells lose all of their human chromosomes, whereas others retain one or more human chromosomes for various lengths of time. A single cell from a population of hybrid cells can be grown into a clone of identical cells and analyzed for the specific human chromosomes it contains. An alternative method for selecting a hybrid cell containing a specific human chromosome involves growing the population of hybrid cells in a special culture medium that selectively kills cells lacking the desired chromosome. These techniques have been used to create a series of cell lines called somatic-cell hybrid panels in which each cell line contains only one copy of one human chromosome in a rodent background.

Libraries made from such cell lines have advantages over libraries made from normal human cells. Because DNA from only one human chromosome is present in the target DNA, all human DNA inserts in the library are known to come from that chromosome. Fur-

thermore, hybrid-cell libraries contain inserts from only one copy of the human chromosome, whereas in libraries made from human cells containing chromosome pairs there is no easy way to determine whether a clone from the library originated from one or the other member of the homologous pair. On the other hand, libraries made from hybrid cells have the disadvantage that the clones containing human inserts may constitute as little as a few percent of the total number of clones, which makes selecting the human inserts from the rodent background very laborious.

Libraries from total cellular DNA have been made in phage, cosmid, and YAC vectors. The use of phage libraries gradually gave way to cosmid libraries, especially for studies of genes too large to be cloned and propagated in λ or plasmid vectors, and for studies that required assembling sets of overlapping clones that spanned large regions of DNA. Cosmids, in turn, were replaced by YACs, and current interests are in improving YAC technology or developing alternate cloning systems that can carry very large inserts. Any of these libraries may be screened for clones of interest. The purpose of screening may be to construct physical maps for small regions around genes or gene families, to construct maps for entire chromosomes, or to select polymorphic markers for use in genetic-linkage mapping (see "Modern Linkage Mapping" in "Mapping the Genome"). Inserts in cosmid or phage clones may also be subcloned into M13 vectors for DNA sequencing.

Library Amplification and Storage

Amplification of a DNA library (that is, growing more copies of the clones) is not as simple and straightforward

as implied in the introduction. The range of insert sizes and the variety of DNA sequences in libraries makes nearly every clone unique; therefore, each host cell has a somewhat different task to perform in replicating its cloned insert. The inevitable consequence is that some host cells grow faster than others, and if libraries are amplified by simply growing more cells, some sequences will be over- or under-represented in the amplified library. This problem is relatively mild in phage libraries, but even they can become distorted in representation if they are amplified too many times. Nonrecombinant phage usually reproduce faster than recombinants, so they rapidly become the most common constituent in an overamplified library. Therefore, phage libraries are best handled by amplifying them only once, by one seeding on a lawn of E. coli cells, and freezing aliquots of the harvested phage particles for future use or for sharing with other laboratories.

In the case of cosmid libraries, it is usually disastrous to grow the clones in close proximity to and therefore in competition with one another. We found that a single amplification of a cosmid library in which 2 to 3 percent of the clones were nonrecombinant produces a library consisting of 40 percent nonrecombinants. Such a result is clearly unacceptable, especially for libraries that are difficult to construct. Unfortunately, the solutions to this problem are labor-intensive. Perhaps the best method is to lightly seed a primary library on agar plates, allow each bacterium to form a small colony, and transfer a portion of each colony with a toothpick into a well in a 96-well microtiter plate. A part of each colony can then be moved to another microtiter plate with a 96-prong hand stamp or by a robot, if one is available. This procedure ensures that each colony will survive, but for a library including the

Libraries from Flow-sorted Chromosomes

Larry L. Deaven

For any kind of genomic-DNA library, subdividing the DNA of the entire genome before library construction is almost always advantageous. The resulting set of libraries includes all of the genomic DNA, but each library is less complex than a single library containing all of the cellular DNA. A natural way to make subsets of human DNA is to make a separate library for each chromosome. To include all of the nuclear DNA in human cells, 24 different libraries are necessary (22 autosomes plus the X and Y chromosomes). The libraries vary in size, the largest (for chromosome 1) being five times as large as the smallest (for chromosome 21).

The most efficient way to make chromosome-specific libraries is to start with flow-sorted chromosomes. Los Alamos scientists pioneered the technology of flow sorting chromosomes as a direct result of the invention and development of flow cytometers at the Laboratory during the 1970s. Figure 1 diagrams flow sorting as we use it in making DNA libraries.

The first libraries made from sorted chromosomes at Los Alamos were from Chinese hamster chromosomes. Those chromosomes are larger and better differentiated from one another by base-pair content than are human chromosomes, properties which make them relatively easy to sort on a flow cytometer. On the basis of that success, we thought it would be feasible to construct certain types of libraries from sorted human chromosomes. The Department of Energy agreed to support the work, and because the scope of the envisioned project was large, we asked our colleagues at Lawrence Livermore National Laboratory if they would join in an effort to make a complete set of chromosome-specific libraries. Our initial discussions in 1983 led to the National Laboratory Gene Library Project, which continues to be a component of the Human Genome Centers at the two laboratories.

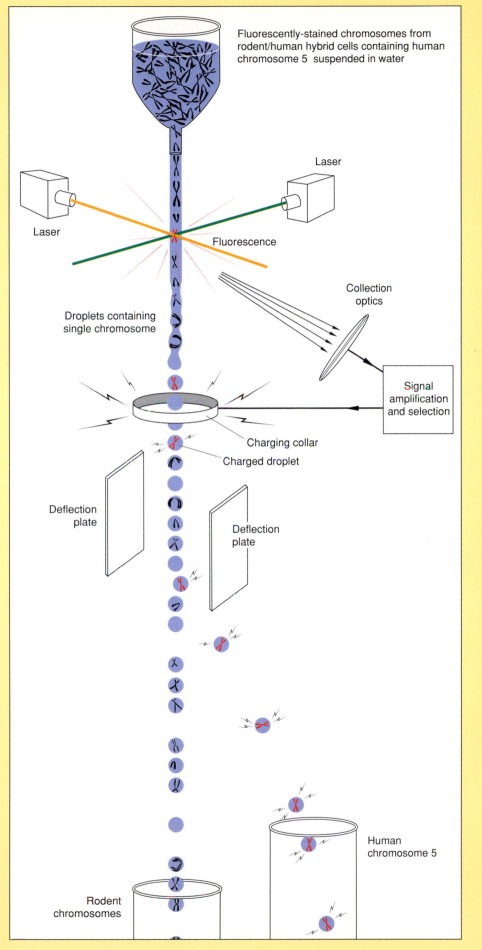

Fluorescently-stained chromosomes from rodent/human hybrid cells containing human chromosome 5 suspended in water

Laser

Laser

Fluorescence

Collection optics

Droplets containing single chromosome

Signal amplification and selection

Charging collar

Charged droplet

Deflection plate

Deflection plate

Human chromosome 5

Rodent chromosomes

Figure 1. Purifying Chromosomes through Flow Sorting

Flow sorting provides a way of separating chromosomes of one type from a mixture. The example in the illustration is the separation of human chromosome 5 from rodent chromosomes all isolated from a rodent/human hybrid cell line. A liquid suspension of metaphase chromosomes is carried through the flow sorter in a narrow stream. The chromosomes have been stained with two fluorescent dyes: Hoechst 33258, which binds preferentially to AT-rich DNA, and chromomycin A_3, which binds preferentially to GC-rich DNA. The stained chromosomes pass through a point on which two laser beams are focused, one beam to excite the fluorescence of each dye. Each chromosome type has characteristic numbers of AT and GC base pairs, so chromosomes can be identified by the intensities of the fluorescence emissions from the two dyes. If the fluorescence intensities indicate that the chromosome illuminated by the lasers is the one desired, the charging collar puts an electric charge on the stream shortly before it breaks into droplets. When droplets containing the desired chromosome pass between charged deflection plates, they are deflected into a collection vessel. Uncharged droplets lacking the desired chromosome go into a waste-collection vessel. The flow instruments used at Los Alamos can analyze 1000 to 2000 chromosomes per second and sort approximately 50 chromosomes per second.

Figure 2.   Phage Cloning Using Sorted Human Chromosomes as Target DNA

The phage vector (Charon 40) used to construct libraries from flow-sorted human chromosomes at Los Alamos contains a *cos* site, a large number of restriction sites, and a removable section consisting of repeat sequences (see Figure 6 in the main text). When the vector is used for cloning, the section of repeat DNA is cut into small pieces and discarded. The removal provides space for insert DNA. The vector consists of a 19-kbp arm and a 9-kbp arm, leaving room for inserts of 10 to 25 kpb. After the vector DNA has been isolated from phage particles, it is digested with the restriction enzymes *Bam*HI and *Nae*I. The eightyfold-repeated sequence constituting the central portion of Charon 40 contains an *Nae*I site, so the central portion is cut into small pieces by the *Nae*I digestion. The *Bam*HI digestion provides cloning sites on one end of each vector arm. Because *Bam*HI and *Sau*3AI produce identical sticky ends, the cloning sites are compatible with the *Sau*3AI sites on the ends of each fragment of partially digested target DNA. When the vector arms are ligated with fragments of target DNA, a concatamer forms that is cut at the *cos* sites to form individual recombinant phage chromosomes. These chromosomes are packaged into phage particles which then infect *E. coli* cells.

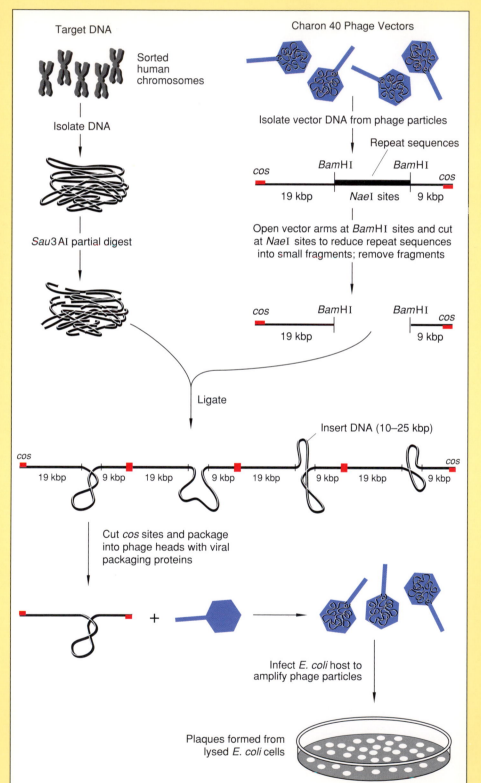

In 1983 the Human Genome Project did not exist. It was too early to seriously consider the construction of a physical map and the sequencing of the entire genome. Genetic mapping, on the other hand, was enjoying a period of unprecedented growth. The theory and methodology of finding genes using DNA markers had been developed, and major efforts were under way to locate human disease genes and to develop high-resolution genetic maps (see "Modern Linkage Mapping" in "Mapping the Genome"). Accordingly our first aim for the library project was to construct a phage library of small DNA inserts for each human chromosome. Small inserts were desirable for two reasons. First, the major challenge in making libraries from sorted chromosomes is to maximize the efficiency of each step in the cloning procedure in order to be able to make large libraries from small amounts of sorted DNA. In 1983, the technology for making small-insert (complete-digest) libraries was more reliable and could start with smaller amounts of target DNA than that for large-insert (partial-digest) libraries, which require cosmids. The second reason was the utility of small-insert libraries to genetic mappers. Repetitive DNA sequences are dispersed throughout the human genome, and the larger the insert, the more likely it is to contain at least one sequence repeated elsewhere. Probes containing repetitive sequences hybridize to many sites in the genome unless the repeat sequence is blocked. Single-copy probes identify only one site, a useful step in genetic mapping.

Our strategy for the first set of libraries made from sorted chromosomes was to digest the chromosomal DNA completely with a six-base cutter and to clone the fragments into a λ-phage vector called Charon 21A. Such a restriction enzyme reduces DNA to fragments having an average length of 4 kbp. However, approximately a third of the DNA is in fragments larger than 9 kbp, the upper limit for acceptance by Charon 21A. To reduce the amount of uncloned DNA, we constructed for each chromosome two libraries using different restriction enzymes; the Los Alamos project used *Eco*RI, while the Livermore project used *Hin*dIII. We estimate that at least 90 percent of the chromosomal DNA is contained in the two libraries together.

Our small-insert libraries were amplified one time, then sent to the American Type Culture Collection in Rockville, Maryland, where they are stored in liquid nitrogen. Samples from the original libraries are available to research groups throughout the world. They have been used extensively as a source of probes for polymorphic markers used in mapping genes, especially genes that can cause diseases. For example, as part of the searches for the defects responsible for cystic fibrosis and Huntington's disease, several hundred probes have been isolated from the chromosome-4 and chromosome-7 libraries and mapped to those chromosomes. Although improved methods now permit the construction of larger-insert libraries, the Los Alamos and Livermore complete-digest libraries are still useful. Over 4000 samples have been sent to research laboratories.

As we were finishing construction of the complete-digest libraries, it became obvious that chromosome-specific libraries with larger inserts were highly desirable. For molecular studies of gene structure and expression, they would have the advantage of

Figure 3. Cosmid Cloning of DNA from Sorted Human Chromosomes

The cosmid vector (sCos 1) contains two *cos* sites for rejoining the linear recombinant molecule after transformation. It also contains two selectable markers [resistance to ampicillin (amp^R) and to neomycin (SV2*neo*)], a number of restriction sites, a plasmid replicon including an origin of replication (ori), and promoter sequences from the T3 and T7 phage. The T3 and T7 promoters are used to generate end probes, as discussed in the section on YACs in the main article. The vector molecule is linearized by cutting with the restriction enzyme *Xba*I, then separated into two cloning arms by cutting with *Bam*HI. After fragments between 35 and 45 kbp in length are ligated to the vector arms, the recombinant DNA molecules thus produced are packaged into phage protein coats. The resulting infectious phage particles insert the recombinant molecules into *E. coli* cells where the molecules cyclize and live as plasmids. To prevent the faster-growing *E. coli* cells from overwhelming the slower ones, each colony is placed in a separate well of a microtiter plate.

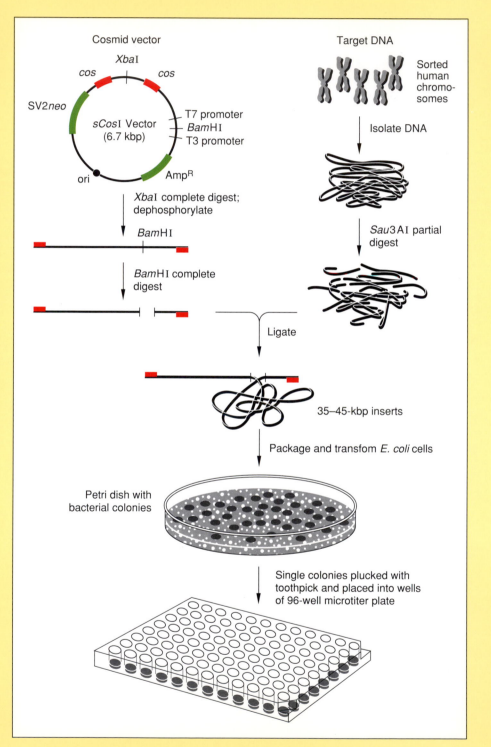

containing whole genes or even groups of genes in a single cloned insert. Moreover, molecular biologists were then discussing and planning the mapping and sequencing of the entire human genome. Large-insert libraries from each chromosome would be a valuable resource for those massive tasks. The entire human genome in a cosmid library can be thought of as a jigsaw puzzle of 75,000 pieces; the chromosome-specific libraries would be 24 puzzles with an average of 3125 pieces in each.

During the years we spent constructing small-insert libraries, significant improvements were made in the efficiency of vector systems capable of carrying large inserts. The most important improvement for our large-insert project was the construction of cosmid vectors with two *cos* sites instead of one. Such cosmid vectors can be cleaved into two cloning arms, each with a *cos* site at one end. The cosmid arms can then be ligated to the partially digested human target-DNA fragments, much as in phage cloning. Each resulting recombinant molecule consists of two cloning arms each ligated to an end of a fragment of human DNA. If the *cos* sites are between 30 kbp and 52 kbp apart, the recombinant molecule can be packaged in vitro to produce infectious phage particles. Using this cloning system, a cosmid library with inserts 35 to 45 kbp in length can be made from less than a microgram of DNA.

The laboratories' joint strategy for the construction of a second set of libraries with larger inserts was to divide the human chromosomes between Los Alamos and Livermore. Each laboratory would construct a partial-digest phage and cosmid library for the chromosomes assigned to it. Los Alamos has made libraries for chromosomes 4, 5, 6, 8, 11, 13, 16, and 17; Livermore, for chromosomes 19, 22, and Y.

Our current work incorporates several changes in the construction and handling of libraries. All chromosomes are sorted from hybrid-cell lines rather than from human cells because of the advantages discussed in the main text. The phage libraries, illustrated in Figure 2, have inserts 10 to 25 kbp long. They are stored as pools of clones in a liquid medium and distributed as samples like the small-insert libraries.

As illustrated in Figure 3, the cosmid libraries are seeded on Petri plates. The libraries are then arrayed, that is, single colonies are transferred to 96-well microtiter plates. Enough colonies are isolated to cover the chromosome five times. A chromosome of average size requires about 5×3125 or 15,625 colonies. The inserts have not yet been characterized, so we do not know whether the DNA in the inserts covers the entire chromosome. When all the colonies have been transferred, we make five to ten copies of each microtiter plate. Sets of microtiter plates are sent to laboratories involved in projects to map the entire chromosome or a major portion of it. In addition, the colonies in one set of plates are allowed to grow to high density, and then the bacteria are removed from each well and pooled. Laboratories interested in isolating one or a few genes on the chromosome can obtain portions of the pooled library.

An advantage of storing a library in a set of microtiter plates is that each clone has an alphanumerically labeled location. The labeling permits all the data on the clones from different laboratories to be combined for analysis. Ideally, all interested laboratories should have copies of the plates; however, distribution of so many copies would be too expensive.

The partial-digest libraries that have been completed are major resources for laboratories constructing physical maps for chromosomes 4, 5, 8, 11, 16, 17, and 19. The libraries are used directly in assembling contigs of cosmids and also contribute to physical mapping with YACs. In order to make a high-resolution map from YAC contigs, each YAC must be subcloned into cosmid or phage vectors, a time-consuming process. A more rapid way to find cosmids that are part of a YAC is to screen an arrayed cosmid library with DNA from the YAC insert. A second major use of the partial-digest libraries is in the isolation of genes for detailed studies of normal and abnormal structure and expression. A third use is the identification of specific chromosomes or parts of chromosomes. Each library is very pure, and the inserts in it can be labeled with fluorescent stains and hybridized in situ to cells or metaphase chromosomes. In interphase cells hybridization reveals the nuclear location of the chromosome represented in the library. In metaphase chromosomes hybridization identifies only the pair of chromosomes that the library represents. If a piece of a labeled chromosome has been broken and has translocated to another chromosome, the translocation is easily visible. The latter application is revolutionizing the detection of chromosomal rearrangements induced by substances that break chromosomes and by diseases like cancer, in which rearranged chromosomes are common.

Although our cosmid libraries are not yet complete, during the past two years we have devoted a substantial portion of our library-construction effort to YAC cloning. We were fortunate in having Mary Kay McCormick join our Center in 1989. Before coming to Los Alamos, she had demonstrated the feasibility of using sorted chromosomes as the source of target DNA in making YACs. To construct a YAC library, we had to overcome two major obstacles. Long pieces of human DNA had to be obtained from sorted chromosomes, and YAC-cloning techniques had to be optimized in order to use the small amounts of DNA available after sorting. Solutions to both problems were found through the skills of dedicated investigators. Chromosome isolation and flow sorting must be accomplished without delay because DNA degradation begins as soon as the chromosomes are extracted from the cells. To sort 1-microgram samples of DNA in a limited time, sorting continues around the clock. The sorted chromosomes are collected in agarose plugs which hold the DNA in the stable agarose matrix and protect it from shear stresses during isolation from the chromosome and digestion with restriction enzymes. The agarose is then melted so that the vector arms and DNA ligase can be mixed in. After ligation the recombinant molecules are fractionated by preparative pulsed-field gel electrophoresis, which concentrates all the DNA fragments longer than 200 kpb into a single band in the gel.

To facilitate transformation, the walls of yeast cells are removed. (Yeast cells without walls are called spheroplasts.) The long recombinant DNA molecules are added to the spheroplasts in the presence of the polyamines spermine and spermidine, which are believed to bind to and condense DNA. To obtain large numbers of recombinant yeast colonies (as many as 2400 have been obtained from 1 microgram of target DNA), all of the above steps must work well. Probably the most frustrating step is transforming the yeast cells. It is difficult to control, it sometimes fails, and because it is the last cloning step, failure means that all the previous work must be repeated.

We have completed two YAC libraries, one for chromosome 16 and one for chromosome 21. Both libraries were made from target DNA completely digested with restriction enzymes that have infrequent cleavage sites. Therefore, how completely the libraries represent chromosomal DNA depends on how uniformly the cleavage sites are distributed along the chromosomes. We will not know the completeness of the representation until we have generated a considerable amount of data on each library. Preliminary results suggest that the YACs made from digests with *Eag*I or with a combination of *Not*I and *Nhe* are clustered near certain chromosomal regions such as the centromere, but that YACs made from *Cla*I digests may be more uniformly distributed. We are attempting to ensure that future YAC libraries have unbiased distributions by making them from partial digests. Other studies of the libraries suggest that the frequency of chimeric inserts is quite low. Fifty-three YAC inserts have been hybridized in situ to chromosome 21. None of them hybridized to more than one region of the chromosome, which would have been evidence of a chimera.

The reasons for the absence of chimeric inserts are not completely clear. We took a number of steps intended to reduce their frequency. As illustrated in Figure 4, chimeric YACs are believed to originate either from ligation of two pieces of target DNA or from recombination between two YACs after they have both transformed the same yeast cell, especially when at least one YAC is incomplete.

To minimize the coligation of target DNA, we added much more vector DNA to the ligation mixture than the restriction fragments could react with. To reduce the possibility of recombination inside yeast cells, we took two precautions. The first was to handle target-DNA restriction fragments so as to minimize breakage. The second was to attempt to limit the possibility that more than one YAC would enter a single spheroplast by diluting the YACs to the point where it was unlikely that two YACs would enter the same spheroplast.

Although sufficient data are not yet available to thoroughly evaluate the chromosome-specific YAC libraries, all evidence to date suggests that they will be a valuable resource for constructing physical maps of chromosomes. The libraries combine the advantages of large insert size and division into subsets of the genome to provide the least complex mapping elements available. They are being used to close the gaps between cosmid contigs in the Los Alamos chromosome-16 map, and they should prove to be excellent sources of fragments for the initiation of maps of other chromosomes. We expect the Library Project now to focus on the construction of large-insert libraries in YACs and other cloning systems under development.

Figure 4. Chimeric YACs

Part A shows two causes of chimeric YACs. The first is that, since target DNAs are all cut with the same restriction enzyme, they can ligate to each other. The resulting chimeric insert can then ligate to vector arms. The second is that if two YACs enter the same yeast cell and their inserts have homologous sequences, they can recombine with each other, producing a chimeric YAC. Recombination is especially likely if one or both of the YACs is incomplete, either because the insert is broken or because it ligated to only one vector arm. Part B shows our solutions to the problem. To limit breaking we keep sorted chromosomes in agarose and handle the DNA carefully. Our target DNA molecules are typically longer than 2000 kbp. Since the restriction digest produces fragments averaging 200 kpb, few fragments have broken ends. Then we add many more vector molecules than insert molecules to the ligation reaction, making ligation between two insert molecules unlikely. During transformation, to reduce the probability that two YACs enter a yeast cell, we add *E. coli* DNA, which is not homologous with human DNA. That step greatly dilutes the YACs while keeping the total DNA concentration high enough to induce transformation.

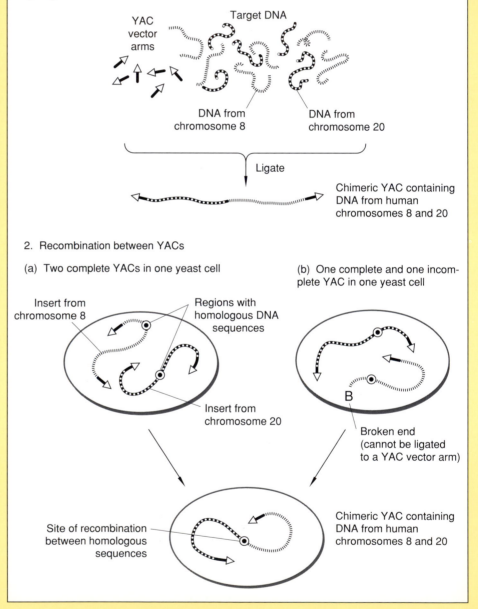

Problem: Production of Chimeric YACs

1. Coligation of target-DNA fragments

During the ligation step in cloning, two fragments of target DNA ligate to each other before ligating to YAC vector arms.

2. Recombination between YACs

(a) Two complete YACs in one yeast cell

(b) One complete and one incomplete YAC in one yeast cell

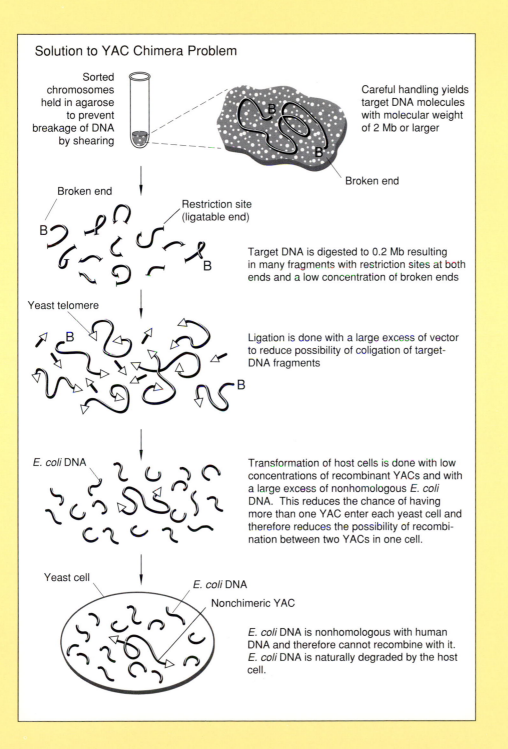

Solution to YAC Chimera Problem

Sorted chromosomes held in agarose to prevent breakage of DNA by shearing

Careful handling yields target DNA molecules with molecular weight of 2 Mb or larger

Broken end

B

B

Broken end

Broken end

Restriction site (ligatable end)

B

B

Target DNA is digested to 0.2 Mb resulting in many fragments with restriction sites at both ends and a low concentration of broken ends

Yeast telomere

B

B

Ligation is done with a large excess of vector to reduce possibility of coligation of target-DNA fragments

E. coli DNA

Transformation of host cells is done with low concentrations of recombinant YACs and with a large excess of nonhomologous *E. coli* DNA. This reduces the chance of having more than one YAC enter each yeast cell and therefore reduces the possibility of recombination between two YACs in one cell.

Yeast cell

E. coli DNA

Nonchimeric YAC

E. coli DNA is nonhomologous with human DNA and therefore cannot recombine with it. *E. coli* DNA is naturally degraded by the host cell.

Library Distribution

The success of the people working in the Library Project has created a need for large-scale duplication of clones in microtiter plates. The Los Alamos portion of the cosmid-library project will require copying over 200,000 clones six to ten times, and our future work in YAC-library construction will produce more clones to be copied. As important as duplicating clones in microtiter plates is making replicas of microtiter plates as spots on nylon membranes, a procedure that provides a convenient way to screen an entire library. A 96-prong stamp is inserted into the wells of a microtiter plate and then gently placed on a membrane. The bacteria collected on each prong are transferred to the membrane. The membrane rests on an agar culture medium from which the bacteria absorb nutrients. The resulting 96 colonies in the form of spots on the membrane can then be screened with a DNA probe. Any spots that hybridize with the probe DNA can be identified and the corresponding clones can be located in the microtiter plate. Those clones can then be selected and regrown for further analysis. We use this screening procedure extensively in our construction of a map of chromosome 16, and we currently use it to share our libraries with other laboratories. For example, an investigator at the Institute of Cytology of the Russian Academy of Sciences is interested in finding inserts that come from a region of chromosome 5. We sent her a set of membranes containing spots from each microtiter well in the arrayed chromosome-5 library. She probed the membranes with her collection of probes from the region she was interested in, and we selected and shipped colonies corresponding to each of the spots that tested positive. Duplicating and shipping copies of the library in microtiter plates is expensive, and we hope that the use of membranes will prove to be a useful alternative.

To help us meet the demands of library duplication, a group of robotics engineers at Los Alamos has constructed a robot capable of accomplishing that task. The robot can choose a microtiter plate from a dispenser, scan the barcode label on the plate, and insert a 96-prong tool into the wells in the plate. The robot then presses the tool against a membrane, transferring spots of bacteria from the prongs to the membrane. Finally it sterilizes the tool, replaces the lid on the microtiter plate, and returns the plate to a stacker. The robot can transfer colonies to the same membrane up to 96 times, each time shifting the position of the tool slightly, and thus can vary spot densities from 576 to 9216 per 22-cm^2 membrane. The robot's versatility is valuable; because denser packing of spots is more efficient but may be harder to read, different densities are suitable for different applications. ∎

Further Reading

L. Scott Cram, Dale M. Holm, and Paul F. Mullaney. 1980. Flow cytometry: A new tool for quantitative cell biology. *Los Alamos Science*, volume 1, number 1.

L. Scott Cram, Larry L. Deaven, Carl E. Hildebrand, Robert K. Moyzis, and Marvin Van Dilla. 1985. Genes by mail. *Los Alamos Science*, number 12.

entire human genome it requires picking 75,000 colonies by hand. Another procedure is to seed the primary library on a series of filter membranes laid on agar surfaces. After colonies form, the original filters can be copied by pressing them against additional filters. This method is somewhat less tedious than the one previously described, but colonies may be lost if they do not transfer and regrow from the master filters.

Yeast colonies must be handled individually and are usually placed in microtiter plates. Since only about 7500 YACs would be needed to cover the human genome, library distribution is much less labor-intensive than for cosmids.

All libraries can be stored indefinitely by freezing them at -70°C. Before the colonies are frozen, they are suspended in their growth medium supplemented with 30 to 40 percent glycerol; the glycerol protects cellular structures from damage by ice-crystal formation.

Problems and Errors in Cloning

The previous discussion of vectors may make cloning seem more straightforward than it is. All cloning systems involve difficulties, especially the newer ones that have not had the benefit of years of testing and improvement. It would be unfair to the people who diligently and carefully perform this work not to describe some of the pitfalls that can be encountered.

A problem common to all cloning systems that has not yet been discussed in detail is the occurrence of unwanted ligations when vector and target DNAs are joined with DNA ligase. Undesirable ligations include the religation of the ends of a linearized plasmid and the joining of two phage or YAC arms. In many cases, such ligations would result in nonrecombinant contaminants of a library, which in some cases would be indistinguishable from recombinants. Another undesirable process is the ligation of two small fragments of target DNA, which may later be cloned as a chimeric insert. The standard practice to avoid these ligations is to treat either the vector or the target DNA with an enzyme called calf intestinal alkaline phosphatase (CIP). This enzyme removes phosphate groups from the 5′ ends of linear DNA. Because DNA ligase cannot join DNA molecules unless the 5′ ends have phosphate groups, undesirable ligations between treated molecules can not happen.

With some phage and cosmid vectors, ligation between vector molecules does not cause problems because the vector DNA is not large enough for proper packaging and therefore a vector religation does not result in a viable nonrecombinant. In those cases the target DNA rather than the vector DNA is treated with CIP. That method is very useful in preventing the formation of chimeric inserts, especially when the target DNA contains small fragments.

Unfortunately, all the CIP must be removed to make the subsequent ligations work efficiently. CIP is removed by digestion with another enzyme called proteinase K, followed by extraction of protein-degradation products with phenol and chloroform. Since those steps require handling the DNA, they increase the risks of shearing and of degradation by nonspecific nucleases (DNA-digesting enzymes that are common contaminants in biochemicals). Therefore CIP treatment is seldom used for the large and consequently fragile fragments needed for YAC constructions. The protocols for CIP treatment must also be carefully controlled because an incomplete treatment would result in a library of questionable value. Furthermore, a batch of CIP that contains nucleases can destroy painstakingly prepared target DNA.

An example of the tricky nature of library construction is the loss of restriction-enzyme specificity, a phenomenon called star activity. Earlier in this article restriction enzymes were described as being specific for one DNA sequence. For some enzymes, this is not completely true. Their specificity may be altered when they are used under altered reaction conditions. These altered conditions include high enzyme concentration, use of manganese instead of magnesium, low concentration of electrolytes, high pH, or the presence of organic solvents such as glycerol. If DNA is digested with *Eco*RI, for instance, under any of these conditions, the enzyme can cleave DNA at sequences that differ from the normal recognition sequence by a one-base substitution. The result of star activity is a library some of whose clones are jumbles of small pieces of vector and insert DNA.

New Directions in Library Construction

Libraries for Constructing STS Markers. An STS library is a chromosome-specific library designed to facilitate identification and cloning of STSs (sequence-tagged sites) from one human chromosome (see "The Polymerase Chain Reaction and Sequence-tagged Sites" in "Mapping the Genome"). The inserts in an STS library are cloned in M13 vectors. Since the M13 cloning system is efficient, STS libraries can be made with very small amounts of sorted DNA or from the DNA in a rodent-human hybrid cell line containing a single human chromosome. The target DNA is digested to completion with one or two frequent cutters, and then it is ligated with M13 double-stranded DNA. The resulting libraries of M13 clones have small (200 to 1000 base pairs) inserts that are in a useful form for the dideoxy chain-termination sequencing method.

After each cloned insert has been sequenced, the sequence is searched for a single-copy sequence of 200 to 300 base pairs that can be used as an STS. The polymerase chain reaction can then be used to locate the clones in a total genomic YAC library that contain the identified STSs. In this approach, a small amount of sorted DNA is used to make an M13-based chromosome-specific library that can provide hundreds of STS markers for each chromosome.

Microdissection Libraries. Micro-dissection libraries are made from a specific region of a chromosome and are usually very small libraries, perhaps containing only a few inserts. The target DNA may be from a single chromosome band or from an area containing a defect such as a visible gap or fragile site. Target DNA may be obtained by fixing a chromosome on a microscope slide and scraping off and collecting an identifiable region. An alternative method is to use a laser to burn away all of the chromosome except the region of interest. The tiny amounts of DNA obtained are usually amplified using PCR and then cloned into a phage vector that accepts small inserts. These libraries are useful as probes to determine which cosmids or YACs from other libraries contain inserts that cover the dissected region. Probes from microdissection libraries have been used effectively to screen chromosome-specific libraries constructed from flow-sorted chromosomes.

cDNA Libraries. The synthesis of a cDNA probe for the human β-globin gene as early as 1975 was made possible by a unique feature of reticulocytes, the precursors of red blood cells. Reticulocytes produce large amounts of hemoglobin and contain very little mRNA other than the globin mRNAs. Therefore the mRNA extracted from human reticulocytes is essentially pure globin mRNAs. Once extracted, the globin mRNAs are reverse transcribed (by the enzyme reverse transcriptase) into cDNAs that hybridize to those clones in a human genomic library that contain all or a portion of each of the human globin genes. Similarly, mRNA extracted from cells of the pituitary gland has been used to isolate the growth-hormone gene.

The abundance of one or a few mRNAs in certain specialized cells makes synthesizing cDNA probes for the corresponding genes relatively easy. However, in most cells some 10,000 genes are expressed at different levels, and the copy numbers of the corresponding mRNAs range from 1 to 20,000. To facilitate screening a library of the cDNAs synthesized from such a population of mRNAs, the cDNAs are cloned in special plasmid or λ-phage vectors in which the cloning site is embedded within the bacterial gene for β-galactosidase. The host bacterial cell "recognizes" the β-galactosidase gene and transcribes not only the β-galactosidase gene but also the foreign cDNA insert. If the insert is in the right orientation and in the same reading frame as the bacterial gene, the result is a fusion protein consisting of part of β-galactosidase attached to part of the polypeptide product of the mRNA. A labeled antibody to the protein product corresponding to a cDNA of interest can then be used to select the clone or clones containing the cDNA of interest. (An antibody to a certain protein binds only to that protein.)

To reduce the labor involved in screening a cDNA library, attempts have been made to reduce the number of different cDNAs present in the target DNA by preparing the target DNA from the mRNAs that are present in one cell type but not in another. The mRNA from cell type 1 is reverse transcribed into single-stranded cDNA, which is then allowed to hybridize with a larger quantity of the mRNA from cell type 2. The cDNA that remains single-stranded corresponds to the mRNA that is present only in cell type 1. A library made from that cDNA contains fewer cDNA species and is therefore easier to screen than a library of the cDNAs corresponding to all the mRNAs present in cell type 1.

More recently attempts have also been made to construct normalized, or equalized, cDNA libraries. The ideal normalized cDNA library would not only be normalized (contain an equal number of clones of each cDNA) but would also be complete (contain all the cDNAs corresponding to all the mRNAs present in any cell of the organism at any time during its life). No complete normalized cDNA library is yet available, but cDNA libraries that are close to being normalized are available for certain human tissues. The procedure for normalizing libraries begins with the synthesis of the cDNAs corresponding to all the mRNAs in a selected tissue and cloning the cDNAs in λ-phage vectors. The cloned inserts are amplified by PCR, denatured, and allowed to renature. Because the abundant cDNA species renature more rapidly than the rare species, the abundances of the cDNA species that remain single-stranded vary by a factor much smaller than the original 20,000. In fact, variation by a factor of 40 has been achieved. An obvious application of a normalized cDNA library is as a source of probes for selecting clones from other libraries and locating genes on physical maps.

The continuing need for reliable and efficient cloning systems capable of propagating inserts larger than 45 kbp (the upper limit for cosmids), has led to the development of several alternatives to YACs, all of which are still being improved. The perfect cloning system for a library, by today's standards, would accept inserts in the range of 200 to 300 kbp. With inserts of that size a library would not need an excessive number of clones to cover the human genome and would still allow genes to be located with a useful degree of precision. The ideal system would have all the features mentioned in the discussion of host cells earlier, particularly low frequencies of chimera formation, clone loss, and deletion of inserts (which are the major disadvantages of YACs). In addition, all human sequences should be clonable in the system, so that libraries can cover the entire genome and any desired region can be located by using an STS.

Cloning systems have evolved steadily since the 1970s and new types of libraries will continue to be developed as new applications arise. The Laboratory has pioneered the construction of chromosome-specific libraries (see "Libraries from Flow-sorted Chromosomes"). That work too is evolving in response to the challenges presented by the Human Genome Project and by the rapid progress of molecular genetics. ■

Further Reading

Stanley N. Cohen. The manipulation of genes. *Scientific American*, July 1975, 25–33.

L. L. Deaven, M. A. Van Dilla, M. F. Bartholdi, A. V. Carrano, L. S. Cram, J. C. Fuscoe, J. W. Gray, C. E. Hildebrand, R. K. Moyzis, and J. Perlman. 1986. Construction of human chromosome-specific DNA libraries from flow-sorted chromosomes. Cold Spring Harbor Symposia on Quantitative Biology 51:159.

Ernst-L. Winnacker. 1987. *From Genes to Clones: Introduction to Gene Technology*, translated by Horst Ibelgaufts. New York: VCH Publishers.

Shelby L. Berger and Alan R. Kimmel, editors. 1988. *Guide to Molecular Cloning Techniques*. Methods in Enzymology, volume 152. San Diego: Academic Press.

J. Sambrook, E. F. Fritsch, and T. Maniatis. 1989. *Molecular Cloning: A Laboratory Manual*, second edition. Cold Spring Harbor, New York: Cold Spring Harbor Laboratory Press.

David A. Micklos and Greg A. Freyer. 1990. *DNA Science: A First Course in Recombinant DNA Technology*. Cold Spring Harbor, New York: Cold Spring Harbor Laboratory Press.

Larry L. Deaven. 1991. *Chromosome-Specific Human Gene Libraries*. In *Encyclopedia of Human Biology*, volume 2, Renato Dulbecco, editor-in-chief. San Diego: Academic Press.

James D. Watson, Michael Gilman, Jan Witkowski, and Mark Zoller. 1992. *Recombinant DNA*, second edition. New York: W. H. Freeman and Company.

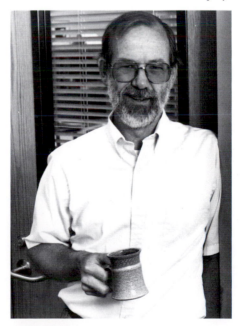

Larry L. Deaven is the principal investigator of the National Laboratory Gene Library Project at Los Alamos and Deputy Director of the Los Alamos Human Genome Center. [See "Members of the Human Genome Center at Los Alamos National Laboratory" for biographical details.]

COMPUTATION *and* the GENOME PROJECT
—*a shotgun wedding*

James W. Fickett

*T*he human genome may be considered a biological "program" written in a largely unknown programming language. Assembling a full description of this complex object and making the description available to all researchers via computer network will require innovation in software engineering. Understanding the structure and function of the genome will require scientific breakthroughs in which computation will play a major role.

Several years ago a marriage of necessity took place between molecular biology and computational science. The bride was attired in an astounding mix of items by her favorite designers. Her makeup was executed by Lambda Head and her coiffure by E. Coli and C. Elegans. She wore a choker by Phage Tail, a bodice by Ribosomes Unlimited, a stomacher by S. Cerevisiae, sleeves and gloves by Chromosomes to Order, a skirt by Microtiter Plate and Petri Dish, and a train fashioned by numerous artisans of Wonderful Life. The groom's attire, starting with his essential boots, is strictly high-tech. The marriage has had its ups and downs, but both partners are starting to learn from one another.

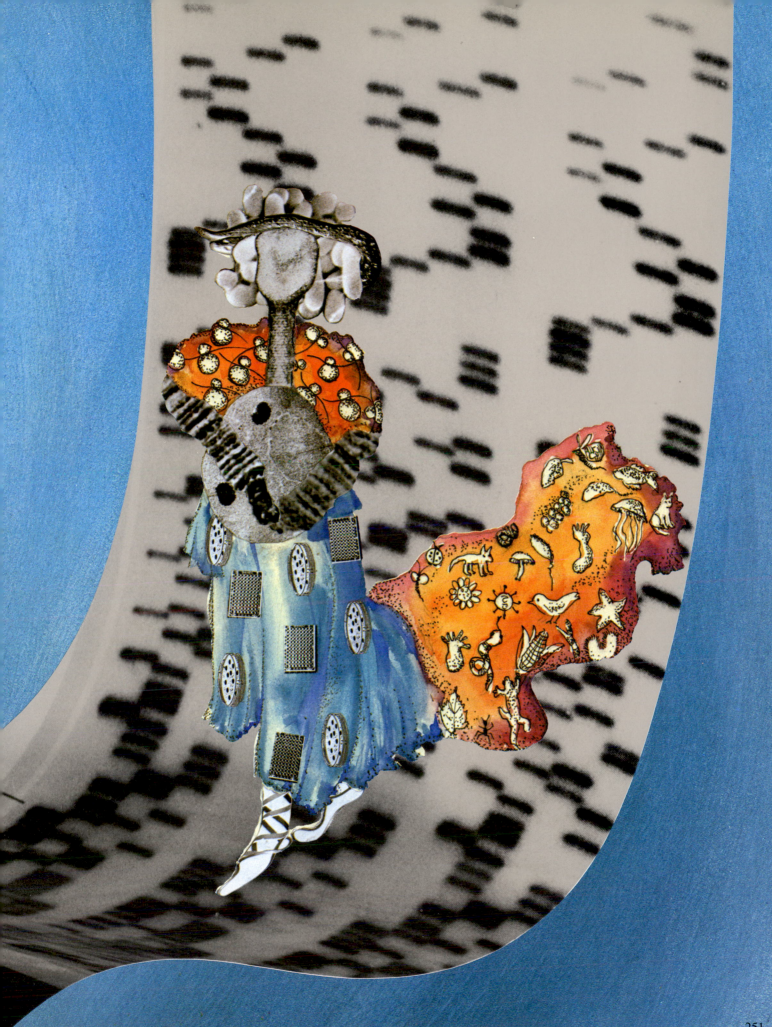

The genome is more than a blueprint

Elsewhere in this issue the nature and function of the human genome are described from a biochemical point of view. We begin by describing the genome in computational terms. Since the DNA polymer is made up of four monomer units, whose standard abbreviations are A, C, G, and T, a DNA molecule may be represented by a character string using only these four letters. The chemical monomers are called nucleotides; the strings are known as nucleotide sequences. The human genome, from this point of view, is a set of 24 character strings (representing 24 chromosomes), with a total length of a few billion letters, that is, with a size of a few gigabytes.

The genome is often called the blueprint for the species. In brief, and very roughly speaking, the genome is a concatenation of genes; each gene contains the plans for a protein; and proteins are the key building blocks of the body. (Essentially all enzymes—biological catalysts—are proteins, much of the structure of the body is protein, and the molecules that are not proteins are made by those that are.) For a description of how a gene is expressed to produce a protein see "Protein Synthesis" in "Understanding Inheritance."

The blueprint metaphor is very useful, but does break down in some respects. A blueprint for a home normally depicts only the home. But the genome, even as a blueprint, does much more. There are enzymes that read genes and make the corresponding proteins, and the genome specifies these (as if a blueprint contained drawings for hammers, nails, and workmen). There are even enzymes for rearranging the genome (as if a blueprint were to specify an independent-minded contractor).

Furthermore, the genome contains many regions that, rather than listing specifications for protein, interact with enzymes in process-control mechanisms. For example, certain enzymes known as transcription factors must bind to control regions near a gene each time that gene is used to produce a protein. Such regions are altogether outside the blueprint metaphor. So it is profitable instead to think of the genome as a program, written in a largely unknown programming language. Within the program are data arrays—the codon triplets that account for the "blueprint" parts of genes. The main program encodes a number of other related programs that act on the main one: a copier, interpreters, and rearrangers. A good part of the main program is concerned with proper communication between the main and related programs.

The goal of the Human Genome Project is an atlas

The final goal is the annotated sequence. The eventual goal of the Human Genome Project is to obtain the full nucleotide sequence of the genome, with each region annotated as to function. From the point of view of the program metaphor, this means obtaining a full, documented listing of the program.

In one sense this goal is only the culmination of a trend. It has become clear over the last two decades that almost any problem in biology can be more easily solved if the underlying genetic specification (that is, the annotated nucleotide sequence) of the relevant biochemistry is known. And because of the revolution in biotechnology, we are now able to see the genetic specification of any organism in as much detail as we wish (and can afford: the current cost of sequencing an average gene is on the order of $10,000, and isolating the relevant genetic material may well cost more). Annotated nucleotide sequences have thus accumulated at an exponentially increasing rate.

However, the Human Genome Project goes far beyond the trend of ever increasing sequence determination, for its aim is not just more sequence. In fact the hallmark of the genome project is an interest in the design and working of the genome as an organic whole.

Obtaining the full sequence and gaining an understanding of its overall organization will require many years and a significant amount of money. What will we gain that could not be had by a piecemeal approach? One example comes from the determination by a European collaboration of the full sequence of yeast chromosome III. (The human genome project includes the study of several model organisms.) One of the surprises in this sequence is that there seem to be many more genes than expected. Since the functions of most of those genes are not yet known, their discovery by other methods would have been long in coming.

On a more fundamental level, through the genome project we will learn a great deal about the programming language in which organisms are specified. The human genome is quite possibly the most complex object yet studied by science, encoding thousands of protein products which, working together in intricate combinations, manage the genetic program, build the human body from scratch, and maintain it for a

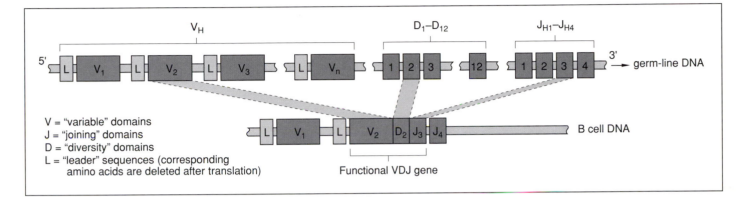

Figure 1. More Complex Genes: The Immunoglobulins

The immune system produces somewhere between a million and a hundred million different immunoglobulins. If each of these protein antibodies were encoded by a separate gene, the genome would have no room to encode anything else. In fact the immunoglobulins are specified in a tiny fraction of the genome. How this is accomplished is an excellent example of "genome programming." A typical immunoglobulin molecule is made up of four protein subunits: two identical "heavy chains" and two identical "light chains." Each of these has a "constant region" to interact with immune-system cells, and a "variable region" that is specific to a particular foreign molecule. The figure shows a schematic diagram of the genetic information corresponding to the variable region of a heavy chain. In germ-line DNA, that is, the DNA inherited from one's parents, there are several hundred V ("variable") domains, followed by twelve D ("diversity") domains, followed by four J ("joining") domains. In lymphocytes (white blood cells) this DNA is rearranged so that a particular V, D, and J region are joined to make an exon for the variable region of the heavy chain. Many thousands of different combinations are produced in different cells. In addition, the rearrangement is somewhat inaccurate, producing more variants. Also, in this region mutations are unusually common, even during the life of one cell, producing still more variation. The light chains are produced by similar mechanisms. Finally, each of the many light chains can pair with each of the many possible heavy chains, so that there are billions of possible immunoglobulins. From these the immune system duplicates and maintains those that turn out to be useful in recognizing foreign molecules.

lifetime. We now know little bits of how this complexity is orchestrated; concentrating on the big picture will teach us much more.

Second, the fully described sequence, like a geographic atlas or a star atlas, is a resource of enduring interest. In a deep sense biology, especially molecular biology, is data-driven. While physics and chemistry deal with general laws, biology, like geography and history, deals in large part with many specific cases. There are generalizations in biology but, while the generalizations of physics and chemistry are close to being exact models from which one can predict the behavior of matter, the generalizations of biology are more in the nature of analogy. They guide the intuition rather than enabling one to predict the behavior of the system.

General principles in biology are frequently implemented by each organism in idiosyncratic ways. There is, for example, a so-called "universal" genetic code by which the nucleotides of genes are translated three at a time into the amino acids of proteins. But many organisms have slightly different codes. Thus, whereas in many areas of science one gathers data to establish a point and, once the point is established, one is done with the data, in biology the data are central and are referred to again and again.

The intermediate goal includes coarser-resolution maps. We are still very far from having the complete sequence. At present only about 6 million nucleotides of human sequence (about 0.2 percent of the total) are known. Furthermore, the cost of determining the

sequence is currently too high (on the order of $1 per nucleotide) to contemplate an immediate drive to obtain the full sequence. Fortunately, much useful information can be obtained without sequencing. Maps of lower resolution than the sequence can be based on various sorts of landmarks—features of a chromosome detectable in some experiment. The distances between such landmarks are typically measured in ways that give one a very rough approximation of the number of base pairs between them. All such maps may be considered to be conceptually built on the (yet unknown) sequence as a coordinate system.

One technique with immediate medical application is linkage mapping. Chromosomes break and recombine fairly frequently as the genetic material

Decades of Nonlinearity: *the growth of DNA sequence data*

Christian Burks, Michael J. Cinkosky, and Paul Gilna

The first nucleotide sequence was published in 1965; it was the sequence of an RNA molecule less than 100 nucleotides long. The methods used were so arduous that until the mid-1970s a person could determine the sequence of only about a hundred bases in a year. Then Maxam and Gilbert in the U.S. and Sanger in England developed new sequencing techniques that were a hundred times faster (see "DNA Sequencing" in "Mapping the Genome"). Figure 1 shows that today biologists are determining the complete sequences of pieces of DNA over 100,000 nucleotides in length. Almost 100,000,000 nucleotides of sequence data have been published—a wealth of information that has formed the basis for many scientific discoveries. How has the enormous and rapidly growing quantity of data been maintained and managed?

As shown in Figure 2a, the rate of sequence-data accumulation was increasing rapidly in the late 1970s. (Data for Figure 2a were compiled from the GenBank database, which includes the publication date and length of each sequence entered.) In response to the growing interest in gathering and analyzing the data, the biology community held several discussions in 1978 on establishing a database facility to collect, organize, and distribute sequence data and annotation about each sequence. For design purposes, the operation of a database can be compared to industrial processes in which a set of input objects is transformed into a set of output objects. In a sequence database, the input is DNA sequences generated by individual laboratories and stored in individual formats with varying amounts of annotation; the output is a collection of DNA sequences stored at a central facility in a uniform format with a precisely defined degree of annotation. For any such process to be workable and efficient, the mechanism for the process must match the volume of the input stream.

During the planning stages for the public sequence databases, how fast did biologists expect the amount of data to grow? Up to 1981 the few recorded projections generally assumed linear growth. Figure 2b shows a linear projection—based on the average annual rate from 1975 to 1977, 25,000 nucleotides per year—for the period up to 1986. (Note that the scale of Figure 2b compresses the previously impressive growth up to 1978.) The linear model predicts that under 300,000 nucleotides of sequence data would have been accumulated by 1986, and that a database project would have had to handle no more than 30,000 in any year. Funding-agency planning and subsequent project proposals to the agencies were based on that linear model. In 1982 the GenBank project, the American sequence database, was established at Los Alamos through a five-year contract with the NIH. (Also in that year a database storing essentially the same information was established at the European Molecular Biology Laboratory; Japan developed a similar institution a few years later.) Because a steady rate of data accumulation was expected, GenBank was staffed with only a few people who were expected to search the literature and enter into a database all the DNA and RNA sequence data that would appear.

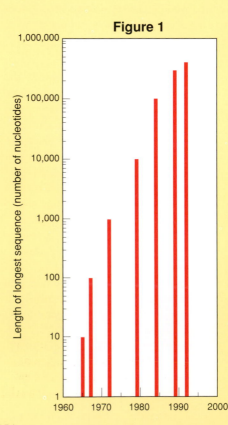

Figure 1

Suppose the community had instead projected exponential growth for the sequence data. Figure 2c shows that if we use the annual rate increase for the years 1975-77 (64 percent per year) to project the accumulation over the period 1978-86, an exponential model predicts an accumulation 15 times that of the model in Figure 2b, and a rate of accumulation orders of magnitude higher. Clearly, in that scenario a database project could not rely on a constant number of staff members each processing data at a constant speed.

What really happened? As can be seen in Figure 2d, the increase of sequence data far outstripped even the exponential model, and completely dwarfed the linear model that was actually used to design GenBank. This created a crisis for the scientific community wanting access to all these data and in particular for the GenBank project, which was responsible for providing access.

In 1986-87, as we planned and developed proposals for the second five-year GenBank contract, we revisited the issue of modeling the growth of sequence data. Figure 2e presents the envelope in which we expected the growth to lie. The lower limit is an extrapolation from the previous three years assuming a constant rate of acceleration. The upper limit is based on the assumption that seven billion bases of sequence, twice the total of the human genome, will be determined by 2005 (consistent with the goals of the Human Genome Project). The rate of acceleration is assumed to increase linearly to bring the curve to that endpoint. With the genome project in mind, we developed a new strategy—and corresponding mechanisms—for the flow of data in and out of the database (see "Electronic Data Publishing in GenBank" below) that we believed would accommodate growth within the projected envelope shown in Figure 2e.

Five years later, Figure 2f shows that actual growth of sequence data has indeed remained within this envelope, and that the accumulation of nucleotide sequence data continues to accelerate. It is worth noting that if the Human Genome Project goals for sequencing are to be met, the rate of sequencing will have to accelerate considerably over the next decade. ■

Further Reading

Walter B. Goad. 1983. GenBank—and its promise for molecular genetics. *Los Alamos Science* 9 (Fall): 52–61.

C. Burks, J. W. Fickett, W. B. Goad, M. Kanehisa, F. Lewitter, W. P. Rindone, C. D. Swindell, and C.-S. Tung. 1985. The GenBank nucleic acid sequence database. *Computer Applications in the Biosciences* 1:225–233.

Christian Burks. 1989. How much sequence data will the data banks be processing in the near future? In *Biomolecular Data: A Resource in Transition*, edited by R. R. Colwell, pp. 17–26. Oxford University Press, England.

Christian Burks. 1989. The flow of nucleotide sequence data into data banks: role and impact of large-scale sequencing projects. In *Computers and DNA*, edited by G. Bell and T. Marr, pp. 35–45. Addison-Wesley, Reading, MA

Michael S. Waterman. 1990. Genomic sequence databases. *Genomics* 6:700–701.

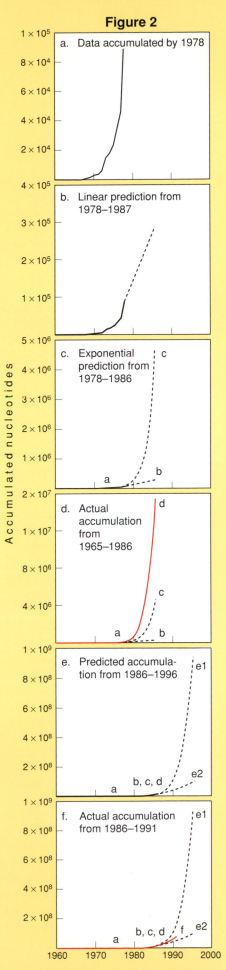

Figure 2

a. Data accumulated by 1978

b. Linear prediction from 1978–1987

c. Exponential prediction from 1978–1986

d. Actual accumulation from 1965–1986

e. Predicted accumulation from 1986–1996

f. Actual accumulation from 1986–1991

Accumulated nucleotides

is passed from parent to offspring, and measuring the frequency with which two traits are inherited together allows one to calculate the probability that the responsible genes are on the same chromosome, and if so, about how far apart they are. Linkage mapping has been used successfully to find the approximate location of several disease genes, as a first step in the process of locating and studying the defect. The cystic-fibrosis gene was recently isolated in this way, leading to a much clearer understanding of the disease.

Thus the intermediate goal of the Human Genome Project is an atlas of maps containing one map for each chromosome. Each map is conceptually an annotated sequence, although the sequences are, at the moment, very sparsely filled in.

A complication in this picture is that most groups currently maintain separate maps for linkage-mapping data, sequencing data, and data resulting from other techniques. This is because of disparities in units of measurement. Distances measured in linkage experiments, for example, are expressed in morgans. (The distance in morgans between two sites is the average number of recombination events between them in one meiosis—one set of cell divisions producing an egg or sperm.) But because frequency of recombination at a particular site on the chromosome depends strongly on the (usually unknown) nucleotide sequence at the given site, distances in morgans do not translate by any fixed formula to distances in nucleotides. Nevertheless, we will show below that it is both possible and profitable to integrate these different views of the chromosome into a single map. As well, differences between individuals (there are several billion human genomes, not one) may be best represented as variants within a single comprehensive map.

Both the creation and communication of maps depend on computational tools

Computation plays a central role in almost every facet of the Genome Project. This may come as a surprise, since biology has not traditionally been as heavily computational as, for example, physics or chemistry. But molecular biology is different from traditional biology, and the Genome Project accentuates the differences. There follow two examples.

Disperse workgroups depend on complex communication. Since maps are of perennial interest, and also grow and change daily, there is a great need for instantaneous communication between the producers and consumers of map information. The need for continuous communication is currently most often seen in working groups spread across several laboratories and engaged in the search for a single disease gene. A good example is found in the consortium of laboratories searching for the genetic defect which leads to Huntington's disease.

In such groups continuous communication is often now maintained by faxing text or drawings of maps. However, maps are rapidly growing too complex to manage in this way. In order to track positional information on thousands of map elements at many levels of resolution, undergoing frequent revisions and additions, one needs highly structured databases linked by computer network to graphical interfaces at many sites. This key computational need will require significant development beyond what is currently available.

In the next section we will discuss the major challenges in information management for the Human Genome Project.

Recognition of significant patterns in sequence data depends on sophisticated analysis. Computation also plays a central role in discovering the language of the genome. Many biologically significant patterns in sequence data are invisible to the eye, but can be detected with the aid of computation.

Such insight comes frequently, but an early example is still one of the prettiest. In 1983 R. Doolittle and his colleagues were comparing newly determined sequences to sequences archived in existing databases, and discovered that the transforming (that is, cancer-causing) protein $p28^{sis}$ produced by simian sarcoma virus was remarkably similar to platelet-derived growth factors (PDGFs), proteins whose function in stimulating cell growth was well known. This discovery suggested the natural hypothesis that the sarcoma (connective-tissue cancer) caused by $p28^{sis}$ results from a malfunction in the normal biochemical pathways for PDGFs. Though the cancers are still imperfectly understood, the hypothesis seems to be sound. It has been shown that in the transformation process $p28^{sis}$ interacts with the normal cellular receptors for PDGFs.

In the final section of the article we will discuss the current state of the art in computer interpretation of sequence data.

```
MLLTSSLHHPRHQMSPGSWKKLIILLSCVFGGGGTSLQNKNPHQPMTLTWQGDPIPEELYKMLSGHSIRSFDDLQRLLQGDSGKEDGAELD
                      MNRCWALFLSLCCYLRLVSAEGDPIPEELYEMLSDHSIRSFDDLQRLLHGDPGEEDGAELD


LNMTRSHSGGELESLARGKRSLGSLSVAEPAMIAECKTRTEVFEISRRLIDRTNANFLVWPPCVEVQRCSGCCNNRNVQCRPTQVQLRPVQ
LNMTRSHSGGELESLARGRRSLGSLTIAEPAMIAECKTRTEVFEISRRLIDRTNANFLVWPPCVEVQRCSGCCNNRNVQCRPTQVQLRPVQ


VRKIEIVRKKPIFKKATVTLEDHLACKCEIVAAARAVTRSPGTSQEQRAKTTQSRVTIRTVRVRRPPKGKHRKCKHTHDKTALKETLGA
VRKIEIVRKKPIFKKATVTLEDHLACKCETVAAARPVTRSPGGSQEQRAKTPQTRVTIRTVRVRRPPKGKHRKFKHTHDKTALKETLGA
```

Figure 2. Sequence Alignment between a Sarcoma Oncogene and a PDGF

The upper sequence is the amino-acid sequence of the precursor of the cancer-causing protein p28^{sis} produced by simian sarcoma virus, as translated from nucleotides 3657 to 4772 of the virus's genome. The lower sequence is that of the precursor to a human protein, c-sis/platelet-derived growth factor 2, as translated from cDNA. Lines between the sequences indicate identical amino acids. The conspicuous similarity between the two proteins suggests that the viral gene originated through incorporation into the virus's genome of human sequence or similar sequence from another primate. Moreover, SIS/PDGF2 promotes normal cell growth and its mRNA has been found in tumors, suggesting that p28^{sis} causes cancer by a mechanism related to the functioning of SIS/PDGF2. (The amino-acid abbreviations are A, alanine; C, cysteine; D, aspartic acid; E, glutamic acid; F, phenylalanine; G, glycine; H, histidine; I, isoleucine; K, lysine; L, leucine; M, methionine; N, asparagine; P, proline; Q, glutamine; R, arginine; S, serine; T, threonine; V, valine; W, tryptophan; Y, tyrosine.)

The Human Genome Project requires advances in information management

Many components of an information-management system for the Genome Project already exist—commercial database management systems (DBMSs), computer networks, and hardware for graphical display—but many of the components specific to biology have yet to be developed. For example, though for fiscal accounting systems the data categories and transactions have been standardized for many years, the language in which an emerging description of the genome is being written changes and expands frequently. Without being comprehensive, we present in this section a few of the key problems and how they are being solved.

Efficiency is a natural focus at the stage of covering ground. In the early stages of a mapping project, when a large portion of the map-to-be is "terra incognita," the main business is simply data acquisition, and a key focus of the project engineers is efficiency in the data-acquisition process.

LANL is placing great emphasis on building a "physical map" of human chromosome 16. A physical map is one which gives access to the DNA of any region, and is made by determining pairwise overlaps among a large number (about 4000 at Los Alamos) of cloned segments of DNA, and then deducing the arrangement of the clones relative to each other and to the chromosome (see "The Mapping of Chromosome 16"). It almost goes without saying that an electronic database is required for efficient information processing in a mapping project the size of that at LANL. To give some idea of the complexity of the information we note that the physical-mapping database at Los Alamos currently tracks the sizes and sources of approximately 100,000 fragments of DNA from chromosome 16, and records over 7,000,000 pairwise positional relationships relevant to the emerging map.

The Los Alamos database is currently implemented in the Sybase Relational Database Management System (DBMS) on a network of Sun workstations. Because the Sybase software handles the network transparently, it appears to each project participant as if all the data were stored and immediately available on his or her own desktop.

SCORE: *a program for computer-assisted scoring of Southern blots*

T. Michael Cannon, Rebecca J. Koskela, Christian Burks, Raymond L. Stallings, Amanda A. Ford, Philip E. Hempfner, Henry T. Brown, and James W. Fickett

The Human Genome Project aims to collect unprecedented (for molecular biology) amounts of information, so the transfer of repetitive tasks to machines is essential. As part of the LANL physical-mapping effort, we have partially automated the task of entering clone-fingerprint data into computers. One aspect of the automation was the development of a simple image-manipulation program called SCORE. This program has improved the accuracy of the data entry and sped up the process by an order of magnitude.

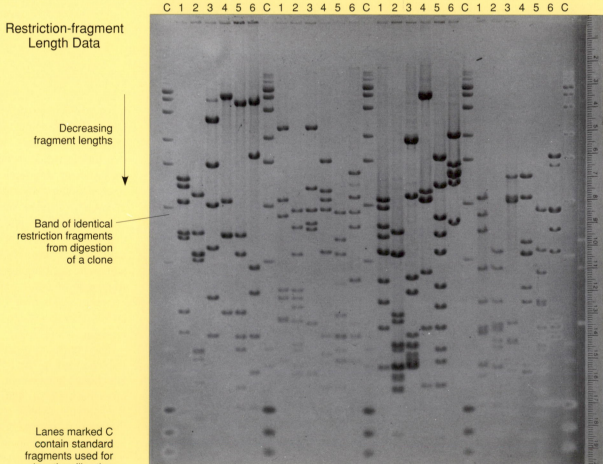

Restriction-fragment Length Data

Decreasing fragment lengths

Band of identical restriction fragments from digestion of a clone

Lanes marked C contain standard fragments used for length calibration

Gel Image

As explained in "The Mapping of Chromosome 16," the Los Alamos physical-mapping project uses clone fingerprints that consist of two kinds of data. The first is a list of the lengths of DNA fragments obtained by digesting a larger cloned fragment with a restriction enzyme and then separating the restriction fragments by length using gel electrophoresis. On the previous page appears a sample photograph of a gel. The gel is divided into vertical lanes, each lane containing all the fragments of one digest of one clone. Every clone is subjected to three digests, so there are three lanes of fragments from each clone. Each fuzzy horizontal band within a lane consists of identical restriction fragments from the digest contained in the lane. The band's vertical position gives the length of the fragments in it.

The second kind of data is a Southern blot of the gel that indicates whether or not (or to what degree) certain repetitive sequences are present in each restriction fragment. The figure below is a blot image produced by hybridization of repetitive sequences to the gel shown on the left (see "Hybridization Techniques" in "Understanding Inheritance"). Bands of fragments produce a signal on the blot image only if they contain the particular repetitive element being tested for.

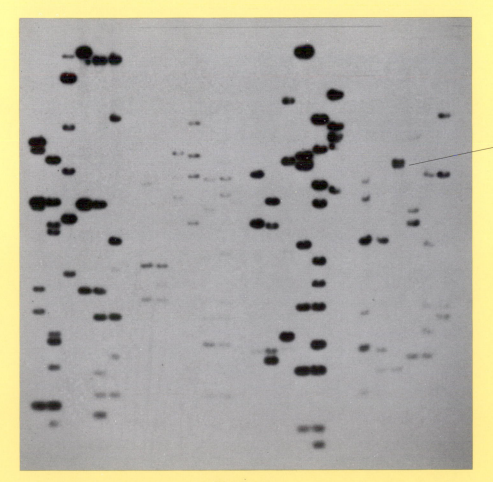

Cot1 Hybridization Data

Strong hybridization signal indicates that the restriction fragments at this position contain relatively long stretches of Cot1 repetitive sequences

Blot Image

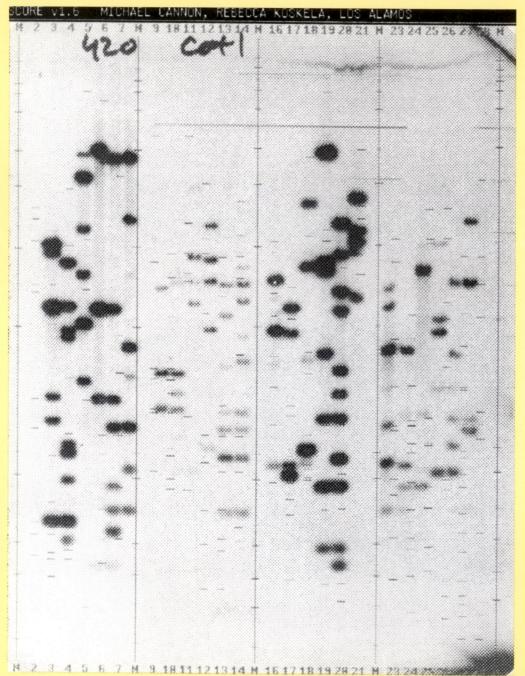

The blot image is used to assign a score to each band indicating the strength of its hybridization signal, a process known as scoring the blot. Therefore the bands on the blot image must be matched with the corresponding bands on the gel image. Formerly the two images were matched by hand, one region at a time. Each fragment was identified manually by numbering the lanes and bands on the photographs. After the scores were assigned, they were typed into our mapping database in a separate operation. Scoring the blot was the most labor-intensive part of fingerprinting. Now we score blots on a scientific workstation using the SCORE program.

Before SCORE is run, the fragment lengths are determined by a commercial image-processing workstation. Another program takes the report from the image processor and stores the lengths in the database. Also, the blot image is digitized using a desktop scanner. SCORE retrieves the fragment lengths from the database and constructs a schematic of the gel image in which the bands are denoted by colored horizontal lines positioned according to their length. The program then superimposes the digitized blot image on the schematic gel image. The figure above shows the two images on the previous pages as stored in the computer and superimposed; they match only approximately.

When the two images are on the screen, the user chooses two points on each image that should be aligned. The program then resizes and moves the digitized blot image to align it with the schematic gel image. The figure at right shows how the user sees the two images overlaid and matched on the computer screen.

At this point the actual scoring takes place. The user points to a band with a mouse, is given a menu of possible scores, and chooses one. Thus the program retains the use of expert human judgement where necessary. SCORE displays the score chosen, next to the band, for the rest of the session (colored letters in the figure). Any score may be revised at any time. If a band shows on the blot image but not on the gel image, the user may add a new fragment to the database. When all fragments have been scored, the program places their scores directly into the database, each score being associated with the proper fragment.

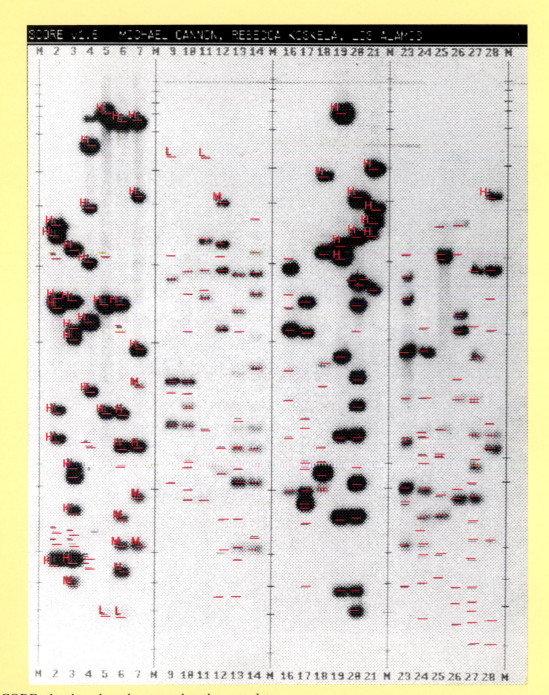

This program has not only cut the time needed for scoring the images by a factor of ten, but it has eliminated typographical errors in data entry. Using SCORE also has the advantage that the complete fingerprint data are in a database, easily accessible by network to the whole group working on the project and readable by the map-construction software, from the moment they are first determined.

For most genome projects, including that at LANL, interface software that translates between internal storage format and the users' intuitive view of the data is developed locally. The accompanying sidebar, "SCORE: a program for computer-assisted scoring of Southern blots," shows one specialized graphical editor which has facilitated rapid and error-free data entry.

Building and maintaining such interface software is itself a formidable task. Efficiency in the software development process is therefore as important as efficiency in the primary task of data acquisition. So although it would be pleasant to have specialized interface software for each data-processing task, there is a need for some more general and less expensive interface. This need is especially acute because experimental techniques and strategies for mapping are constantly changing as biotechnology advances, so that specialized software often has a rather short lifetime.

This need for a general and inexpensive interface has been met by a "database browser" developed by Robert Sutherland at Los Alamos. Someone using the browser sees any of a set of similar screens, one for each type of object in the database. (Types of objects include clone, clone overlap, and DNA sequence.) An example of a data screen is shown in Figure 3. All the screens follow the same style, making the browser easy to learn. Each one lists both the attributes of the current object, and also the other kinds of objects related to the given one. One can retrieve data either by filling in known attributes and asking the software to complete the form, or by following links from one object to related ones. Thus the browser provides access to all data in the database without requiring the user to know a specialized query language.

The current version of the browser is quite easy to maintain, because all the screens are derived from a template set of forms and procedures, in a relatively straightforward way. Nevertheless, every time the database structure changes (a not infrequent occurrence, as experimental methods and strategies change) some custom programming is needed. A new version of the browser is planned, in which the browser software itself will be capable of reading the database structure and configuring itself to match. We think the new version will be invaluable to other laboratories newly setting up mapping efforts, enabling them to put in place a rudimentary data-management system very quickly.

Map definition is a natural focus at the stage of mature results. In the fourteenth century, when maps were mostly local, it was possible to make reasonable maps assuming the earth was flat. In the age of exploration, however, the science of map making came to depend on a clearer understanding of the shape of the earth, and on an analysis of the distortion resulting from projecting a spherical surface onto flat paper. Similarly, now that the Genome Project has accumulated mapping data that cover several large regions of the genome fairly densely, it is time to consider carefully just what genome maps are and how we should go about constructing them.

It might seem as if a one-dimensional map of a DNA molecule should be trivial, or at least that it should be simpler than a geographic map. But in fact genome maps are more complex than geographic maps in at least three important ways. Two of these—the use of incommensurable units of distance and the variation among six billion humans—have already been mentioned.

The third is a high level of ambiguity in the data. Given two known points on the earth's surface, it is straightforward to estimate the distance between them. But given two genes or two fragments of cloned DNA, it is typical to go to considerable trouble only to estimate the probability that they are adjacent. Distance relationships are probabilistic not only because the mapping experiments give only partial information,

Figure 3. The Clone Screen in the Database Browser
Attributes of the clone include, for example, the name of the project using it and the clone insert length. Related objects include sequences, for example; if the user highlights "sequence" at the right of the form, and then clicks on the button "follow link," any sequences derived from this clone will be retrieved.

but because copies of many genes and other sequences occur more than once in the genome with only small differences. Since all physical-mapping methods depend on sequence similarity to determine whether two pieces of DNA are identical, mapping experiments sometimes indicate overlap where there is none. Derivation of a consensus map from fuzzy, probabilistic data is one of the more interesting and important challenges in the Genome Project.

Map construction is an optimization process based on fuzzy objectives. Probably because of the analogy to more familiar geographic maps, investigators often see the map-building process as fundamentally incremental. That is, at any given stage of map construction, one takes as given the map as it stands so far, and looks for the best way to add new data to the existing structure. Even in the apparent exceptions to this practice, as when a committee attempts to reconcile two contradictory maps, one can observe a fundamentally incremental approach—to save as much as possible of an existing structure and add new, or contradictory, data in as conservative a way as possible.

But recognition is growing that map construction requires a global, non-incremental procedure. The reason is simple—as long as the data are probabilistic, it is likely that parts of the map as constructed so far are wrong, so that the entire map needs to be reconsidered when new data come to light. (For example, among those pairs of DNA clones which have a 0.9 probability of overlap, we expect, by definition, one pair out of ten not to overlap.) Therefore one should treat map construction as an optimization problem. Adopting this point of view, one takes all the probabilistic statements about positions as a large set of objectives which a "good" map should fulfill, and attempts to reconcile them all

simultaneously, as well as possible, in a consensus map. Calculating an explicit fitness for maps, rather than relying on intuition is, though mathematically routine, a novel idea for many physical-mapping groups. The definition of a good criterion for fitness is a difficult problem; it will probably not be solved in a standardized way for some time.

As input to the optimization problem, it is important to correctly state the objectives. That is, whereas current procedure is often to interpret raw experimental data by placing a new point on the map directly, there should be an intermediate step of recording the results of the experiment alone—an overlap between two clones, say, or a localization of some clone to the region between two known genetic markers—with realistic ambiguity in position and probability.

For the optimization itself, a number of techniques might be applied, including linear programming, simulated annealing, and genetic algorithms. We (the author, M. Cinkosky, and D. Sorensen) have adapted genetic-algorithm techniques to develop an optimization algorithm for assembling physical maps. We chose the genetic-algorithm techniques because the overlap data often contain apparent contradictions and genetic algorithms are known to be robust in the face of such data, and also because the map objectives are not naturally stated as linear equations or inequalities. The input to our algorithm can be clone-overlap data from any kind of experiment, as long as the data fit into the categories of overlap likelihoods, estimated overlap extents, and estimated clone lengths. For computational efficiency, the input clones must be divided into *a priori* contigs in which each clone is connected to the others by a chain of overlaps all having probabilities greater than 0.5. The genetic algorithm then searches

for an arrangement of the clones in a contig which fits the experimental data well, but does not try to determine the overall arrangement of the contigs on the chromosome. The algorithm is called GCAA, for Genetic Contig Assembly Algorithm. Figure 4 illustrates GCAA as it is used in LANL's chromosome-16 mapping project.

A genetic algorithm operates by a simulation of evolution. GCAA begins by constructing a population of a few hundred different arrangements of the clones assigned to an *a priori* contig. In each arrangement, called a GCAA-chromosome, every clone is randomly assigned a length close to its measured length. Every clone is also assigned a position to the right of an arbitrary starting point. The analogy to evolution is that GCAA-chromosomes "mate" and produce "children" whose characteristics are determined by a process resembling genetic recombination. Then only the "fittest" GCAA-chromosomes survive to mate in future generations.

GCAA calculates the fitness of each GCAA-chromosome by checking how well it corresponds to the data, with discrepancies from the most certain data points given the most weight. Three separate measures of fitness are computed: one for the overlap probabilities, one for the overlap lengths, and one for the clone lengths. For the overlap-likelihood and clone-length data, discrepancies from the most certain data points are given the most weight.

In the core of the algorithm, the following procedure is carried out repeatedly: GCAA selects a "tournament" of four GCAA-chromosomes at random. The two chromosomes whose clones have the most disparate positions then "mate" and produce two "children." In each child of the mating, some of the clones are positioned as in one parent, and the other clones have their arrangement taken from the other parent.

Computation and the Genome Project

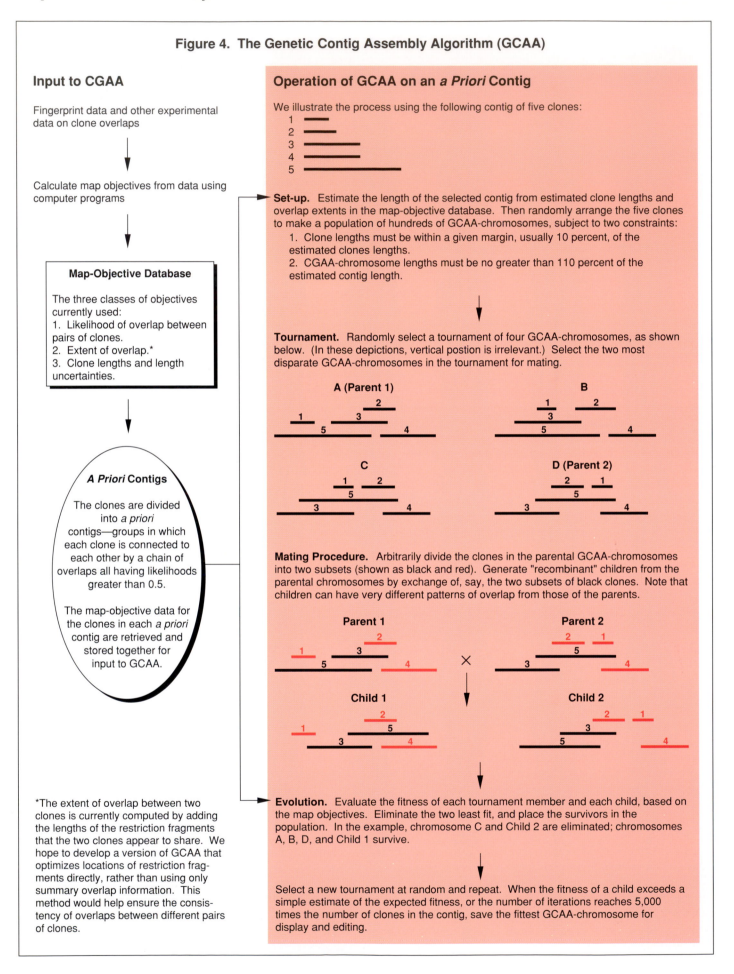

Figure 4. The Genetic Contig Assembly Algorithm (GCAA)

Input to CGAA

Fingerprint data and other experimental data on clone overlaps

Calculate map objectives from data using computer programs

Map-Objective Database

The three classes of objectives currently used:
1. Likelihood of overlap between pairs of clones.
2. Extent of overlap.*
3. Clone lengths and length uncertainties.

A *Priori* Contigs

The clones are divided into *a priori* contigs—groups in which each clone is connected to each other by a chain of overlaps all having likelihoods greater than 0.5.

The map-objective data for the clones in each *a priori* contig are retrieved and stored together for input to GCAA.

*The extent of overlap between two clones is currently computed by adding the lengths of the restriction fragments that the two clones appear to share. We hope to develop a version of GCAA that optimizes locations of restriction fragments directly, rather than using only summary overlap information. This method would help ensure the consistency of overlaps between different pairs of clones.

Operation of GCAA on an *a Priori* Contig

We illustrate the process using the following contig of five clones:

Set-up. Estimate the length of the selected contig from estimated clone lengths and overlap extents in the map-objective database. Then randomly arrange the five clones to make a population of hundreds of GCAA-chromosomes, subject to two constraints:
1. Clone lengths must be within a given margin, usually 10 percent, of the estimated clones lengths.
2. CGAA-chromosome lengths must be no greater than 110 percent of the estimated contig length.

Tournament. Randomly select a tournament of four GCAA-chromosomes, as shown below. (In these depictions, vertical postion is irrelevant.) Select the two most disparate GCAA-chromosomes in the tournament for mating.

Mating Procedure. Arbitrarily divide the clones in the parental GCAA-chromosomes into two subsets (shown as black and red). Generate "recombinant" children from the parental chromosomes by exchange of, say, the two subsets of black clones. Note that children can have very different patterns of overlap from those of the parents.

Evolution. Evaluate the fitness of each tournament member and each child, based on the map objectives. Eliminate the two least fit, and place the survivors in the population. In the example, chromosome C and Child 2 are eliminated; chromosomes A, B, D, and Child 1 survive.

Select a new tournament at random and repeat. When the fitness of a child exceeds a simple estimate of the expected fitness, or the number of iterations reaches 5,000 times the number of clones in the contig, save the fittest GCAA-chromosome for display and editing.

The mating scheme is described in more detail in Figure 4.

After carrying out the mating, GCAA evaluates the fitnesses of the two child chromosomes. If some child's overlap and overlap-extent scores are both greater than or equal to those of any of the original four members of the tournament, then that child replaces the least fit original member. (If both scores of the two chromosomes are equal, the clone-length score breaks the tie—its only function in the whole procedure.) The remaining four chromosomes are returned to the pool, and a new tournament is selected. The process is repeated thousands of times, after which the fittest GCAA-chromosomes, for most *a priori* contigs, agree quite well with the data. In practice, experienced users can often improve the output of the genetic algorithm by making small changes. However, few if any people could start from scratch with a sizable number of objectives and produce a result that needed only minor changes.

GCAA has been successfully used at Los Alamos to construct or improve large portions of the chromosome-16 physical map. At the current time, the strategy for completing the map is based on extending contigs in a highly directed way by "walking off the ends" (see "The Mapping of Chromosome 16"). Thus it is particularly crucial right now that we have a computational method to deduce as well as possible the correct arrangement of the clones in all contigs.

New data on the chromosome-16 map are, of course, accumulating daily. So it is essential to be able to apply GCAA in real time. At Los Alamos, H. Brown has built a graphical interface called map_ed for the GCAA algorithm which allows a user to retrieve map objectives from the database, run GCAA, and display or print the resulting map. Thus as new information accumulates, it is always possible to see its effect on the emerging map. Map_ed is being replaced by a more versatile system called SIGMA (discussed below).

Integration: one map is better than many maps. In everyday life one occasionally needs to use several maps of a region at one time, for example a state highway map, a map of a national forest, and a contour map of part of the forest. Each map is at a different scale and has different information, so all are needed.

The same situation obtains with genome maps, but while handling separate geographic maps is only inconvenient, with genome maps the map-construction process (which of course is foundational) is made much less accurate by having the data collected and arranged piecemeal. In fact, separate maps are all intertwined and all incomplete, and any one can be better assembled with information from all the others.

Many current map-management systems have no graphical component at all. Of course this considerably lessens usability. The two systems that do have a graphical interface (Encyclopedia of the Mouse, developed under the leader-

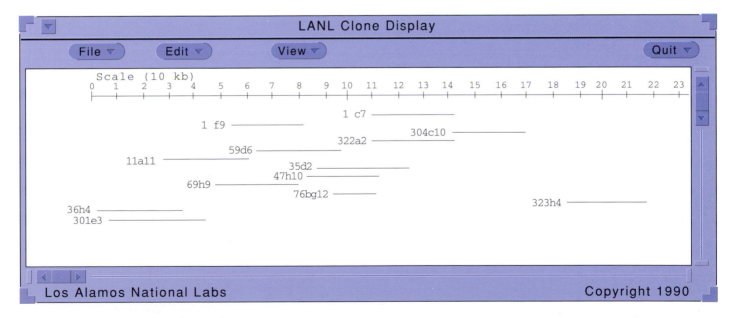

Figure 5. A Screen in Map_ed

Given the number of a starting clone, map_ed deduces the *a priori* contig containing that clone, retrieves the corresponding objectives from the database, and computes the map of the contig using GCAA. The map is displayed and may be edited, printed, and saved.

ship of J. Nadeau of Jackson Laboratory in Maine, and ACEDB, developed by J. Thierry-Mieg of the Centre National de la Recherche Scientifique in France and R. Durbin of the Molecular Research Council in Britain) manage a set of related maps in a graphical electronic "book," but do not integrate all the data for one chromosome into a single map.

We have developed a map-management system (described in "SIGMA: System for Integrated Genome Map Assembly") that gives a more integrated approach in two senses. First, map fragments given in different units are all stored as part of a single map structure, with a screen display that can be switched from one unit to another. And second, the experimental results, as summarized in the map objectives, are stored along with the map, so that the map can be evaluated or revised on the basis of the original data at any time. SIGMA has a graphical interface in the spirit of Computer-Aided Design/Manufacturing systems, in that it represents and allows manipulation of the data in a way that is close to the human conceptual model.

In the stage of widespread application, Electronic Data Publishing makes communication efficient. Getting information from producer to consumer can easily cost more, in time, energy, and money, than generating the information in the first place. This is partly due to the massive amounts of information in the modern world. But it is also due to an increase in the number of places one must look: the number of possible pairwise interactions among N people is proportional to N^2. The modern information explosion creates a widespread need for a network infrastructure which makes saving, finding, and retrieving data as cheap as possible.

A case in point is GenBank, an international collection of nucleotide sequence data managed at LANL for the last decade. The exponential growth of GenBank, described in "Decades of Nonlinearity: The Growth of DNA Sequence Data," has been due in part to the spread of sequencing as a singularly effective means of enquiry, and also to continual improvements in the efficiency of sequencing techniques. As sequencing became more efficient, GenBank had also to continually improve the efficiency of the data-entry process, or else merely collecting the data would have taken an ever increasing share of the community's resources.

GenBank pioneered in making use of the whole community's expertise to greatly increase the efficiency of the data-collection effort. How this was accomplished is described in "Electronic Data Publishing in GenBank."

The main issue in retrieval is availability. Currently many people in the GenBank user community are retrieving data from copies of GenBank updated by hand on local machines—copies that are often months out of date. These users fail to benefit from the rapid entry of newly available data into the central GenBank master copy. However, the same software that enabled us to implement the Electronic Data Publishing paradigm allowed us to easily log all changes to the database and send the resulting logs to so-called satellite copies of the database, thus updating those copies automatically. This mechanism provides a means by which an arbitrary number of copies of GenBank around the world can be brought up to date daily.

Even more difficult than keeping many databases and database copies up to date is the problem of selection and retrieval: data are only available if one can find them. For the average user it is a significant problem to find out which database(s) might contain the needed data, and then finding out how to query the relevant database(s). The problem is compounded when the answer to a user's question is spread across a number of related databases—for example map information for a gene might be found in the Genome Data Base at Johns Hopkins University, the sequence of the gene in GenBank, and related literature listed in MedLine at the National Library of Medicine.

This suggests that a key current need in information management is to make a large number of disperse and independently maintained databases appear to users as a single collection with a single query language.

Both academic computer scientists and commercial vendors have made inroads on actually integrating multiple databases, each with some autonomy, into what appears to users as a single virtual collection. However at present the multiple databases must all be managed by the same vendor's software for this to be a workable solution.

At present several groups in the molecular-biology community do provide partial solutions to this problem. One approach, implemented, for example, in the Chemical Substances Information Network system developed by the Computer Corporation of America, the National Library of Medicine, and Bolt Beranek and Newman Laboratories, is to make a smart piece of interface software that incorporates a great deal of knowledge about many individual databases. The difficulty is that as the world changes this kind of software requires a great deal of expensive maintenance. Another, more common, approach is to import copies of many databases to a single machine, and convert them all to a single format. Here, again, updating the collections and maintaining the format conversion-software is a continuing difficulty.

In data collection, Electronic Data Publishing led to a great increase in efficiency by decentralizing responsibility

SIGMA: *system for integrated genome map assembly*

Michael J. Cinkosky, James W. Fickett, William M. Barber, Michael A. Bridgers, and Charles D. Troup

Ｗith high-quality road maps available at stores everywhere, it is easy to forget just how much effort went into the production of the first accurate geographical maps. Even maps only a few hundred years old contain glaring errors, such as the early maps of North America that show California as an island. However, when one considers how difficult it was to obtain accurate information on which to base those maps, one can understand why the maps were so inaccurate. The human genome is at present about as difficult to explore as that early wilderness was.

Although biologists have for some time been able to examine small regions in great detail, they are only now developing the experimental techniques that will allow the generation of reasonably detailed maps of each chromosome. Even now, data on the lengths of map elements and the distances between them are too fragmentary to use in building precise maps of entire chromosomes. In fact, with fragmentary data coming from many different types of experiments where even the units of measurement are incompatible, the present situation is remarkably similar to that of early cartographers who relied on the (doubtless contradictory) reports of numerous travelers returning from the area being mapped.

Unlike early explorers, however, biologists today can bring the power of computers to bear on the problem. To this end, we are producing a special-purpose tool for building accurate genome maps called SIGMA (System for Integrated Genome Map Assembly). SIGMA applies several modern ideas including object-oriented databases, optimization theory, genetic algorithms, and interactive computer graphics.

Building maps in SIGMA involves two basic activities: collecting information and drawing working maps (representations of the structure of the genome that are in reasonable agreement with experimental data). At the heart of the SIGMA system is an object-oriented database that stores all the data used in the map-building process, including all of the (potentially inconsistent) data on which the maps are based.

Maps in SIGMA can be constructed either automatically (by routines discussed below) or by users. The primary interface to SIGMA is the interactive graphical map editor shown in the figure on the next page. With this editor, users can see the positions assigned to map elements and change the positions to build or improve maps. The editor works like computer-aided drafting and design tools to let users easily view and edit the map without requiring them to understand the structure of the database in which the map is stored. Furthermore, because the software was

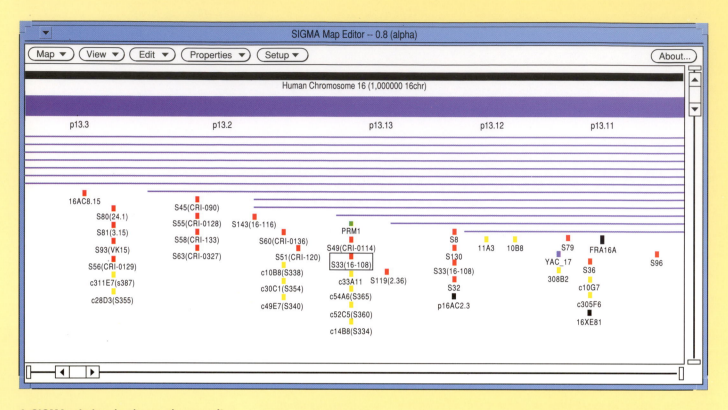

A SIGMA window is shown above as it might appear on a user's computer screen. The window contains the SIGMA map canvas, here showing a portion of a map of human chromosome 16. The display includes several different types of map elements: chromosome bands (thick bars at the top of the canvas), chromosome fragments from hybrid-cell lines (thin blue lines), anonymous DNA markers from the Genome Data Base (red bars), cosmid clones from the Los Alamos mapping effort (orange bars), YACs (blue bars), genes (green bars), and fragile sites (black bars). (The clones and fragile sites are not drawn to scale in this view because they would be too small to see.)

designed explicitly for genome maps, users have a wide choice of styles in which maps can be displayed, depending on the particular question of interest.

One problem in integrating genome maps is that conversions between the various units employed vary from one region of the chromosome to another and are even non-linear. In SIGMA, the different scales are integrated by dividing the map into regions of arbitrary size in which users can specify linear conversions between various units. For instance, in one part of the chromosome a centimorgan (the unit of genetic distance) may be set equal to a million base pairs, while in another part a centimorgan may correspond to half a million base pairs. Users can freely change the units in which the map is displayed. In the figure above the chosen linear scale is spatial distance along a metaphase chromosome as observed under a microscope. Therefore SIGMA shows element lengths and inter-element distances given in base pairs, say, according to the conversion between base pairs and spatial distance assigned for the part of the chromosome in which the elements lie.

SIGMA handles the problem of fragmentary data by treating the map-assembly process as an optimization problem. In optimization theory, one is presented with a number of (possibly inconsistent) statements that should be true about a solution to a particular problem. These statements, perhaps in conjunction with estimates of their certainty, are called "objectives". The goal is the generation of one or more solutions that satisfy the objectives as well as possible.

For genome maps, an objective is typically either a statement about a single element in the map (such as, "This YAC is about 400,000 base pairs long"), or a statement about the positional relationship between two elements (such as, "These two clones probably overlap by about 10,000 base pairs"). Even a map of only modest complexity can be based on literally millions of such objectives, far more than a human can sensibly handle. SIGMA, on the other hand, easily tracks this quantity of information and can help users find maps that meet the objectives as closely as possible. The figure opposite shows the user's view of how SIGMA manages objectives.

SIGMA: Element Properties

Type: ▽ Cosmid Clone

Name: S33

Description: from Los Alamos flow-sorted library

Left End: 0.03548   Right End: 0.3551

Objectives

Min. Length: 28500 ▽ bp   Max. Length: 4100   bp

Relationships:

Cell Line CY18 (Contained Within -.98)
Cell Line N-BH8B (Contained Within -.98)
Cell Line N-TH2C (Contained Within -.98)
Cell Line CY 14 (Contained Within -.98)
Cell Line CY15 (Does Not Overlap -.98)
Cell Line CY185 (Does Not Overlap -.98)
Cell Line CY165 (Does Not Overlap -.98)
Cell Line CY160 (Does Not Overlap -.98)

Relationship: ▽ Contained Within   Likelihood: .98

Min. Dist: ___ ▽ bp   Max. Dist: ___ bp

Source: ▽ Hybridization

(Apply)   (Reset)

SIGMA includes special optimization routines to automate map assembly. (The routines currently use only objectives concerning clone lengths, clone-overlap probabilities, and lengths of overlaps, which are the data used in constructing contig maps.) The optimization is performed by algorithms inspired by natural genetics, called "genetic algorithms". (See the discussion of genetic algorithms in the main text.) Whether a map was made by the optimization routines or by hand, SIGMA can automatically evaluate how well it fits the objectives. Thus the user can edit the map interactively, seeing how each change affects the map's agreement with the data.

As the map grows and new data become available, the collection of map objectives grows. Old objectives are never discarded unless a user explicitly deletes them. Because the objectives can be passed along to other users as part of a map, subsequent users of the map have access to all the information on which it is based, allowing them to make their own judgements about the correctness of the conclusions. This ability is very important when one laboratory's data appear to conflict with prior results from another group. Instead of being limited to the final product of the earlier work, the second team can look "inside" the map, examining the assumptions on which the map is based to find the specific causes of discrepancies.

Finally, SIGMA was designed from the beginning to be used with Electronic Data Publishing (see the sidebar "Electronic Data Publishing in GenBank" immediately following). Not only can users easily share data with other SIGMA users, but they can prepare submissions to the public mapping databases with just a few keystrokes. ∎

To demonstrate how SIGMA handles map objectives, one element, clone S33, has been selected in the map canvas; consequently its properties appear in the Element Properties Window (left). That window displays, in addition to the type, name, and description of the element, the graphical coordinates of the element in the canvas and some of the objectives involving the element. The first two objectives shown give the minimum and maximum lengths of clone S33 consistent with experiment. The objectives that follow state relationships inferred from experiments in which clone S33 was· hybridized with a panel of hybrid-cell lines, each containing only a portion of chromosome 16. For each hybrid-cell line that the clone hybridized with, an objective has been created indicating that the clone lies within that chromosome fragment. For each hybrid-cell line that the clone did not hybridize with, an objective has been created indicating that the clone and that chromosome fragment do not overlap. All those objectives have been assigned a 0.98 probability of being correct, based on the uncertainty of the experiments. Finally, the last two distances in the window are the maximum and minimum values of the distance between the left endpoint of the clone and the left endpoint of the highlighted hybrid-cell line. (If the two elements overlapped, the length of the overlap would be given; if they did not touch, the distance between them would be given.)

Electronic Data Publishing in GenBank

Michael J. Cinkosky, James W. Fickett, Paul Gilna, and Christian Burks

Improvements in DNA-sequencing technology in the mid-1970's enabled researchers around the world to determine the exact sequence of nucleotides in samples of DNA much more easily than before (see "Decades of Nonlinearity: The Growth of DNA Sequence Data" above). Computers were the most convenient way to handle the large quantities of sequence data discovered using the new methods. Furthermore, since many people became interested in applying computer technology to interpreting those data, the data needed to be readable by computers. To meet those needs, Walter Goad created the Los Alamos Sequence Library in 1979, which in 1982 became GenBank.

Like many scientific databases at that time, GenBank was designed as a curated data repository. For its first several years of operation, the data were collected from published articles containing DNA sequence data in figures. The sequence data and related annotation (for example, information about the function and structure of the sequence) were typed into a computer and formatted into complete database entries, which were then distributed to users in both electronic and printed form.

The limitations of this style of operation became obvious fairly early. The volume of data being generated continued to grow dramatically. It became increasingly difficult for the database staff to keep up with the flow of data, and the delay between publication of an article and appearance of the data in the database grew accordingly. At the same time, the data were becoming increasingly important to biologists, which aggravated the problem of slow turn-around time for data processing.

Another problem was that a growing body of data would never, as the situation stood, appear in the database because it would never appear in print. Journals were already beginning to limit the amount of space that they would devote to printing nucleotide sequences; therefore, authors began omitting "uninteresting" sequence data (such as introns and other non-coding regions) from their papers. For computational biologists, however, those data are potentially of great interest and not having them in the public database would severely hinder some types of studies. Furthermore, in 1986 both the DOE and NIH began to talk about the Human Genome Project. If undertaken, that project would result in the generation of at least a thousand times the quantity of data that was already in the database, and probably far more. It was becoming critical to develop a different approach to building and maintaining the database.

Electronic Data Publishing

Reconsidering the problem made it clear that sequence data and results based on those data should be handled by completely separate communication methods. Whereas scientific results needed peer review and an essentially free-form medium like the printed page, sequence data needed a largely automatic form of quality control and a highly structured, electronic format to be useful. To meet this need, we created what we call Electronic Data Publishing.

In Electronic Data Publishing, the originators of the data retain responsibility for the data in much the same way that they retain responsibility for the contents of published articles. Rather than being communicated primarily through journal articles, the data are deposited directly into an electronic database, and a separate article referring the reader to the appropriate database entries is published in a traditional journal. The database staff provides tools to help the originators get their data into the database, as well as software to provide automatic checks on the quality and integrity of the data.

To speed the transition to this new model, we enlisted the aid of many of the editors of the journals in which most of the sequence data were appearing. Because they were as acutely aware of the problems as we were (they were particularly interested in reducing the number of pages devoted to the printing of sequence data), many agreed to require submission of the data to the database before a paper discussing the data could appear in their journals. Within a year we were receiving a significant percentage of our data in electronic form before the related article appeared in print.

Table 1. Divisions of GenBank				
Division	Number of entries (June 1992)	Change in number of entries since March 1992	Number of bases (June 1992)	Change in number of bases since March 1992
Bacteriophage	779	18	1,102,766	-13,880[1]
Other viruses	7,750	1,238	11,883,566	1,007,715
Bacteria	7,965	760	13,732,370	1,290,821
Organelles	2,241	130	3,721,811	409,921
Plants and fungi	6,196	682	10,713,664	1,436,907
Invertebrates	6,079	868	8,422,573	977,127
Rodents	12,737	909	13,942,988	964,730
Primates	15,996	1,257	17,258,180	1,620,375
Other mammals	2,660	215	3,537,274	355,010
Other vertebrates	3,250	276	3,915,314	342,341
RNA	2,698	162	1,517,776	134,686
Unannotated	1,649	-360[2]	1,532,138	-297,009[2]
Synthetic[3]	1,282	27	857,738	42,302
Total	**71,282**	**6,220**	**92,165,158**	**8,270,506**

Implementation of the Electronic Data Publishing model also required the development of a large software system with several major components. First, we designed and built a relational database to store the data in a far more structured manner than was practical with our original ASCII-text database format. Then we built an interactive, window-based interface to this database, called the Annotator's WorkBench, which enables people to work directly on the contents of the database. We also worked with the European Molecular Biology Laboratory and the DNA

[1]As part of our curation of GenBank, we often combine duplicated sequence data into a single representation. In the Bacteriophage division between January and March 1992, the amount of data submitted was less than the amount of duplicate data merged, so the net change during that period was a decrease.

[2]The Unannotated division of the database was formerly used to distribute data quickly by releasing them to the public in raw form prior to the more detailed work of annotation. No data have been added to this division for some time. We continue to relocate sequences from this division to their appropriate taxonomic division through annotation, resulting in a decrease of the amount of data classed as unannotated.

[3]Synthetic DNA includes such laboratory-constructed DNA as short oligonucleotide probes, cloning vectors, expression vectors, synthetic genes, etc., which cannot readily be considered as originating from single taxonomic species.

Table 2. Amount of Sequence Data from Well Studied Organisms

Organism	Bases sequenced	Number of genome equivalents sequenced	Percent of total data in database
C. elegans (nematode)	0.54×10^6	0.007	0.7
E. coli (bacterium)	2.81×10^6	0.597	3.6
S. cerevisiae (yeast)	2.95×10^6	0.203	3.8
D. melanogaster (fruit fly)	3.02×10^6	0.018	3.9
M. musculus (mouse)	6.89×10^6	0.002	8.9
H. sapiens	13.44×10^6	0.005	17.4

Databank of Japan to develop systems for sharing data, so that researchers need enter data into only one of the three databases. Finally, we created a format for automatically processable database submissions and wrote software to aid in the preparation of these submissions, which is distributed freely to anyone requesting it. Data submitted in that format are run directly into the database, where the database staff can easily use validation software that we have written to check the data for biological consistency. (As a simple example, the software checks that exons do not contain stop codons).

The impact of these changes on our operation has been dramatic. We now receive about 95 percent of our data directly from researchers, mostly in automatically processable form. In 1984, we processed sequences containing approximately 1.38 million nucleotides. At that time, it was taking, on average, more than one year from publication for data to appear in the database at a cost of approximately $10 per base pair. In 1990, we processed 10 times as much data (about 14.1 million nucleotides) with an average turn-around time of two weeks at a cost of roughly $0.10 per base pair. Further, we have been able to maintain this performance since 1990, despite the fact that the rate of submissions has more than doubled to 30 million base pairs per year in the first half of 1992.

A brief survey of the contents of GenBank indicates the extent of sequence data and the areas in which biologists have been particularly interested. Table 1 shows the contents as of release 72 (June 1992) broken down by taxonomic and other categories of origin. Approximately half the data are from expressed regions, the rest being primarily introns and sequences immediately upstream and downstream of genes. A new development is the submission of thousands of rough sequences, each a few hundred base pairs long, from human cDNAs (see pages 136–139 in "Mapping the Genome").

About 2850 organisms (including viruses) are represented in GenBank. The only completely sequenced genomes are from viruses and cell organelles (mitochondria and chloroplasts), ranging in size from a few hundred base pairs for certain plant viruses to more than 200 kilobase pairs for the cytomegalovirus. Table 2 gives information (as of December 1991) on the organisms to which the most sequencing effort has been devoted. (The heading, "number of genome equivalents," means the ratio of the number of bases sequenced from that organism to the number in its genome, without the subtraction of any duplications in the database.) In one notable recent change, the amount of sequence in the database from the nematode *Caenorhabditis elegans* increased by a factor of about 7.7 between December 1988 and December 1991, 2.5 times larger than the increase of the database as a whole. ■

for the data. The idea of using computer networks to decentralize information management and place responsibility for different tasks wherever these tasks may most efficiently be placed, we term Commonwealth Informatics. We think Commonwealth Informatics will be an important strategy for many aspects of managing information in the next decade.

For retrieval from multiple databases, Commonwealth Informatics would be implemented by building multi-database access software that depends on a single protocol for integrating databases across the network, while leaving the connection between the multi-database access system and the individual databases up to the team at each database site (for example, GenBank and GDB). Aside from the software development, the only centralized component of this retrieval scheme is an index to the available databases and the kinds of information in each. A first step in this direction is the Listing of Molecular Biology Database (LiMB), a database of databases currently maintained by G. Redgrave under the direction of C. Burks at Los Alamos.

We are beginning to learn to read the genetic program

As DNA sequence accumulates and is made widely and flexibly available by means of networked databases, significant progress is being made in learning to read the genetic programming language. The fundamental question is this: given the sequence of some region of the genome, can we discern where the genes are, under what conditions they are expressed, and what the function of the products might be?

Even very simple and partial answers to these questions have great practical importance. For example, until a few years ago diabetes was treated with either porcine or bovine insulin, available as by-products of the meat industry. Now human insulin is routinely made by means of a synthesized gene implanted in a genetically altered bacterium. (Though this artificial human insulin is widely used, not everyone agrees that it is an improvement over animal insulin. Some studies indicate that artificial human insulin produced in genetically engineered plants may un-dergo more human-like post-processing of the protein product than artificial insulin produced in bacteria.) While the protein products of the synthetic bacterial gene and the natural human gene are identical, the two genes are quite different. In fact, the natural human gene would not even function in a bacterial cell. The human gene has two introns; because bacteria cannot excise introns, the synthetic gene must have none. The human gene has control elements that turn on the gene only when needed. The bacterial version has a control element that maintains maximum production levels at all time. Even the codons that are used in the synthetic gene, while specifying the same sequence of amino acids as those in the natural gene, have been chosen to maximize the rate of production. The design and implementation of this synthetic gene is made possible by a very incomplete, but still very powerful, understanding of the bacterial programming language.

Again, many genetic diseases are far better understood now than they were only a few years ago, because the region of the genome in which the defect lies has been located and the cause of the disease studied directly. Sickle-cell anemia results from a single-nucleotide change in the alpha hemoglobin gene (a 0.0000000002 percent change in the genome). The gene whose corruption

Intron

Natural gene	...GCA GAG GAC CTG CAG G GTGAG...GGCAG TG GGG...
Artificial gene	...GCT GAA GAC CTT CAA GTG GGT...
Common product	... Ala Glu Asp Leu Gln Val Gly...

Figure 6. Comparison of Part of the Natural and Artificial Human Insulin Genes
The regions of the natural gene just preceding and just following the second intron are shown, along with the corresponding part of the artificial gene. The intron has been deleted in the latter. Note also that the two genes have different sequences, but the same protein translation.

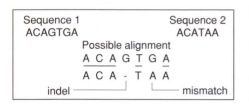

Figure 7. A Simple Alignment
Shown is one possible alignment between the two sequences ACAGTGA and ACATAA. In order to match bases near each end, a deletion has been introduced in the second sequence (shown by '-'). A horizontal line between the two sequences indicates a matching base; a space indicates a mismatch.

causes cystic fibrosis was located in 1989, and the change in function of the encoded protein is now being elucidated. Several specific forms of gene therapy, in which the defective region of the genome is repaired, are being tested in clinical trials. One important component of elucidating and treating genetic defects is the computational technology for analyzing sequence data to find and interpret genes.

The tool most used for analyzing sequence data is calculation of similarity. When a gene is newly sequenced it is very desirable to discover its biochemical means of action. The state of our knowledge does not allow us to predict the enzymatic activity of a protein from its sequence, but we often can shed important light on the function of a newly sequenced gene by comparing it with all other known sequences (as one who is just learning a foreign language can guess at the meaning of a phrase by comparing it with similar sounding known phrases). If there is a similarity to some gene that has already been studied, anything known about the biochemistry of the previously sequenced gene may help decipher the workings of the newly sequenced one. Of course, such comparison normally suggests

hypotheses and further experiments, rather than completely elucidating the function of the sequence.

There are a number of difficulties in finding meaningful alignments between pairs of sequences. At the root of these difficulties is the fact that biologically meaningful alignments contain both mismatches and indels (short for "insertions or deletions"). Figure 7 gives a simple example of an alignment; a longer example without indels appeared in Figure 2.

The most basic alignment algorithm is the so-called dynamic-programming algorithm, first described in print by S. Needleman and C. Wunsch, and still widely used in several variations. The purpose of this algorithm is to find that alignment which has the lowest cost, where the cost is the number of mismatches times a preset mismatch penalty, plus the number of indels times a preset indel penalty. If the sequences are $A = a_1 a_2 \ldots a_M$ and $B = b_1 b_2 \ldots b_N$, the algorithm proceeds by calculating inductively all optimal alignments between initial segments of A and initial segments of B. That is, let A_m be the string consisting of the first m characters of A (where $1 < m < M$), and B_n be the string consisting of the first n characters of B (where $1 < n < N$). Then the algorithm calculates the best alignment between every A_m and every B_n by extending shorter alignments one base at a time. The scores of those alignments can be laid out in an $M \times N$ matrix in which the (m, n) element, in the $(m + 1)$st column and $(n + 1)$st row, is the optimal score for aligning the first m characters of the first (top) sequence with the first n characters of the second (side) sequence. Figure 8 shows such a matrix.

The first alignments constructed are the trivial ones between the A_m's and the empty sequence as well as those between the B_n's and the empty sequence; their

scores are the costs of deleting those segments, which are the indel penalty times m or n respectively. Those scores appear in the top row and left column of the matrix in Figure 8. The remaining alignments and their scores are calculated as follows. The best alignment between A_m and B_n is the best of these three possibilities, all based on previously calculated alignments between shorter sequences: (1) the best alignment of A_{m-1} with B_{n-1}, followed by a match or mismatch of a_m with b_n, or (2) the best alignment of A_m with B_{n-1}, followed by the deletion of b_n, or (3) the best alignment of A_{m-1} with B_n, followed by the deletion of a_m. Constructing all the alignments of initial segments results in calculating the best alignment of A with B as the culmination of the process. Figure 8 shows how the process aligns the sequences in Figure 7.

Quite different optimal alignments may result, depending on whether untranslated gene (nucleotide) or translated protein (amino acid) sequences are compared, and depending on what scoring scheme is used. Current consensus is that the most functionally meaningful alignments between related genes are found by aligning protein sequences with a scoring scheme that takes into account chemical similarity between different amino acids.

Speed is a major concern in searching databases for similar sequences. When a sequence is newly determined, the investigator will normally want to compare it to every sequence in GenBank, both to find out if the DNA fragment has been sequenced before, and to try to discover the function of the DNA sequenced by comparison with other, related, sequences (from the same or different organisms). The straightforward dynamic-programming algorithm described above would, if applied to a typical sequence of 1000 bases, take on the order of a day on the fastest general-purpose single-processor computers. Faster response time is very desirable, so considerable effort has gone into accelerating comparison between a single "query" sequence and a database.

Specialized hardware can greatly increase the speed of searching a database. For example the problem is almost trivially parallelized: R. Jones of Thinking Machines has written algorithms, for the CM2 connection machine with 64,000 processors, that split the database among the processors so that each one only does a few comparisons. In another direction, T. Hunkapillar of the California Institute of Technology has implemented the dynamic-programming algorithm in hardware, producing the so-called BISP (Biological Information Signal Processing) VLSI chip. The BISP chip is not yet widely available, but is reported to be capable of comparing a query sequence (of any length) against a database at the rate of 12,000,000 database nucleotides per second. This makes database access, rather than algorithm speed, the rate-limiting step for most applications.

Databases are most often searched on personal computers and workstations. Thus another approach that has been extensively pursued is to narrow the search and make detailed searches only in promising areas. First the database is pre-indexed by making a so-called "hash table" of all "words" (subsequences) of a given length (typically 4-10). Then each time the program is run, all locations in the database of all words of the chosen length from the query sequence are found using the hash index. Finally, where there are promising "clumps" of matches, more detailed comparisons are made using the dynamic-programming algorithm. W. Pearson (U. Virginia) and D. Lipman (National Library of Medicine) pioneered this approach with an algorithm called FASTA.

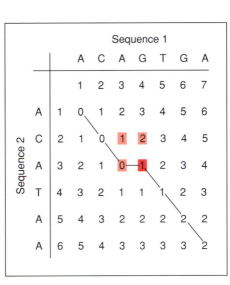

Figure 8. An Illustration of Dynamic Programming

The two sequences are those shown in Figure 7, and the scoring scheme is the simple one where the cost of both mismatches and indels is 1. The matrix shows the scores of all optimal alignments of initial segments of the two sequences. The first row and first column of the matrix give the trivial initialization scores, equal to the costs of simply deleting the corresponding initial segments. The matrix is then filled in one row at a time, from top to bottom and left to right. The induction step described in the text may be illustrated with the matrix cell containing a 1 boxed in red [the (4, 3) element]. The value of 1 in this cell is calculated on the basis of the values in the (3, 2), the (4, 2), and the (3, 3) cells (all highlighted) as follows. The best score for aligning ACAG of the top sequence with ACA of the side sequence must logically include one of three shorter alignments: (1) An alignment of ACA from the top sequence with AC from the side sequence. The best score of such an alignment is 1 [in the (3, 2) cell]. (2) An alignment of ACAG from the top sequence with AC from the side sequence. The best score of such an alignment is 2 [in the (4, 2) cell]. (3) An alignment of ACA from the top sequence with ACA from the side sequence. The best score of such an alignment is 0 [in the (3, 3) cell]. In case 1 the rule given in the main text calls for extending the alignment of ACA with AC to an alignment of ACAG and ACA by a mismatch of G with A, which would give a score of 2 for the boxed element. In case 2, the alignment between ACAG and AC is extended to an alignment between ACAG and ACA by a deletion of the A at the end of the second sequence, giving a score of 3. Finally, case 3 requires a deletion of G from the first sequence, resulting in a score of 1. The best of these three scores is 1, so this is what appears in the box. Once the matrix is full, the program chooses the best score along the right and bottom edges, and works backwards through the matrix to find what shorter alignments gave rise to this best score. The black line shows the set of best shorter alignments, and hence the best alignment, for these two sequences. Given the scoring system used, the best alignment is that shown in Figure 7.

An even faster algorithm called BLAST (Basic Local Alignment Search Tool) has been developed by S. Altschul, W. Gish, W. Miller, E. Myers, and D. Lipman, at the National Library of Medicine, Pennsylvania State University, and University of Arizona. BLAST first compiles a list of the words in the query sequence, then expands it to include all words "near" these—that is, such that the score of a no-gap alignment with one of the words in the query sequence meets a certain cutoff—and then uses the hash table to find promising sequences for more detailed analysis. On such sequences BLAST extends the word matches to longer segment matches, but does not perform the full dynamic-programming algorithm. Running with typical parameters on a Sun Sparcstation, BLAST can search GenBank in about twenty seconds. With these algorithms there is always a chance of missing an unusual alignment that does not fall within the initial pre-screening criteria. However, most investigators consider the trade-off of sensitivity for speed to be quite acceptable.

The amount of sequence data will continue to grow rapidly. However with accompanying advances in hardware, and with refinements of current algorithms, it appears that comparing new sequences with the corpus of known data will remain practical, and an important source of insight.

Finding genes. The central functional component of the genome is the gene, which may be defined in computational terms as a pattern imposed on the DNA sequence, resulting in a protein (or, sometimes, RNA) product. (See "The Anatomy of a Gene" in "Understanding Inheritance.") At the present time there is no sure way, either experimental or computational, to locate all the genes in a DNA sequence. However computational techniques can provide a very useful starting point in locating likely candidates for genes. The techniques are particularly well developed for finding genes coding for RNA that is not translated into protein. For instance, G. Fichant and C. Burks of LANL have developed a highly effective algorithm for finding tRNA genes. The rest of this discussion will refer only to the more complex problem of finding protein-coding genes.

Computer recognition of genes is not a simple problem. As far as we understand at the moment, there are no simple, local, key patterns that one can use to detect the presence of genes. For example, every triplet of bases that occurs as a codon in genes (where it stands for a particular amino acid; see "The Genetic Code" in "Understanding Inheritance") also occurs many millions of times outside of genes, with no meaning that we yet recognize. Thus solving the gene-recognition problem depends on integrating information from a number of clues spread out over thousands of bases of sequence.

In the long run, as we seek to understand how the genome works, our hope is to know how the cell recognizes genes. That is, we want to know what the enzymes are that control gene expression and how they recognize control sites on the DNA. Much progress has been made in elucidating the control of transcription and translation of genes in prokaryotes (simple one-celled organisms without nuclei). But the control of gene expression in humans is much more complicated, and the computer recognition of human control elements is still in its infancy.

There is, however, another approach. While we do not yet know enough about DNA-protein interaction to recognize genes the way the cell does, we can recognize certain patterns in a gene region that are side-effects of the way the gene is built. The simplest pattern is called an open reading frame. Reading frames are the six possible ways in which any stretch of DNA can be interpreted as a string of codons, depending on which strand is read and on whether a given base is interpreted as the first base of a codon, the second, or the third. A reading frame is said to be open in a region where it contains no stop codons, which are the triplets of bases that signal the end of translation of mRNA into protein. (See "The Genetic Code" and "Protein Synthesis" in "Understanding Inheritance.") In most organisms the stop codons on the sense strand of a gene are TAG, TAA, and TGA. (The sense strand has a base sequence equivalent to that of the mRNA.) Figure 9 shows the three reading frames of one strand of a viral sequence; stop codons are marked.

Since the genes of prokaryotes (and bacterial viruses) are uninterrupted, the protein-coding portions of their genes must lie in long continuous open reading frames. Most prokaryotic genes consist of at least fifty codons, and more typically hundreds, which do not

include any stop codons. On the other hand, an entirely random sequence of bases contains stop codons on average about once in twenty-one triplets in each reading frame. Therefore long open reading frames in prokaryotic and bacteriophage genomes are likely to contain genes. The third reading frame in Figure 9 is an example.

To find genes in eukaryotic genomes, one must look for more subtle patterns, mainly because eukaryotic genes are divided into exons (protein-coding regions) separated by introns (non-coding regions). Long open reading frames are still good candidates for exons, but some exons are as short as ten base pairs. Moreover, eukaryotic genomes contain long open reading frames that are not expressed. Therefore attention has turned to sequence patterns that distinguish coding from non-coding sequence. In the main, these patterns arise because coding sequences obey what are called codon preference rules. In most cases the same amino acid can be specified in genes by any of several synonymous codons. This latitude in choice of codon seems to be exploited systematically, in such a way that different bases are more common in different codon positions. For example T occurs more often at the second position of codons than at the first or third. The periodicity arising from these preferences is strikingly illustrated in the autocorrelation functions of the individual bases. Figure 10 shows the autocorrelation functions for the occurrences of T in coding and non-coding regions.

A variety of statistical techniques can be used to detect the nonrandom choice of triplets in coding regions. Such measurements can give an algorithm which, on a sample of about 150 bases of sequence, can differentiate protein coding from noncoding regions about 95 percent of the time.

The translated sequence starting from position 1

5214   5184
5' CGC CTC GGC CTC TGA GCT ATT CCA GAA GTA GTG AGG AGG CTT TTT TGG AGG CCT AGG CTT
   Arg Leu Gly Leu End Ala Ile Pro Glu Val Val Arg Arg Leu Phe Trp Arg Pro Arg Leu

5154   5124
   TTG CAA AAA GCT TTG CAA AGA TGG ATA AAG TTT TAA ACA GAG AGG AAT CTT TGC AGC TAA
   Leu Gln Lys Ala Leu Gln Arg Trp Ile Lys Phe End Thr Glu Arg Asn Leu Cys Ser End

5094   5064
   TGG ACC TTC TAG GTC TTG AAA GGA GTG CCT GGG GGA ATA TTC CTC TGA TGA GAA AGG CAT 3'
   Trp Thr Phe End Val Leu Lys Gly Val Pro Gly Gly Ile Phe Leu End End Glu Arg His

The translated sequence starting from position 2

5213   5183
5' GCC TCG GCC TCT GAG CTA TTC CAG AAG TAG TGA GGA GGC TTT TTT GGA GGC CTA GGC TTT
   Ala Ser Ala Ser Glu Leu Phe Gln Lys End End Gly Gly Phe Phe Gly Gly Leu Gly Phe

5153   5123
   TGC AAA AAG CTT TGC AAA GAT GGA TAA AGT TTT AAA CAG AGA GGA ATC TTT GCA GCT AAT
   Cys Lys Lys Leu Cys Lys Asp Gly End Ser Phe Lys Gln Arg Gly Ile Phe Ala Ala Asn

5093   5063
   GGA CCT TCT AGG TCT TGA AAG GAG TGC CTG GGG GAA TAT TCC TCT GAT GAG AAA GGC ATA 3'
   Gly Pro Ser Arg Ser End Lys Glu Cys Leu Gly Glu Tyr Ser Ser Asp Glu Lys Gly Ile

The translated sequence starting from position 3

5212   5182
5' CCT CGG CCT CTG AGC TAT TCC AGA AGT AGT GAG GAG GCT TTT TTG GAG GCC TAG GCT TTT
   Pro Arg Pro Leu Ser Tyr Ser Arg Ser Ser Glu Glu Ala Phe Leu Glu Ala End Ala Phe

5152   5122
   GCA AAA AGC TTT GCA AAG ATG GAT AAA GTT TTA AAC AGA GAG GAA TCT TTG CAG CTA ATG
   Ala Lys Ser Phe Ala Lys Met Asp Lys Val Leu Asn Arg Glu Glu Ser Leu Gln Leu Met

5092   5062
   GAC CTT CTA GGT CTT GAA AGG AGT GCC TGG GGG AAT ATT CCT CTG ATG AGA AAG GCA TAT 3'
   Asp Leu Leu Gly Leu Glu Arg Ser Ala Trp Gly Asn Ile Pro Leu Met Arg Lys Ala Tyr

Figure 9. A DNA Sequence in Three Reading Frames

The nucleotides numbered 5243 to 5062 of the genome of the simian virus SV40 are shown. (The strand depicted is the one known to be the sense strand in this region.) Also shown are the three possibilities for the translation of the sequence, each using a different reading frame, or division of the sequence into triplets of nucleotides. In this part of the SV40 genome, the first two reading frames depicted contain many stop codons (translated as "END" and highlighted), so the region does not code for proteins when read in those frames. In the third reading frame (boxed), on the other hand, there is a long region without stop codons—a promising candidate to be a protein-coding region. In fact, experiments have demonstrated that the sequence shown does include the beginning of a gene, whose translation starts with the highlighted ATG codon. (In the great majority of mRNAs, translation starts with AUG, corresponding to ATG in the sense strand of the DNA and to methionine in the protein product.) (Adapted from a figure by Maxine Singer and Paul Berg. *Genes and Genomes: a Changing Perspective.* Mill Valley, CA: University Science Books, 1991.)

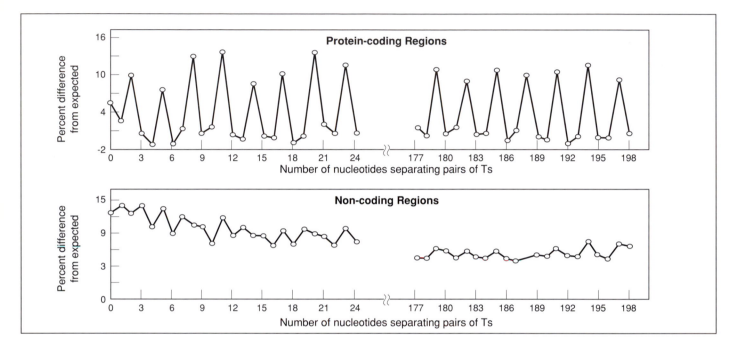

Figure 10. Periodicity of T Due to Codon Preference Rules
For each value of the separation *n*, the number of occurrences of the pattern T . . . T, with *n* nucleotides between the two T's, was counted. Plotted is the percent difference of that number from the number of such pairs expected if nucleotides occurred at random. Results are shown for all the coding sequences (a) and all the non-coding sequences (b) in GenBank when this study was performed (1982). Since T occurs preferentially at the second codon position, in coding regions the percent difference at *n* = 2, 5, 8 . . . is noticeably large. T's separated by two nucleotides, for instance, are at corresponding positions in consecutive codons. No such pattern appears in non-coding regions. Results for the other bases and for pairs of unlike bases show similar differences between coding and non-coding regions.

Research continues to find ever more accurate discrimination methods. R. Farber, A. Lapedes (both of Los Alamos), and K. Sirotkin (National Institutes of Health) report that a single-layer neural net reading each group of six consecutive bases can differentiate exonic from intronic sequences 180 bases long with a sensitivity well over 99 percent. With accuracies of 95 percent and sensitivities of 99 percent already in hand, the main hindrance to further development may soon be the accuracy of the databases. Though every care is taken by both investigators and database staff to make annotation both complete and correct, it is quite possible that the database annotation as to whether regions are coding or non-coding, by which these algorithms are measured, contains errors or omissions of a few percent.

All known algorithms depending on codon preference (so-called region methods) are rather poor at picking out the precise endpoints of coding regions. Thus current emphasis in this field is shifting towards combining region methods with recognition methods for biochemically active sites of transcription and translation initiation, intron splicing, etc. Two such systems have now been described in print and publicly disseminated: GM (for Gene Modeler), written by C. Fields (National Institutes of Health) and C. Soderlund (Los Alamos), and GeneID, written by R. Guigo (Los Alamos), S. Knudsen (University of West Florida), N. Drake (Tufts University) and T. Smith (Brown University).

Both of these programs analyze many different patterns over a large stretch of sequence, integrate the results, and present the user with a number of possible ways in which a gene or genes might be encoded in the sequence. The state of the art is that programs can suggest possible genes, and that the real genes in the region are likely to be at least variants of the ones proposed. It is not possible at present to predict the precise form of the gene or the conditions under which it is expressed.

Prediction of structure and function of proteins. Current techniques for the interpretation of sequence data are almost universally of what one might call a linguistic nature: they depend on the existence or frequency of certain simple patterns of letters in the DNA-sequence string. However it is not to be forgotten that the basis for all the effects of DNA in the living cell is the three-dimensional shape and charge distribution of biomolecules. In the long run, our understanding of the biochemistry of DNA, and therefore of the principles underlying the DNA programming language, will depend on our ability to relate the nucleotide sequence of DNA, and amino-acid sequences of protein, to the three-dimensional molecules of life. The promises of this infant science, a part of structural biology, are great, but remain mostly in the future.

Summary

The information gained from the Human Genome Project will reside in a very large database listing and describing the program for constructing and running the human body. With the development of new information-management techniques this information will be efficiently gathered from, and distributed to, a loosely coordinated and global community of scientists. Analysis tools are being developed to read the genome program and describe its functionality. While our knowledge of the biological programming language, and the tools we have to interpret it, are both at an early stage, they are also both very powerful, giving daily fundamental new insights into the workings of cells, organs and organisms, and leading to more powerful biotechnology. ∎

Acknowledgments

I am grateful for insightful remarks from Christian Burks, Michael Cinkosky, Doug Sorensen, David Torney, and the editors.

Further Reading

S. F. Altschul, W. Gish, W. Miller, E. W. Myers, and D. J. Lipman. 1990. Basic Local Alignment Search Tool. *Journal of Molecular Biology* 215:403-410.

M. Cinkosky, J. Fickett, P. Gilna, and C. Burks. 1991. Electronic data publishing and GenBank. *Science* 252:1273-77.

R. F. Doolittle, editor. 1990. *Methods in Enzymology* 183. San Diego: Academic Press. (A special issue of the journal devoted to sequence-analysis methods)

G. A. Fichant and C. Burks. 1991. Identifying Potential tRNA Genes in Genomic DNA Sequences. *Journal of Molecular Biology* 220:659-671.

R. Guigo, S. Knudsen, N. Drake, and T. Smith. 1992. Identification of genes in DNA sequences. *Journal of Molecular Biology*, in press.

A. Gupta, editor. 1989. *Integration of Information Systems: Bridging Heterogeneous Databases.* New York: IEEE Press.

J. Holland. 1975. *Adaptation in natural and artificial systems.* Ann Arbor, Michigan: University of Michigan Press.

J. R. Lawton, F. Martinez, and C. Burks. 1989. Overview of the LiMB database. *Nucleic Acids Research* 17:5885-5889.

S. G. Oliver *et al.* 1992. The complete DNA sequence of yeast chromosome III. *Nature* 357:38-46.

M. L. Pearson and D. Söll. 1991. The human genome project: a paradigm for information management in the life sciences. *The FASEB Journal* 5:35–39.

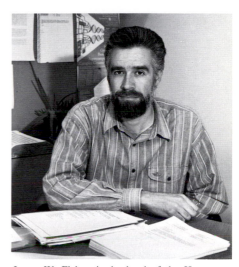

James W. Fickett is the head of the Human Genome Information Resource and section leader for Genome Analysis and Informatics. [See "Members of the Human Genome Center at Los Alamos National Laboratory" for biographical details.]

Rapid DNA Sequencing Based On Single-Molecule Detection

by Lloyd M. Davis, Frederick R. Fairfield, Mark L. Hammond, Carol A. Harger, James H. Jett, Richard A. Keller, Jong Hoong Hahn, Letitia A. Krakowski, Babetta Marrone, John C. Martin, Harvey L. Nutter, Robert R. Ratliff, E. Brooks Shera, Daniel J. Simpson, Steven A. Soper, and Charles W. Wilkerson

It is no secret that faster and cheaper DNA-sequencing techniques must be developed to make large-scale sequencing projects possible and to provide a routine tool for diagnostic medicine. Current methods are probably a hundred to a thousand times too slow and at least a hundred times too expensive for routine use (see pages 142-159 in "Mapping the Genome"). Several years ago, a group of us set out to find a better way.

Concluding that gel-based techniques could never achieve the required speed or sequence long stretches of DNA in one pass, we considered a variety of radically new potential methods, some more realistic than others. Ultimately we settled on a scheme that we believed might provide the needed high speed and low cost.

The method involves a combination of technologies from several fields, including molecular biology, enzymology, chemistry, and physics. In concept the method is simple. We would take a single strand of DNA, and starting from one end, remove and identify one nucleotide at a time. Building on Los Alamos expertise in flow cytometry, we intended to suspend the selected DNA strand in a gently flowing stream of water, which would carry the nucleotides to a detector after they were cleaved from the strand. The nucleotides would be removed in order, and if we avoided scrambling that order during the detection process, the sequence would be obtained immediately.

We knew that enzymes (called exonucleases) exist that sequentially remove one nucleotide at a time. Those enzymes can cleave several hundred or more nucleotides from DNA each second. Enzymology was a key element in our method—if nature had not provided those enzymes, our approach would have been unworkable.

Identification of the cleaved nucleotides posed a difficult problem since nature had no ready solution. Laser-excited fluorescence of a dye molecule attached to a nucleotide seemed to be the most likely method for detecting one nucleotide at a time. Such sensitivity had never before been achieved for a molecule in solution, surrounded by trillions of others. But a long history of ultrasensitive detection experiments by our group and others, demonstrating ever increasing sensitivity, encouraged us to believe that new insight and a few tricks might bring us to the ultimate sensitivity limit. After some considerable effort, single-molecule detection was achieved.

281

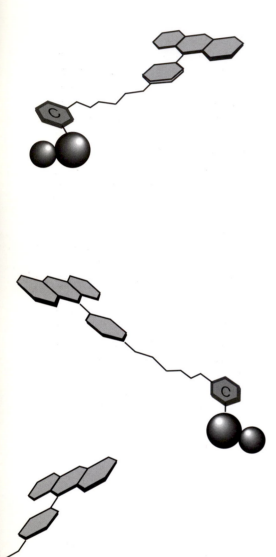

to synthesize pieces of DNA using as raw materials nucleoside triphosphates (dNTPs) bound to dye molecules; the template would be a strand of DNA that we want to sequence (see "DNA Replication" in "Understanding Inheritance"). If no errors occur during synthesis, the dye-labeled strand we created would have a sequence exactly complementary to the template DNA. Thus the sequence of the template would be revealed by sequencing the labeled strand.

A separate technical problem was how to select only a single dye-labeled DNA molecule and suspend it in the flowing water. Using optical traps, in which counter-propagating laser beams hold small objects, seemed like a possibility. Then perhaps the DNA strand could be attached to a tiny bead that would serve as a handle by which the laser beams could hold it.

We estimated that, once we put all these components together, we would be able to obtain rough sequence at the rate of hundreds of bases per second and to sequence tens of thousands of bases consecutively, surpassing by orders of magnitude the performance of current technology.

The Progress and the Problems

The past two years have brought progress in developing some of the techniques we need to make our sequencing scheme a reality. We have chemically attached highly fluorescent dyes to nucleoside triphosphates and used them to synthesize 7000-base DNA strands in which all the C and U nucleotides on one strand were labeled. (Uracil substitutes for the very similar thymine in these experiments.) We are working on replicating longer strands because one of the great potential strengths of our

method is the ability to provide long stretches of sequence data in a single pass. (We hope to sequence entire cosmid clones, about 40,000 bases long; gel-based methods can sequence fewer than 1000 bases at a time.) In addition, we have demonstrated that various exonucleases cleave DNA in which all the nucleotides of one type on one strand are labeled, albeit the cleavage is slower than normal. Much of the biochemistry and enzymology is being developed with the help of an industrial partner, Life Technologies, Inc. (LTI), under a Cooperative Research and Development Agreement.

Our plan calls for synthesizing strands in which all the nucleotides are labeled, but if synthesis with all four species of labeled nucleotides continues to prove difficult we could fall back on using only two labeled nucleotide species at a time. By making DNA with each of the six combinations of two labeled nucleotides (that is, a strand with labeled A and C only, one with labeled A and G only, and so forth) and carrying out the rest of our procedure for each strand, we would determine the complete sequence.

To suspend DNA in flowing water we may first attach it to a microscopic bead. Therefore we need to determine automatically whether a bead is attached to exactly one fluorescently labeled DNA molecule. We have identified single DNA molecules by the visual appearance of their fluorescence under a microscope, but we have not yet automated the process. We have also used flow sorting to select beads attached to DNA molecules based on their fluorescent brightness; we are working on increasing the sensitivity so that we can reliably identify single DNA molecules. All our identification experiments use stained DNA molecules that fluoresce roughly as brightly as labeled DNA molecules

But detection of a nucleotide is not enough. We must identify which of the four possible types of nucleotides, A, C, G, or T, is passing through the detector. For identification we planned to attach a distinctive fluorescent dye molecule to each type of nucleotide. The color of the attached dye's fluorescence would provide the identification. We needed to work out how to chemically attach the labels to each base of the DNA, making sure that the dyes did not impede the cleavage reaction. Our approach was of the size we plan to sequence. Construction of an adequate optical trap or development of another way to manipulate the beads remains to be done. Among the standard alternatives to optical trapping are making the bead out of a magnetic material and manipulating it with magnetic fields as well as using mechanical means such as micropipettes.

The detection of single dye-labeled nucleotides is the last step in our scheme, and there we have achieved an important success. We have been able to detect single dye molecules and dye-labeled nucleotides dissolved in water. Further, we have now developed techniques that allow us to distinguish single molecules of one dye from molecules of another by the difference in the color of their fluorescence. As discussed in the following sidebar, "Single-Molecule Spectroscopy in Solution," detection of individual molecules in solution may also find applications in fields other than sequencing.

The nucleotides must be detected in the order in which they were cleaved. However, in the distance between the suspended DNA molecule and the detector, molecular diffusion may scramble the order in which the nucleotides pass through the beam. We are trying to devise designs for the flow and the attachment of the DNA that minimize this problem.

Developing our rapid-sequencing method involves several technological advances. Although none of the parts is ready yet for inclusion in the overall scheme, we have made great progress and continue to be optimistic about overcoming the remaining obstacles because no fundamental principles stand in the way, only difficulties that can be overcome with ingenuity.

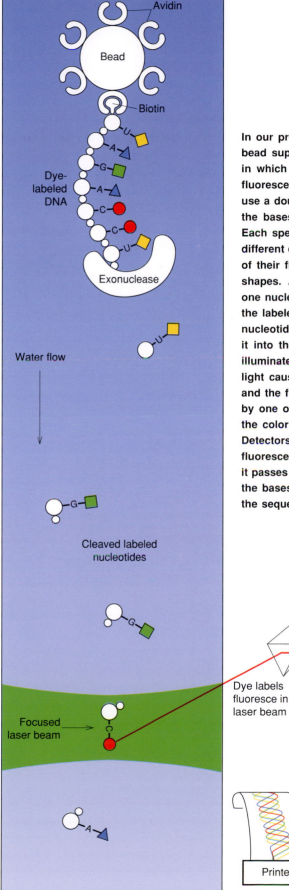

In our projected sequencing method, a bead supports a single strand of DNA in which each base is labeled with a fluorescent dye molecule. (We could also use a double-stranded molecule in which the bases on one strand are labeled.) Each species of base is labeled with a different dye, depicted here with the colors of their fluorescence and with different shapes. An exonuclease enzyme cleaves one nucleotide at a time from the end of the labeled DNA strand. Once a labeled nucleotide is cleaved, flowing water carries it into the detection volume, which is illuminated by a laser beam. The laser light causes the dye label to fluoresce and the fluorescence signal is registered by one of four detectors, depending on the color of the fluorescence emission. Detectors measure the frequency of the fluorescent light, identifying each base as it passes through the beam. The record of the bases going through the beam gives the sequence of the DNA.

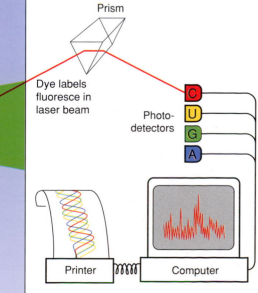

1. Dye-labeled Nucleotides

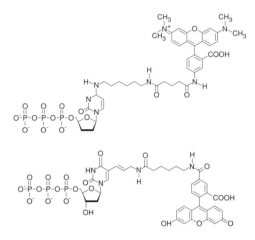

2. Synthesis of Dye-labeled DNA

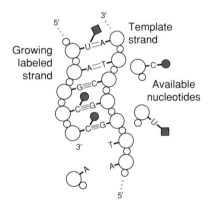

5'
3'
Template strand
Growing labeled strand
U A
A T
G≡C
C≡G
C≡G
T
A
A
5'
Available nucleotides
C
U

3. Biotin-Avidin Attachment of DNA to a Bead

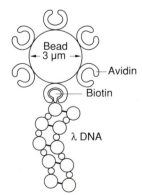

Bead 3 μm
Avidin
Biotin
λ DNA

Current Status

We are working on the various components of the project individually. The figures and captions on the next two pages outline both the current status of each component and some of the challenges that remain.

1. To make labeled DNA, we need four species of nucleoside triphosphates (dNTPs), each species labeled with a different fluorescent dye. We have experimented with several commercially available dye-labeled nucleotides, two of which are shown. The first is dCTP linked to tetramethyl rhodamine (commercially available); the second is dUTP linked to fluorescein (synthesized by Life Technologies, Inc.). Since our replication and cleavage experiments work with only some of the labeled nucleotides we have tried, we expect to construct many new ones to find four with which our full scheme can succeed. Those labeled nucleotides will be developed by LTI.

2. To synthesize labeled DNA strands, we will replicate a template strand of DNA using the labeled nucleotides. In collaboration with LTI, we have made DNA molecules about 7000 bases long in which all the C's and U's on one strand are dye-labeled. (The template is the genome of the M13 phage.) The figure is a schematic "snapshot" of DNA replication in which the C's and U's available in the reaction have dye labels, indicated by circles and squares. We determined the completeness of the replication by gel electrophoresis of the product; we are in the process of testing the fidelity.

3. Next we must attach a labeled strand of DNA to a solid support in order to hold it in flowing water. Working with unlabeled DNA strands, we have studied two standard ways of attaching DNA strands to beads about 3 microns in diameter. In one method the beads are glass and so the DNA binds electrostatically. In the other (shown schematically) a polystyrene bead is coated with avidin, a biotin molecule is attached to the 5′ end of the labeled DNA strand, and the tight binding between avidin and biotin attaches the DNA to the bead. The electrostatic attachment method does not interfere with digestion of DNA by an exonuclease. Since that method involves contact between the DNA and the bead at many points, whereas the biotin-avidin method only involves contact at the last base of the DNA, we expect that the biotin-avidin method will not interfere with exonuclease cleavage either.

4. Since the attachment step just described may be performed by mixing beads into batches of labeled DNA, we need to be able to identify beads carrying exactly one DNA molecule, and then move one of those beads into a stream of water and hold it in position there. We have learned to identify under a microscope single fluorescently stained λ DNA molecules (about 48.5 kbp long) not attached to beads. The objects we identified are confirmed to be λ DNA by chemical tests and by length measurements with gel electrophoresis. The method involves some computer assistance; we have begun work on automating it fully. With an alternative method, flow sorting, we have distinguished beads carrying one to three fluorescently stained

DNA molecules from other fluorescent objects. The sensitivity of that method needs to be improved so that we can be confident of identifying single molecules. We have not yet tested ways of manipulating and suspending single beads, but hope to use one of the techniques mentioned in the main text.

5. Once a DNA molecule is suspended in the stream of water, an exonuclease will cleave bases one by one from the labeled DNA. Working with LTI at their laboratories, we tested the exonuclease cleavage of DNA in which one species of base is labeled. (The DNA was produced in our replication experiments.) All six exonucleases we studied digested the DNA. Some of the exonucleases act on single-stranded DNA, others on double-stranded. Four of the enzymes are polymerases or components of polymerases. (Most polymerases include a part that acts as an exonuclease, apparently to proofread replication.) We studied one enzyme, the polymerase made by the T7 phage, in more detail. The enzyme completely digested 300-base DNA strands made with rhodamine-labeled C or rhodamine-labeled U (but degradation of strands made with fluorescein-labeled U was incomplete). The completeness of the digestion was determined by gel electrophoresis of the reaction products, which showed no fragments longer than one base. The cleavage rates under the conditions we used were around 10 to 20 nucleotides per second, two to five times slower than rates for unlabeled DNA. (To measure cleavage rates, we stop the reaction at various times by adding chemicals that "poison" it, and determine the size of the undigested portion by gel electrophoresis or other methods.) We are continuing to search for enzymes and reaction conditions that give rapid and complete cleavage.

6. In the final step a stream of water will carry the labeled bases one by one through a laser beam, where each base will be identified by the laser-induced fluorescence of its dye label. We have not yet constructed a prototype flow system. The flow must not change the order of the cleaved bases and must ensure that each base passes through the detection volume of about 10^{-12} liters. As described in "Single-Molecule Spectroscopy in Solution", we have succeeded in detecting single dye molecules and dye-labeled nucleotides, and in distinguishing single molecules of two species of dyes (shown as circles and triangles). We need to make the detector capable of distinguishing four species, and to improve the accuracy of detection and identification from about 65 percent to at least 99 percent to be adequate for DNA sequencing. ∎

Further Reading

J. H. Jett, R. A. Keller, J. C. Martin, B. L. Marrone, R. K. Moyzis, R. L. Ratliff, N. K. Seitzinger, E. B. Shera, and D. J. Simpson. 1989. High-speed DNA sequencing: An approach based upon fluorescence detection of single molecules. *Journal of Biomolecular Structure and Dynamics* 7: 301–309.

S. A. Soper, L. M. Davis, F. R. Fairfield, M. L. Hammond, C. A. Harger, J. H. Jett, R. A. Keller, B. L. Marrone, J. C. Martin, H. L. Nutter, E. B. Shera, and D. J. Simpson. 1991. Rapid DNA sequencing based on single molecule detection. *Proceedings. SPIE: The International Society for Optical Engineering* 1435: 168.

J. D. Harding and R. A. Keller. 1992. Single-molecule detection as an approach to rapid DNA sequencing. *Trends in Biotechnology* 10: 55.

5. Cleavage of labeled DNA

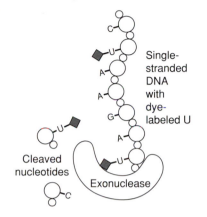

6. Single-molecule Detection

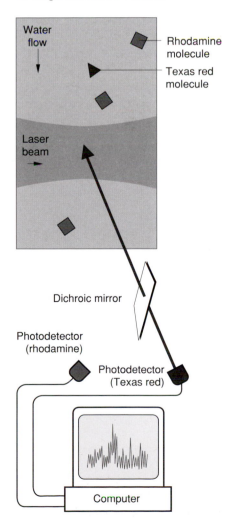

Single-Molecule Spectroscopy in Solution

Steven A. Soper, Lloyd M. Davis, and E. Brooks Shera

Detecting minute concentrations of chemicals in liquid environments has many applications. Consequently for over a decade scientists have been pushing the limits of detection sensitivity to lower and lower chemical concentrations. The Los Alamos plan for rapid DNA sequencing, described in the preceding pages, calls for the ultimate sensitivity—detection of single molecules. This article reviews the first technique used to accomplish that feat.

The technique involves measuring the fluorescence emission of a molecule as it passes through a laser beam. In addition to identifying the molecule, such spectroscopic measurements can reveal information about that molecule's chemical or physical surroundings, and thus single molecules may be used as probes to explore biological processes and structures at a microscopic level.

Physical Basis for Detection

Our detection method is applicable to fluorescent dye molecules, or to any molecules, such as nucleotides, that have been labeled with fluorescent dyes. The molecules, in solution, pass through a rapidly pulsed laser beam of such a wavelength that the dye can absorb the light. The solution must be so dilute that only one fluorescent molecule at a time passes through the beam. As each molecule passes through, many extremely brief pulses of light illuminate it; each pulse may cause the molecule to emit a fluorescence photon. Thus while in the beam each molecule produces a short burst of photons. We ascertain when a fluorescent molecule is in the beam by detecting some of the individual fluorescence photons that make up the burst and discriminating them from other photons that reach the detector.

Figure 1a illustrates both the process of fluorescence and other processes that compete with it. The processes begin when a molecule in its ground electronic state absorbs a photon and is thereby excited to a higher electronic state. (Our experiments use photons of visible light that excite the molecule to the first excited singlet state.) Fluorescence occurs when the molecule then quickly relaxes to a slightly lower energy through changes in its rotational and vibrational motion, and finally returns to the ground electronic state by emitting a photon. The photon emitted in the transition from the first excited singlet state to the ground state is called the fluorescence photon. A molecule is said to be fluorescent if it has a high probability of returning to the ground state by that path rather than by the other paths shown in Figure 1a. That probability is called the fluores-cence quantum yield. As Figure 1b shows, the frequency (and energy) of the fluorescence photon is lower than that of the absorbed photon. The average difference, called the Stokes shift, is roughly the same for most organic dyes. For example, a dye we often use, rhodamine 6G, is excited by green light and emits yellow fluorescence.

Once the molecule returns to the ground state, by any path, it is again available for excitation. However, absorption of a photon does not always bring about a reversible process. Sometimes absorption causes the molecule to undergo photobleaching, an irreversible change into a different chemical species, after which the molecule can no longer fluoresce and often cannot absorb light of the frequency of the absorbed photon. (The same process causes the fading of dyed materials exposed to sunlight.) If photobleaching occurs, the production of fluorescence photons stops even if the molecule is still illuminated. The probability that an excited molecule will bleach instead of returning to its original state is called the photobleaching efficiency (though in our work photobleaching is a source of inefficiency).

For single-molecule detection, an important feature of fluorescence is that the time between the excitation of the molecule and the emission of a

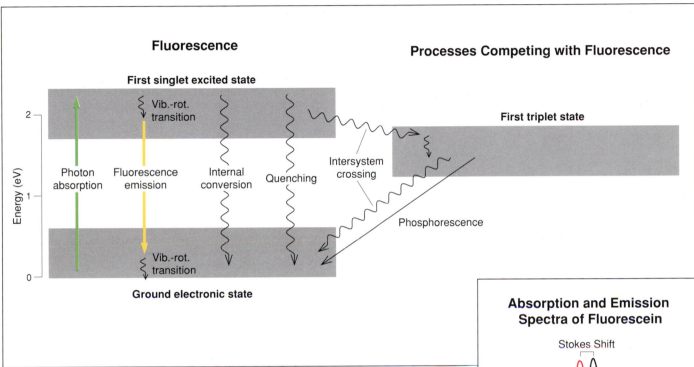

Fluorescence

Processes Competing with Fluorescence

First singlet excited state

Vib.-rot. transition

Photon absorption

Fluorescence emission

Internal conversion

Quenching

Intersystem crossing

First triplet state

Phosphorescence

Energy (eV)

Vib.-rot. transition

Ground electronic state

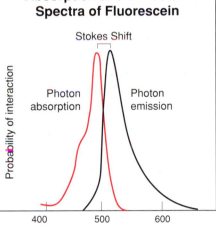

Absorption and Emission Spectra of Fluorescein

Stokes Shift

Photon absorption

Photon emission

Probability of interaction

Photon wavelength (nanometers)

Figure 1. (a) Fluorescence of a Dye Molecule

An energy-level diagram of a dye molecule showing the processes involved in fluorescence, as well as those that compete with fluorescence. In all cases the first step is absorption of a photon (green arrow), which causes the molecule to make a transition from its ground electronic state (a singlet state for most organic molecules) to the first excited singlet state. (Each electronic state is shown as a continuous band because within each such state are many closely spaced rotational and vibrational levels, which overlap one another when the molecule is in solution.) The excited molecule may return to the ground state in several ways, one of which is fluorescence. When undergoing fluorescence, the molecule first loses energy by a rapid series of rotational and vibrational transitions (wavy arrow), remaining in the same electronic excited state. The molecule then makes an electronic transition to some level within the ground electronic state (yellow arrow), emitting a photon—the fluorescence photon. Finally the molecule relaxes to a low-lying level within the ground electronic state by further vibrational and rotational transitions (wavy arrow). The average time from photon absorption to fluorescence emission is called the fluorescence lifetime. Most organic fluorescent dyes have lifetimes of a few nanoseconds. Processes that compete with fluorescence are indicated by lighter arrows. A molecule in the first singlet excited state can decay to the ground state without fluorescing. The energy is converted either into heat (internal conversion) or into the excitation of a molecule of another species (quenching). Another possibility is that the molecule can decay (without emitting a photon) to an excited triplet state (intersystem crossing). After a time that for organic dyes is much longer than the fluorescence lifetime, the molecule decays to the ground electronic state, with or without photon emission. (Photon emission in a transition from the first triplet state is called phosphorescence, and has a much longer lifetime than fluorescence.)

(b) The Stokes Shift

The probabilities of photon absorption and fluorescence emission as functions of wavelength for a typical fluorescent dye (fluorescein). Note that the emission curve peaks at a longer wavelength than the absorption curve. The difference between the two peaks is the Stokes shift. The fluorescence photon has a lower energy than the absorbed photon because some of the molecule's excitation energy is converted into heat though rotational and vibrational transitions.

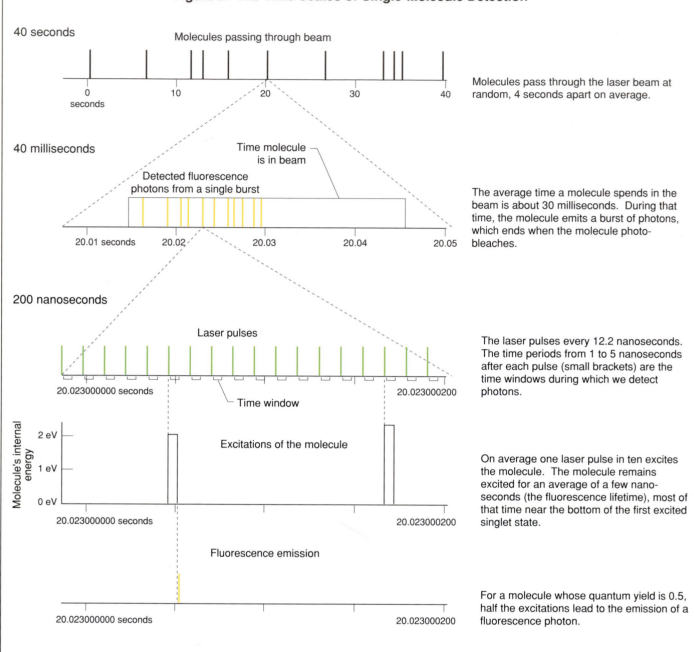

Figure 2. The Time Scales of Single-Molecule Detection

40 seconds

Molecules passing through beam

Molecules pass through the laser beam at random, 4 seconds apart on average.

40 milliseconds

Time molecule is in beam

Detected fluorescence photons from a single burst

The average time a molecule spends in the beam is about 30 milliseconds. During that time, the molecule emits a burst of photons, which ends when the molecule photobleaches.

200 nanoseconds

Laser pulses

The laser pulses every 12.2 nanoseconds. The time periods from 1 to 5 nanoseconds after each pulse (small brackets) are the time windows during which we detect photons.

Time window

Molecule's internal energy

Excitations of the molecule

On average one laser pulse in ten excites the molecule. The molecule remains excited for an average of a few nanoseconds (the fluorescence lifetime), most of that time near the bottom of the first excited singlet state.

Fluorescence emission

For a molecule whose quantum yield is 0.5, half the excitations lead to the emission of a fluorescence photon.

fluorescence photon is usually finite—and long enough to measure. That time difference follows an exponential probability distribution whose average is called the fluorescence lifetime. The dyes we use have fluorescence lifetimes of a few nanoseconds. Timing is crucial to the design of our experiments on single-molecule detection. Figure 2 illustrates the relevant time scales. The flashes of light from our laser last about 0.07 nanoseconds and repeat every 12.2 nanoseconds.

Since the duration of the laser pulses is much shorter than the fluorescence

lifetime, each pulse can bring about fluorescence at most once, thus producing at most one photon. The time between pulses is much longer than the fluorescence lifetime, so a molecule that absorbs a photon is practically certain to return to the ground state and be ready for another excitation by the time the next pulse arrives. Therefore, in principle, every pulse could cause the molecule to emit one fluorescence photon. Since our apparatus detects individual photons, we can take advantage of the interval between the arrival of the laser pulse and fluorescence to dis-

tinguish between fluorescence photons and photons produced by scattering of light from the laser pulse, as will be described below in the discussion of background light.

Signal Strength from Single Molecules

For the fluorescence signal to be detectable, its strength (the number of photons the signal comprises) must be large enough to be distinguished from photons produced by background sources. To make the simplest estimate of the signal strength, we recall that the molecule can produce one photon, but no more, for every pulse that illuminates it. In our apparatus the molecules' transit time through the beam is about 30 milliseconds, so with the laser pulsing at 12-nanosecond intervals we might expect a molecule with a large quantum yield to emit a burst of 2,400,000 photons—provided that the laser is powerful enough to excite the molecule with each flash and that photobleaching does not occur. Actually, the laser intensity we use is so low that typically a molecule will be excited by only about one laser pulse in ten. Even so, we might expect about 240,000 photons. However, photobleaching practically always stops the emission of photons before the molecule leaves the beam, thereby greatly reducing the size of the signal. The average number of excitations a molecule endures before bleaching is the reciprocal of the photobleaching efficiency, which for rhodamine 6G dissolved in water is 1.8×10^{-5}. Accordingly each rhodamine 6G molecule is excited, on average, 56,000 times before it photobleaches (so a more powerful laser would not increase the signal). Of those excitations, the fraction that induces fluorescence is by definition the fluorescence quantum yield. The quantum yield of rhodamine 6G is 0.45, so on average, a rhodamine 6G molecule is expected to produce about 25,000 fluorescence photons.

Our photon detector records about one photon of every thousand emitted, so we might hope to see 25 photons from one molecule. (Our group has recently obtained a detector that should do ten times better than our present equipment.) For more precise estimates of the signal size, we constructed an elaborate Monte Carlo computer simulation of our experiments that includes all the physics and photochemistry that significantly

affect our detection ability. Of the processes not yet mentioned but included in the simulation, the most important is diffusion, or random motion, of dye molecules, through which they can move into or out of the beam. The results from the simulation suggested that a typical signal would contain 10 to 15 photons. The simulation also proved to be very helpful in designing our experiment and quickly optimizing such experimental conditions as the flow rate and the size of the detection volume.

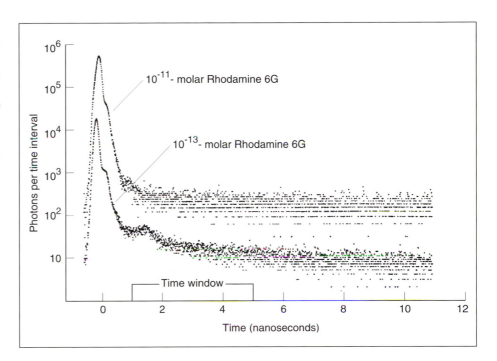

Figure 3. The Basis for Time-gated Detection of the Fluorescence Signal
The plotted data were accumulated during experiments in which laser pulses illuminated two dye solutions with different concentrations of R6G: 10^{-11} molar and 10^{-13} molar. The graph shows the number of detected photons as a function of the time interval (measured from the time of excitation) in which they were emitted. During the first nanosecond, the light intensity is independent of the dye concentration and therefore must be due mainly to light scattered from the laser pulse. After 1 nanosecond, the light intensity decreases exponentially and is proportional to the dye concentration, as one would expect from fluorescence emission. After about 5 nanoseconds, minor background sources with long lifetimes (perhaps from the glass in our apparatus) start to compete with the more quickly decaying fluorescence signal. Therefore to minimize the contribution from the background, we count only photons emitted in the time window shown, between 1 and 5 nanoseconds after each pulse.

Reducing the Background

Detection of light from single molecules in solution is difficult because the number of background photons is far larger than the number of photons in the fluorescence burst. Most background photons are laser photons that have undergone either Raman scattering from water molecules, Rayleigh scattering primarily from small-scale fluctuations in the density of the water, or reflection from surfaces of water and glass in the equipment. A smaller source of background is laser-induced fluorescence of impurities in the water. Light from Rayleigh scattering and reflection has the same color as the green laser light, so we can block most of it by placing a color filter in front of our detector. For example, we can use a filter that reflects green light but transmits yellow fluorescent light from rhodamine 6G. The color filters are made of thin layers of various colorless materials deposited on a clear glass support. By means of optical interference, the filters reflect all but one photon in a million at the frequency of the laser light while transmitting about 60 percent of the fluorescence photons.

The light from Raman scattering can be from a hundred to a thousand times more intense than a typical fluorescence signal. Some of that light has the same color as the fluorescence emission of the molecule, so it can not be eliminated by filtering. However, photons scattered from a laser pulse are nearly simultaneous with the pulse, whereas fluorescence photons are likely to be emitted well after the pulse. The time dependences of light from those two sources are shown in Figure 3 (previous page), a plot of the light intensity (versus time) obtained when a pulsed laser beam illuminated solutions of rhodamine 6G containing two different concentrations of the dye. The height of the initial light-intensity peak is independent of the dye concentration, so most of the photons constituting that peak are background photons. On the other hand, the light intensity at later times depends strongly on the concentration; therefore, much of the light at later times must come from the dye molecules, presumably from fluorescence. With these considerations in mind, we reduce the background by counting only those photons produced after the bright laser pulse is over but while the probability of emission of a

fluorescence photon is still relatively high, a procedure called time gating. The time window during which we record photons is shown in Figures 2 and 3. Ignoring photons emitted outside that window causes a small loss of signal, but decreases the number of accepted background photons by a factor on the order of a thousand.

Together, time gating and color filtering reduce the background intensity reaching the detectors by a factor of roughly a billion. Consequently, we can see the faint fluorescence signal from a single dye molecule even though tens of trillions of surrounding water molecules are illuminated by the laser. By the same token, we detect fluorescence from impurities in the water, so they are an important source of background. We minimize their effect, first, by purifying the water as much as possible and, second, by minimizing the volume of water illuminated by the laser and monitored by our detectors.

Identification by Color

For many applications, including high-speed DNA sequencing, merely detecting each dye molecule that passes through the laser beam is not sufficient; we also need to distinguish different types of molecules. Because the molecules are detected by their fluorescence emission, it is natural to distinguish molecules of different chemical species by observing some spectroscopic property such as the color of their fluorescence emission. The emitted photons of different colors can be separated by using a glass prism to bend the light in different directions according to color. However, in our set-up, it is more efficient to use color filters and color-selective (dichroic) mirrors, which, like the color filters described earlier, work by thin-film

interference. Each type of molecule we want to detect is assigned its own photodetector, which is shielded by a color filter that transmits light of that molecule's emission wavelength but reflects light from molecules of other types in the solution. In principle, every dye molecule that passes through the beam can be identified by noting which detector signals its presence.

A fluorescent dye molecule absorbs and emits light over a range of wavelengths (as shown in Figure 1). Consequently, to be readily distinguishable by fluorescence color, different dyes must have emission spectra whose peaks are well separated in wavelength, by at least some tens of nanometers. Since the Stokes shift is roughly the same for most organic molecules (about 20 nanometers), it is difficult to find two dyes that absorb efficiently at the same wavelength but fluoresce at wavelengths far enough apart to be distinguishable. Therefore we need a different laser to excite each species of dye—a complication in designing the experiment.

Apparatus for Spectroscopy

Figure 4 shows the apparatus we have developed for a demonstration of spectroscopy on single molecules. Two lasers, one activated by the other, provide two colors of excitation light in synchronized pulses so that we can observe two types of molecules in one solution. Since dyes and dye-labeled nucleotides behave the same way in the experiment and labeled nucleotides must be made specially, we have used the dyes rhodamine 6G and Texas red in our experiments to date. Water containing an extremely low concentration of dye molecules flows through a glass tube, called the flow cell. Laser light is focused into a very narrow beam that

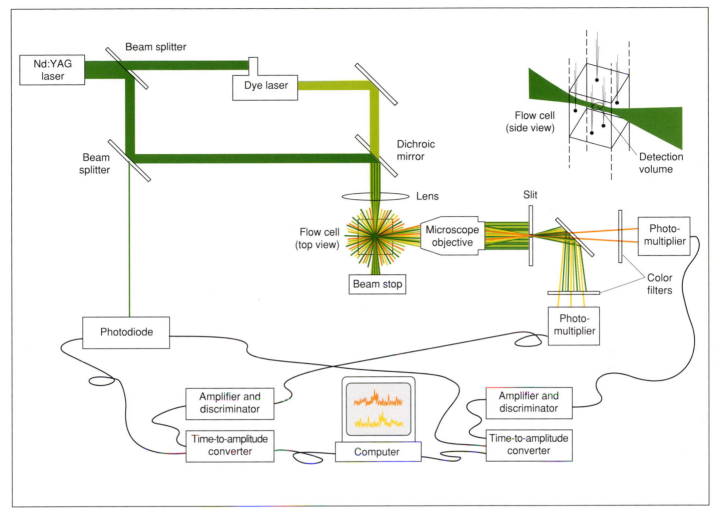

Figure 4. Apparatus for Single-Molecule Spectroscopy

The figure schematically illustrates the optics for delivering two pulsed laser beams to a flow cell containing fluorescent dye molecules of two different kinds as well as the apparatus for detecting fluorescence signals emitted by the two dyes, rhodamine 6G and Texas red. A mode-locked neodymium:YAG laser produces pulsed green light (532 nanometers). Part of the light is deflected by a beam splitter toward a dye laser and causes that laser to produce yellow light (585 nanometers, a wavelength that can excite the dye Texas red) pulsed with the same frequency as the green light that stimulates it. To generate a start signal for time-gated detection of the fluorescence signal, another beam splitter sends a small fraction of the original green light to a photodiode. Various lenses and mirrors (most of them not shown) direct the rest of the green laser light and all the yellow laser light to a dichroic mirror. A delay in the path of the green light synchronizes the green and yellow light pulses. The dichroic mirror combines the two beams into one by transmitting yellow light and reflecting green light. Then a lens focuses the combined beam into the detection volume within the glass flow cell (inset). As an extremely dilute solution of the dyes flows through the cell, the laser light induces the emission of fluorescence light from dye molecules. Some of the laser light is also scattered from the water in the flow cell. To detect the fluorescence signal, a microscope objective (which subtends about 2 percent of the total solid angle) collects light from the flow cell and focuses it on an opaque plate with a slit. Only light that comes from the detection volume, a small fraction of the water illuminated by the beam (about 10^{-12} liters), passes through the slit. This arrangement minimizes background light from outside the detection volume, including fluorescent impurities. Likewise if light comes from other directions (meaning that it is background) the edges of the slit block it. Light emerging from the slit continues to another dichroic mirror that reflects the long-wavelength light, including the orange fluorescence from Texas red, toward one detector, while transmitting the yellow fluorescence from rhodamine 6G to the other detector. Color filters in front of each detector transmit only photons in the expected frequency range for fluorescence of the appropriate dye. As explained in the text, the photomultiplier tubes produce current pulses for about 5 percent of the incident photons. The pulses are then amplified, and small pulses, which probably result from random instrumental noise, are filtered out by discriminators. Next pulses from photons that were not emitted during the time-gating window are rejected. The necessary time-keeping is performed by time-to-amplitude converters (TACs). A TAC begins measuring time at an electrical start signal produced by the photodiode each time a flash of green laser light reaches it. Then every time the TAC receives an electrical pulse from the photomultiplier, which indicates the arrival of a photon from the detection volume, it generates an output pulse whose peak voltage is proportional to the time since the start signal. Other electronic components accomplish the time gating by transmitting only those pulses whose voltage indicates that the corresponding photons were emitted inside the time-gating window.

Figure 5. Computer Processing of the Data

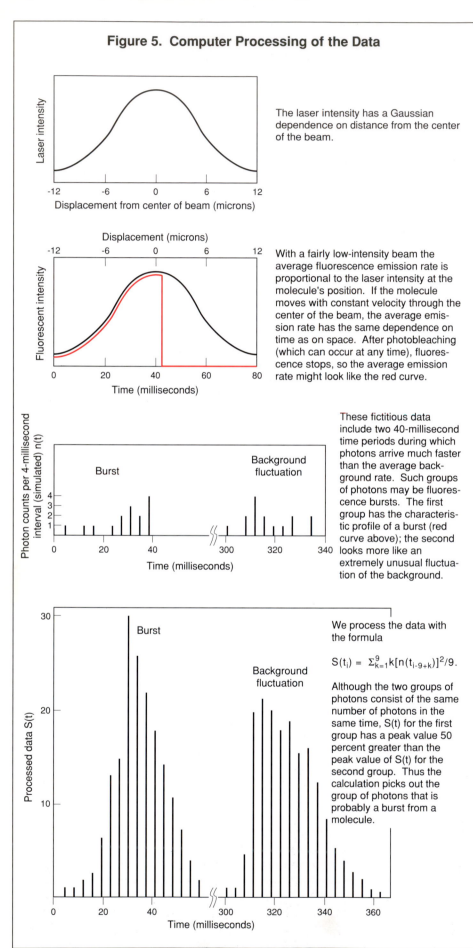

The laser intensity has a Gaussian dependence on distance from the center of the beam.

With a fairly low-intensity beam the average fluorescence emission rate is proportional to the laser intensity at the molecule's position. If the molecule moves with constant velocity through the center of the beam, the average emission rate has the same dependence on time as on space. After photobleaching (which can occur at any time), fluorescence stops, so the average emission rate might look like the red curve.

These fictitious data include two 40-millisecond time periods during which photons arrive much faster than the average background rate. Such groups of photons may be fluorescence bursts. The first group has the characteristic profile of a burst (red curve above); the second looks more like an extremely unusual fluctuation of the background.

We process the data with the formula

$$S(t_i) = \Sigma_{k=1}^{9} k[n(t_{i-9+k})]^2/9.$$

Although the two groups of photons consist of the same number of photons in the same time, S(t) for the first group has a peak value 50 percent greater than the peak value of S(t) for the second group. Thus the calculation picks out the group of photons that is probably a burst from a molecule.

passes through the flow cell, where it causes the dye molecules to fluoresce, and produces background light through scattering processes. A fraction of the light from the flow cell falls on lenses, which focus that light onto a plate with a slit. Light emanating from the detection volume, a very small volume around the focal point of the laser beam, passes through the slit. A dichroic mirror directs light of the color produced by rhodamine 6G to one photodetector while sending light of the color produced by Texas red to the other detector. At the detector, each photon of the selected wavelength passes through a color filter and strikes the cathode of a photomultiplier tube where it can produce a free electron by the photoelectric effect. Electric fields accelerate the electron toward the anode, causing it to jar other electrons loose from solid structures of the tube, which in turn are accelerated and jar still more electrons loose. Thus about one photon in twenty that strikes the cathode gives rise to a current pulse large enough for the rest of the electronics to discriminate it from noise in the detector. As indicated in Figure 4, electronic components measure the time, relative to the most recent laser flash, at which each photon arrives at the detector, and reject photons that do not arrive during the time-gating window.

Figure 5 outlines the computer data processing that distinguishes fluorescence bursts emitted by molecules of each type from the background photons that reach the detector. The distinguishing feature of a fluorescence burst is the time dependence of the rate at which photons are detected. Typically the rate increases as the molecule moves toward the center of the laser beam, where the laser light is most intense, then drops abruptly when photobleaching occurs. Though random fluctuations in the background

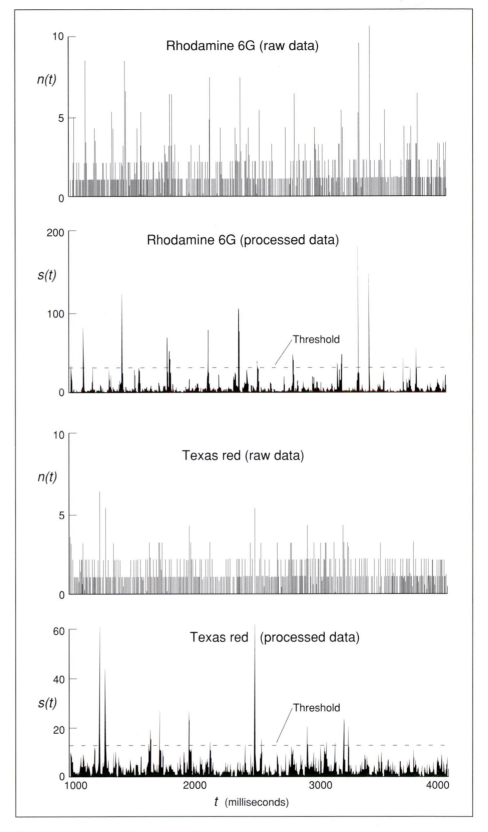

may occasionally produce many photons in a short time, they are unlikely to duplicate the characteristic time profile of a fluorescence burst. Every few milliseconds, the computer program calculates a function $S(t)$ that depends on the detection rate of the photons that arrived at the detector during the previous few dozen milliseconds. The function's value is large when the temporal pattern of incoming photons is typical of a fluorescence burst, but smaller when photons arrive in other patterns. If many photons arrive in rapid succession but their rate of arrival does not increase with time as in a burst, the value of $S(t)$ calculated from those data will be smaller than that for a typical burst. We record the presence of a molecule when the value of $S(t)$ exceeds a set threshold.

Experimental Results for Single-Molecule Detection

We used the apparatus shown in Figure 4 with solutions of single dyes, and more recently with a solution of rhodamine 6G and Texas red, both diluted to 10^{-14} molar. In the latter experiment the flow speed through the detection volume was about 290 microns per second. Figure 6 shows raw and processed data for both dyes. Peaks in the processed data above the thresholds (dotted lines) are interpreted as signals from dye molecules. Thus we are able to detect and distinguish individual dye molecules of two types in a mixed solution.

Computer processing does not eliminate all errors. We set the thresholds so that the false-positive rate in experiments with no dye present is no more than 0.01 per second. In an experiment with only rhodamine 6G we saw 87 percent of the dye molecules (calculated by comparison with the

Figure 6. Single-Molecule Discrimination of Two Dyes

The apparatus depicted in Figure 4 was used to detect and distinguish two different dye molecules, R6G and Texas red. The upper pair of graphs shows raw data $n(t)$ and processed data $S(t)$ from R6G. All peaks in $S(t)$ higher than a threshold marked by the dotted line were interpreted as indications of fluorescence bursts from R6G molecules. Use of the threshold restricted the false-positive rate to 0.01 per second. The lower graphs show the analogous data for the same time period from Texas red.

estimated rate at which molecules pass through the detection volume). Since the optimum chemical conditions for reducing photobleaching of rhodamine 6G are incompatible with those for Texas red, when we ran experiments with both dyes we detected 79 percent of the rhodamine 6G molecules and 54 percent of the Texas red molecules that flowed through the detection volume. (Improvements in the apparatus, such as our new photomultipliers, should soon allow much better efficiencies.) These experimental results agree approximately with our Monte Carlo prediction of the rate at which we should detect single molecules. The agreement gives us confidence that we understand the photophysics of single molecules in solution.

Identification by Lifetime

Spectroscopic properties other than emission wavelength can be used to distinguish different types of molecules. Fluorescence lifetime is convenient for us to measure. It is particularly useful because molecules of different types usually have different lifetimes, as do molecules of any one type in different chemical environments. As stated above, fluorescence lifetime is the average amount of time that a molecule remains excited before returning to the ground electronic state through the emission of a fluorescence photon, and the individual times from excitation to emission are random and follow an exponential probability distribution.

The standard way to measure a fluorescence lifetime is to excite a concentrated solution of a dye with a pulse of light and observe the exponential decay in intensity of the light that the many dye molecules produce. (An exponential-decay curve in data from essentially the same experiment

appears in Figure 3.) On the other hand, to determine the average lifetime of a single dye molecule, we must re-excite that molecule many times and measure the time to fluorescence following each excitation. Our apparatus is already set up to observe the individual times between excitation and fluorescence, denoted ΔT, since that measurement is required to implement the time gating described earlier. Because the resulting sample of individual ΔT values is small, it is more efficient to calculate the lifetime from the data by taking the mean of the time differences between excitation and fluorescence than to fit the data to an exponential distribution (as shown by Peierls in 1935).

The main purpose of our experiments was to demonstrate the feasibility of measuring the fluorescence lifetimes of single molecules with enough precision to discriminate between chemical species. Therefore we took steps that are incompatible with certain applications of lifetime measurements, such as high-speed sequencing. In particular, to maximize the number of fluorescence photons from each molecule, we reduced photobleaching by using methanol as the solvent and extended the time window almost to the next laser pulse. We also used a low flow speed so that each molecule would remain in the beam longer. The solvent moved so slowly, in fact, that the length of time the

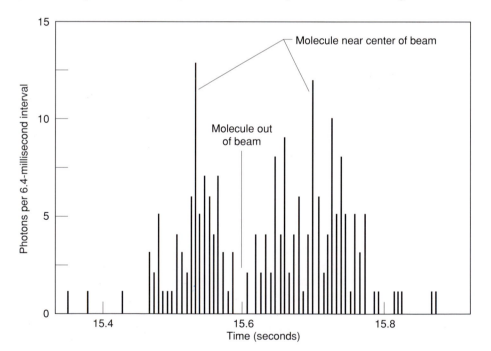

Figure 7. Photons from a Single Molecule

The bars represent the number of photons detected in 6.4-millisecond time intervals during a measurement of the fluorescence lifetime of a single molecule. The profile of the burst differs from the typical profile of fluorescence bursts shown in Figure 5 because the lifetime experiment differed from our color-discrimination experiments in having a much slower flow and reduced photobleaching. Those conditions allow molecules to wander randomly into and out of the beam while still fluorescing; the data shown suggest that a molecule entered and left the beam twice.

molecules stayed in the detection volume was determined more by diffusion than by the flow. Bursts often exhibited multiple peaks as a molecule wandered into, out of, and back into the beam. To ensure that every burst, even those with multiple peaks, came from a single molecule, we made the dye so dilute that during experiments lasting several minutes, only a few dye molecules passed through the detection volume. Between bursts, the photon detection rate was low and approximately equal to the background rate.

Figure 7 shows a typical burst consisting of about 200 photons from a Texas red molecule (compared to 10 to 15 photons in our color-discrimination experiments). From those data we can determine the fluorescence lifetime of the molecule with an accuracy of $200^{-1/2}$ or 7 percent, sufficient to distinguish many species of dyes.

Figure 8 gives the ΔT values for each of the photons that made up the burst shown in Figure 7. Since time gating is still necessary to reduce the background, we must ignore photons emitted shortly after the laser pulse. We can still determine the average lifetime of each molecule by measuring ΔT from the beginning of the time window rather than from the time of the laser pulse, because the lifetimes have an exponential distribution. Accordingly we ignore the ΔT values less than 0.7 nanoseconds and subtract 0.7 nanoseconds from all the larger values. Then the average of the values in Figure 8 is a reasonably accurate measurement of the fluorescent lifetime of that molecule. (We make a small correction for our inability to record ΔT values greater than 11 nanoseconds, when the next laser pulse begins to interfere. In principle the background makes another correction necessary, but in this case the expected background in the short duration of a burst is negligible.)

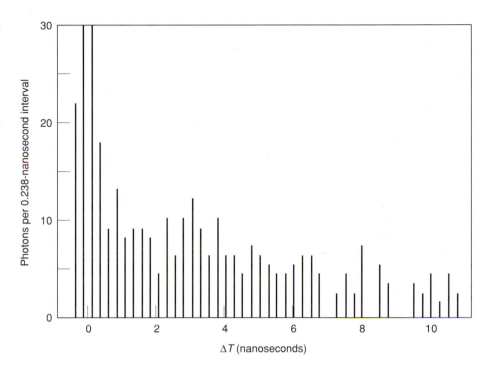

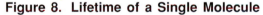

Figure 8. Lifetime of a Single Molecule
The data are from the same photon burst shown in the previous figure, but here the vertical bars give the number of photons whose emission times (measured from the previous excitation time) fell in each 0.238-nanosecond interval of ΔT. (We have not used time gating so that we can show times less than 1 nanosecond after the laser pulses, where a contribution from Raman scattering, too large for the scale of this graph, is present.) With only about 200 photons, the data follow the expected exponential distribution very roughly, but still give a reasonably accurate value for the average lifetime.

From the data plotted in Figure 8, we computed the lifetime of the molecule that produced that burst to be 4.5±0.3 nanoseconds, in agreement with the value 4.17±0.01 nanoseconds measured on bulk solutions of Texas red. Lifetimes computed for all the individual bursts clustered near the known value. Our measurements are the first determinations of fluorescent lifetimes for single molecules in solution. In future experiments such measurements could be used to identify the molecular species that produced the burst by comparison to values previously measured from bulk samples of the dye. In rapid sequencing, identification by lifetime has

the advantage that one might use related dyes with similar spectra but different lifetimes, and thus one would need only one laser and one photomultiplier.

With proper experimental design, two or more independent spectroscopic properties, such as lifetimes and emission spectra, could be measured simultaneously on each passing molecule. It might also be possible eventually to measure other quantities such as photobleaching efficiency and the molecule's effectiveness at absorbing photons. Knowledge of two or more parameters would be useful in cases where the value of a single parameter is insufficient to make a definitive identification.

Other Applications of Spectroscopy

We have discussed single-molecule spectroscopy primarily from the point of view of identification of molecular species, as when a dye molecule is attached as an identification tag to a nonfluorescent molecule, for example a DNA base. However, data collected by observing individual molecules can reveal features that are not evident in the average behavior of a group. For example, in a group of dye molecules, one in fifty might be bound to another molecule that diminishes its quantum yield, causing the average yield to be slightly less than the true value. A bulk experiment would reveal only the average value, whereas the true yield as well as the statistics underlying the decreased average would be readily accessible using single-molecule spectroscopy.

Moreover, to the extent that spectroscopic properties are modified by the immediate environment of a molecule, measuring those properties can supply information about that environment on a microscopic scale (provided the environment changes little in the time needed for the measurement). For example, fluorescence lifetime can be used to measure distances on the atomic scale. An excited fluorescent molecule (donor) can lose its excitation energy to a nearby acceptor molecule if the donor's range of emission energies overlaps the acceptor's range of absorption energies. (See the depiction

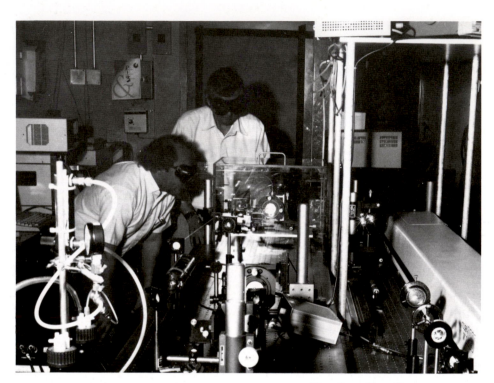

of quenching in Figure 1.) Such energy transfer reduces the fluorescence lifetime of the donor. Because the probability of energy transfer depends strongly on the distance r between donor and acceptor (as r^{-6}), measurement of the donor's fluorescence lifetime provides a measurement of its distance from the acceptor. We hope to use this molecular-level "yardstick" to determine distances that are inaccessible by other means, particularly in biological systems. Such potential applications, as well as the promise of rapid DNA sequencing, will maintain our interest in developing single-molecule spectroscopy. ∎

Further Reading

R. Peierls. 1935. Statistical errors in counting experiments. *Proceedings of the Royal Society (London)* A149:467.

E. B. Shera, N. K. Seitzinger, L. M. Davis, R. A. Keller, and S. A. Soper. 1990. Detection of single fluorescent molecules. Chemical Physics Letters 175:553–557.

S. A. Soper, L. M. Davis, and E. B. Shera. 1992. Detection and identification of single molecules in solution. Accepted for publication in *Journal of the Optical Society of America* B.

Members of the Human Genome Center at Los Alamos National Laboratory

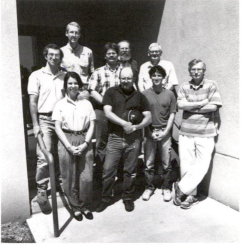

Rapid Sequencing
Row 1: B. Marrone, H. Nutter, J. Schecker, B. Shera.
Row 2: P. Goodwin, P. Ambrose, D. Keller.
Row 3: C. Wilkerson, J. Martin.

Mapping and Libraries ▼
Row 1: C. Lemanski, J. Graeber, M. Campbell, D. Robinson,
E. Campbell, L. Clark, N. Brown, J. Buckingham, K. Dennison,
D. Grady, N. Doggett, E. Hildebrand, B. Lobb, D. Bruce,
W. Erickson. *Row 2*: L. Deaven, J. Longmire, J. Fawcett.
Not pictured: L. Deusing, A. Ford, J. Gatewood, J. Jett, M. Jones.

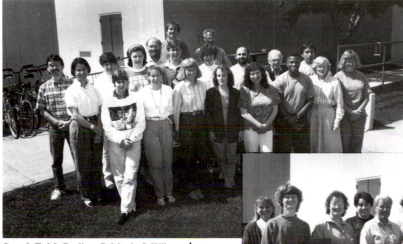

Row 1: E. McCanlies, C. Munk, J. Wilson, ▲
M. McCormick, P. Schor, D. McRae, J. Tesmer,
L. Meincke. *Row 2*: E. Martinez, B. Marrone,
L. Saunders, J. Meyne, M. Wilder, T. Riley,
K. Shera, B. Rappaport, B. Wagner, C. Naranjo.
Row 3: B. Moyzis, B. Ratliff.
Not pictured: J. Spuhler, R. Stallings, S. Thompson.

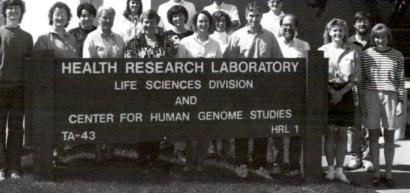

Robotics
Left to right: P. Medvick, T. Beugelsdijk, J. Fowler,
D. Trimmer, J. Roybal, R. Roberts.
Not pictured: B. Hollen, M. Kozubal, L. Stovall.

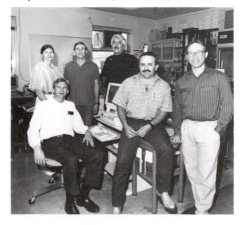

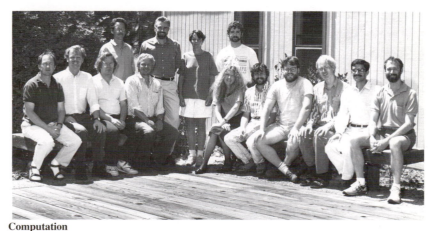

Computation
Left to right: P. Gilna, M. Cinkosky, M. Bridgers, G. Keen, R. Pecherer, J. Fickett, C. Macken,
G. Fichant, R. Sutherland, Y. Quentin, G. Redgrave, C. Troup, M. Ijadi, W. Barber.
Not pictured: G. Bell, C. Burks, M. Engle, E. Fairfield, M. Mundt, D. Sorensen, D. Torney.

E. Morton Bradbury received a B.S. in physics and a Ph.D. in biophysics

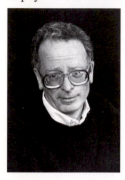

from King's College, University ofLondon, in 1955 and 1958, respectively. After completing his postdoctoral research at Courtauld Research Laboratory, he was appointed head of the Department of Molecular Biology at Portsmouth (England) Polytechnic in 1962, where he remained until his appointment at University of California, Davis, in 1979. He became leader of the Life Sciences Division at Los Alamos National Laboratory in 1988. Bradbury's research has been devoted to understanding whether chromosome organization and chromosome structure are involved in determining how a cell looks and behaves; the structure and function of active chromatin; and the process by which chromosomes condense prior to cell division. In pursuing his investigations, Bradbury has combined the results of measurements derived from the use of a wide range of techniques, including optical spectroscopy, nuclear magnetic resonance, x-ray diffraction, electron diffraction, and neutron diffraction. The recipient of numerous awards and honors, Bradbury has also chaired a number of scientific organizations, including the British Biophysical Society, the International Council for Magnetic Resonance in Biology, and the Neutron/Biology Committee of the Institut Laue Langevin. In addition, Bradbury is a member of HERAC and a member of the HERAC subcommittee on structural biology.

Michael J. Cinkosky joined the GenBank project at the Laboratory in 1984, after

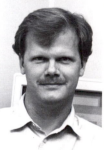

earning a B.A. in liberal arts from St. John's College in Santa Fe. He is currently one of the principal investigators for the GenBank project as well as lead designer of the SIGMA genome-map editor being produced by the Human Genome Information Resource at Los Alamos.

Larry L. Deaven earned B.S. and M.S. degrees in genetics from Pennsylvania

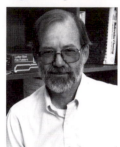

State University in 1962 and 1964, respectively. He studied cell biology and cytogenetics at the University of Texas M. D. Anderson Hospital and Tumor Institute and received a Ph.D. in biomedical sciences in 1969. In 1971 he joined the Laboratory where he utilized flow cytometry and chromosomal-banding analysis to study the chromosomal rearrangements and changes in DNA content found in the cells of many tumors. He also studied the types of chromosomal damage and ensuing cellular effects induced by products and by-products of energy research and development. In 1983 Deaven became the principal investigator of the National Laboratory Gene Library Project at Los Alamos. The project has produced over fifty different human-DNA libraries from flow-sorted chromosomes. Over 2500 copies of those libraries have been distributed to human-genome research laboratories throughout the world. In 1981 Deaven received the Commemorative Medal of Achievement from the University of Texas M. D. Anderson Hospital and Tumor Institute for his work in cytogenetics and cell biology, and in 1987 he received a Distinguished Performance Award from the Laboratory for his work on DNA-library construction. Outside the Laboratory Deaven enjoys growing flowers, especially species and cultivars of the genus *Clematis*.

Norman A. Doggett earned his B.A. in chemistry from North Carolina State University in 1980 and his Ph.D. in pathology from the University of North Carolina at Chapel Hill in 1986. For three years Doggett was a postdoctoral research fellow in the Department of Genetics at Columbia University. In 1989 he joined the Life Sciences Division of Los Alamos National Laboratory as a staff scientist in the Genetics Group. His major research interests include human-genome organization, physical mapping, and molecular genetic approaches to finding disease genes. Currently he is one of the principal investigators in the project to complete a physical contig map of human chromosome 16 and is a principal investigator of a Laboratory-funded effort to clone the gene for Batten's disease.

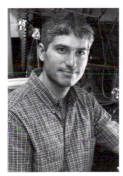

James W. Fickett earned his Ph.D. in mathematics from the University of

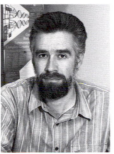

Colorado in 1979 and, after teaching for one year at Texas A&M University, joined the Laboratory's Theoretical Biology and Biophysics Group as a postdoctoral fellow in 1980. He worked until 1987 on the GenBank project, managing the release process and directing most of the software development. In 1986 he and Michael Cinkosky planned the restructuring of GenBank that was to implement the Electronic Data Publishing paradigm. In 1982 he developed TESTCODE, an algorithm for recognition of genes in DNA sequences, which has been incorporated into a number of commercial software packages for sequence analysis. He headed the Human Genome Information Resource in 1987 and again from 1989 to the present and has been section leader for Genome Analysis and Informatics since 1989.

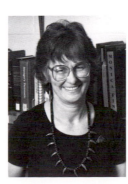

Monica Fink
Administrative Assistant

Carl E. Hildebrand received his M.S. in biophysics in 1968 and his Ph.D. in biophysics in 1970 from Pennsylvania State University. His dissertation focused on the effects of hydrostatic pressure on bacterial protein synthesis using cell-free protein synthesizing systems. After a postdoctoral appointment at Los Alamos National Laboratory, Hildebrand joined the staff of the Laboratory's Genetics Group where his studies were directed toward biochemical

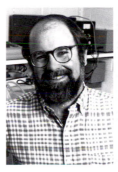

and molecular genetic analyses of the response of rodent and human cells to trace metals. Hildebrand was appointed deputy leader of the Genetics Group in 1983. The following year he won a National Research Service Award and was appointed a senior fellow at the Daniel W. Nebert, M.D., Laboratory of Developmental Pharmacology in Bethesda, Maryland. In 1984 he resumed his duties as deputy leader of the Genetics Group and, concurrently, served as associate leader of the Life Sciences Division. In 1989 he was appointed the leader of the Genetics Group. He now serves as a principal investigator in developing the human-genome physical-mapping project and as scientific advisor in the Genomics and Structural Biology Group.

James H. Jett received his B.S. and M.S. in physics from the University of New 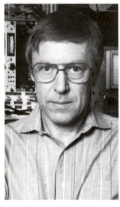 Mexico and, after serving a stint in the U.S. Navy, earned his Ph.D. in nuclear physics from the University of Colorado at Boulder in 1969. In 1969 he received a postdoctoral appointment in the Physics Division at Los Alamos National Laboratory and later became a staff member of that division. Since 1972 he has been a staff member in the Laboratory's Life Sciences Division. His interests include developing data-analysis and data-interpretation techniques for flow-cytometric and biological data, and developing applications of flow techniques to chromosome analysis and sorting. He has conducted analyses of prophage induction in *Haemophilus influenzae* by ultraviolet light. In addition, he has participated in the design, development, and programming of a computer-based in-vitro radiation-measurement system and contributed to the chromosome-16 mapping effort. Jett has been an Adjunct Associate Professor of Cell Biology at University of New Mexico School of Medicine since 1985.

Richard A. Keller earned his B.A. in chemistry from Allegheny College in 1956 and his Ph.D. in chemical physics from the University of California, Berkeley, in 1961. After teaching a short time at the University of Oregon, Keller worked at the National Bureau of Standards in Washington, D.C. until 1976, when he joined the staff of Los Alamos National Laboratory. He has been leader of the Rapid DNA Sequencing Project since 1988. Keller's research interests are in the development and characterization of new laser-based analytical techniques. His group has been responsible for the detec- 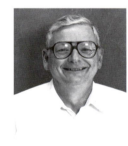 tion of small numbers of atomic species by resonance fluorescence, for the development of intracavity absorption spectroscopy, and for the development of optogalvanic spectroscopy. Current projects include resonance ionization mass spectrometry, laser-induced fluorescence of mass-selected ions, and detection of single molecules in fluid solution by an adaption of flow cytometry. Keller was made a Laboratory Fellow in 1983.

John C. Martin received his B.A. in physics from Drury College in 1965 and 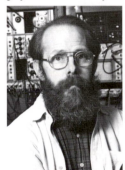 joined Los Alamos National Laboratory in 1966. He is a staff member in the Cell Growth, Damage, and Repair Group of the Life Sciences Division. His research interests include developing biological applications of fluorescence-detection instrumentation, performing chromosome and DNA analysis and sorting, measuring fluorescence decay, detecting single molecules, and developing rapid DNA-sequencing techniques and fluorescence DNA imaging. In addition to having been awarded numerous patents for his work, Martin received two RD-100 awards and the Los Alamos Patent of the Year Award in 1992 for inventing a method of rapid base sequencing of DNA and RNA. Martin has written extensively for various refereed scientific journals.

Robert K. Moyzis is director of the Center for Human Genome Studies at Los 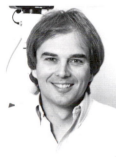 Alamos National Laboratory and is internationally known for his pioneering work on human genome organization. His discovery of the human telomere is a landmark in the history of our understanding of chromosome structure and function. Moyzis is the driving force behind the successful physical-mapping effort at Los Alamos and continues to balance his research and administrative responsibilities in the genome center. He serves on numerous committees that oversee the DOE and NIH Human Genome Project, including the DOE Human Genome Coordinating Committee and the joint NIH-DOE Human Genome Advisory Committee. Moyzis received his B.A. in biology and chemistry from Northeastern Illinois University in 1971 and his Ph.D. in molecular biology from Johns Hopkins University in 1978. Following postdoctoral and faculty appointments in the biophysics division at Johns Hopkins, he moved to Los Alamos National Laboratory in 1983. From 1984 to 1989 Moyzis was the leader of the Laboratory's Genetics Group, assuming his current position as center director in 1989.

E. Brooks Shera received his M.S. in physics from the University of Chicago in 1958 and his Ph.D. in nuclear physics from Case Western Reserve University in 1962. After a postdoctoral appointment at Argonne National Laboratory where he studied beta decay, Shera joined the Physics Division of Los Alamos National Laboratory in 1964. He carried out the first experiments that used slow neutrons to study the Mössbauer effect and pioneered the coincidence method to deduce nuclear energy levels from the gamma radiation that follows neutron capture. When intense beams of muons became available from the Laboratory's LAMPF accelerator, he led an international collaboration that made uniquely precise measurements of nuclear sizes and shapes by studying the spectra of x rays from muonic atoms.

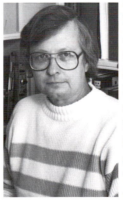 He was elected Fellow of the American Physical Society in 1982. Several years ago he became interested in the contributions that physics could make to molecular biology. This interest led to work on techniques for identifying proteins and eventually to development of methods for high-speed DNA sequencing. While not completely forsaking nuclear physics, his main interest is the application of imagination and "classical" and table-top physics to biological problems.

Raymond L. Stallings earned his M.S. from Texas A&M University in 1978 and 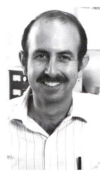 his Ph.D. from the University of Texas Graduate School of Biomedical Sciences in 1981. After appointments as a research associate at the University of Texas System Cancer Center and as a postdoctoral fellow at Los Alamos National Laboratory, he joined the faculty of the University of Texas, Houston, in 1985. Stalling's early research interests emphasized the mapping, dissection, and analysis of the Chinese hamster genome. He also taught courses in human and somatic-cell genetics at the University of Texas Health Science Center Graduate School of Biomedical Sciences, and in 1987 he became a special member of the faculty of that institution. Also in 1987 he joined the staff of the Life Sciences Division of Los Alamos National Laboratory. He is currently an Associate Professor of Human Genetics at the University of Pittsburgh. Stallings is a member of the American Association for the Advancement of Science and the American Society of Microbiology.

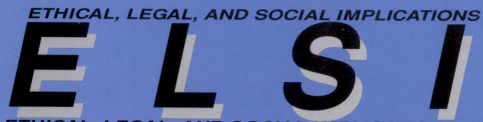

ETHICAL, LEGAL, AND SOCIAL IMPLICATIONS
E L S I
ETHICAL, LEGAL, AND SOCIAL IMPLICATIONS

Gerald Friedman and Richard Reichelt

ERIC JUENGST

NANCY WEXLER

*T*he Human Genome Project is providing a flood of scientifically valuable genetic information. That information promises advances in diagnosis, in prevention, and later in therapy. At the same time, the new knowledge also promises to intensify current health-care problems and bring up perplexing new ethical issues. History demonstrates that genetic information can be misused; in the United States, the most infamous examples were the compulsory-sterilization programs in the early part of the twentieth century. A current, less extreme example is the denial of insurance coverage to a family simply because one member has a genetic disorder—even when the disorder can be inexpensively treated.

Preparing for Changes

The National Institutes of Health (NIH) and the Department of Energy (DOE) have recognized the need to prepare for the social impacts of the Human Genome Project. They have created, as an integral part of the project, a program for studying its ethical, legal, and social implications (ELSI). In fiscal year 1992 $2 million from the DOE (3 percent of its genome budget) and $5 million from the NIH's National Center for Human Genome Research (5 percent of the center's budget) were set aside for the ELSI program.

The research funded by ELSI grants is intended to be useful for policymaking related to genetics. ELSI grants also fund education in the science and the social implications of the genome project. A joint NIH-DOE working group has been established to help pursue those goals and advise the sponsoring agencies. Members of the ELSI Working Group have offered advice to the Equal Employment Opportunity Commission (EEOC) and to Congress.

The ELSI program is a first for federally supported scientific research. Traditionally, researchers in the natural sciences concentrated on their investigations and allowed society to interpret and use the results as it chose. Now for the first time a research effort includes a structure in which "hard" scientists, social scientists, health-care workers, legal experts, and philosophers discuss the implications of present and potential scientific results.

The ELSI Working Group has identified four high-priority issues for study: fairness, privacy, delivery of health care, and education. In the context of genetics, fairness means freedom from discrimination on the basis of genotype. Privacy means an individual's control of the generation and disclosure of genetic information about himself or herself. Delivery concerns practices of the physicians, counselors, and laboratories that generate and provide genetic information. Education means helping policymakers, health-care professionals, biologists, and social scientists as well as the general public become aware of the new knowledge and of the problems and opportunities that it creates. In practice, many specific issues fall into more than one of those categories.

Nancy Wexler, president of the Hereditary Disease Foundation and a leading participant in the search for the Huntington's-disease gene, has chaired the ELSI Working Group since its inception. Recently she summarized the situation and the group's mission.

> I've heard people say—including people in Congress and even some scientists—that the public can be hurt by genetic information. It's true that in the past that information has been used against people. But genetic information itself is not going to hurt the public; what could hurt the public is existing social structures, policies, and prejudices against which information can ricochet. We need genetic information right now in order to make better choices so we can live better lives. We need the improved treatments that will eventually be developed using genetic information. So I think the answer is certainly not to slow down the advancing science, but to try, somehow, to make the social system more accommodating to the new knowledge.

Fairness and Discrimination

Employment or insurance coverage have reportedly been denied to people identified as having a genetic disorder or as being at risk for genetic disease. Sue Levi-Pearl, the scientific liaison for the Tourette Syndrome Association (TSA) and a member of the ELSI task force on insurance, recently described discriminatory practices that she has encountered.

I've had many opportunities to share the concerns, triumphs, and heartaches of those people with Tourette syndrome and other inherited disorders. While many affected families view recent and imminent scientific breakthroughs with hope, they also view the possibility of new genetic tests with despair. People with inherited disorders know firsthand the ways in which genetic-test results can be misused.

Tourette syndrome is an involuntary-movement disorder. The life spans of affected individuals, unlike the lifespans of people with cystic fibrosis or Tay-Sachs disease, are the same as those of the general population. The disorder has a wide range of expression—from mild tics that disappear in childhood to more severe motor and vocal tics that last a lifetime. Recent data suggest that the vast majority of those affected have mild cases that *never* require medical attention. Yet the typical profile of someone with a confirmed diagnosis is an employed, healthy person in his mid-twenties who takes an inexpensive generic medication—and still cannot obtain health insurance. The two-word explanation for denial of coverage is "Tourette syndrome," and that's it. I can testify that our organization, TSA, receives scores of such reports every day.

Do insurers understand the variable expression of Tourette syndrome? Absolutely not. People with poorly understood genetic conditions are often rendered uninsurable because an insurer *suspects* the possibility of significant medical expenses.

One recent case concerns a successful, self-employed architect who called TSA in desperation. After his child was diagnosed with a mild case of Tourette syndrome, the architect and his family lost their medical insurance. The insurance company had determined that the child's inherited, and therefore pre-existing, condition would inevitably lead to a brain tumor and require costly medical reimbursement. That medical misinformation was then entered into a large database consulted by the insurance industry, thereby guaranteeing the architect could not obtain insurance at any price. Gone are the days when only you and your physician "knew." Laws protecting the confidentiality of genetic information must be enacted now. These sorts of problems will be exacerbated in the future because our country's health-care system is already in crisis. If some program of national insurance is not federally mandated, we will soon face a national disaster in health care.

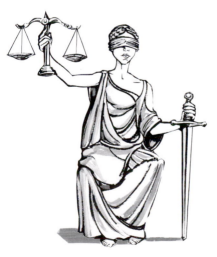

What choices remain for the uninsured families afflicted with genetic diseases? A representative from the National Organization for World

305

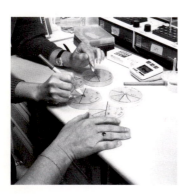

Diseases recently suggested two desperate options: (1) move to Canada, or (2) get a divorce, claim desertion, and become eligible for Medicaid.

The issues are equally complex and worrisome in the area of employment discrimination. Due to the unusual nature of the symptoms, many talented, qualified people with Tourette syndrome have a hard time obtaining employment. The recently confirmed genetic basis of the disease has only compounded the problem. Even a job candidate with mild symptoms could possibly have children with Tourette syndrome and eventually cause high medical expenses for an employer. The employer may say, "Why bother? This person is carrying the wrong genes."

Fairness issues also arise because of differences in culture and societal power between ethnic groups. Recently Troy Duster, director of the Institute for the Study of Social Change at the University of California at Berkeley, talked about some of his concerns at an ELSI Working Group meeting.

I've been asked to comment on the topic of genetics and racial discrimination. Let me begin with a caricature: On one side are Human Genome Project scientists, busily uncovering and disclosing genetic markers and sequencing the genome; on the other side is a society, which is completely homogeneous with respect to ethnicity, race, and class, neutrally receiving the information. I paint this picture because it seems implicit in the funding allocations of the Human Genome Project—97 percent to the uncovering, mapping, and sequencing of the genes and 3 percent to the ethical, legal, and social implications. Thus the assumption behind the project is that scientific discovery is 97 percent of the problem while dissemination and consumption is only a very small issue. But since every society is complex and stratified, the rosy picture of people receiving and responding to genetic information without regard to their strong social differences is untenable.

Indeed, we know from social research over the last two decades how important these social differences can be in populations at greatest risk for a genetic disorder. Certain ethnic groups have seized ownership of information about a genetic disease, controlling the information flow and screening process. Other groups have either rejected the information outright, or received an incomplete, fragmented picture of the disease. For example, screening for Tay-Sachs disease in the United States was controlled and influenced by people of Ashkenazic Jewish descent. The result was an effective, voluntary screening program. At the other extreme were the sickle-cell anemia tests that occurred in Greece in the 1970s: there was no shared notion of sickle-cell anemia being a societal problem; rather, the disease was perceived as the problem of a few individuals and family members. Differing from those two examples was the testing for sickle-cell anemia in America, which was politicized as the disease of blacks. In this case, African-Americans did not control the mandatory screening programs that were put into place. Test results were then used as pretexts for discriminatory employment policies. As with the screening programs in Greece, the genetic information ended up being rejected, but for different reasons.

Ethnic perceptions of medical information are crucial. In the early 1960s Irving Zola studied the way different groups describe their disease symptoms to physicians. Some ethnic groups tend to be stoical, almost nonverbal; other ethnic groups tend to express themselves forcefully, even exaggeratedly. In another study the anthropologist Debra Woo examined the ways different groups react to mental-health problems. She observed the Chinese have low rates of contact with the mental-health system, not because they have few mental-health problems, but because of a cultural concept called *pao tin*—taking care of one's own—that makes people less likely to seek help from outside establishments.

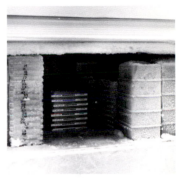

Thus, we see different groups responding to health problems in starkly different ways. It is clear genetic information shouldn't simply be dropped into the social realm without a delicate understanding of these dynamics. To do so—especially if the affected group is at the bottom of the social order, with few resources for understanding the information and its implications—is irresponsible.

Few states have laws governing the use of genetic information by employers and insurers. The most important Federal law that implicitly forbids some kinds of genetic discrimination is the Americans with Disabilities Act (ADA) of 1990. That act provides employment protections for people who have disabilities but are nevertheless qualified to do a job. Specifically, the ADA prohibits employers from discriminatory practices in hiring, firing, and promoting people who are disabled for any reason, including genetic illness; people who have a history of illness that does not affect their present ability to work; and people who are perceived as if they were disabled—for example, a severely burned person who is shunned in the workplace. The ADA took effect in July 1992 for all companies with twenty-five or more employees, and will take effect in July 1994 for all companies with fifteen or more employees.

Although the ADA clearly protects people disabled by an expressed genetic disorder, it may not cover a carrier of a genetic disorder. A carrier of an autosomal (not sex-linked) disorder, such as sickle-cell anemia or cystic fibrosis, has one defective gene and one normal gene; such a person does not have the disease caused by the defective gene. If two such carriers have children, on average one-fourth of their children will inherit a defective gene from each parent and therefore have the disease. From an employer's point of view, hiring a carrier means risking higher medical-benefits costs because the carrier has a chance of having children who will need expensive medical treatment. Although the risk is small, an employer might refuse to hire such a person even though he or she is capable of doing the job. There is no evidence that employers are not hiring carriers, but the economic incentives to do so will increase as genetic screening becomes more widespread and less expensive.

Other areas not addressed by the ADA are discrimination against people with late-onset genetic disorders such as Huntington's disease and adult polycystic kidney disease, and against people whose genotypes indicate increased risk of later illnesses. The EEOC has not yet provided regulatory guidance on the applicability of the ADA to people with genes for late-onset disorders. It has stated that additional legislation may be necessary to extend the act to cover genetic predispositions. In 1991, members of the ELSI Working Group sent a recommendation to the EEOC and testified before Congress on the need to strengthen legal protection against workplace discrimination based on a person's genotype.

In addition to its activities in the employment area, the ELSI Working Group has created an Insurance Task Force to explore potential uses of genetics by the insurance industry and possible means of protecting against unfair discrimination. The task force is chaired by two members of the working group and includes representatives of the insurance industry, corporate benefit plans, academia, and voluntary health organizations.

A commonly expressed fear is that insurers will require genetic tests or will obtain test results. Then they could either deny coverage or charge high premiums to those with genetic diseases or propensities to disease. Insurance carriers have the opposite worry: "adverse selection" by insurance applicants based on information about themselves that is not shared with insurers. For example, a person may receive a battery of genetic tests, discover that he or she has a gene that causes a late-onset disease, and then buy increased health insurance on anticipation of greater health-care costs. Another person may discover that his or her risks are comparatively low and buy less health insurance. Such practices could increase the demand for reimbursement of health-care expenses while reducing insurers' ability to spread the cost across the population. Both problems will get worse as the effects of more genes are discovered. Insurers insist that they should have all the information known to the policyholder. Such an arrangement might discourage people from having themselves tested, since policy-holders may want to avoid knowing about risks that they would be forced to disclose. Eventually, the ELSI Insurance Task Force hopes to recommend health-insurance reforms that balance the interests of insurance companies and consumers.

Privacy

Many people believe that their medical records, including genetic data, should be between them and their physicians. However, medical data are often obtained by third parties—employers, insurers, even the Medical Information Bureau, an information resource for the entire insurance industry. Likewise many people assume that personal data about them will not be generated without their consent. However, with genetic testing that assumption is not always correct—for instance, information about a person's genes can be deduced from information about his or her relatives, sometimes with great certainty. Thus there are many unresolved issues relating to the generation and disclosure of genetic information.

Some privacy questions raised by genetic testing arise from many people's desire not to know genetic information about themselves, especially when tests are subject to error and therapies are not available. For example, when people at risk for Huntington's disease were informed of a free predictive test, only about 10 percent took advantage of the opportunity to take the test. The desire not to know can lead to privacy conflicts in families. For instance, as Huntington's disease usually has a late onset, a young adult might want to be tested although his or her at-risk parent does not have symptoms and does not want to know. If the person tested has the disease gene, the parent must have it as well, so the child's test could provide the parent with unwanted information. Another conflict occurs when parents want their child tested, since the child might later prefer not to know the result. At present, testing

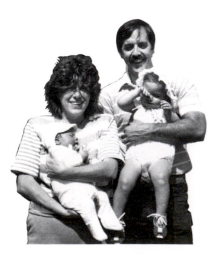

centers only test adults who can provide informed consent, feeling that parents should not know the genetic status of their minor children without the children's informed consent.

Under the aegis of the ELSI Working Group, a Genetic Privacy Collaboration of ELSI grantees and contractors is analyzing privacy issues from several perspectives. In addition, the DOE's ELSI program will concentrate its research funds on studies of privacy issues. One area to be covered is the development of guidelines for genetic databanks. Some state forensic laboratories store genetic "fingerprints" from convicted felons by which they may be identified later (for instance from genetic fingerprints determined from blood or semen found at a crime scene). The Defense Department has announced that it will maintain a bank of tissue samples from every member of the armed forces for use in identifying the remains of people killed in combat. Scientific laboratories maintain pedigree data on research subjects. At present there are no general standards for the protection of information in those databanks.

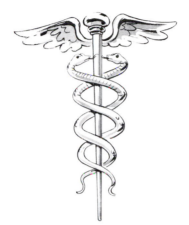

Another research topic is distinguishing genetic information that should be kept confidential or even not generated except at the request of the person involved from genetic information that must be disclosed for valid public-health reasons. The conflicts between privacy and public health related to genetics have some resemblances to the conflicts related to AIDS.

The Genetic Privacy Collaboration will also determine attitudes and expectations of the public and of various subgroups regarding the privacy of genetic information. Investigators will analyze the social-science literature, study public opinion by surveys and other methods, and compare genetic-screening programs in different states and involving different ethnic groups.

ELSI-supported research will also include legal and philosophical studies of the right to privacy in the context of genetic information. The studies will be of use to the states that are currently considering laws to protect genetic data and to Congress if it takes up such legislation. Foreign approaches to safeguarding genetic privacy will be analyzed as well. The European Community and several individual European countries have adopted measures that may serve as models for action in the United States.

Our society is only now beginning to address the topic of genetic privacy. As the ELSI privacy task force and other national privacy study groups analyze and discuss these issues, the limits of genetic privacy and possible ways to protect it should become clearer.

Currently, our society faces a challenge in bringing genetic knowledge into the medical mainstream so that the greatest number of people will reap the benefits. A common decision based on genetic information is whether to abort an embryo that has a genotype associated with a disease. A pregnant woman facing that decision and thus confronting the moral and personal issues of abortion may need accurate information—for instance, the error rate of the test. The symptoms of some genetic diseases, such as fragile-X syndrome, range from severe to practically

Delivery of Genetic Services

unnoticeable. Therapies are available for some diseases; for others therapies seem imminent. Genetic knowledge will be of such magnitude and such medical import that professional genetic counselors—people trained in special master's-degree or clinical-nursing programs—wonder if they will be able to meet the demand for information. Dianne Bartels, the administrative director of the Center for Biomedical Ethics at the University of Minnesota, outlined some of the concerns raised at an NIH/ELSI conference on genetic counseling in the United States.

Counselor education will become more challenging as information flows in from the Human Genome Project. The massive amounts of information may be beyond the capacities of a single person to assimilate, creating the need for various subspecialties. How will genetic counselors be taught in the future? Who will teach them? Are the current two-year master's-degree programs adequate? These are just a few of the questions that are being raised about counselor education.

There are also urgent questions about how much information a counselor should impart to a client. Genetic counselors believe it is in the client's interest to have *all* of the available facts. This leads to a kind of Joe Fridayism—just the facts, Ma'am—that is potentially devastating for the client. Someone may discover, for example, that his father is not really his father during a routine screen for Huntington's disease. Clearly, there are limits to the factual model for counseling.

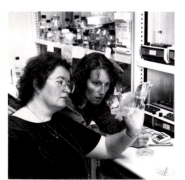

Another issue that stretches this model is finding the XYY karyotype, an abnormal chromosome combination that was once considered to be positively linked to violent, criminal behavior in adult males. The basis for the now-discredited link was a series of studies on a highly select population of XYY males—namely those imprisoned for various crimes. As far as I know, no studies of XYY among the general population have convincingly linked it to violent behavior. But some genetic counselors are telling clients, "It may not be good science, but XYY has been linked to criminal or sociopathic behavior. Genetics textbooks say that XYY males are tall, have acne, and may have learning disabilities. Most people with XYY have no symptoms." How is a client supposed to make a reproductive decision given that information? I would challenge geneticists and genetic counselors to address what is *relevant* genetic information for clients.

The current standard for the profession is to present information in a "non-directive, value-neutral way" and in a manner that "preserves client autonomy." Essentially this means the counselor shouldn't project his or her values onto the patient. But does this standard work in a practical sense? A patient with a high cholesterol level isn't told by his doctor, "Your cholesterol is 350. It could kill you, so gather some information on cholesterol and make whatever decision you want." The doctor's advice will be much more directive; it is likely to include recommendations about treatments or lifestyle changes that can ameliorate the illness. Those in the genetic counseling profession, however, still cling to the "nondirective counselor and autonomous patient" model—I believe this model is increasingly untenable.

We are swiftly reaching the ethical limits of client autonomy. Some clinics and laboratories refuse to give out information about the gender of unborn children. Nevertheless, a recent study shows that 60 percent of genetic counselors will either do, or refer, screening for sex selection. Some clients are saying, "People get abortions for no reason at all—why can't I have an abortion because I want a girl?" Many clinics and genetic counselors respond that gender is not a medical problem to be addressed by genetic testing. Decisions need to be made on who formulates policy: individual labs and clinics, legislatures, or the clients themselves.

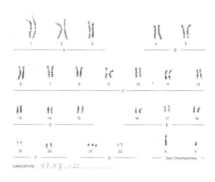

We need to conduct more research on what genetic counselors are taught and how they actually respond in clinical situations. Pilot programs on counseling norms—with their societal and ethical implications—could yield important insights as to how counselors ought to be educated. Also, we need to address the information-surfeit problem and what the counselor's role will be in the future. Will counselors specialize to address specific diseases? Will they continue to work in academic centers, in private practices, or in primary practice offices?

Demand for counselors may increase as more tests for genetic diseases are found in the course of the Human Genome Project. At present there are only about 1500 trained genetic counselors in the United States. A multitude of known genetic disorders may require the training of many more professionals who can interpret tests, answer questions, provide counseling, and direct people to treatment services.

To address ways of effectively delivering genetic information to the public, the DOE and NIH are funding a National Academy of Sciences/National Institute of Medicine study on "Assessing Genetic Risks." A second major initiative is a pilot project on cystic-fibrosis testing. Cystic fibrosis is a potentially severe disorder that, until recently, usually resulted in death in early adulthood. About 1 in 2500 North American white children has the disease, implying that about 1 in 25 people in that group carries a defective gene. Although the gene has been isolated and a test has been developed, testing for carriers on a large scale would bring up difficulties. One problem arises from the existence of many disease-causing mutations of the gene, each of which must be tested for individually. Current tests detect only certain mutations that together account for 85 to 90 percent of the total number of cystic-fibrosis carriers. Thus a negative result does not guarantee that the person tested does not carry a defective gene. Also, the frequencies of the disease and of the various mutations differ according to ethnic group. Furthermore, although any doctor could send a blood sample to a laboratory and receive a result, some might be unable to effectively explain that result to patients or to prevent potential psychological trauma. Faced with so many uncertainties, physicians are not routinely testing for cystic fibrosis. Instead, the National Center for Human Genome Research, the National Institute of Child Health and Human Development, and the National Center for Nursing Research are jointly supporting pilot programs to determine whether, under what circumstances, and how such tests should be administered.

Eric Juengst, director of the NIH ELSI program, stated in a press release of October 1991,

Whether clinical testing for cystic fibrosis carrier status should become more routine is still very much an open question. . . . The underlying goal of these studies is to help determine whether testing services should remain focused on members of families already at risk, or whether it is feasible to offer the test more widely in an ethically acceptable manner.

The cystic-fibrosis pilot project aims at supplying health-care professionals with much-needed information about how to maximize a patient's understanding of the test results and to protect privacy. Seven research teams are conducting three-year studies intended to define the best methods for educating and counseling individuals who want to be tested for cystic fibrosis. Several of the studies will survey attitudes toward and understanding of testing among physicians and various populations in the lay public. Others will try out and evaluate strategies for pre-test education and post-test counseling. Such research is a first step toward building a flexible health infrastructure able to take advantage of genetic breakthroughs in the future and to respond to the needs of patients and members of their families who have concerns about genetic information.

Education

The public needs information on both the social issues and the underlying science of the genome project in order to decide the questions that are arising. Providing information to people whose work requires an understanding of genetics is even more important. Many instances of the problems described earlier—unfair insurance practices, discriminatory hiring policies, and inadequate delivery of genetic information—are driven by ignorance. For example, advances in genetics are showing that certain former diagnoses actually labeled two or more diseases. Thus a physician trained in the old school to diagnose neurofibromatosis by certain symptoms, for example, may not realize that what was once considered a single disease is two diseases, each with its own genetic signature, its own symptoms (slightly different from the other's), and its own treatment. Therefore the ELSI program is supporting projects that study ways of bringing information to medical professionals as well as to life-science and social-science researchers and to government officials.

Another aspect of education is the training of scholars studying issues arising from the genome project. Accordingly, the ELSI program includes postdoctoral fellowships for research-oriented training. The fellowships are open to biomedical scientists working on such topics as sociology, ethics, and law and to doctors in the humanities working on science relevant to the genome project. Also, to support research on ELSI topics, the DOE maintains at Los Alamos National Laboratory a library of relevant books and articles and a database indexing the library. Database services—for example, listings of publications selected according to author, key words, and source, or sorted chronologically—are available on request. A bibliography of those materials, containing more than 2600 entries, was published by the DOE in May 1992, and is also available.[*]

---

[*] Requests for the bibliography or for database searches should be sent to Michael R. Roth or Michael S. Yesley, MS A187, Los Alamos National Laboratory, Los Alamos, NM 87545. Telephone: (505) 667-3766. Fax: (505) 665-4424. Electronic mail: ROTH_MICHAEL_R@OFVAX.LANL.GOV or YESLEY_MICHAEL_S@OFVAX.LANL.GOV.

Finally, the ELSI program is intended to help the public understand the issues that have been outlined in this article. Therefore the program has commissioned surveys of public knowledge and attitudes. It has also initiated several public-education efforts. For example, the Colorado Biological Sciences Curriculum Study has prepared a genetics module that can be included in a typical high-school biology course. The module is five to six days long and includes exercises in both hands-on science and ethical analysis. All fifty-five thousand high-school science teachers in the United States will be given the opportunity to include this module in their biology classes. Since many students take biology as their high-school science requirement, the module should be highly effective in getting genetics and related ethical issues into the mainstream. In addition, the ELSI program provided a grant to the New York television station WNET to prepare a television documentary called "The Future of Medicine." The ten-part series dramatizes the impact of genetics on medicine.

Leaders of the ELSI project regard education as a field of paramount importance. Nancy Wexler has discussed both immediate concerns in the education of health-care workers, and the long-term goal of public education and public involvement in decision-making.

> Genetics just has not been well taught in many universities. It has been chopped up into pieces and added to lots of different disciplines as an after-thought. We need to think more creatively about improving the curriculum as a whole. We also need to think about helping helping people already working in health care who want more genetic education. I think it's un-likely that every single doctor is going to go out and buy a genetics book. I must say that having patients who ask questions is definitely the best mo-tivation to learn, because doctors want to be able to answer their patients responsibly and intelligently. Nobody wants to have to say, "I haven't a clue, and furthermore I don't feel like finding out." A public that develops a hunger for answers will goad all of us in medical research and practice to try to do a better job.

> If you compare society's handling of genetic knowledge to making a movie, then what we in ELSI can do is help write the script. If the movie is going to be made, the public must act as the producers. They have to help raise the money and hire the cast and get it going. If you don't have a script then you don't have a movie—but if you don't have a producer your movie will never be made. The public must be partners every step of the way. ■

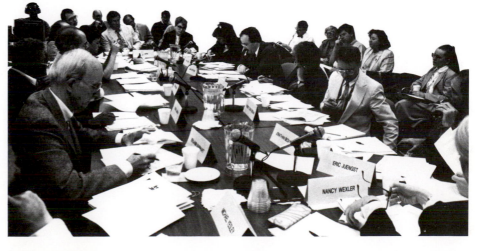

The authors thank Michael Yesley and Nancy Wexler for valuable dis-cussions.

An invitation to genetics in the 21st Century

At the moment of conception, the genetic blueprint of a new life comes into being. It is an intricate message differing in slight but crucial ways from one human being to another. So far molecular biologists have decoded only a tiny fraction of this set of instructions; we live for the most part in ignorance of how our genetic inheritance will influence the course of our lives. The goal of the Human Genome Project, a fifteen-year, international research effort, is to read the entire contents of that message and to provide the tools for deciphering the genetic differences among us. Are we ready as individuals and as parents for the emergence of this new knowledge? Are we ready as a society? As a species?

At the invitation of Leon Botstein, president of Bard College, and with the sponsorship of Los Alamos National Laboratory, some of the leading participants in the Genome Project gathered at Leon's home on December 5, 1990, to answer questions about the goals and ethical implications of the project. *Los Alamos Science* offers this presentation not because the questions were all-inclusive or the answers definitive but because the issues raised, both philosophical and practical, will become more pressing as information from the Genome Project accumulates. We hope to stimulate discussion among you, your family, and your friends as we prepare to consider and act upon the resulting information with wisdom, compassion, hope, and openness.

Leon Botstein: Ladies and gentlemen, let me welcome you. The topic this evening is the Human Genome Project, and my role is to explain the format of the discussion and to introduce the panel. This is an unusual opportunity to participate in a discussion about an important issue with the people who *ought* to know what it's all about. First, David Botstein will give a somewhat brief introduction to the Project, in which he will state its goals, its history, and why he thinks it's necessary. Then, each of the panel members will be given the opportunity to make an opening statement. After that, the floor will be open to questions from the audience. I'm certain that this is not a particularly reticent panel, so there's no need for me to moderate—but rather, perhaps, to adjudicate.

Now I will introduce the panelists. David Baltimore is President of Rockefeller University. He, along with Howard Temin and Renato Dulbecco, won the Nobel Prize for the discovery of reverse transcriptase. I can't refrain from mentioning that he is a graduate of Swarthmore College, a small liberal arts college like Bard College. Next, my brother, David Botstein, Chairman of the Genetics Department at Stanford and a long-time member of the faculty at MIT. He invented the use of DNA markers and is one of the initiators of the Human Genome Project. Next is James Dewey Watson, who, together with Francis Crick and Maurice Wilkinson, won the Nobel Prize for discovering the structure of DNA. Dr. Watson is Director of the Human Genome Initiative of the National Institutes of Health and also the author of a classic book on the character of scientific discovery—*The Double Helix*. Also here tonight is Robert Moyzis, Director of the Center for Human Genome Studies at Los Alamos National Laboratory and the discoverer of the human telomere, a

special DNA sequence that makes up the end of every human chromosome. Finally, Nancy Wexler, President of the Hereditary Disease Foundation and an Associate Professor at the Department of Neurology and Psychology at Columbia Presbyterian Medical College. Nancy is Chairman of the Department of Energy–National Institutes of Health joint working group on the ethical, legal, and social issues of the Human Genome Project, the group known as ELSI. I think there could not be a more distinguished and appropriate panel for this discussion.

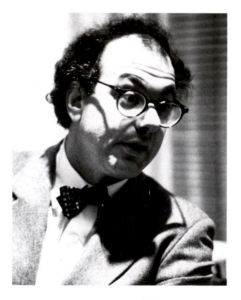

There are many questions which were put forth by a variety of people interested in the Human Genome Project. What are the goals of the Project? What has been achieved and what might be achieved in twenty years? What are the main scientific arguments against the Project, what are the scientific arguments for the Project, and how important is it compared with other scientific projects? What are the obstacles to its success? How do scientists share the results of this project? How likely is it that the technology coming from this project will be available to physicians, hospitals, and

clinics? What positive effects might come from the resulting technology? Will there be a revolution in health care? What could prevent us from taking full advantage of such benefits? What are the social effects? Why might it lead to greater social inequality, or conversely, to greater homogeneity? Is there a valid concern with respect to eugenics? Can we influence the human gene pool? Will this project affect our view of ourselves? What myths will be challenged by this research? What theological questions might be invoked by this work? Is there some issue of responsibility which might lead us not to pursue this project? Does the individual own the rights to his or her own genome? What are the legal implications? Finally, do people really want to know about their genetic inheritance? These questions are probably more than enough to generate considerable controversy. I turn the floor over to you, David.

David Botstein: One of the challenges we have not yet fully met is explaining to people who are not directly involved in the Human Genome Project what we are doing and why we are doing it. As a result, a considerable amount of misunderstanding has arisen. My purpose in this introduction is not to give you a hyper-rapid education in biology, but instead to introduce a few of the basic terms and to present the fundamental ideas around which this project is based.

First, and I'm sure most of you know this, our genes are made of DNA. It has been clear for about fifty years that, to the first approximation, all of a person's inherited characteristics are specified by the DNA of the fertilized egg. Therefore, to *understand* the entire message encoded in a person's DNA is to know everything about his or her inheritance. I did not say *transcribe* or *put on optical disk*. I said *understand*,

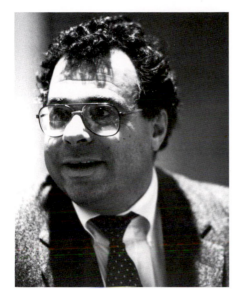

and a complete understanding of the message is a long way off. The big deal about a person's DNA—aside from the fact that it encodes all the information for making the person—is that it contains an extremely large number of paired nucleotide bases—six billion. Simply determining the base sequence of all that DNA is a big technical problem. In fact, determining the base sequence of *any* segment of DNA is one of the triumphs of modern biology.

For about ten years people have been able to sequence a little bit of DNA here, and a little bit there. That is, they've been able to determine the sequence of nucleotide bases for a relatively small number of genes. We know that the sequences of most genes specify proteins and that the proteins do the work in the cell. In general, however, we don't know how a particular gene and the particular protein it encodes determine a visible or measurable inherited characteristic. In this soup of six billion base pairs, the average gene, the average coding sequence for a protein, is only one thousand base pairs long, and we estimate that the human genome contains between 50,000 and 100,000 genes. So

we have a very complicated technical task, first in trying to find all those genes and then in trying to understand what they do. In the last ten years it has become clear that we have the technical means to at least begin to write down the sequence of all the base pairs in the human genome. The question is: Why do it? Much of the opposition to the Human Genome Project is based on the fact that just knowing the sequence of base pairs doesn't mean anything in itself. The genetic code lets you turn the base sequence of a gene into the amino-acid sequence of a protein, but even that doesn't mean anything by current technology. It's as if you had a row of hieroglyphics and a way of transcribing them into Urdu—but you don't understand or speak Urdu. That's pretty much the situation we're in.

The next question is: How can we give meaning to the proteins that are derived from the genes? Sometimes there is a way because we've been collecting information about genes and proteins for a long time. We know globin. It's a protein that has been studied for fifty years; it carries oxygen in the blood. We know insulin, a protein that regulates the sugar in the blood. We know the sequences of the genes for these proteins. The functions of these proteins have been studied in lower organisms, such as bacteria, yeast, and mice, and a huge amount of research and manipulation has been done on these organisms. So when people found the human cystic-fibrosis gene and looked at its sequence, they said, "Aha!" because the sequence looked like the sequence of a gene that had been studied in a number of other organisms. It's called the multidrug-resistance gene, and there is a substantial literature—several hundred papers—surrounding it. When people found the neurofibromatosis gene, they again said, "Aha!" because its sequence is related to a well-known oncogene, or

cancer-causing gene, and much of the biochemistry of the oncogene has been worked out in great detail. In fact, the relationship between the two genes gave a logical explanation as to what might cause neurofibromatosis tumors. So to make the discovery of genes meaningful as well as easy, we need to know the sequences of genes in experimental organisms. Yeast, for example, has genes that are very similar to those of higher organisms. However, even though the yeast genome is 250 times smaller than our own, the yeast genome has been only partially sequenced.

> *We have the technical means to at least begin to write down the sequence of all the base pairs in the human genome. The question is: Why do it?*

The first proponents of the Human Genome Project proposed simply to go ahead and sequence the entire human genome with the current technology. Many people, including me, were appalled by this proposal because—it was stupid. A framework with which to interpret all those sequence data did not exist, and the technology then current was so slow that the job would have taken somewhere between thirty thousand and sixty thousand man-years. The Project would have wiped out biology in the same way that the space shuttle wiped out planetary astronomy. In response to this proposal, the National Research Council formed a committee that included opponents and proponents, and we drafted a set of three propositions. The first was that we begin *not* by blindly sequencing the human genome but instead by making physical maps of it, maps similar to but on a larger scale than those that helped us find the cystic-fibrosis and neurofibromatosis genes so quickly. Included in the first proposition were proposals to improve sequencing technology so as to make it faster as well as to apply current sequencing techniques to model organisms so that we might again say "Aha!" as the human genome is being sequenced. It was also suggested that we make more detailed genetic-linkage, or co-inheritance, maps. Second, we proposed some kind of oversight by scientists of this new endeavor so that it would be neither entirely undirected research nor your Stalinist we-tell-you-what-to-do research. It's somewhere in between. It's both application-oriented and goal-oriented, but individual creativity is still applicable. And third, we proposed that a fairly substantial portion of the money be spent studying the ethical, legal, and social implications of the Project as a means of preventing us from outrunning our own thoughts and, more to the point, from outrunning those of society regarding the use of this information in ways that will benefit humankind.

Nancy Wexler: I have heard many people ask, "Can we really afford to do this project—not only in terms of the expense in time, energy, and money but also in terms of the costs for us as a society? Can we afford the ramifications of having this genetic information made available to the individual, to our insurance companies, to our employers?"

The genotype of each person here contains genetic messages indicating that at some point you are likely to develop cancer or that you are prone to heart disease, diabetes, or some other disorder. No doubt several of you have children with genetic disorders. Many of us know people with schizophrenia, or leukemia, or Alzheimer's disease, all

of which have a genetic component. If, however, just as we might visit a fortune teller to have our palms read, we could

If . . . just as we might visit a fortune teller to have our palms read, we could go out and have our DNA read . . . would we really want to know our genetic futures . . . ?

go out and have our DNA read and predictions made accordingly, would we really want to know our genetic futures and the genetic futures of our offspring? Would we want to run the risk of having others know? If the health-insurance industry could predict our futures from the results of genetic testing, would we be able to get adequate insurance policies? Could we be turned down for coverage entirely? Or, if we applied for a new job, could the employer evaluate and eliminate our applications on the basis of genetic information, saying, "No, I'm sorry. You are predisposed to developing certain kinds of cancer, and we can't afford to hire you because you are too likely to increase our insurance costs." Worries such as these are not unfounded. It is a simple fact that discrimination is often economically driven, and people are concerned about what will happen to their lives when genetic information becomes available.

On the other hand, those of us who have been working in the field of genetic disease for a long time and who are engrossed in efforts toward finding treatments and cures, feel strongly that the question is not whether we can afford to do this project but rather

whether we can afford *not* to do this project. Genetic diseases are like deadly assassins. If you are in a family at risk, you know the assassins are there, but you have no way of finding them and no way of hiding from them. The Genome Project will provide ways of finding those assassins and methods for pinning them down. It will find the lethal genetic killers as well as the genes for life–crippling disorders such as obesity and alcoholism. We'll be learning about the genes that are unique to humans and the many, many genes that we share with other species. This information will expand our understanding of our genetic heritage and enable us to have greater control over our individual lives and, eventually, better diagnoses and treatments for our genetic disorders.

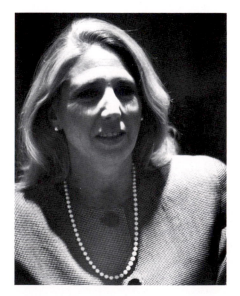

There is, of course, the potential for serious misuse of genetic information both in the manner in which it is delivered to the individual and the way in which it is received by society. So, as we proceed with the Genome Project, we want to anticipate potential problems and concerns. Therefore, the DOE and NIH formed a joint working group on the ethical, legal, and social implications of the Project. This group, informally known as ELSI, is working to develop programs and legislation to ensure that genetic information is used wisely and to the advantage—not the detriment—of the individual and society as a whole. Unfortunately, many of the concerns and issues that ELSI hopes to anticipate and address are already with us. The present situation with respect to health insurance is very disturbing. Thirty-seven million people don't have any health insurance, and fifty million are underinsured. So we need to consider *now* what will happen when the Genome Project makes possible the diagnosis of more and more genetic disorders. The high visibility of the Genome Project is, in effect, throwing a spotlight on existing problems of discrimination and social stigmatism. People are beginning to realize that almost all of us are at risk in some fashion or another, and that knowledge can give us a new impetus toward solving these problems.

Bob Moyzis: It's always a pleasure to be invited to talk about this project, one that I feel is arguably the most exciting in the history of science. We're talking about nothing less than unraveling the complete package of genetic information present in each one of your cells. In addition to accelerating the pace of identifying the genes responsible for known genetic diseases, the new information will help us to identify the genes involved in disorders like heart disease and cancer. The genetic components of these complex yet common disorders are largely indecipherable with current technology. The Human Genome Project will change that. It will form the basis for identifying many of the genes that cause the diseases that afflict mankind. As well as addressing these worthwhile pragmatic goals, this project will provide the intellectual framework for the next century of

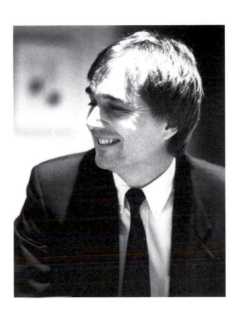

biological understanding. We may finally understand processes as diverse as the development of a human embryo from a single fertilized egg and the

Given the benefits that are going to come out of this project, not in two hundred years but probably in our lifetimes, . . . it's essentially unethical not to pursue it.

mechanisms underlying complex human behaviors. To paraphrase what our next speaker, Jim Watson, has been quoted as saying, given the benefits that are going to come out of this project, not in two hundred years but probably in our lifetimes, I feel it's essentially unethical not to pursue it.

Jim Watson: I will explain my role in leading the NIH component of the Human Genome Project. After we

recommended that the Project should go ahead and proposed a sum of money that would allow the work to be completed in a reasonable amount of time, my first

Who would want to have the rest of his life predicted if it can't be changed?

task was to assure Congress that the scientific community wanted the Project, believed it would work, and felt confident that it wouldn't be another Hubble telescope—that it was a project whose success was insured if we could get the money. The second task was to spend the money wisely. So I drafted a group of first-class scientists as advisors to the Project. I am the nominal head of the NIH component, but the real leadership comes from the advisors, who meet in formal session twice a year. We have also put together a staff of administrators within the National Institutes of Health who are really very good. People thought our project would be fun to administer. The third task, and the most important, was to persuade a group of younger people to actually *work* on the Project. We needed very bright people to put these maps together. One initial complaint was that this project's lab work was for people you wouldn't want to go to dinner with because they would have to be dull. On the contrary, the Project appeals to bright people because, if they skillfully choose their region of the genome, they may get to work on an interesting disease gene. The people working on the Project are as good as any other group working in molecular biology today. We're giving out a number of ordinary grants, but we've decided that a few people need to get a lot of money if the Project is going

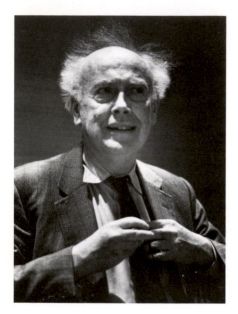

to be done effectively. The Project is almost in good shape from a funding standpoint. We didn't get all the money that was initially proposed, but I think we've got enough money to fund most of the good people. We've assembled a group of highly imaginative people who are committed to the Project, and I'm actually feeling relaxed about it. The initial objections about the Project being *big* science and *unnecessary* science have been overcome. The next problem we are going to face is that of having developed predictive capabilities without having developed the cures. Who would want to have the rest of his life predicted if it can't be changed? As we find out how to predict diseases, we also have to find out how to do something about treating and curing them. That's the way to make the Project worthwhile in the best sense.

David Baltimore: I have the reputation of being a critic of the Genome Project, a role I'm not particularly comfortable with because most of what's going on is, to my mind, very appropriate and very exciting. But I can comment on it from

a somewhat larger point of view because I'm neither a member of the Project nor a part of an advisory group nor a recipient of any grants. The Human Genome Project is now a great concern for all of modern biology because the maps being made will help find *all* genes, not only those that cause disease, but those that do all the normal things. To a large extent, we are what we are because of our genes. In order to discover all the genetic blueprints that determine what we are and to understand how we came to be what we are, we need the Human Genome Project. But this project as it stands today is a very small piece of modern biology. The Genome Project is being funded at $100 million a year, whereas *$8 billion* a year of NIH money is spent on health research. Molecular genetics, modern genetics, molecular biology—all of these words subsume an incredible ability, evolved over the last fifteen years, to gain an understanding of the workings of all of the systems of the body. The Genome Project will help to bring together disparate attempts in laboratories around the world to find out

> ## We have lived with a myth about ourselves for a very long time, and that myth is that we are all equal, all the same.

how kidneys work, how livers work, how a fertilized egg develops into a human being—or into a tree sloth. I support the Human Genome Project in its *human* focus because there are a whole range of things that are particularly human, and we have to study them within our own DNA if we are ever going to understand our learning

processes, our behavioral processes, and ultimately our ability or inability to work together to form a society. In a broad sense the Human Genome Project represents an attempt to do all of these things.

There are, inevitably, ethical problems arising out of the works of modern biology, but they don't necessarily relate to the Genome Project alone. We are

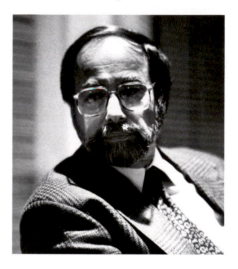

delving into ourselves. We have lived with a myth about ourselves for a very long time, and that myth is that we are all equal, all the same. It's a myth with very potent political and social implications and a myth we ought to believe as long as we have nothing else to believe in. The Genome Project is going to teach us that we are not all the same, that we are all different in ways we could never have understood before. We are going to have to come to terms with the fact that we are all born with different talents and tendencies. It is my belief that knowledge brings freedom and that knowledge of ourselves will bring us freedom from potential disease, from the potential inability to learn, and from the potential inability to cope with certain aspects of modern society. We need to know not just what it is that makes us human beings, but what makes us *particular*, *individual* human beings, and the Genome Project is a piece of the development of that understanding, a piece we need to support. When we contemplate the ethical challenges that lie ahead, we need to examine not only the Human Genome Project, which is a paper tiger in many ways, but also the overall capabilities of modern biology. I ask you to consider whether you agree with me that this kind of knowledge represents freedom.

Questions & Answers

Question: From a layman's point of view, one of the most interesting things about this massive science project, perhaps unlike others in the past, is that it is taking on from the very beginning the questions of its own implications for human beings. How are you going to examine the legal, ethical, and social aspects of this project?

Nancy Wexler: Jim Watson is responsible for initiating the formal structure within the Human Genome Project to anticipate and address those issues. The development of such a program made some people nervous. They said, "Well, the ethical issues will take care of themselves as we go along." But Jim thought those issues should be explored and addressed as an integral part of the Genome Project. So he went ahead and created a working group that is now jointly sponsored by the Department of Energy and the National Institutes of Health. Both organizations have designated a portion of their total budgets for the Genome Project for the examination of the ethical, legal, and social implications of the Project, thereby creating the largest biomedical-ethics budget anywhere in the country.

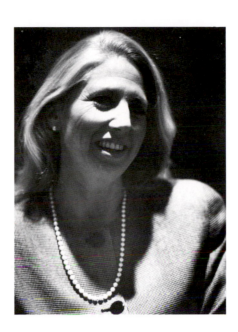

The funds are being used to support a large number of activities. The joint NIH-DOE ELSI working group, which meets four times a year, hopes to stimulate public discussion as well as help develop policy options that assure that the knowledge the Project generates will be of maximum benefit to individuals and to society. ELSI has identified four high-priority areas for program activities: quality and access in the use of genetic tests; fair use of genetic information by employers and insurers; privacy and confidentiality of genetic information; and public and professional education. We've organized conferences and workshops, and we are supporting a variety of research projects related to this topic. We are looking at existing legislation and perhaps will develop model legislation and model policy. The visibility of the Genome Project has meant that certain penchants for discrimination have been opened to public scrutiny in a way they have never been before.

Bob Moyzis: I think it's important to emphasize that by setting aside a

percentage of the genome budget for ELSI activities, we will not be able to miraculously decide all of the ethical issues associated with this project. We hope instead to catalyze exactly the type of discussion we are having tonight. We all hope that society as a whole will come to a realistic and positive consensus on the solutions long before the problems are permitted to materialize. We live in a democracy. All of us should be involved in deciding how we want to deal with the inevitable problems.

Question: You have suggested that studies of DNA will reveal ethnic differences, personality differences, psychological proclivities, and so on. Is that true? Will such studies reveal why two brothers, for example, David and Leon Botstein, have gestures that are very similar?

David Botstein: Frankly, we don't know the answer to that question. Maybe our gestures are our mother's

> *Genetic facts don't change your rights. The idea that we are all equal means we all have equal rights, not equal abilities.*

gestures, and we learned them from her, or maybe we inherited them from her—right now we can't tell. I think, however, that we are going to find out that in some cases our behavior is inherited and in other cases it is not, and we have to learn to live with that fact. Common sense already tells us that. But in my view genetic facts don't change your rights. The idea that we are all equal means we all have equal rights, not equal abilities. The fact is I could never have been a professional basketball player—I simply wasn't tall enough.

Leon Botstein: *That's not the reason.*

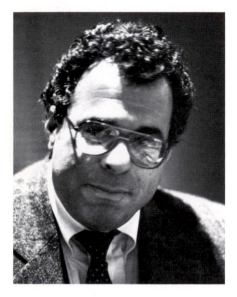

David Botstein: That was among the very many reasons. On the other hand, certain skills or abilities are easily improved by training. Take running, for example. Even unselected people can run. They may run much more slowly than their potential, but if they train hard, eat the right stuff, and learn how to get down on the blocks and anticipate the starter's gun, they will run faster. It will be extremely difficult to sort out the genetic component of such skills even if we are able to follow all of the genes involved. Some people will be very smart or very athletic because they study or train, and others will be up at the same level due to natural talent. Separating the two components is not a matter of genetic technology alone. It's difficult, and for some abilities it's never going to happen. So while we will be able to figure out the genetic component for a lot of these personal traits, it's very unlikely that we will be able to

predict with certainty whether a person will be smart or be a fast runner without regard to factors such as education and training.

Question: In his opening statement David Baltimore said the knowledge resulting from the Genome Project will bring freedom, but knowledge also brings responsibility and choice. Suppose prenatal testing reveals a genetic propensity toward alcoholism or low IQ or something else that the parents may simply not want to settle for even though it is not a disease. Will the parents be allowed to say, "We do not want this being ever to come into existence"? Can society eventually determine that certain qualities disappear? We can already do that to some extent, but if it's a question of IQ, what will happen?

David Baltimore: There is no question that along with knowledge and the freedom of choice will come very difficult social and political questions that have major moral aspects and that don't have a right or wrong answer. As our knowledge of human genetic variability deepens, the opportunity to avoid more and more traits in our offspring will present itself. It is very

> *By understanding the inheritance of an individual, we can help that individual develop his or her maximum potential.*

doubtful that we will see the disappearance of specific traits, but individuals will have a wider range of choices. To me, it is much more important that by understanding the inheritance of an

individual we can help that individual develop his or her maximum potential. This may mean tailoring the individual's education both to take advantage of strengths and to compensate for weaknesses. It may mean counseling an individual to take directions in life that build on inborn capabilities.

Jim Watson: I would prefer to trust the individual rather than the state in that sort of decision. Some people feel very strongly that sex selection shouldn't be allowed, but I would have compassion for parents who already had eight boys and wanted a girl. I would personally be very frightened by any political control that took the power away from parents. I shudder at the thought of state control over this issue. The laws would necessarily be imperfect.

David Botstein: I would like to point out the following simple-minded numerical facts about designing the make-up of future generations. When you pass on traits, you pass them on in a binary way. The father's sperm decides whether an offspring will be a boy or a girl. That means half the fertilized eggs will be boys, so if you choose boys you already have only half of the fertilized eggs to choose from. If you make another binary choice, you have a quarter of the eggs to choose from. If you have yet another binary choice, it's an eighth. If the array of basketball-playing genes is thirty, then only one out of over a billion of the embryos has them all, and that's a prohibitively low fraction. So choosing a genotype for anything complicated is, in principle, extremely impractical. It's just not likely to happen. The moral problem is there whenever you choose one embryo over another, but this business of specifically designing your offspring in one fashion or another—forget it!

Leon Botstein: David, the popular myth is not so much being able to choose among embryos but being able to make changes in a given embryo.

David Botstein: Genetic information will permit you to identify, in part, what's going to happen to an individual. That's a prerequisite to manipulation, but it's not nearly sufficient, and manipulation, at least manipulation of egg and sperm cells, is very, very far away. What you can do is choose from among the available embryos and, as I said, it's unlikely that there will be much of that. In fact, I expect there will be none.

Jim Watson: I'd like to make a point. Eugenics is supposed to be a bad word that we sort of equate with Hitler. It says we are trying to determine or change the nature of the human germ plasm. The most repulsive aspect about the eugenic efforts both in this country and, in particular, in Germany is that eugenic choices were made by the state, often on the basis of very incomplete knowledge. In this country we had a sterilization program that involved about twenty thousand women who were judged to be feeble-minded solely on the basis of their being prostitutes. This program was carried out in the 1920s and 1930s, and the people who were sterilized had no choice in the matter. The matter went to the Supreme Court, where a decision was made in favor of the sterilization program. The jurist most responsible for the decision was Oliver Wendell Holmes, who said that the state had the right to improve its future citizens. Then when we saw what happened in Germany, we decided that eugenics was extremely bad. On the other hand, to say that you can't really make choices to eliminate a gene for Duchenne's muscular dystrophy, to say that you want to perpetuate that gene for your descendants, is to be *mad*. That gene brings total and abso-

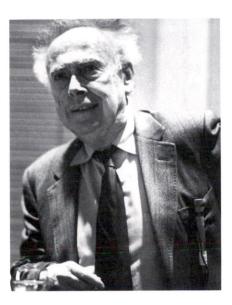

lute agony upon your descendants. If you have the option of having children without that gene, you might certainly want to choose that option. That's my opinion. Likewise, if you know you are a member of a cancer-prone family, and there are means by which you can have children who would not possess this trait, I think you as parents should have the opportunity to make that choice. I think it would be absolutely dangerous for anyone else, especially the state, to make such decisions. To say that parents must perpetuate things that bring only

No one should be allowed to prevent us from improving our own individual lives and the lives of our children.

agony upon themselves and their offspring appears to me to be terribly immoral. No one should be allowed to prevent us from improving our own individual lives and the lives of our children.

Question: David Baltimore pointed out the myth of equality. But we're fortunate that in our political system, in our culture, in our institutional arrangements, we try to assure equality of opportunity in a wide variety of ways. But there is another kind of myth deep in our Western culture, and that is the notion that we are volitional animals, that we have a capability to choose how we act, appropriately or inappropriately. I do not object to the Genome Project on this ground, but it seems that we are heading toward challenging a fundamental precept of our society as we unfold the dynamics of behavior by means of our growing understanding of genetic inheritance. I wonder whether some of the opposition to the Genome Project might stem from a fear that the results of the Project will show that we are not in fact volitional animals and do not really have free will.

Jim Watson: I have not met anyone who does not believe he has free will, the ability to make choices. But we will not really know what that means until we understand how our brains function, and that is a long way off. Nevertheless, if we eventually do understand how they function, I will be very surprised if we feel any differently. If you are born into a given political or cultural tradition, there are pressures to stay in that tradition. My political views are pretty similar to my parents' political views, and so traditions are passed on. We might say that I don't really have the freedom to be a Republican, but actually I do. So I don't think the Genome Project is going to touch the free-will issue.

Question: When you say that the gene that causes cystic fibrosis is somehow abnormal, I think we are all with you. But in the case of behavioral or learning processes, how do you decide what the healthy or normal gene is? Is there a way of defining normal by more valid means than merely by accepting society's viewpoint?

David Botstein: That's a good question. I don't know what's normal. In dealing with species other than ourselves, we have an operational definition of normal. Normal is what you find out in the wild. It's called wild type. If you catch a fly and it has certain characteristics, that's wild type, that's normal. Any differences are not called mutations or diseases, they're called polymorphisms, a neutral term, right? The point is that when people die horrible deaths due to their genetic content, we say disease, but we might simply view it as a variation of what you would call wild-type human.

David Baltimore: You say there are normal and polymorphic variants, but that's not really correct. There is no normal. They are all polymorphic variants.

David Botstein: That's right. I stand corrected.

David Baltimore: I learned it from you so I know it's right. There is a range of variations we consider normal and there are those outside that range that we consider abnormal. Things like cystic fibrosis are clearly diseases, but we have to be very conscious of the fact that in any gene we will see a very wide range of variation and that most of that variation is normal.

Nancy Wexler: Even in terms of a single disease the variation can be very great, and variations in the symptoms and progression of the disease make counseling very difficult. For example, one child with cystic fibrosis will die at age four and another will still be living at age fifty. It's hard to consider options

and make choices when the effects of the disease are so unpredictable.

Bob Moyzis: That's an important point. One of the more immediate impacts of this project that we all hope to see is a more individualized approach to health care. Complex human diseases like heart disease, for example, are likely to

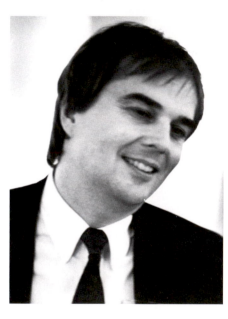

be the result of a combination of many genes. Nevertheless, you are treated like the generic human being, and the doctor tells you the fifteen things that you should do to lower your cholesterol. The new information will free us from this idea that we're all the same, and you'll get much more individualized medical treatment. In five or ten years you will be able to walk into your doctor's office and the doctor will take a little bit of blood, get an analysis of a variety of genes, and be able to personalize your treatment. Maybe you will be able to eat all the eggs that you want because it's probably not going to matter whatsoever, but you better avoid, say, jogging ten miles per day because it's probably going to kill you. I say

probably because for complex things like heart disease, it is doubtful that we will ever be able to say with real certainty that if you do this or that you'll be free of the disease.

Question: You said you have received a great deal of funding for this very difficult technical project, but I think the ethical aspects are even more difficult. I'm interested in knowing how they will be addressed. How will they be funded and how is that money going to be spent?

Nancy Wexler: The efforts to evaluate the ethical, legal, and social implications of the Genome Project are as much a part of the Project as the efforts to construct the maps. ELSI's activities go hand in hand with the development of the basic science because it's critical that our discussions, workshops, research and conference grants, and efforts toward

It's unlikely that we'll see many people going into their obstetrician's or gynecologist's offices to sort through embryos and pick out their favorites.

policy development be grounded in the capabilities and limitations of both current and future technology. David's calculations show that it's unlikely that we'll see many people going into their obstetrician's or gynecologist's offices to sort through embryos and pick out their favorites. People talk about these kinds of horror stories, but technically and practically, I doubt it will be our top problem. At this point we are trying to clarify the issues and assess the most salient ones through discussions of the kind we're having right here. What are people really concerned about? What do people see as the issues for them? Are there issues of which we are unaware? A group of seven research teams around the country, managed by ELSI, has undertaken a three-year study to evaluate the benefits of making a test for the cystic-fibrosis gene available to the public. The study will also develop and assess methods for educating and counseling people who want to be tested for this gene. We hope the findings will supply health-care professionals with strategies that maximize a person's understanding of genetic testing as well as record-keeping and disclosure policies that will best protect the individual against breaches of confidentiality, stigmatism, and discrimination. ELSI has also established an Insurance Task Force working toward developing guidelines

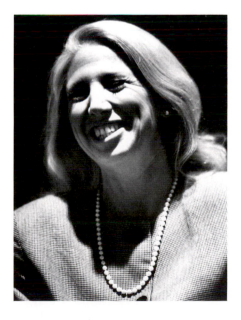

for insurance policy by 1993, and we have commissioned a White Paper to delineate policy options in the area of genetic testing relative to insurance and

employment. Funding also goes toward individual research grants, conference grants, and post-doctoral fellowships designed to address the entire range of ethical, social, and legal implications of the Project. The ELSI Working Group has carefully evaluated the Americans With Disabilities Act and outlined suggestions for the improvement of the Act relative to genetic issues such as discrimination and privacy. ELSI also sponsors public outreach meetings in order to encourage community discussions. We hope to educate the public and stimulate community interest and involvement in the process of shaping future policies.

Question: You have a lot of big names working on this project, and they have drawn an enormous amount of funding, congressional and otherwise. How will this project affect other areas of science where funding might be somewhat reduced?

Jim Watson: The money spent on the Genome Project is going to make other aspects of biological science more efficient by bringing them out from under an umbrella of complete ignorance, similar to the one that shrouded cancer research before the discovery of oncogenes. A lot of money is now being spent on trying to alleviate terrible medical conditions. People go to Congress, and Congress votes money in an attempt to help. For example, one of the best things we can do to address the problem of aging is to try to find the genes that predispose one to Alzheimer's or other forms of abnormal aging. By doing that we'll gain real scientific clues as to what is going on and what we can do to help.

Question: First, could you share with us the three or four most difficult confidentiality questions related to the Genome Project? Second, I can imagine a time

when boy meets girl and there's an added dimension, the genetic cost. The two might be a perfect match until they check to see if they have matching cystic-fibrosis cards. Is that where we're headed, everybody carrying around their own genetic ID card? Third, Dr. Watson, you said everyone has free will, but does everyone have the same capacity to exert their will? And is that capacity detectable through genetic testing? Is it associated with a gene? And if it is associated with a gene, then what does that mean for those who don't have the capacity to exert their will?

Jim Watson: You have cited several ethical problems that need to be addressed, but the most critical of them—and you referred to it indirectly—is what I call genetic injustice. DNA replication

> *No matter how it may upset the insurance companies and the employers, confidentiality has to be a guaranteed right.*

isn't perfect, so some people are born with genes that do not work properly. People are either slightly disabled or greatly disabled depending on what gene function is impaired and the extent of that impairment. Everyone knows that people are different from one another, and it's been convenient to ascribe those differences to our environments, to the fact that we didn't have certain opportunities in our childhood, or we didn't have a good education, or we didn't see a doctor when we should have, and so on.

In our rational society we think we can pass laws to correct the inequalities resulting from man's environment. We can do away with poverty. We can do away with all the things that clearly make people unequal. But now we know that certain kinds of inequality come from our genes. A paper on early-onset breast cancer identifies a gene on the short arm of chromosome 17 that predisposes women to breast cancer.

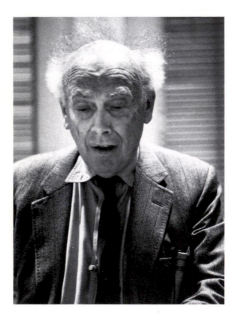

Women who inherit that gene are going to have a much greater probability of having breast cancer than other women. That's terribly unjust, there's nothing nice about it, but it's true. How do we cope with that inequality? Do we tell people to have tests so they can find out if they have that gene? Do people really want to know? Would it be better if everyone thought they were equal, that it's God's will if they get cancer?

Some call New Jersey the Cancer State because of all the chemical companies there, but in fact, the major factor is probably your genetic constitution. If you were lucky enough to have both your parents live to be one hundred, you're probably going to live a long life. Basically the inequality comes from our

genes, and what we have to do is try to find cures and treatments so that we can circumvent the inequalities.

Our knowledge of some diseases is improving so quickly that such hopes are not completely unrealistic. In other cases, science won't be able to come to the rescue. In those cases genetic information *must* be confidential. We shouldn't be stamped as unequal due to our genetic heritage. No matter how it may upset the insurance companies and the employers, confidentiality has to be a guaranteed right. For example, no presidential candidate should be able to say, "*I* will let my genes be seen by everyone," thereby forcing his opponent to come out with what might be construed as damaging genetic information. The need for confidentiality is paramount. We must try to treat and cure as much genetic inequality as we can, but it exists and we've got to live with it.

David Botstein: Jim proposes to make genetic information so confidential that nobody but the individual can know anything. The better solution would be to have health insurance guaranteed for everyone. Then the injustice of having the wrong genes would not be compounded by the injustice of not having any health care, which is where we seem to be heading in this country. If we solve the insurance problem, then I believe there will be no pressure for genetic testing. Usually health insurance is the issue.

Nancy Wexler: We as Americans feel that we are *legally* entitled to greater confidentiality than is actually granted us by law. We're now looking at the extent to which existing laws protect against violations of confidentiality. The genetic privacy issue is complicated because laws vary from state to state just as record-keeping methods and

disclosure policies vary from one health-care provider to another.

Another complication arises from the fact that our genomes are inherited from our parents and passed on to our children. That simple fact means that *personal* information about one individual's genome will often yield information about that individual's parents, siblings, or children. It's like pulling a thread on a sweater—one tug and a whole string of aunts, uncles, and cousins begins to unravel. We want the use of genetic testing to be a positive development in a health-care environment where privacy is assured, but there may be situations where absolute respect for an individual's genetic privacy could be detrimental to their relatives' health. ELSI is working to develop policies that will help satisfy questions about the ownership and control of genetic information as well as matters of consent to disclosure and use of such information. It's a complex issue, but we need to keep in mind the fact that the real attraction of the Genome Project lies in the hope that by understanding disease genes we can develop treatments. Before we had the

It's like pulling a thread on a sweater—one tug and a whole string of aunts, uncles, and cousins begins to unravel.

ability to detect disease genes, the only way a couple could find out whether they had the *matching cards* mentioned earlier was to *have* an affected child, and then they had that agony to face. One of the benefits of having a genetic test for breast cancer, for example, is that it allows for early detection and treatment and the ability to save many, many lives.

David Baltimore: The questions about confidentiality and testing may be the most difficult issues facing us at this time. In the long run, however, I expect this concern will probably dissipate and eventually disappear. As we learn more, we will discover that all of us have some deleterious aspects in our inheritance, and the only means of having a work force at all will be to dismiss the concept of the perfect person for the perfect job. However, I hope that long before we come to that conclusion, we will have put the responsibility not on the individual but on the insurance companies and the employer. We have health insurance so as to share health risks, and one of the rights an individual has is the right to work in the profession of his or her choice. I'm uncomfortable about psychological testing, and I am *very* much opposed to genetic testing as a basis for granting or denying employment or insurance.

Question: Who will take care of the confidentiality of the genes of an embryo? Is it possible to protect it? If it's possible in the United States, is it also possible in India or Argentina?

David Botstein: The problems in India and Argentina are very serious, and I doubt that any massive amount of genetic screening will be done. Many countries still have trouble getting *vaccinations* done.

Nancy Wexler: Nevertheless, let's recognize the fact that they had to pass a law in India against sex selection because parents were using genetic screening to avoid having female offspring.

David Botstein: That sort of problem is self-correcting.

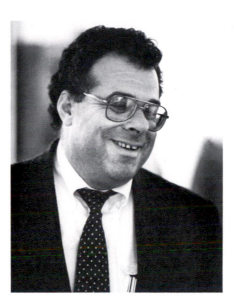

Nancy Wexler: Yes! It's *definitely* self-correcting. Most geneticists never intended their scientific work to be used for anything other than the detection of serious diseases. In certain situations, however, it is necessary to institute laws or use social policy to prevent *other* people from using scientific knowledge for purposes beyond those which the geneticists had envisioned.

Question: If we use genetic information to select against certain disease genes, such as cystic fibrosis, by choosing the good eggs and avoiding the bad ones, will our gene pool be depleted?

> ### The question is: Can you eliminate genes from the population? The answer is: No.

David Botstein: The question is: Can you eliminate genes from the population? The answer is: No. There is a simple numerical argument. Cystic

fibrosis is a recessive disease, so only people with two CF genes, we call them homozygotes, are affected with the disease. But most CF genes are in *hetero*zygotes, people with one normal gene and one CF gene. These people are carriers, but they exhibit no adverse symptoms and therefore are not selected against. Since they are not selected against—and why should they be?—the CF gene will always remain within the population.

Question: Would that be true for dominant genes as well?

David Botstein: No, it is not true for dominant genes. But there are very few prevalent dominant genes for serious diseases except those that are *new* mutations. Dominant disease genes tend to fall by the wayside because of their dominance. People who are afflicted with the worst dominant diseases usually don't live long enough, or they're simply unable, to bear offspring.

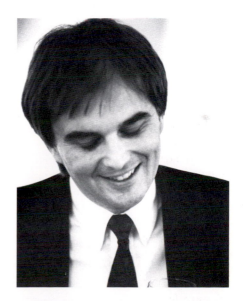

Bob Moyzis: The question concerning the gene pool raises a very critical point, namely, that all species, humans included, benefit from great genetic diversity. It is essential for our survival and future adaptability. Although some have imagined that genetically homogeneous societies would have advantages, true homogeneity would be a death sentence. Environments change, including social environments, and a species that cannot adapt will be eliminated. No matter how much we learn about the human genome over the next hundred years, there will always remain many things that we do not understand or cannot predict, such as who will be a great artist. It's not clear we will ever figure out the genetic components of complex human traits such as creativity. If you select against a particular gene, you may be eliminating something else that we deem valuable but the origins of which we don't yet understand.

No matter how much we learn about the human genome over the next hundred years, there will always be many things that we do not understand or cannot predict.

Jim Watson: A case in point might be the genes which predispose people to manic-depressive psychosis—finding those genes is an objective of the Project. We want to find a treatment that will be better than lithium since some cases don't respond to it, nor to any known drug. We're thinking the Project may be the best way of finding out what goes wrong. On the other hand, we might want to pause and wonder what our society would be like *without* manic-depressives—

Nancy Wexler: The room would be empty!

Jim Watson: It is a disease which can bring great suffering, but it can also bring great fortunes. Manic-depressives can do things that others say cannot be done. So it's a case where it's not obvious that we're dealing with a *bad* gene.

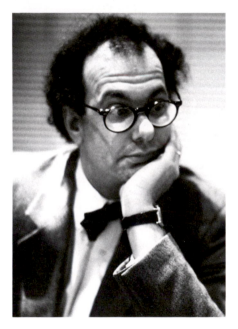

Leon Botstein: We would almost certainly lose our great poets.

Question: Suppose you find a genetic propensity for something like aggression, which affects other people as well as the individual. How would you cope with that? Do you leave all of society naked and exposed to a person who might be dangerous?

Jim Watson: I think that's the sort of ethical question that you can't really deal with until you've shown that such a genetic propensity exists. Even if you could, how would you use the information? Most good scientists, for example, are terribly aggressive.

Question: I am not really completely comfortable with the scientific aspects of what we have discussed, but it seems to me that there are really two issues. One we would all vote for, namely, the issue of diseases; and one we would all vote against, that is, the issue of personality traits, such as IQ. We're spending this country's fortunes so as to make learning about our genes a lot easier. Are we going to learn more about these somewhat vague personality traits or more about these lethal diseases?

It seems . . . that there are really two issues. One we would all vote for, namely, the issue of diseases; and one we would all vote against, that is, the issue of personality traits, such as IQ.

David Botstein: I believe we will understand diseases much earlier than personality traits because diseases are much better defined. We haven't really defined personality traits precisely enough to correlate them with genetic information. So diseases will probably come first.

Question: Do you suspect the ethical considerations will have to broaden in order to be relevant to other cultures and other societies? Tonight, the answers about confidentiality seem to relate back to our society, which values individual rights and has insurance. But the transfer of this technology to cultures that don't have notions of individual rights,

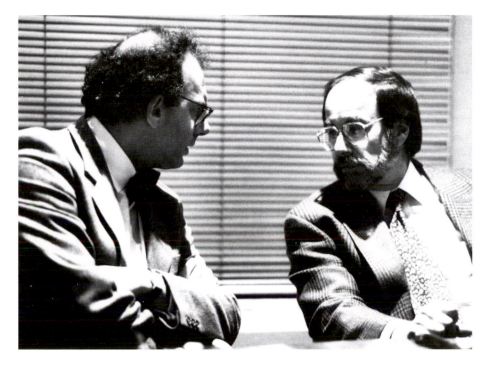

much less insurance for individuals, might have very serious repercussions.

Nancy Wexler: That is an important issue. People are concerned about giving diagnostic probes to China, for example. Should we give diagnostic testing capabilities to countries where counseling is not likely to accompany the tests and where confidentiality rights are not guaranteed? Through an international organization called the Human Genome Organization, which has an ethics working group, we try to collaborate with other countries in order to emphasize the importance of providing those services and protections.

Question: What is the time frame in which you hope to accomplish the Genome Project?

David Botstein: The high-resolution genetic-linkage map and the sequences of some of the model organisms are both parts of our five-year goal, as is a great majority of the physical map.

The human-genome sequence itself is, essentially, not one of the five-year goals. The expectation is that it will be completed in approximately fifteen years.

Jim Watson: Within the next five to ten years we want to get all the tools needed by the disease-gene hunter, the person who wants to find, say, the Alzheimer's gene. We are in a hurry to get them. That's our impatience. We say in five years, maybe ten, the last bits of that resource will be put together. We are in a hurry. ∎

Photos by G. Steve Jordan, New York

Glossary

allele Any one of the variations of a gene or a polymorphic DNA marker found in the members of a species. Numerous alleles of a given gene or polymorphic DNA marker may exist, but an individual eukaryote possesses at most two alleles of the gene or polymorphic DNA marker.

Alu sequence A DNA sequence about 300 base pairs long that is repeated, one copy at a time, almost 2 million times along the DNA molecules of the human genome. Sequences similar to the Alu sequence are dispersed throughout other mammalian genomes. The function of such repeated sequences is not known.

amino acid An organic compound consisting of a hydrogen atom, an amino group ($-NH_2$), a carboxyl group ($-COOH$), and a "side chain" bonded to a carbon atom. Each of the more than eighty known amino acids contains a different side chain. Twenty of the known amino acids serve as the building blocks of proteins.

autosome Any chromosome of a eukaryotic organism other than a sex chromosome. The human genome includes forty-four autosomes as twenty-two homologous autosome pairs. Compare **sex chromosome**.

bacteriophage Also called phage. Any one of the viruses that infect bacteria. The genomes of certain phages have been modified to serve as cloning vectors. Fragments of foreign DNA with lengths between about 12,000 base pairs and about 22,000 base pairs are cloned in vectors derived from the genome of the λ (lambda) phage.

base sequence See **sequence**.

biosynthesis Formation of chemical compounds by a living organism.

cDNA (complementary DNA or copy DNA) A single-stranded DNA segment whose sequence is complementary to that of a messenger RNA and thus consists of sequences complementary to the protein-coding sequences that appear on the sense strand of the protein gene from which the messenger RNA was transcribed. cDNAs are synthesized in vitro by reverse transcription of messenger RNAs extracted from cells and are used as hybridization probes for protein genes.

centimorgan The unit of genetic distance, a measure of how frequently two genes on the same chromosome are separated by crossing over and therefore not inherited together. A distance of 1 centimorgan between two genes means that they have a 1 percent chance of not being inherited together. In humans 1 centimorgan corresponds roughly to a physical distance of 1 million base pairs. Compare **genetic distance**.

centromere 1. The DNA sequence within a eukaryotic chromosome to which fibers of the mitotic spindle attach during mitosis and meiosis. Centromeres are essential to the proper parceling out of chromosomes to daughter cells and gametes. 2. The region of attachment between the two identical eukaryotic chromosomes formed by DNA replication. The centromeric region of a chromosome is the constricted region seen along a metaphase chromosome when viewed with an optical microscope; despite the name, the centromeres of many chromosomes are not centrally located. See pages 10–11.

chimera A recombinant clone each member of which contains segments of a genome that are noncontiguous in vivo.

chromatin The complex of DNA and five proteins (histones) that is the major component of eukaryotic chromosomes.

chromosome Any one of a certain species-specific number of threadlike cellular structures, each containing a DNA molecule. Every cell of every member of a eukaryotic species possesses the same number of chromosomes, each of which is confined within the cellular nucleus and contains a linear DNA molecule. The chromosomes within a eukaryotic cell are visible with an optical microscope only when they have become condensed in preparation for cell division. In contrast, every member of any prokaryotic species possesses only one chromosome, which contains a circular rather than a linear DNA molecule, is not confined within a nucleus, and is never visible with an optical microscope.

chromosome banding pattern A pattern of alternating dark and light transverse regions (bands) formed on a fully condensed chromosome by appropriate chemical treatment and staining. Such banding patterns are the means for unambiguously distinguishing the different pairs of homologous chromosomes of an individual eukaryote, and the different bands along a single chromosome are used to identify different regions of the chromosome. See page 11.

classical genetics The study of inheritance based on the concept of the gene as a discrete unit of heredity, data about the transmission of genes from one generation to another, and the behavior of chromosomes rather than on the molecular details of genes and chromosomes. Compare **molecular genetics**.

clone 1. A population of genetically identical unicellular organisms (in this publication *Escherichia coli* or *Sac-charomyces cerevisiae*) or viruses (here phages) arising from successive replications of a single ancestral unicellular organism or virus. 2. A recombinant clone. 3. The fragment of foreign DNA contained in each member of a recombinant clone. 4. A population of identical cells arising from the culture of a single cell of a certain type, such as a human fibroblast or a rodent-human hybrid cell containing a full set of rodent chromosomes and a single human chromosome.

cloning See **molecular cloning**.

cloning vector A relatively short length of DNA into which a DNA fragment to be cloned is inserted. The resulting recombinant vector can be replicated by a host cell by virtue of certain DNA sequences contained within the cloning vector.

codon 1. A triplet of adjacent ribonucleotides along a messenger RNA. Sixty-four such RNA codons are possible. The RNA codon AUG is always the first codon in a messenger RNA to be translated (into the amino acid methionine) and is therefore called the START codon. Each of three other RNA codons signals the cessation of translation of a messenger RNA and is called a STOP codon. Each of the remaining sixty RNA codons is translated into one of the other nineteen amino acids that appear in proteins. 2. The triplet of adjacent deoxyribonucleotides that must appear within the sense strand of a protein gene if transcription of the template strand of the gene is to yield a given RNA codon. The DNA codon corresponding to a given RNA codon is generated simply by replacing each U in the RNA codon by T. See **genetic code**.

complementary base pair Either of the two pairs of bases A and T or C and G. A is said to be the complement of T and vice versa, and C is said to be the complement of G and vice versa. The succession of hydrogen bonds between complementary base pairs is the glue that holds DNA in its natural double-stranded configuration. (Another complementary base pair is the pair A and U, the RNA analogue of T.)

complementary DNA See **cDNA**.

complementary sequences The sequences of two single-stranded nucleic-acid segments (either two single-stranded DNA segments or one single-stranded DNA segment and an RNA segment) are said to be complementary if each base in the 5′-to-3′ sequence of one segment is the complement of the corresponding base in the 3′-to-5′ sequence of the other segment. For example, the DNA sequence 5′-GTAGC-3′ is complementary to the RNA sequence 3′-CAUCG-5′, and the two strands of a chromosomal DNA molecule are complementary along the entireties of their lengths. Two single-stranded nucleic-acid segments with complementary sequences can hydrogen bond to each other.

contig A set of overlapping cloned DNA fragments all members of which have been arranged in the same order that the fragments are found along a chromosomal DNA molecule in vivo. A contig map is a physical map made up of contigs. See pages 118–119.

cosmid A synthetic cloning vector possessing desirable features of plasmid and λ-phage cloning vectors. Fragments of foreign DNA with lengths between about 33,000 base pairs and about 47,000 base pairs can be cloned in cosmids.

crossing over A natural process that produces new combinations of the genetic information present on the DNA molecules within two homologous chromosomes by effecting the exchange, during meiosis, of corresponding regions of the DNA molecules. See page 32.

cytogenetics The study of the inheritance of traits by combining methods of both cytology and genetics. The discovery of microscopically visible chromosomes and advances in optics, microscopy, and cytochemistry have given the field of cytogenetics a prominent place in the study of chromosome number and morphology in both normal and diseased states.

cytology The study of the structure, behavior, reproduction, and pathology of cells.

cytoplasm The substance of a eukaryotic cell between the cellular membrane and the nuclear membrane.

denature To separate DNA into its constituent single strands.

deoxyribonucleotide See **nucleotide**.

diploid chromosome set The species-specific set of chromosomes found in all the cells of a multicellular organism except its gametes. The diploid chromosome set of most species contains an even number of chromosomes because the chromosomes occur as homologous pairs or in the case of those species that possess sex chromosomes, of homologous pairs of autosomes and a pair of homologous or nonhomologous sex chromosomes. One member of each chromosome pair is inherited from each parent. The diploid chromosome set of any human normally contains forty-six chromosomes. Compare **haploid chromosome set**.

DNA (deoxyribonucleic acid) A double-stranded polymer consisting of a roughly random sequence of four deoxyribonucleotide pairs. Species-specific and individual-specific genetic information is encoded in the order of the deoxyribonucleotide pairs (usually called simply base pairs) along the chromosomal DNA molecule or molecules of an organism. See pages 40–41.

DNA fingerprint Any observable characteristic of a chromosomal DNA molecule or a fragment thereof that can be used to identify a particular individual of a species, a particular recombinant clone, or a particular product of a polymerase chain reaction.

DNA library A collection of recombinant clones. Each member of each recombinant clone in a library contains the same fragment of foreign DNA, as an insert within a recombinant vector, and all the foreign-DNA fragments within all the members of all the recombinant clones in the library originated from the same source.

DNA replication The process by which a parent chromosomal DNA molecule is converted into two daughter DNA molecules, each identical to the parent DNA molecule and each consisting of one strand of the parent DNA molecule and one newly synthesized strand. The two daughter DNA molecules are bound to each other along their centromeric regions and together are called a sister-chromatid pair. See pages 42–43.

DNA sequence A fragment of DNA with a particular, although not necessarily known, sequence.

dominant allele A variant of a gene that determines which variant of the trait specified by the gene is exhibited by an individual eukaryote when only one copy of the allele is present in the

genome of the individual. Compare **recessive allele**.

enzyme A protein that acts as a catalyst in a biochemical reaction. A few biochemical reactions are now known to be catalyzed by RNA molecules rather than by proteins. Such catalytic RNA molecules are called ribozymes.

eukaryote Any species or any individual of a species that is a member of the taxonomic kingdom Protoctista, Fungi, Animalia, or Plantae. A eukaryote, whether unicellular or multicellular, is characterized by the presence within the cytoplasm of numerous specialized organelles (see page 8), by the existence of a membrane-bounded nucleus enclosing genetic material organized into multiple chromosomes, and by an elaborate mechanism of cell division involving a mitotic spindle (see page 14–15). In addition, sexual reproduction, a mechanism for increasing the genetic diversity of a species, is common among eukaryotes. Compare **prokaryote**.

exon A protein-coding region of a gene, that is, a base sequence that is translated according to the genetic code into an amino-acid sequence of the gene's protein product. Most protein-coding genes in eukaryotes consist of a series of exons interrupted by introns. Compare **intron**.

flow cytometry A method for sorting cells according to the amount and/or chemical composition of their constituent DNA. The method has been adapted to sorting metaphase chromosome. See page 237.

gamete An ovum or a sperm. Gametes are produced by meiosis of special cells of multicellular organisms and contain a haploid set of chromosomes.

gel electrophoresis A method for separating fragments of DNA or RNA by length. The method involves migration of the DNA fragments through a gel (a porous, semisolid medium) under the influence of an electric field. See pages 55–56.

gene A segment of DNA that contains the information necessary for the controlled biosynthesis of some "gene product." A protein gene contains the infomation necessary for the biosynthesis, by transcription and translation, of a protein or one of the constituent polypeptides of a protein. An RNA gene contains the information necessary for the biosynthesis, by transcription, of an RNA molecule other than the RNA molecules that are translated into proteins or constituent polypeptides. Any individual eukaryote possesses two copies of almost every gene. The two copies may be identical, or they may differ sufficiently to cause some observable difference in the characteristics of the individual. In either case one copy of the gene is located at some position along the DNA molecule within one member of a homologous chromosome pair; the other copy is located at the same position along the DNA molecule within the other member of the homologous chromosome pair. Genes are parceled out to daughter cells and to gametes as predicted on the basis of the observed behavior of chromosomes during mitosis and meiosis.

gene expression Conversion of the information in a gene to a gene product (see **gene**). The rate at which a gene is expressed varies in response to external stimuli and, in the case of multicellular organisms, with cell type and developmental stage.

gene regulation Control of the rate at which a gene is expressed. The primary mechanism of gene regulation is control of transcription initiation. See page 64.

genetic code A listing of the amino acid or translation signal specified by each of the sixty-four possible codons. See page 48.

genetic distance A quantity that can be roughly correlated with the physical distance between two genes that are located on the same chromosome. The genetic distance between two such linked genes is defined as the probability of the occurrence, during a single meiosis, of crossing over at any point along the segment of DNA between the two genes. The method used to determine a genetic distance, called linkage analysis, requires the existence of at least two alleles for each of the two genes and is applicable not only to linked variable genes but also to linked polymorphic DNA markers. The unit of genetic distance is the centimorgan. See pages 34–35 and pages 86–99.

genetic-linkage map A map showing the genetic distances between pairs of linked variable genes or polymorphic DNA markers.

genetics See **classical genetics, molecular genetics**.

genome The totality of the DNA contained within the single chromosome of a bacterial species (or an individual bacterium) or within the diploid chromosome set of a eukaryotic species (or an individual eukaryote). The human genome, for example, consists of approximately 6 billion base pairs of DNA distributed among forty-six chromosomes. Sometimes the term "the human genome" is used to refer instead to the approximately 3 billion base pairs of DNA within the twenty-two different human autosomes and the human X and

Y chromosomes. The term "genome" is also applied to the genetic material of a virus, which may be either DNA or RNA.

genotype The pair of alleles of a variable gene possessed by an individual, or the pairs of alleles of any number of variable genes possessed by an individual. The genotype of an individual is a primary determinant of the individual's phenotype.

GT sequence The tandem repeat (5'-GT)$_n$, where n is variable and ranges from 15 to 30. The GT sequence is repeated about 100,000 times throughout the human genome; its function is not known.

haploid chromosome set The species specific set of chromosomes found in all the gametes produced by a multicellular organism and consisting of one (randomly selected) member of each homologous chromosome pair possessed by a eukaryotic species and, if both males and females of the species possess a pair of sex chromosomes, of one (randomly selected) sex chromosome. Thus the haploid chromosome number of most organisms is one-half of its diploid chromosome number. A human gamete normally contains twenty-three chromosomes. Compare **diploid chromosome set**.

heterozygous Possessing one copy of each of two different alleles of a gene or a polymorphic DNA marker. Compare **homozygous**.

homologous chromosomes Chromosomes that, during metaphase, are indistinguishable in size, location of centromere, and banding pattern. The homology of a pair of metaphase chromosomes is due to a very high degree of similarity in the order of the deoxyri-

bonucleotide pairs along their constituent DNA molecules. See pages 10–11.

homologous sequences Two molecules or segments of DNA (or RNA) are said to have homologous sequences if a high percentage of the corresponding base pairs (or bases) in their sequences are identical. For example, many genes of *Mus musculus* and *Homo sapiens* have homologous sequences.

homozygous Possessing two copies of the same allele of a gene or a polymorphic DNA marker. Compare **heterozygous**.

hybridization Hydrogen bonding of two single-stranded segments of DNA with complementary sequences or of one single-stranded segment of DNA and one segment of RNA with complementary sequences. Hybridization is the basis of a technique for identifying, among many different DNA fragments, those fragments that contain a DNA segment of interest. The technique requires the availability of a probe for the segment of interest. See pages 61–63.

in-situ hybridization Hybridization between a free segment of DNA (or RNA) and an intact chromosomal DNA molecule. In-situ hybridization is the basis of a technique for determining the location of a fragment of DNA along an intact chromosomal DNA molecule or the location of an intact chromosomal DNA molecule within the cellular nucleus. See pages 61–63.

interphase The entirety of the eukaryotic cell cycle except the mitotic phase. Because the chromosomes within a cell are not condensed during interphase, the genes along the chromosomal DNA molecules are accessible to transcription. Therefore, most of the biosynthetic activities of a cell, including DNA replication, occur during interphase. The transition from interphase to the mitotic phase is signaled by the condensation of duplicated chromosomes into microscopically visible structures. See page 9.

intron A region of a protein gene that separates one exon of the gene from another. The introns of a protein gene are transcribed but are excised from the RNA transcript before it is translated. Very few prokaryotic protein genes contain introns, whereas many eukaryotic protein genes contain at least one intron. Introns also occur in genes coding for ribosomal RNAs and some transfer RNAs. See page 64. Compare **exon**.

karyotype A display of the set of chromosomes extracted from a eukaryotic somatic cell arrested at metaphase. The chromosomes are banded and photographed through an optical microscope, and the micrographs of individual chromosomes are arranged by hand into a standard array of homologous chromosomes and sex chromosomes (provided the cell originated from a species possessing sex chromosomes). A karyotype is helpful in revealing chromosomal abnormalities that are symptomatic of various disorders. See page 11.

linked genes Two or more genes that reside on the same chromosome of a eukaryotic organism. The classical method for determining whether two genes are linked requires that both genes have dominant and recessive alleles and involves detecting statistically significant deviations from Mendel's law of independent assortment for the co-inheritance of the trait variants specified by the alleles of the two genes. See pages 86–93.

locus The position on a chromosome or on its constituent DNA molecule of a gene or other DNA landmark.

map See **genetic-linkage map** and **physical map**.

meiosis The type of cell division undergone by the precursors of gametes. Meiosis involves two successive divisions of nuclear matter, and each gamete produced possesses a haploid chromosome set. See page 15.

messenger RNA (mRNA) An RNA molecule formed by transcription of the template strand of a protein gene and removal from the resulting primary transcript of any introns present. A messenger RNA serves as a template for translation. See pages 45–47.

metaphase The stage of mitosis or meiosis in which the fully condensed duplicated chromosomes (sister-chromatid pairs) are aligned along the equatorial plane of the dividing cell. See pages 14–15.

metaphase chromosome 1. A fully condensed duplicated chromosome (sister-chromatid pair), or, in other words, a sister-chromatid pair in the configuration it assumes during metaphase of mitosis or meiosis. 2. Either one of the fully condensed sister chromatids in a metaphase chromosome. See pages 14–15.

mitotic spindle The apparatus that directs the motion of chromosomes during mitosis and meiosis.

mitosis The type of cell division by which a unicellular eukaryote reproduces asexually or by which a multicellular organism increases in size and replaces dead cells. The daughter cells produced by mitosis are genetically identical to the mother cell. See page 14.

molecular cloning The production of many identical copies of a DNA fragment by inserting the fragment into a cloning vector and propagating the resulting recombinant vector in a host cell.

molecular genetics The study of the molecular details of the regulated flow of genetic information among DNA, RNA, and proteins and from generation to generation. Compare **classical genetics**.

mutagen Any of a wide variety of agents, including certain types of radiation, certain chemicals, and infecting viruses, that can cause mutations in the genome of an organism.

mutation Any alteration in the base sequence(s) of the constituent DNA molecule(s) of the genome of an organism. Some mutations are caused by external mutagens; others are caused by natural mechanisms such as crossing over or the incorporation of foreign DNA into a genomic DNA molecule. Any nonlethal mutation is transmitted to successive generations of a cell, but only mutations in the DNA of gametes or their precursors are transmitted to successive generations of a multicellular organism.

nematode Any member of a group of worms with unsegmented bodies. The nematode *Caenorhabditis elegans* is the only multicellular organism for which the lineage of every cell has been traced and for which the interconnections among all the neurons have been determined. Furthermore, a physical map covering 95 percent of the *C. elegans* genome has been constructed, and a project to sequence its entire genome is under way.

nucleic acid The generic name for DNA or RNA.

nucleotide The generic name for the building blocks of DNA and RNA. A deoxyribonucleotide (or DNA nucleotide) consists of a phosphate group attached to a deoxyribose residue, which in turn is attached to the residue of one of four nitrogenous organic bases (adenine, cytosine, guanine, or thymine). A ribonucleotide (or RNA nucleotide) consists of a phosphate group attached to a ribose residue, which in turn is attached to the residue of one of four nitrogenous organic bases (adenine, cytosine, guanine, or uracil). Neighboring nucleotides along a strand of DNA or RNA are linked by a covalent bond between an oxygen atom in the phosphate group of one nucleotide and the 3′ carbon atom in the sugar residue of the other nucleotide. See pages 40–41.

oligonucleotide A segment of single-stranded DNA synthesized in vitro and usually containing at most a few tens of deoxyribonucleotides. Oligonucleotides serve as hybridization probes and as the primers required in a polymerase chain reaction.

phage See **bacteriophage**.

phenotype The variant of a heritable trait exhibited by an individual, or the variants of any number of inheritable traits exhibited by an individual. The genotype of an individual cannot in general be deduced from its phenotype. Compare **genotype**.

physical map A map showing physical distances (in base pairs) between landmarks along a chromosomal DNA molecule, such as genes, restriction sites, RFLPs, and sequence-tagged sites. The lowest-resolution physical map of a human chromosomal DNA

molecule is a chromosomal banding pattern; the highest-resolution map, the sequence of deoxyribonucleotide pairs along its entire length, will probably not be available for some time. The physical maps to be produced by the Human Genome Project are contig maps (see **contig**), which are of intermediate resolution.

plasmid Small, circular DNA molecules found in and replicated by various bacterial species, including *E. coli*. Engineered plasmids are used as cloning vectors. Fragments of foreign DNA about 4000 base pairs long can be cloned in plasmids.

polymerase An enzyme that catalyses the template-directed linking (polymerization) of the precursors of deoxyribonucleotides or ribonucleotides. A DNA polymerase catalyzes the basic chemical reaction of DNA replication: the synthesis of a strand of DNA with a sequence complementary to that of a template strand of DNA. The reaction requires the pre-existence of a "primer," a very short strand of DNA or RNA bound by complementary base pairing to the template strand. See page 43. An RNA polymerase catalyzes the basic chemical reaction of transcription: the synthesis of an RNA molecule with a sequence complementary to that of one strand (the template strand) of an RNA gene or a protein gene. No primer is required. See page 46.

polymerase chain reaction (PCR) An in-vitro process for producing many millions of copies of a DNA fragment. The process involves successive repetitions of a series of reactions and, when applied to a sample containing many different DNA fragments, can amplify one selected fragment. See pages 128–130.

polymorphic DNA marker A region along a chromosomal DNA molecule of a eukaryotic species whose sequence varies among a population of the species. The alleles of a polymorphic DNA marker are inherited in just the same fashion as are the alleles of a variable gene. Analysis of the co-inheritance of a variable gene on some chromosomal DNA molecule and polymorphic DNA markers on the same chromosomal DNA molecule helps to pinpoint the location of the gene. See pages 94–99.

polypeptide Also called polypeptide chain. A string of amino acids linked by peptide bonds. The term "polypeptide" is not exactly synonymous with the term "protein" because some proteins are composed of more than one polypeptide.

probe A labeled stretch of single-stranded DNA (or RNA) whose sequence includes the complement of one strand of a DNA sequence of interest. Such a probe is required for using hybridization to detect the presence of the DNA sequence of interest in a sample containing many different DNA sequences. See pages 61–63.

prokaryote Any species or any individual of a species that is a member of the taxonomic subkingdom Eubacteria of the kingdom Prokaryotae. Prokaryotes are almost invariably unicellular and are characterized by the absence of a membrane-bounded nucleus, the absence of organelles other than ribosomes, a genome consisting of a single closed loop of DNA, and a mechanism of cell division that does not involve a mitotic spindle. Furthermore, mechanisms for exchange of genetic information among members of a prokaryotic species are rare. Compare **eukaryote**.

promoter The portion of a gene to which RNA polymerase must bind before transcription of the gene can begin.

protein A biological macromolecule composed of at least one polypeptide. The numerous different proteins specified by the genome of an organism play different roles in its maintenance and reproduction and, in the case of a multicellular organism, in its development from a single cell. Some proteins catalyze the chemical reactions that occur in cells; others provide mobility or mechanical support; others defend against foreign substances; others generate and transmit nerve impulses; and others control cell division and differentiation.

recessive allele A variant of a gene that determines which variant of the trait determined by the gene an individual exhibits only when it is present on both members of a homologous chromosome pair. Compare **dominant allele**.

recombinant clone A clone of a recombinant cloning vector, or, in other words, a clone of a vector than contains a fragment of foreign DNA.

recombinant DNA molecule A stretch of DNA than includes DNA from more than one source and can be replicated by a host cell without being incorporated into the genome of the host cell. Examples are recombinant plasmids and recombinant phage genomes.

repetitive DNA A collective term for all the DNA sequences that occur more than once in the genome of an organism. Prokaryotes possess no or very little repetitive DNA, whereas many eukaryotes possess a great deal. Roughly a third of the human genome, for example, is repetitive DNA. The functions of a few repeated human DNA sequences are known; the functions of

most are still a matter of speculation. See **Alu sequence, GT sequence, satellite DNA**.

restriction enzyme (type II restriction endonuclease) A protein capable of binding to any occurrence of a specific short DNA sequence and of catalyzing the cleavage of both DNA strands within or near that sequence. The discovery of restriction enzymes helped precipitate the recombinant-DNA revolution. See pages 52–54.

restriction fragment Any DNA fragment produced by the action of a restriction enzyme.

restriction site Any occurrence of the DNA sequence to which a restriction enzyme binds.

reverse transcription The synthesis of a strand of DNA from a template strand of RNA. The sequence of the synthesized DNA strand is complementary to the sequence of the RNA template strand. Reverse transcription, which is catalyzed by the enzyme reverse transcriptase, is the first step in the reproduction of certain viruses, including the virus that causes AIDS, and is also the reaction by which cDNAs are synthesized in vitro.

RFLP (restriction-fragment-length polymorphism) A type of polymorphic DNA marker that results in differences among individuals in the lengths of the restriction fragments that originate from the polymorphic region.

ribosomal RNA (rRNA) The RNA molecules found in ribosomes.

ribosome A cellular organelle involved in translation. A ribosome effects the synthesis of a protein or a polypeptide by catalyzing the linkage, in the order specified by a messenger RNA, of the

amino acids carried by transfer RNA molecules. A ribosome contains a relatively small number of different RNA molecules and a large number of different proteins. See page 47.

RNA (ribonucleic acid) A single-stranded polymer consisting of a sequence of linked ribonucleotides (see **nucleotide**). Numerous different RNA molecules constitute the bulk of the cellular nucleic acid and play different roles. Messenger RNAs, ribosomal RNAs, and transfer RNAs are involved in protein synthesis; others are components of the spliceosomes involved in RNA splicing; a few are known to act as catalysts; and one is known to be involved in the transport of newly synthesized proteins to their ultimate destinations within the cell.

RNA splicing The process by which an RNA molecule transcribed from the template strand of a gene is rid of any introns it may contain. The product of splicing is a messenger RNA or the mature form of some other type of RNA. See page 45.

satellite DNA Any of the tandem repeats found at the centromeric and telomeric regions of the chromosomal DNA molecules of many eukaryotes.

sequence Also called base sequence. 1. A listing of the deoxyribonucleotide pairs within a DNA molecule or segment in the order they appear along the DNA molecule or segment in vivo. 2. A listing of the ribonucleotides within an RNA molecule or segment in the order they appear along the RNA molecule or segment in vivo. The process by which such sequence data are obtained is called sequencing. See pages 151–159.

sex chromosome Males of some species, including all mammals, possess two chromosomes that are not homologous to each other or to any other chromosomes the males possess. However, one of those exceptional chromosomes is homologous to both members of a homologous chromosome pair possessed by the females of such a species. Any one of those three homologous chromosomes is called an X chromosome. The other exceptional male chromosome is called a Y chromosome. Collectively the X and Y chromosomes are called sex chromosomes because one or the other is involved in determining maleness (possession of testes). The Y chromosome of a mammal is easily distinguished from its much larger X chromosome and is the sex chromosome that determines maleness. On the other hand, the Y chromosome of the fruit fly *Drosophila melanogaster* is comparable in size to its X chromosome and is not the sex chromosome that determines maleness. Although the X and Y chromosomes of a male are not homologous, the two do pair up during meiosis and one or the other is parceled out to each sperm.

sister-chromatid pair The two identical chromosomal DNA molecules formed by replication of a single chromosomal DNA molecule. The binding of the members of a sister-chromatid pair along their centromeric regions accounts for the X shape of metaphase chromosomes.

somatic cell Any cell of a multicellular organism other than gametes or the precursors of gametes.

Southern hybridization A hybridization technique in which the fragments to be interrogated with a hybridization probe have been length-separated by gel electrophoresis and transferred from the gel to a nylon nitrocellulose filter. The filter containing the length-separated

fragments is sometimes called a Southern blot. See page 63.

STS (sequence-tagged site) A short (200 to 300 base-pair long) segment of a chromosomal DNA molecule whose sequence has been determined and is known to be unique because the STS can be selectively amplified by a particular polymerase chain reaction. A set of STSs located on a chromosomal DNA molecule helps to integrate the genetic-linkage and physical maps of the chromosomal DNA molecule. See pages 130–134.

telomere 1. Either terminus of a eukaryotic (and hence linear) chromosome. 2. The DNA sequence that terminates either end of a eukaryotic chromosomal DNA molecule.

transcription The biosynthesis of an RNA molecule from a DNA template strand. The sequence of the synthesized RNA molecule is complementary to the sequence of the DNA template strand. See page 46.

transduction The phage-mediated transport of genetic information from a member of a bacterial strain or species to a member of the same or a different strain or species.

transfer RNA (tRNA) Any one of a group of small RNA molecules that are involved in translating the sequence of codons along a messenger RNA molecule into a sequence of amino acids along a polypeptide. See page 47.

transformation The process by which a plasmid cloning vector enters an *E. coli* host cell or a yeast artificial chromosome enters a yeast host cell.

translation The linking of amino acids

carried by transfer RNA molecules in an order specified by the order of the codons along a messenger RNA molecule. The product of translation is a protein or a polypeptide. See page 47.

translocation The transfer of a segment of a chromosome from its usual location to a new location on a homologous chromosome or a nonhomologous chromosome. Translocations are often symptomatic of disease and can be detected as changes in the banding patterns or morphologies of metaphase chromosomes.

virus Any of numerous and varied submicroscopic organisms that are incapable of reproduction outside a host cell. The structure of viruses is remarkably simple: each consists of a genome, which may be either DNA or RNA, and a protein body that not only protects the genome but also facilitates entry of the genome into a host cell. Almost all living organisms are susceptible to attack by viruses.

wild type An individual of a species that exhibits the variants of inheritable traits that are typical of a natural population of the species.

YACs (yeast artificial chromosome) 1. A linear recombinant DNA molecule that is replicated as a yeast chromosome by a yeast host cell because it contains, in addition to a fragment of foreign DNA, a yeast centromere, a yeast origin of replication, and two yeast telomeres, one at each end. Fragments of foreign DNA with lengths up to 1 million base pairs can be cloned as YACs. 2. The vector arms to which the ends of a foreign DNA fragment are ligated to form a YAC.

zygote The single cell formed by fertilization of an ovum by a sperm.

Art Credits for *Los Alamos Science*, Number 20

Original Art

Cover painting, Gloria Sharp
pages 0–1, David R. Delano
page 3, David R. Delano
pages 68–69, Steve Elder
page 173, Jim Cruz
pages 250–251, Gloria Sharp
pages 280–281, Gloria Sharp
pages 302–303, David R. Delano

Photography

page 6, *Los Alamos Science* file
page 7, *Los Alamos Science* file
page 10, *Los Alamos Science* file
page 11, *Los Alamos Science* file
page 40, Mel Prueitt, CN91–3979
page 56, *Los Alamos Science* file
page 63, *Los Alamos Science* file
page 66, John Flower, 92–109–015
page 67, Mel Prueitt, CN91–3979
pages 72–178, Margo Bennett and Steve Jordan, *Los Alamos Science* file
page 132, 92–372
page 169, 89–1478
page 177, John Flower, 88–114–008
pages 182–217, *Los Alamos Science* file
page 218, John Flower, RN92 150–002
page 249, John Flower, 92–110–14
pages 252–278, *Los Alamos Science* file
page 279, John Flower, 92–110–62
page 296, RN91–1938
page 297 (top to bottom), John Flower, 92–112–028; John Flower, 92–112–009; John Flower, 92–112–001; Henry Ortega, RB92–039–005; John Flower, 92–112–016
page 298 (left to right), John Flower, 88–114–005; John Flower, 92–110–66; John Flower, 92–110–24
page 299 (left to right), John Flower, PUB-92–111–20; John Flower, PUB-92–110–62; John Flower, PUB-92–110–05; John Flower, PUB-88–111–3
page 300 (left to right), John Flower, PUB-88–103–6; John Flower, PUB-88–108–14; John Flower, PUB-88–104–6
page 301 (left to right), John Flower, PUB-88–112–6; John Flower, PUB-88–105–19; John Flower, PUB-88–110–11
pages 302–303, Public Affairs Office, 91–161–26; Family photo, Pete Sandford; John Flower, PUB-92–110–51; John Flower, RN91–136025; PhotoBank, Inc., 92–378; PhotoBank, Inc., 92–372; John Flower, 92–110–41; John Flower, 92–110–11, John Flower, 92–110–06; Public Affairs Office, 911617
page 306, John Flower, 92–110–11
page 307, John Flower, 92–110–41
page 308, Pete Sandford
page 310, John Flower, 92–110–06
page 311, *Los Alamos Science* file
page 313, Public Affairs Office, 911617
pages 314–329, Steve Jordan, New York, *Los Alamos Science* file

Index

A

Aberrations, of chromosomes, 36. *See also* Mutations

Abortion, genetic information and, 309, 311, 322

ACEDB, 266

Acquired immune deficiency syndrome. *See* AIDS

Acute nonlymphocytic leukemia (ANLL), 182, 185, 206, 208, 212, 213

Adenine
DNA and, 38–41
RNA and, 48

Agarose gel, 55, 56

Agassiz, Jean Louis, 25

AIDS (acquired immune deficiency syndrome), 77, 138, 336. *See also* Autoimmune diseases

Alanine, codons for, 48

ALDOA deficiency, 185

Algorithms. *See* Computation; Software

Alkaptonuria, 37

Allele(s)
blending of, 20
defined, 19, 20, 22, 330
distance between pairs. *See* Genetic distance
dominant, 18–20, 22, 332
pairing of, 20, 22
recessive, 19, 20, 22, 336

α-globin gene, 224

Alpha satellite DNA, 187, 211

Altschul, S., 275

Alu
inter-Alu PCR, 133, 196, 198, 199, 203–204
repeats, 51, 186, 187, 330

Americans with Disabilities Act (ADA), 307–308, 325

Amino acids
codon preference rules, 276–278
codons for, 44, 45, 48, 64
defined, 330
listed, 48
protein structure and, 39, 44, 165
protein synthesis and, 45–48

Aminoacyl synthetases, 47

Aminoacyl-tRNAs, 46–47

Ampicillin-resistance genes, 224, 225

Amplifying
DNA, 58–60, 128–134
DNA libraries, 219–220, 235

Anaphase, defined, 14–15

Anemia, 185. *See also* Sickle-cell anemia

Aneuploidy, 80, 214

Animalcula, 4

ANLL (acute nonlymphocytic leukemia), 182, 185, 206, 208, 212, 213

Annotator's WorkBench, 271

Antibiotic resistance
genes for, 223–226
recombination and, 232
See also specific antibiotics

Anticipation, defined, 212

Anticodons, defined, 46–47

APRT deficiency, 185

Aquinas, Thomas, 3

Arginine, codons for, 48

Aristotle, 3–4

Asexual reproduction
of bacteria, 13
of single-celled eukaryotic organisms, 14

Asparagine, codons for, 48

Aspartic acid, codons for, 48

Autoimmune diseases, 139. *See also* AIDS; Immune receptor loci; Immunoglobulins

Autosomal chronic granulomatous disease, 185

Autosomal dominant Mendelian disorders, 26, 98

Autosomal recessive Mendelian disorders, 26–27

Autosomes, defined, 11, 12, 330

Avery, Oswald Theodore, 38

B

*Bacillus amyloliquefaciens. See Bam*HI

Bacon, Roger, 3

Bacteria
asexual reproduction of, 13
cell cycle of, 9
as host cells, 232
plasmids, 58–60, 220, 224–226, 232, 335
See also Bacteriophages; *Escherichia coli*; λ phages; Restriction enzymes

Bacterial transduction. *See* Transduction

Bacteriophages
defined, 37–38, 226–228, 330
libraries of, 226–228, 231–235, 241, 247
M13, 152, 156, 231–232, 235, 247–248, 284
ordering of genes on genetic maps of, 49
Phage Group, 37–38
See also λ phages

Baker's yeast. *See Saccharomyces cerevisiae*

Balding, David, 135, 190

Baltimore, David
on ELSI, 320–322, 324, 327
on mapping, 78
on revolutionizing biology, 78
on sequencing, 78, 80
vita, 180

*Bam*HI, 54, 225, 226, 238

Banding pattern, of metaphase chromosomes, 11, 33, 36, 169, 177, 330

Barber, William M., 267–269

Bartels, Dianne, 310–311

Bases
defined, 38–40
illustrated, 40–41
number in human genome, 71
See also Complementary base pairs

Basic local alignment search tool (BLAST), 275–276

Batten's disease (CLN3), 185, 207

Beadle, George Wells, 37

Benzer, Seymour, 45

Berg, Paul, vii, 277

β-globin gene, 219–220, 224, 248

Beth, T., 135

Beugelsdijk, Tony, 199

Biological information signal processing (BISP) chip, 275

Biology
advances in, technology and, 75–76
computation and, 256–257
current state of, 149–150
graduate students, 84, 110, 149
revolutionizing
general, 70, 83, 84, 85, 150, 168, 319
human multigenic-trait analysis, 78–80, 84, 320–322
human variable-trait analysis, 73–74, 78–79, 320–326
mapping and, 78, 79
sequencing and, 142
See also Cell biology; Structural biology

Biomedical community
chromosome 16 and, 185, 206

Biomedical community (*continued*)
individualized health-care delivery and, 82, 324
physical mapping and, 206
providing tools for, 82, 141, 150, 164
See also Diseases
Biophysics, 149
Biosynthesis, defined, 330
Biotechnology. *See* Technology development; Technology transfer
BISP (biological information signal processing) chip, 275
BLAST (basic local alignment search tool), 275–276
Blending
of alleles, 20
inheritance, 28
Blood cells
cell cycle of, 9
electron micrograph of, 7
pairing of different alleles and, 20
See also Anemia; Hemoglobin; Hemophilia
Blotting, defined, 63. *See also* Southern hybridization
Bohr, Niels, 149
Botstein, David
on disease-gene isolation, 76–77, 328
on ELSI, 321–322, 323, 324, 326, 327, 328
on gene-pool depletion, 327
on goals of Human Genome Project, 316–318
on informatics, 160, 161, 162, 163
on Mendel, 72
on model organisms, 78
on multigenic traits, 78, 328
on polymorphic DNA markers, 73, 76–77, 94
on protein function, 77
on revolutionizing biology, 79
on sequencing, 71, 79–80, 81
on STS markers, 123, 125–126
on student interest in genome field, 84
on technology development, 146, 147
on time line for Human Genome Project, 328, 329
vita, 180
Botstein, Leon, 315–316, 322–323, 328
Boveri, Theodor Heinrich, 12, 16, 28
Bradbury, E. Morton, 169–177, 298
Bread mold, 37

Breast cancer, 185, 208, 326–327
Brenner, Sydney, 44, 75
Breuning, Martijn, 207
Bridgers, Michael A., 267–269
Bridges, Calvin Blackman, 28, 30
Brown, Henry T., 258–261, 265
Bulbar muscular atrophy, 212
Burks, Christian
on DNA sequence data growth, 254–255
on electronic data publishing in GenBank, 270–272
listing of molecular biology database (LiMB) and, 273
on SCORE, 258–261
tRNA algorithm of, 276

C
Caenorhabditis elegans, embryonic lineage of, 106–107, 334. *See also Caenorhabditis elegans* genome; Nematodes
Caenorhabditis elegans genome
physical mapping of, 106, 107, 108, 109, 184, 185, 334
sequence data for, 272, 334
Calf intestinal alkaline phosphatase (CIP), 247
California Institute of Technology
genetic-linkage mapping technology, 126–127
immune receptor loci sequencing, 81, 139
interdisciplinary approach, 148
sequencing technology, 144, 145
Callen, David, 133, 193, 207
Cancer, 74, 185, 208, 319, 326–327
Canines, domestication of, 2
Cannon, T. Michael, 190, 258–261
Cantor, Charles, 184
Capillary-gel sequencing, 144
Cardiomyopathy, familial hypertrophic, 185
Cataracts, 185, 212
cDNA
defined, 138, 220, 330
gene density and, 136
gene expression and, 138–139
Human Genome Project goals, 137, 139
libraries of, 136, 138, 220, 233, 248–249
limitations of, 139
sequencing, 136–139
Cell biology, rise of, 4–5, 12–13, 16
Cell cycle, defined, 9

Cell division, discovery of, 5, 12. *See also* Meiosis; Mitosis
Cells
eukaryotic, 8–10
examples of, 6–7
germ-line cells, 15
plant, 8
somatic, 5
See also Gametes
Cell theory, 5
Centimorgans, defined, 31, 92, 330
Centre d'Etude du Polymorphisme Humain (CEPH), 140–141
Centromeres
defined, 10, 80, 168–169, 330
illustrated, 14, 15, 168
repetitive DNA sequences of, 188, 211, 213–214
Centrosomes, defined, 14–15
CETP deficiency, 185
Chargaff, Erwin, 39
Charon 21A, 239
Charon 40, 229, 238
Chase, Martha, 38
Children, genetic uniqueness of, 13, 16
Chimeras, defined, 330
Chimeric YACs, 105, 195–196, 231, 232, 243–245, 247
Chloroplasts, defined, 8
Cholinesterase gene inactivation, 212
Chromatin, 164–165, 170–176, 330
Chromatosomes, 170–173
Chromosome 1, number of base pairs, 184
Chromosome I (yeast), physical mapping of, 120–121
Chromosome III (yeast), sequencing of, 151, 252
Chromosome 4, physical mapping of, 111, 242
Chromosome 5, physical mapping of, 111, 206, 216–217, 242
Chromosome 7, physical mapping of, 111, 195
Chromosome 8, physical mapping of, 242
Chromosome 11, physical mapping of, 242
Chromosome 14, genetic-linkage mapping of, 127
Chromosome 16
aneuploidy of, 214
disease-gene isolation on, 185, 204–208, 211–213
future plans, 206

genetic-linkage mapping of, 93, 202–206
length of, 169
libraries for
    cosmids, 182, 184, 242
    YACs, 132–133, 135, 184, 195–196,
        206, 242–243, 246
number of base pairs, 184
number of cosmid clones to represent, 185
packing ratio of linear DNA molecule in
    metaphase, 169
photomicrograph of, 182–183
physical mapping of, 182–206
    assembling contig map, 191–193, 263,
        264, 265
    cytogenic breakpoint (hybrid-cell)
        map, 193–194, 202–205
    cytogenic map, 202–205
    disease-gene isolation and, 185, 204–
        208, 211–213
    flow-sorted chromosome libraries and,
        242
    gap closure, 132, 195–203, 206, 243
    genetic-linkage mapping and, 202–
        203, 204–206
    high resolution of, 204–206
    Human Genome Project goals, 206
    illustrated, 191–192, 194, 200–202,
        205
    information management for, 161,
        257, 262
    low-resolution mapping, 193–194,
        202–206
    overlap detection, 188–191, 193, 195,
        234–235
    overview of, 105, 111, 182–185
    reasons chromosome 16 selected for
        mapping, 183–184
    repetitive-sequence fingerprints and,
        186, 188–192, 193
    restriction-fragment fingerprints and,
        191–193
    strategy for, 185–186
    STS-content map, 206
    STS markers and, 131–133, 135, 195–
        197
    verifying map, 193–194, 200–201,
        203–204
    YACs and, 132–133, 135, 184, 195–
        203, 206, 242–243
repetitive DNA on, 182, 183, 186–187,
    203–204, 206, 211–213
uniqueness of, 211

Chromosome 17, physical mapping of, 242
Chromosome 19
    diseases and, 212
    physical mapping of, 105, 111, 242
Chromosome 21
    in-situ hybridization on, 112
    physical mapping of, 105, 111–113
    YAC libraries for, 195–196, 243
Chromosomes, 10–11, 168–177
    aberrations (rearrangements) of, 36
    aneuploidy of, 80, 214
    artificial, 42. See also YACs
    autosomes, 11, 12, 330
    centromeres
        defined, 10, 80, 168–169, 330
        illustrated, 14–15, 168
        repetitive DNA sequences of, 188,
            211, 213–214
    chromatin, 164–165, 170–176, 330
    chromatosomes, 170–173
    crossing over of. See Crossing over
    defined, 10–11, 168, 330
    diploid set, 5, 10, 12–13, 15, 331
    discovery of, 5
    DNA loops of, 169–170, 172–177
    equal segregation of, 13, 16, 19, 22
    euchromatin, 188
    flow-sorted, 195–196, 236–246
    function of, 10, 164–165, 169, 176–177
    haploid set, 5, 12, 13, 15, 333
    heterochromatin, 188
    histones, 10, 169, 170–173, 175, 177
    illustrated, 8, 10–11
    independent assortment of, 13, 16, 21,
        22, 25, 31, 86
    inversions of, 36
    length of human, 50, 92, 93
    mapping. See Genetic-linkage mapping;
        Physical mapping
    metaphase
        banding pattern of, 11, 33, 36, 169,
            177, 330
        defined, 10, 14, 15, 334
        DNA loops of, 169–170, 172–176
        homologous, 10, 12–13, 333
        karyotypes of, 11
        micrographs of, 10–11, 168, 188
        morphological differences of, 12
        nonhomologous sex chromosomes, 11–
            12
        packing ratio of linear DNA molecule
            in, 169

protein scaffold of, 169–170
sister-chromatid pairs, 14–15, 168–
    169, 174, 337
supercoiling of DNA and, 172, 173,
    174–176
visibility of, 10, 14, 36
nondisjunction of, 30–31
nucleosome core particles, 170–175
nucleosomes, 170–175
number for various species, 12, 112
number of human base pairs per chromo-
    some, 184
polytene, 36
protein scaffold of, 169–170
sex chromosomes, 11–12, 336–337
shape of, defined, 33
structure of, 10, 164–165, 168–177
telomeres
    defined, 40, 63, 80, 168–169, 337
    discovery of, 63
    repetitive DNA sequences of, 186,
        187, 211
    replication of, 42
    vertebrates share same telomeric
        sequence, 63
translocations of, 36, 337
See also DNA; DNA libraries; Genes;
    Meiosis; Mitosis; Specific
    chromosomes
Chromosome theory of heredity, birth of,
    28–30
Chromosome X. See X chromosome
Chu, Steve, 146
Cinkosky, Michael
    on contig assembly and analysis, 192,
        263
    on DNA sequence data growth, 254–255
    on Electronic Data Publishing in Gen-
        Bank, 270–272
    on SIGMA, 267–269
    vita, 298
CIP (calf intestinal alkaline phosphatase),
    247
cis elements, 64
ClaI, 206, 230, 243
Clam egg, electron micrograph of, 7
Classical genetics, 28–31, 33, 36, 330
Classical linkage mapping, 86–93
    anchoring a map, 36
    defined, 31, 73, 86
    disease-gene isolation and, 73, 94
    Human Genome Project goals, 73

Classical linkage mapping (*continued*)
   limitations, 73, 93, 94
   x-ray-induced mutations and, 33
Class II restriction endonucleases. *See*
      Restriction enzymes
Class II retrotransposons, 187
CLN3 (Batten's disease), 185, 207
Clones
   defined, 330–331
   storing, 124, 126, 131
   STS markers and, 110, 123, 124, 131
Cloning, 58–60, 219–232
   artifacts of, 144
   calf intestinal alkaline phosphatase (CIP)
         and, 247
   defined, 49, 58–60, 219–224, 334
   E. coli-based, 224–228, 229, 231–232
   efficiency of, 82
   historical background, 221–224
   host cells, 232
   Human Genome Project goals, 82, 221
   ideal insert size for libraries, 248–249
   lifetime of cloning systems, 124
   polymerase chain reaction vs., 60, 128
   problems and errors of, 247
   purpose of, 58, 112, 219
   technology improvements for, 221
   yeast-based, 228–231
   See also Cloning vectors; DNA libraries
Cloning vectors
   defined, 58, 114, 220, 331
   types of, 224–232
   See also Bacteriophages; Cosmids; λ
         phages; Plasmids; YACs
Codon preference rules, 276–278
Codons
   anticodons, 46–47
   computational description of, 252
   defined, 44–45, 48, 64, 331
   START codon, 48, 64, 331
   STOP codons, 48, 276, 331
Cohesive ends. *See* Sticky ends
Co-inheritance
   defined, 20, 73, 86
   disease and, 74
   Mendelian experiments, 20–21
   See also Genetic-linkage mapping
Collinearity hypothesis, 45
Color blindness, 26
Commonwealth Informatics, 273
Communication networks. *See* Computer
      networks

Complementary base pairs
   defined, 38–40, 331
   illustrated, 40–41
   number in each turn of double helix, 175
   number in human DNA molecule, 112,
      168
   number per human chromosome, 184
Complementary DNA. *See* cDNA
Complementary sequences, defined, 40,
   331
Computation, 160–163, 250–279
   BLAST (basic local alignment search
         tool), 275–276
   Commonwealth Informatics, 273
   databases and
      browsing, 262
      designing future, 141, 160–163
      integrating multiple, 266, 273
      speed of searching, 163, 274–276
      updating, 266
   dynamic-programming algorithm, 274–
      275
   Electronic Data Publishing and, 266,
      269, 270–272, 273
   FASTA, 275
   GCAA (Genetic Contig Assembly Algo-
         rithm), 192, 263–265
   GeneID, 278
   gene location and interpretation and,
         162, 273–274, 276–278
   genetic algorithms, 263
   genetic programming language, 252–
      253, 273–274, 278
   GM (gene modeler), 278
   human genome described in computa-
         tional terms, 252–253, 256
   Human Genome Project goals, 141, 160–
      163, 257
   importance to Human Genome Project,
      250, 256–257
   interface software and, 262, 265
   molecular biology and, 256–257
   networking and, 256, 266, 273
   physical map assembly and, 162, 192,
      263–265
   region methods, 278
   SCORE (Southern Blot scoring), 190,
      258–261, 262
   sequencing and
      assembly of sequences, 162–163
      data management, 254–255, 266,
         270–276

   pattern recognition, 162, 256, 257
   similarity analysis, 162, 274–276
   SIGMA (system for integrated genome
         map assembly), 265, 267–269
   single-molecule spectroscopy in solution
         and, 292–294
   See also Databases; Software
Computer networks, 256, 266, 273. *See
   also* Electronic Data Publishing
Computers, DNA technology development
   and, 150
Concatamers, 226, 227
Confidentiality, genetic, 304, 308–309,
   312, 318, 326–327
Contigs, 98–99, 103–104, 108–110, 113–
   122
   branching, 109, 122
   for *Caenorhabditis elegans*, 106–109,
      184–185, 334
   for chromosome 16, 131–133, 185–206
   collecting clones for, 114–115
   constructing maps
      incremental approach, 108–109, 115–
         122, 185–206, 263
      optimization approach, 118, 192, 263–
         265, 268–269
      with SIGMA (system for integrated
         genome map assembly), 265–
         269
      by STS-content mapping, 125, 195,
         206, 216–217
   with cosmid clones, 103–105, 111, 119,
      125, 184–206
   defined, 98, 103–104, 113, 331
   disconnected, 103–104, 108–122, 196–
      203
   disease-gene isolation and, 74, 76–78,
      98–99, 106, 111, 204–206
   for *Escherichia coli*, 121, 184–186
   fitness criterion for, 263
   gap closure
      by fingerprinting, 119, 121
      by walking, 121–122, 143, 195, 234–
         235, 265
      with YACs, 103–104, 132–133, 195–
         203, 206, 243
   genetic-linkage maps and, 98–99, 111,
      120, 126, 142, 202–206
   illustrated, 99, 113, 119, 120
      for chromosome 16, 191, 192, 194,
         200–202, 205
   with λ-phage clones, 103–104

low-resolution, 125, 195, 206, 216–217
overlap detection
overview of, 103
repetitive-sequence fingerprints and,
109–110, 186, 188–191, 193
restriction-fragment fingerprints and,
57, 108, 110, 115–119, 125, 186
STS markers and, 110, 122–123, 125,
131–133, 135, 195
problems with, 103–105, 108–109, 122
for *Saccharomyces cerevisiae*, 106–109,
119–121, 123–124, 184–186
time required for mapping, 103, 108–
109, 122, 186
verifying maps, 120–121, 193–194,
200–201, 203–204
with YAC clones
cosmid clones and, 104, 111
gap closure and, 103–104, 132–133,
195–203, 206, 243
importance of, 103–104, 110
improving YAC cloning techniques
and, 195–196
problems with, 105
size of, 103–105, 110, 122
STS markers and high-resolution contigs, 132–133, 135
STS markers and low-resolution contigs, 125, 195, 206, 216–217
See also Physical mapping
Copy DNA. *See* cDNA
Copying DNA. *See* Amplifying; Replicating DNA
Copy number, fractionation by, 50–52
Corn. *See Zea mays*
Corneal opacities, 185
Correns, Karl Erich, 16
Cosmids
chromosome-specific libraries and, 239–
242
cloning with, 228, 235, 239–242, 247–
249
defined, 58–59, 115, 228, 331
libraries of, 182, 184, 228, 241–242,
247
physical mapping with, 103–105, 111,
119, 125
chromosome 16 and, 182, 184–206
YACs and, 104, 111
cos sites, 226–228
Costs
of cystic-fibrosis-gene isolation, 79

of Human Genome Project, 82, 85, 103,
318
of sequencing cDNA, 139
of sequencing DNA, 61, 139, 151, 159,
252–253, 281
of STSs, 125
See also Funding
*Cot*1 DNA, 187–190, 193
Counseling, genetic, 309–312, 324
Cox, David
on disease-gene isolation, 79
on ELSI, 179
on genetic-linkage mapping, 73, 82
on physical mapping, 82, 103, 105, 110,
111
on sequencing, 82, 142
on STS markers, 127
on technology development, 142, 150
on tools for scientific community, 84
vita, 180
Crick, Francis Harry Compton
DNA structure discovered by, 38–39
genetic code and, 44
on protein synthesis, 45–46
on repetitive DNA, 211
Cri du chat syndrome, 217
Crossing over
defined, 15, 31–32, 88, 331
discovery of, 33–34
frequency of, 31, 73, 88, 92
genetic-linkage mapping and genetic distance and, 31–35, 73, 88–93
genetic uniqueness and, 14, 31
illustrated, 15, 32, 88
probability variability of, 91–93
Cuénot, Lucien Claude, 36–37
Cysteine, codons for, 48
Cystic fibrosis
contig of YAC clones containing gene
for, 195
cost to isolate gene for, 79
described, 311
discrimination against carriers of, 307
frequency of, 311
genetic-linkage mapping and, 256
inheritance of, 26–27, 86
isolation of gene for, 79, 273–274
length of gene for, 50
multidrug-resistance gene and, 77, 317
polymorphous DNA markers and, 74
small-insert libraries and, 239
testing program for, 178–179, 311–312

unpredictability of, 324
verifying gene for, 142
Cytogenic breakpoint maps, for chromo-
some 16, 193, 194, 202–205
Cytogenic maps, for chromosome 16, 202–
205
Cytogenics, defined, 33, 331
Cytology, defined, 331
Cytomegalovirus genome, sequencing of,
151
Cytoplasm, defined, 331
Cytosine, 38–41, 48

D
Dangers, of recombinant organisms, 232
Darwin, Charles, 3, 25, 28
Databases
Annotator's WorkBench, 271
browsing, 262
for chromosome 16, 161, 257
Commonwealth Informatics, 273
developing new, 141, 160–163
Electronic Data Publishing and, 266,
269, 270–273
GenBank, 254–255, 266, 270–276
genetic databank guideline development,
308
Genome DataBase (GDB), 160, 162
Human Genome Project goals, 141, 160–
162
inaccessibility of data in existing, 160, 266
integrating multiple, 266, 273
Listing of Molecular Biology Database
(LiMB), 273
for physical mapping, 161–163, 257,
260–262, 267–269
public access to, 160, 163
retrieval from, 163, 266, 275
for sequencing data, 163, 254–255, 266,
270–276
speed of searching, 163, 274–276
updating, 266
Daughter cells, defined, 14
Davis, Lloyd M.
on rapid DNA sequencing, 280–285
on single-molecule spectroscopy in solution, 286–296
Davis, Ronald W., 94
ddNTPs (dideoxynucleoside triphosphates),
156
Deaven, Larry L.
on DNA libraries, 218–235, 247–249

Index

Deaven, Larry L. (*continued*)
 on libraries from flow-sorted chromosomes, 236–246
 vita, 249, 298
Delbruck, Max, 37
DeLisi, Charles, 71
Democritus, 4
Denaturation, defined, 42, 51, 331
Deoxyribonucleic acid. *See* DNA
Deoxyribonucleoside triphosphates (dNTPs), 42–43, 156, 282, 284
Deoxyribonucleotides. *See* Nucleotides
Department of Energy (DOE)
 "Assessing Genetic Risks" study, 311
 ELSI and, 167, 304, 309, 312, 318–319
 five-year plan for Human Genome Project, 74
 funding for Human Genome Project, 82, 141, 143
 Health and Environment Research Advisory Committee workshop and report, 71
 inaccessibility of data at, 160
 number of genome centers, 83
 sequencing without doing biology and, 81
Development, study of, 79–80, 166–167
Dideoxy chain termination (Sanger) sequencing method, 151–153, 156–158, 232, 247–248, 254
Dideoxynucleoside triphosphates (ddNTPs), 156
Dihybrid, defined, 20
2,8-dihydroxyadenine, in APRT deficiency, 185
Dinucleotide repeats. *See* GT repeats
Diploid chromosome set, defined, 5, 10, 12–13, 15, 331
Discrimination, genetic. *See* ELSI (ethical, legal, and social implications)
Diseases
 aneuploidy and, 80
 computational technology and, 274
 ethical, legal, and social issues. *See* ELSI
 gene isolation for
  on chromosome 16, 185, 204–208, 211–213
  computational techniques for, 276–278
  *Cot*1 hybridization and, 193
  curing disease and, 77–78
  genetic-linkage mapping and, 73–74,

76–79, 94–99, 111, 142, 204–206, 256
 Huntington's Disease, 111, 142
 physical mapping and, 74, 76–78, 98–99, 106, 111, 204–206
 sequencing technology and, 142
gene regulation and, 165–166
Human Genome Project goals, 25, 72–74, 76–79, 97–99, 106, 142–143, 318–319
Mendelian disorders, 25–27, 72–73, 86, 98
from recombinant organisms, 232
repetitive DNA and, 211–212
STS markers and, 124, 126
testing programs for, 178–179, 308–309, 311–312, 326–327
See also Biomedical community; *specific diseases*
Distance, genetic. *See* Genetic distance
Diversity, genetic, factors increasing, 31, 32
DNA (deoxyribonucleic acid)
 alpha satellite, 187, 211
 Alu repeats, 51, 186–187, 330
 amplifying, 58–60, 128–134
 chromatin, 164–165, 170–171, 330
 as chromosome component, 10
 cloning. *See* Cloning
 codons for amino acids, 44–45, 48, 64, 331
 *Cot*1, 187–190, 193
 defined, 40–41, 331–332
 denaturation of, 42, 51, 331
 exceptional nature of DNA molecules, 39
 flexibility of, 171
 fractionation of fragments of
  by copy number and repetitive DNA, 50–52
  by length. *See* Gel electrophoresis
 fragmentation of
  length of fragments, 50, 52–53, 103–104
  location of breaks, 41
  mechanical, 52
  with restriction enzymes, 52–54, 114, 221–223, 336
  symbolic representation of fragments, 41
 gel electrophoresis of. *See* Gel electrophoresis

genetic information flows from DNA to RNA to protein, 45–46
as genetic material, early support for, 38
hybridization of. *See* Hybridization
illustrated, 40–41, 67
L1 repeats, 187
length of human, 39, 50, 168
negative supercoiling of, 175–176
number of base pairs in each turn of double helix, 175
number of base pairs in human DNA molecule, 112, 168
number of human DNA molecules, 112
patenting sequence fragments, 139, 163
polymerase chain reaction (PCR) and. *See* Polymerase chain reaction
polymorphisms of, 73–74, 94, 324
See also Polymorphic DNA markers
probes. *See* Probes
protein synthesis and, 38–40, 44–47
reading frames, 276–277
recombinant. *See* Recombinant DNA molecules; Recombination
renaturation of, 51–52
repetitive, 50–52, 109–110, 186–187
 amount of, 50, 211
 on chromosome 16, 182–183, 186–187, 203–204, 206, 211–213
 classes of, 186–187
 defined, 50–51, 109–110, 211, 336
 discovery of, 51
 diseases and, 211–212
 function of, 65, 109, 211, 336
 renaturation and, 51–52
replication of
 defined, 39, 42–43, 332
 histone acetylation and, 171, 175
 illustrated, 42–43
 interphase and, 9
 lysine acetylation and, 171
 nucleosome supercoil and, 174
 origins-of-replication base sequence and, 42
 semiconservative nature of, 39
RNA compared to, 44
sample preparation for, 50, 58
satellite repeats, 186–191, 193, 211, 336. *See also* GT repeats
sense strands, 45–46, 48, 64, 276
sequencing. *See* Sequencing DNA
stereoscopic image of, 67
structure of, 33, 38–41

344

STSs. *See* STSs (sequence-tagged sites)
supercoiling of, 172–176
telomeres
    defined, 40, 63, 80, 168–169, 337
    discovery of, 63
    repetitive DNA sequences of, 186–187, 211
    replication of, 42
    vertebrates share same telomeric sequence, 63
template strands, 44–45, 64
transcription of
    defined, 44–46, 64, 337
    histone acetylation and, 171, 175
    illustrated, 46, 64
    lysine acetylation and, 171
    nucleosome supercoil and, 174
    reverse, 46, 138, 336
uncoiling of, 171, 174
Watson and Crick and, 38–39
See also cDNA; Chromosomes; Genes
DNA fingerprints, defined, 332. *See also* Repetitive-sequence fingerprints; Restriction-fragment fingerprints
DNA libraries, 218–235
    amplifying, 219–220, 235
    bacteriophage, 226–228, 231–235, 241, 247
    cDNA, 136, 138, 220, 233, 248–249
    from cellular DNA, 232–235
    chromosome-specific
        for chromosome 16
            cosmids, 182, 184, 242
            YACs, 132–133, 135, 184, 195–196, 206, 242–243, 246
        for chromosome 21, 195–196, 243
        creators of, 114, 184, 195
        from flow-sorted chromosomes, 195–196, 236–246
        STS markers and, 195, 247–248
    constructing, 224–235
    contig maps and, 114–115
    cosmid, 182, 184, 228, 241–242, 247
    defined, 60, 114–115, 220–221, 224, 332
    for *Drosophila melanogaster*, 223–224
    duplicating for distribution, 246
    E. coli-based cloning and, 224–229, 232–233
    from flow-sorted chromosomes, 195–196, 236–246
    historical background, 221–224

host cells, 232
hybrid-cell, 235
ideal cloning system for, 249
large-insert (partial-digest), 239–242
locations of, 114
microdissection libraries, 248
National Laboratory Gene Library Project, 114, 184, 236
new directions in, 247–249
plasmid, 224–226, 247
problems and errors in cloning and, 247
purpose of, 114, 221
restriction enzymes and, 221–223
screening, 221, 232–235, 246
small-insert (complete-digest) libraries, 239
steps in preparing, 115
storing, 241–242, 247
for STS marker construction, 247–248
types of, 220–221, 224, 239–242
walking and, 234–235
YAC
    average insert size, 231
    chimeras in, 231
    for chromosome 16, 132–133, 135, 184, 195–196, 206, 242–243, 246
    for chromosome 21, 195–196, 243
    from flow-sorted chromosomes, 133, 195–196, 242–246
    overview of, 184, 228–231
    pooling scheme for PCR-based screening, 132–133, 135, 197
    storing, 247
    STS markers and, 132–133, 195
    See also Cloning
DNA ligase, 59, 114, 222–223
DNA loops, 169–170, 172–177
DNA polymerases
    function of, 39, 42–43, 335
    nucleosome core particles and, 171
    proofreading capability of, 42
DNA sequences
    defined, 332
    patenting, 139, 163
    See also Sequencing DNA
dNTPs (deoxyribonucleoside triphosphates), 42–43, 156, 282, 284
DOE. *See* Department of Energy
Doggett, Norman A.
    on chromosome 16 mapping, 182–210

on chromosome 16 repetitive DNA, 211–215
on polymerase chain reaction and STSs, 128–134
vita, 299
Domestication, of animals and food plants, 2
Dominant alleles, 18–20, 22, 332
Donis-Keller, Helen, 127
Doolittle, R., 256
Downstream, defined, 64
Down syndrome, 30
Drake, N., 278
Drosophila melanogaster
    classical genetics and, 28–30, 33, 36
    development of, 166–167
    DNA library for, 223–224
    eye color experiments, 29–30
    gene regulation in, 167
    genetic-linkage mapping and, 33–35
    homeobox genes, 166
    number of chromosomes, 12
    salivary gland cells, polytene interphase chromosomes of, 36
    segmentation genes, 166
    sex chromosomes, 12
    x-ray-induced mutations in, 33
Duchenne muscular dystrophy, 27, 50, 77–78
Duplicating DNA. *See* Amplifying; Replicating DNA
Durbin, R., 266
Duster, Troy, 306
Dynamic-programming algorithm, 274–275

E
*Eag*I, 243
E. coli. *See* Escherichia coli
*Eco*RI
    defined, 52–54, 57, 59, 221–223
    repetitive-sequence fingerprints, 188–191
    restriction-fragment fingerprints, 57, 116–119
    restriction-site maps, 57, 119
    star activity and, 247
Education
    in genetic information
        overview of, 304
        professional, 312, 313
        public, 167, 178, 304, 311, 312, 313
    See also Graduate students
Eggs. *See* Gametes

Electronic Data Publishing, 266, 269, 270–273

Electrophoresis. *See* Gel electrophoresis

ELSI (ethical, legal, and social implications), 167, 178–179, 302–313
  abortion, 309, 311, 322
  Americans with Disabilities Act, 307–308, 325
  carriers of diseases, 307
  cystic fibrosis pilot studies, 178–179, 311–312
  delivery of genetic services, 304, 309–312, 324
  education
    overview of, 304
    professional, 312–313
    public, 167, 178, 311–313
  employment discrimination, 178, 305–308, 318, 327
  eugenics, 322–324, 327–328
  fairness and discrimination issues, 167, 178–179, 304–308, 318–319
  free-will issue, 323, 325–326
  funding for, 167, 304
  gene-pool depletion, 327–328
  genetic counseling, 309–312, 324
  genetic databanks, 309
  genetic testing, 178–179, 308–309, 311–312, 326–327
  Human Genome Project goals, 141, 167, 178–179
  human variability issues, 320, 323–326
  insurance industry
    discrimination by, 303, 305–308, 318, 327
    genetic testing and, 178, 308, 318, 327
    increases in genetic information unwelcome by, 167, 178
    Insurance Task Force, 308
    laws affecting, 307
  international issues, 327–329
  legal issues, 307–309
  library for, 312
  privacy issues, 304, 308–309, 312, 318, 326–327
  purpose of, 167, 178–179, 303–304, 318–319, 321, 324–325
  racial and ethnic discrimination, 306–307
  sex selection, 311, 322, 327
  types of issues addressed, 167, 178, 304
  what needs to be studied, 178–179

See also Hazards, of recombinant organisms

Embryonic cells, cell cycle of, 9

Employment discrimination, genetic information and, 178, 305, 306–308, 318, 327

Encapsulation theory, 4

Encyclopedia of the Mouse, 265–266

Endonuclease restriction enzymes, type II. *See* Restriction enzymes

Endonucleases, defined, 54

Endoplasmic reticulum, defined, 8, 74

Engineering, DNA technology development and, 147

Enhancers, defined, 64

Entelechy, 3

Enzymes
  aminoacyl synthetases, 47
  defined, 37, 252, 332
  DNA replication and, 39, 42
  exonucleases, 281, 285
  micrococcal nuclease, 170
  one gene-one enzyme hypothesis, 37
  polymerases, 335
  protein synthesis and, 46–47
  purpose of, 252
  reverse transcriptase, 138, 187, 336
  topoisomerase II, 170
  See also DNA polymerase; Restriction enzymes; RNA polymerase

Epigenesis, 4

Epithelial cells, cell cycle of, 9

Equal segregation of chromosomes, 13, 16, 19, 22

Escherichia coli
  cloning and, 49, 58–60, 218–220, 224–229, 232
  electron micrograph of, 6
  extensive study of, 37
  generation time of, 60
  as host cell, 152, 232
  illustrated, 218–219
  ordering of genes on genetic maps of, 49
  penicillin and study of, 76
  plasmids, 58–60, 220, 224–226, 232, 335
  See also Bacteria; Bacteriophages; Cosmids; *Eco*RI; *Escherichia coli* genome; λ phages

Escherichia coli genome, physical mapping of, 121, 184–186

Ethical implications. *See* ELSI

Ethidium-bromide visualization technique, 55, 188–190

Ethnic discrimination, genetic information and, 306–307

Euchromatin, defined, 188

Eugenics, 322–324, 327–328

Eukaryotes
  asexual reproduction of single-celled, 14
  cells
    components of, 8, 10
    cycle of, 9
    protein synthesis in, 45–47
  defined, 5, 332
  gene isolation in, 276–278
  linearity of DNA molecules in, 33, 330
  prokaryotes vs., 45–47, 49, 334
  protein genes, 64–65
  repetitive DNA in, 50–52

Europe, investment in large-scale projects by, 140–141

Evolution
  theory of, 25, 28
  understanding, as Human Genome Project outcome, 166, 193

Exons
  defined, 45, 64, 332
  identifying, 137, 276, 278
  percentage of human genome, 80
  See also cDNA

Exonucleases, 281, 285

Expression, of genes, 65, 138–139, 164–166, 276, 332

F

Fairfield, Frederick R., 280–285

Fairness issues, genetic. *See* ELSI

Familial hypertrophic cardiomyopathy, 185

Familial Mediterranean fever (FMF), 185, 207–208

Farber, R., 278

FASTA, 275

Femaleness, X chromosome and, 12

Fibroblasts, 6, 9

Fichant, G., 276

Fickett, James W.
  on computation and the Human Genome Project, 250–253, 256–257, 262–266, 273–279
  contig assembly and analysis and, 161–162, 192
  on Electronic Data Publishing in GenBank, 270–272
  on SCORE, 258–261

on SIGMA, 267–269
vita, 279, 299
Fields, Chris, 162, 278
Fingerprints, defined, 332. *See also*
    Repetitive-sequence fingerprints;
    Restriction-fragment fingerprints
Fink, Monica, 299
Five-year goals (Human Genome Project),
    140–141, 150, 329. *See also* Human
    Genome Project, goals/outcomes of
Flow cytometry, defined, 332
Flow-sorted chromosomes, libraries from,
    195–196, 236–246
Fluorescence quantum yield, 286, 289
Fluorescence visualization techniques
    for gel electrophoresis, 55, 159, 188–190
    for in-situ hybridization, 62–63, 112
    for single-molecule-detection method,
        282–283, 286–295
FMF. *See* Familial Mediterranean fever
Ford, Amanda A., 258–261
Foreign issues. *See* International issues
Fractionation of DNA fragments
    by copy number and repetitive DNA,
        50–52
    by length. *See* Gel electrophoresis
Fragile X site, 211
Fragmentation of DNA
    length of fragments, 50, 52–53, 103–104
    location of breaks, 41
    mechanical, 52
    with restriction enzymes, 52–54, 57–58,
        75, 221–223
    symbolic representation of fragments, 41
Franklin, Rosalind, 39
Free will, genetic information and, 323,
    325–326
Friedman, Gerald, on ELSI, 302–313
Frischauf, Anna-Maria, 207
Fruit fly. *See* Drosophila melanogaster
Funding
    for ELSI, 167, 304
    for Human Genome Project, 82, 85,
        140–141, 143, 320
    See also Costs

G

G_1 phase, of interphase, 9, 14
G_2 phase, of interphase, 9, 14
Gaertner, Joseph, 17
Galas, David
    on chromosome structure, 164–165, 168
    on disease-gene isolation, 79

on dispersed nature of Human Genome
    Project, 83
on ELSI, 167, 178
on informatics, 160–163
on physical mapping, 105, 140
on revolutionizing biology, 84–85
on sequencing
    cDNA, 136–137
    technology for, 143–145
on technology development, 143–145,
    150
vita, 180
Galileo, microscope and, 4
Galton, Francis, 28
Gametes
    chance and, 19–20
    defined, 5, 332
    discovery of cellular nature of, 5
    meiosis and, 13, 15
    Mendelian genetics and, 18–19
Garden pea. *See Pisum sativum*
Gardiner, Mark, 207
Garrod, Archibald Edward, 37
GCAA (Genetic Contig Assembly Algo-
    rithm), 118, 192, 263–265
GDB (Genome DataBase), 160, 162
Gel electrophoresis
    with agarose gel, 55–56
    defined, 53, 55–58, 332
    examples of, 56
    hybridization and, 62–63
    with polyacrylamide gel, 55, 153, 157–
        158
    pulsed-field, 55–56, 58, 104, 184
    visualization techniques
        autoradiograms, 63, 189, 190
        fluorescence, 55, 159, 188–190
Gel-transfer hybridization. *See* Southern
    hybridization
GenBank, 254–255, 266, 270–272, 273,
    274–276
GeneID, 278
Gene Library Project, 114, 184, 236
Gene Modeler (GM), 278
Gene-pool depletion, 327–328
Generations, defined, 17–18
Genes
    alleles
        blending of, 20
        defined, 19–20, 22, 330
        distance between pairs. *See* Genetic
           distance
        dominant, 18–20, 22, 332

        pairing of, 20, 22
        recessive, 19–20, 22, 336
    antibiotic-resistant, 223–224
    chromosome rearrangements and, 36
    collinearity hypothesis, 45
    composition of, 38–39, 64
    computer recognition of, 276–278
    current state of knowledge about, 65
    defined, 16, 18, 22, 65, 276, 332
    density of, cDNA and, 136
    discovery of, 16, 72
    distance between. *See* Genetic distance
    evolution of, 61
    expression of, 65, 138, 139, 164–166,
        276, 332
    function of, 36–37, 39, 61, 274
    homeobox, 166
    housekeeping, 65
    introduction of term "gene," 18, 22
    isolating
        on chromosome 16, 185, 204–208,
           211–213
        computational techniques for, 276–278
        *Cot*1 hybridization and, 193
        genetic-linkage mapping and, 73–74,
           76–79, 94–99, 111, 142, 204–
           206, 256
        for Huntington's disease, 111, 142
        physical mapping and, 74, 76–78, 98–
           99, 106, 111, 204–206
        sequencing technology and, 142
    "jumping," 187
    length of human, 50, 71
    linked, 86, 334. *See also* Genetic-linkage
        mapping
    mapping. *See* Genetic-linkage mapping;
        Physical mapping
    master, 166
    Mendel and, 16, 18
    for Mendelian traits, 73
    number of human genes, 65, 136–137,
        170
    one gene-one enzyme hypothesis, 37
    outstanding questions about, 65
    promoter segment of, 46, 64, 164–165,
        335–336
    protein, 64–65, 136–139, 164–165,
        276–279
    regulation of, 64–65, 79–80, 164–166,
        177, 276, 332–333
    sense strands, 45–46, 48, 64, 276
    template strands, 44–45, 64
    See also Chromosomes; DNA; Mutations

Genetic code
  defined, 48, 333
  organism-independence of, 48
  protein synthesis and, 45–46, 48
Genetic Contig Assembly Algorithm
    (GCAA), 118, 192, 263–265
Genetic continuity, law of, 5
Genetic counseling, 309–312, 324
Genetic databanks, developing guidelines
    for, 308
Genetic distance
  defined, 31–32, 73, 92–93, 333
  determining, 34–35
  physical distance and, 92–93
  recombination fractions and, 31–35, 91–
    92
Genetic diversity, factors increasing, 31–32
Genetic information, flows from DNA to
    RNA to protein, 45, 46. *See also* ELSI
Genetic-linkage mapping
  of chromosome 14, 127
  of chromosome 16, 93, 202–206
  classical, 86–93
    anchoring a map, 36
    defined, 31, 73, 86–93
    disease-gene isolation and, 73, 94
    first map created, 33
    Human Genome Project goals, 73
    limitations of, 73, 93, 94
    x-ray-induced mutants and, 33
  defined, 333
  for model organisms, 77–78, 141
  modern (with polymorphic DNA mark-
    ers), 94–99
    acceleration of search for markers, 99,
      133–134
    automated techniques for, 126–127
    base-sequence variation and, 94–96
    of chromosome 16, 93, 202–203
    constructing maps, 97, 112–113
    definition of markers, 73–74, 94, 335
    development of markers, 73, 94
    disease-gene isolation and, 73–74,
      76–79, 94–99, 111, 142, 204–
      206, 256
    existing maps for human genome, 127
    finding markers, 96, 126–127
    Human Genome Project goals
      atlas of chromosome maps, 256
      disease-gene isolation, 72–74, 76–
        79, 97–99
      emphasis on, 71, 73–74, 76, 78–
        79, 82, 97

    kit of 150 polymorphic markers, 84,
      127
    polymorphic DNA markers with
      STSs, 74, 97, 99, 126, 140,
      141
    importance of, 73–74, 76–79, 94, 97
    informativeness of markers, 98, 100–
      102, 134
    kit of 150 markers, 84, 127
    physical mapping and, 98–99, 111,
      120, 126, 142, 202–206
    restriction fragment length polymor-
      phisms (RFLPs), 96–97
    STS markers and, 126–127, 133–134,
      141
    universal language for, 123
  of *Mus musculus* genome, 137, 141
  radiation-hybrid mapping, 111
  and revolutionizing biology, 78–79
  single-copy probes and, 239
Genetic Privacy Collaboration, 309
Genetics
  birth of science of, 28
  classical, 28–31, 33, 36, 330
  Mendelian, 16–27, 72
  molecular
    defined, 334
    rise of, 36–39, 44, 49
    techniques of, 49–53, 57–62
  terminology of, 18–19
  See also Heredity
Genetic testing, 178–179, 308–309, 311–
    312, 326–327
Genome DataBase (GDB), 160, 162
Genomes
  defined, 333
  evolution of, 61, 65
  function of, 61, 65
  molecular genetics techniques and, 65
  See also Cytomegalovirus genome; *Esche-
    richia coli* genome; *Homo sapiens*
    genome; λ-phage genome; *Mus mus-
    culus* genome; *Saccharomyces cere-
    visiae* genome
Genotypes
  defined, 19, 22, 333
  independent inheritance of, 21
  introduction of term "genotype," 19
  probability of, 19–20
Germ-line cells, defined, 15
Gilbert, Walter, 71, 75, 147, 151, 254. *See
    also* Maxam–Gilbert sequencing
  method

Gilna, Paul, 254–255, 270–272
Gish, W., 275
Glossary, 330–337
Glutamic acid, codons for, 48
Glutamine, codons for, 48
Glycine, codons for, 48
Glycogen-storage disease, 185
GM (Gene Modeler), 278
Goad, Walter, 270
Goals. *See* Human Genome Project, goals/
    outcomes of
Golgi apparatus, defined, 8
Graduate students
  interest in genome field, 84, 110
  molecular-biology, 84, 149
Grady, Deborah, 206, 216–217
GRAIL, 137
Granulomatous disease, autosomal chronic,
    185
Gray, Joe, 208
Greeks, on heredity, 3–4
Green, Eric, 135, 195
Grew, Nehemiah, 4
Growth-hormone gene, 248
GT repeats, 51, 186, 187, 188–191, 193,
    211, 333
Guanine, 38–41, 48
Guigo, R., 278
Gusella, Jim, 142

H
H1, 170–173, 175
*Hae*III, 54
*Haemophilus aegyptius. See Hae*III
*Haemophilus influenzae. See Hind*II
Hahn, Jong Hoong, 280–285
Haldane, J. B. S., 92, 137
Haldane's mapping function, 92
Hall, Ben, 107
Hammond, Mark L., 280–285
Hamsters, hybrid-cell lines, 235
Haploid chromosome set, defined, 5, 12–
    13, 15, 333
Harger, Carol A., 280–285
Harvey, William, 2, 4
Hazards, of recombinant organisms, 232
HDL, elevated, 185
Heart disease, 319, 324
Hemoglobin
  disorders of, chromosome 16 and, 185
  normal and sickle, 39, 44
  See also Blood cells; Sickle-cell anemia
Hemolytic anemia, 185

Hemophilia, 27, 212
Hempfner, Philip E., 258–261
Heredity, 1–67
    chromosomes and, 10–11, 28, 36
    co-inheritance, 20–21, 73–74, 86
    crossing over and, 15, 31–32, 88, 331
    diseases and. *See* Diseases
    eukaryotic cell components and, 8
    eukaryotic cell cycle and, 9
    genetic distance and, 34–35
    historical perspective
        cell biology, 4–5, 12–13, 16
        chromosome theory of heredity, 28–30
        classical genetics, 28–31, 33, 36
        early ideas, 3, 17
        evolution, theory of, 25, 28
        Mendelian genetics, 16–27, 72
        molecular genetics, 36–39, 44, 49–53, 57–62
        overview of, 2, 4
    humans as inheritance study subjects, 25, 35
    meiosis and, 15
    Mendelian disorders and, 25–27, 72–73, 86, 98
    mitosis and, 14
    nondisjunction and, 30–31
    uniqueness of, 13, 16, 31–32
    unlinked traits and, 86
Hershey, Alfred Day, 37–38
Heterochromatin, defined, 188
Heterozygous, defined, 19, 22, 333
High-density lipoprotein (HDL), elevated, 185
Hildebrand, Carl E.
    on chromosome 16 mapping, 182–210
    on informativeness of polymorphic DNA markers, 100–101
    vita, 299
*Hin*dII, 54
*Hin*dIII, 56, 188–191
Hippocrates, 3
Histidine, codons for, 48
Histones
    acetylation of, 171, 175
    as chromosome component, 10, 169, 170–173, 175, 177
    octamers, 170, 172
HIV. *See* AIDS
Hollen, Bob, 199
Holmes, Oliver Wendell, 323
Homeobox genes, 166

Homologous chromosomes, defined, 10, 12–13, 333
Homologous sequences, defined, 333
Homo sapiens
    genetic uniqueness of individuals, 13, 16, 31, 32
    higher apes vs., gene regulation and, 65
    as inheritance study subjects, 25, 35
    karyotype of, 11
    See also Homo sapiens genome
Homo sapiens genome
    computational description of, 252
    current state of knowledge about, 65, 70
    defined, 71, 112, 124, 252, 333
    development of humans and, 79–80, 166–167
    function of, 81, 137, 252
    length of chromosomes, 92–93
    length of DNA molecules, 50, 93, 112, 168
    length of genes, 71
    molecular-genetics techniques and, 65
    mouse genome and, 65, 136–137, 139, 167
    multigenic-trait analysis and, 78–80, 84, 320–322, 328
    non-protein-coding regions, significance of, 80–81
    number of base pairs in, 168, 184
    number of bases in, 71
    number of chromosomes in, 12, 112
    number of genes in, 65, 136–137, 170
    outstanding questions about, 65
    repetitive DNA in, 50, 109–110, 186–187, 211
    sequencing of
        percentage sequenced, 253
        whole vs. part
            economics of, 80, 139
            meaninglessness of argument, 139
            stupidity of sequencing whole, 71, 78, 317–318
            technological limitations on sequencing whole, 71, 80, 142–143, 151
            value of sequencing part, 81, 139, 142
            value of sequencing whole, 80–81, 151, 252, 253
    variable-trait analysis and, 73–74, 78–79, 320–326
    See also Diseases; Human Genome Proj-

ect; *specific chromosomes; specific diseases*
Homozygous, defined, 333
Homozygous dominant, defined, 19, 22
Homozygous recessive, defined, 19, 22
Homunculi, 4
Hood, Leroy
    on funding for Human Genome Project, 85, 140–141
    on informatics, 162
    on sequencing
        and biology, 71, 81–83
        cDNA, 139
        technology for, 143–145
    on STS markers, 126–127
    on technology development, 143–145, 147–148
    vita, 180
Hooke, Robert, 4
Horowitz, Norman Harold, one gene-one enzyme hypothesis, 37
Host cells, 232
Housekeeping genes, 65
House mouse. *See Mus musculus*
Hsu, T. C., 11
Human genome. *See Homo sapiens* genome
Human Genome Center, members of, 297–301
Human Genome Organization, 329
Human Genome Project
    as analytical science, 74–75
    basic justification for, 78, 81
    coordination required for, 83, 111, 136, 150
    cost of, 82, 85, 103, 318
    criticisms of
        boring science with no useful outcome, 71, 74–75, 82–85, 106, 110, 164–167
        creativity of individual researchers compromised, 83
        loss of control, 79, 83
        money taken away from other projects, 70, 82, 85, 325
        sequencing whole vs. part of genome
            economics of, 80, 139
            meaninglessness of argument, 139
            stupidity of sequencing whole, 71, 78, 317–318
            technological limitations on sequencing whole, 71, 80, 142–143, 151

Human Genome Project (*continued*)
    value of sequencing part, 81, 139, 142
    value of sequencing whole, 80–81, 151, 252, 253
  distributed nature of, 83, 111, 124–125, 136
  efficiency of, 79, 82
  funding for, 82, 85, 140–141, 143, 320
  goals/outcomes of
    cDNA, 137, 139
    chromosome structure and function, 164–165
    cloning, 82, 221
    complex biological questions become addressable, 78–81, 84, 164–167, 320–322, 328
    development studies, 79–80, 166–167
    disease-gene isolation, 25, 72–74, 76–79, 97–99, 106, 142–143, 318, 319
    ethical, legal, social issues, 141, 167, 178–179
    evolutionary understanding, 166, 193
    five-year goals, 140–141, 150, 329
    freedom, 321–322
    gene expression and regulation, 164–166
    general benefits, 70, 83–85, 150, 168, 319
    genetic-linkage mapping
      atlas of chromosome maps, 256
      for disease-gene isolation, 72–74, 76–79, 97–99
      emphasis on, 71, 73–74, 76, 78–79, 82, 97
      kit of 150 polymorphic markers, 84, 127
      polymorphic DNA markers with STSs, 74, 97, 126, 140, 141
    genome function, 137
    health-care delivery individualized, 82, 324
    informatics, 141, 160–163, 257
    infrastructure creation for doing science, 74–76, 84, 164–167
    model organisms, 77, 78, 81, 141
    multigenic-trait analysis, 78–80, 84, 320–322, 328
    overview of, 70, 141, 316–318
    physical mapping
      for disease-gene isolation, 74, 76–79, 98–99, 106

    emphasis on, 71, 74, 76, 78–79, 82, 140–141, 221
    process described, 98–99, 103–111
    STS markers, 123, 125, 132
    protein structure and function, 165
    research training, 141
    sequencing
      long-term goals, 70, 72, 142–143, 151, 255
      model organisms, 77–78, 81, 141
      short-term goals, 71, 79, 81–82, 141, 256
      technology development, 74, 80, 82, 141–145
    serendipitous discoveries, 74–75
    STSs (sequence-tagged sites), 123, 125, 130–131, 132, 141
    technology development
      automation, 127, 146, 150
      cloning, 221
      interdisciplinary challenges, 146–150, 160–163
      mapping, 74, 140, 149
      outlook for, 75, 82, 141
      sequencing, 74, 80, 82, 141–145
    technology transfer, 84, 127, 141, 150
    tools for scientific community, 84, 127, 141, 150, 160
    variable-trait analysis, 73–74, 78–79, 320–326
  importance of, 70–71, 74–76, 79, 81–82, 84
  initial proponents of, 71, 103
  moral obligation to proceed with, 318, 319
  overview of, 70–85, 141, 316–318
  priorities of, 74, 79, 97–98, 113, 221
  problems with, 70–71, 74, 110
  size of, 83, 111, 150
  staff of, 319–320
  time line for, 82, 85, 103, 122, 329
  uniqueness of, 83–84
Humans. *See Homo sapiens*
Hunkapillar, Tim, 148, 275
Huntington's disease
  communication among labs working on, 160, 256
  discrimination against, 307
  gene isolation for, 111, 142
  inheritance of, 26, 86
  small-insert libraries and, 239
  testing for, 308
Hybrid-cell libraries, 235

Hybrid-cell maps, 193–194, 202–205
Hybridization, 61–63, 95–96, 112–113
  automated robotic gridding device for, 199, 218–219, 246
  defined, 61, 333
  in-situ
    defined, 62–63, 333
    outdated technology used for, 146
    uses for, 61–62, 104, 111–113, 121
    single-molecule-detection method vs., 145
  Southern
    defined, 61–63, 337
    robots for, 140
    SCORE program, 258–262
    uses for, 61–62, 95–96, 190
Hybridization sequencing, 145
Hybrids, defined, 17
Hydrogen bonds, of DNA, 38, 40–41
Hypercholesterolemia, 26
Hypertrophic cardiomyopathy, familial, 185

I

Immune receptor loci, sequencing, 81, 139
Immunoglobulins, 253
Indels, 274
Independent assortment, of chromosomes, 13, 16, 21–22, 25, 31, 86
Informatics, Human Genome Project goals, 141, 160–163, 257. *See also* Computation; Databases; Software
Informativeness, of polymorphic DNA markers, 98, 100–102, 134
Infrequent cutters, 58
Ingram, Vernon Martin, 44
Inheritance. *See Heredity*
Insertional activation, 225
Inserts, defined, 58
In-situ hybridization
  defined, 62–63, 333
  outdated technology used for, 146
  uses for, 61–62, 104, 111–113, 121
Insulin, natural vs. artificial human genes for, 273
Insurance industry
  discrimination by, 303, 305–308, 318, 327
  genetic testing and, 178, 308, 318, 327
  increases in genetic information unwelcome by, 167, 178
  Insurance Task Force, 308
  laws affecting, 307

Inter-Alu PCR, 133, 196, 198–201, 203–204
Interdisciplinary approach
    at California Institute of Technology, 148
    for Human Genome Project technology development, 146–150, 160–163
International issues, genetic information and, 327–329
Interphase
    defined, 14, 333–334
    discovery of, 9
    DNA synthesis and, 9
    illustrated, 9, 14
    naming of, 9
    visibility of chromosomes during, 36
Interspersed tandem repeats, 51
Introns
    defined, 45, 64, 334
    eukaryotes vs. prokaryotes and, 49, 334
    identifying, 278
    percentage of human genome, 80
Inversions, defined, 36
Isoleucine, codons for, 48

J
Jackson Labs, 137
Jacob, 3
Jacob, François, 37
Janssen, Zaccharia, 4
J-detector pooling scheme, 135
Jett, James H., 280–285, 300
Johannsen, Wilhelm Ludwig, 18, 22
Johns Hopkins, Genome DataBase (GDB), 160, 162
Jones, R., 275
Jong, Peter de, 198
Juengst, Eric, 311–312
"Jumping" genes, 187
Junk DNA. *See* Repetitive DNA
Juvenile-onset neuronal ceroid lipofuscionosis, 185

K
Kaiser, Rob, 148
Kanamycin-resistant genes, 223
Karlen, Sam, 162
Karyotypes, 11, 334
Kastner, Dan, 208–209
Keller, Richard A., 280–285, 300
Khorana, Har Gobind, 44, 48
Kidney disease, polycystic (PKD1), 26, 185, 207, 307
Knudsen, S., 278

Koelreuter, Josef Gottlieb, 17
Koskela, Rebecca J., 258–261
Kouprina, Natasha, 105
Krakowski, Letitia A., 280–285

L
L1 repeats, 187
λ-phage genome
    described, 226
    *Eco*RI restriction-fragment fingerprint of, 53, 57
    *Eco*RI restriction-site map of, 57
    wildtype, 228, 229
λ phages
    Charon 21A, 239
    Charon 40, 229, 238
    chromosome-specific libraries and, 238–239, 241
    cloning with, 226–228, 235, 238, 239, 241
    defined, 226
    deriving new vectors from wildtype phages, 228–229
    first use of, 228
    host cells for, 232
    illustrated, 219
    insert length of, 59
    libraries of, 226–228, 232–235, 241, 247
    lytic life cycle of, 227
    physical mapping with, 103–104
    See also λ-phage genome
Lander, Eric, 162, 186, 193
Lapedes, A., 278
Larionov, Vladimir, 105
Lawn, defined, 226
Lawrence Livermore National Laboratory
    National Laboratory Gene Library Project, 114, 236
    physical mapping projects, 105, 111, 241
Laws
    genetic continuity, 5
    Mendel's laws, 16, 72
        equal segregation, 19, 22
        independent assortment, 21–22, 25, 31, 86
Lederberg, Joshua, 37, 76
Leeuwenhoek, Antoni van, 4, 75
Legal implications. *See* ELSI
Lenz, H., 135
Leucine, codons for, 48
Leukemia, acute nonlymphocytic (ANLL), 182, 185, 206, 208, 212–213
Levi-Pearl, Sue, 305

Libraries, ELSI library, 312. *See also* DNA libraries
Life Technologies, Inc., 282, 284–285
LiMB (listing of molecular biology database), 273
Linkage groups, defined, 91–92
Linkage mapping. *See* Genetic-linkage mapping
Linkage phases, defined, 87
Linked genes, defined, 86, 334. *See also* Genetic-linkage mapping
Lipman, D., 275
Lipofuscionosis, juvenile-onset neuronal ceroid, 185
Listing of Molecular Biology Database (LiMB), 273
Livermore. *See* Lawrence Livermore National Laboratory
Locus, defined, 334
Los Alamos National Laboratory
    GenBank (sequence library), 254–255, 266, 270–276
    Human Genome Center, members of, 297–301
    National Laboratory Gene Library Project, 114, 236
    physical mapping projects, 105, 111, 241
    See also Chromosome 5; Chromosome 16; Chromosome 21
Luria, Salvador Edward, 37
Lysine
    acetylation of, 171
    codons for, 48

M
M13, 152, 156, 231–232, 235, 247–248, 284
Magnus, Albertus, 3
Maize. *See* Zea mays
Maleness, Y chromosome and, 12
Malpighi, Marcello, 4
Manic-depressive psychosis, 328
Map_ed, 265
Mapping. *See* Genetic-linkage mapping; Physical mapping
Mapping function, 92
Markers. *See* Polymorphic DNA markers
Marner's cataract, 185
Marrone, Babetta, 280–285
Martin, John C., 280–285, 300
Master genes, 166
Mathematical problems, 149, 162–163
Maxam, Allan, 151, 254

Maxam-Gilbert sequencing method, 152–155, 158, 254

*Mbo*I, 54, 95–96

McCormick, Mary Kay, 105, 195–196, 242

McKusick, Victor, 72

Medical community. *See* Biomedical community; Diseases

Mediterranean fever, 185, 207–208

Medvick, Pat, 199

Meiosis
crossing over during. *See* Crossing over
defined, 13, 15, 334
discovery of, 13
equal segregation of chromosomes during, 13, 16, 19, 22
illustrated, 15
independent assortment of chromosomes during, 13, 16, 21–22, 25, 31, 86
nondisjunction during, 30–31
phases of, 15

Mendel, Gregor Johann, 16–25
Galton, Francis, vs., 28
influences on, 28
laws of, 16, 72
equal segregation, 19, 22
independent assortment, 21–22, 25, 31, 86
selective breeding experiments of, 17–25
theory of inheritance, 18–19, 22–24

Mendelian disorders, 25–27, 72–73, 86, 98

Mendelian traits, 25, 73

Mental retardation, 211

Messenger RNA (mRNA)
cDNA and, 138, 248
defined, 45, 334
protein synthesis and, 44–47
See also Codons

Metallothionein gene family, mapping of, 206

Metaphase, defined, 14–15, 334

Metaphase chromosomes
banding pattern of, 11, 33, 36, 169, 177, 330
defined, 14–15, 334
DNA loops of, 169–170, 172–176
homologous, 10, 12–13, 333
karyotypes of, 11
micrographs of, 10–11, 168, 188
morphological differences of, 12
nonhomologous sex chromosomes, 11–12
packing ratio of linear DNA molecule in, 169
protein scaffold of, 169–170

sister-chromatid pairs, 14–15, 168–169, 174, 337
supercoiling of DNA and, 172–176
visibility of, 10, 14, 36

Metaphase I, defined, 15

Metaphase II, 15

Methionine, codon for, 48

Methyltransferases, 221, 232

Micrococcal nuclease, 170

Microdissection libraries, 248

Microsatellite repeats, 186, 187, 211. *See also* GT repeats

Microscopes, early use of, 4

Microtubules, defined, 14–15

Miescher, Johann Friedrich, 16

Miller, W., 275

Minisatellite repeats, 186–187

Mitochondria, defined, 8

Mitosis
cell cycle and, 9
defined, 12, 14, 334
discovery of, 12
illustrated, 14
phases of, 14
See also Interphase

Mitotic spindle, defined, 14–15, 334

Model organisms, mapping and sequencing of, Human Genome Project goals, 77–78, 81, 141

Mold, bread, 37

Molecular biology. *See* Biology

Molecular cloning. *See* Cloning

Molecular genetics
defined, 334
rise of, 36–39, 44, 49
techniques of, 49–53, 57–62

Monod, Jacques Lucien, 37

Moraxella bovis. *See Mbo*I

Morgans, defined, 31, 92, 256

Morgan, Thomas Hunt, 28–31, 33–35, 91

Mouse. *See Mus musculus*

Mouse genome. *See Mus musculus* genome

Moyzis, Robert K.
on ELSI, 167, 321, 324
on five-year goals of Human Genome Project, 74, 140
on gene isolation, 74, 77–78, 103–104, 106, 319
on gene-pool depletion, 327–328
on genetic-linkage mapping, 71–72, 74, 82, 140
on informatics, 160–163
on Mendelian genetics, 72

on physical mapping
approach to, 109–111
distributed effort of, 111
emphasis on, 71, 74
funding for, 82
intrinsic interest of, 106
problems with, 104
theoretical approaches to, 149
YAC chimeras and, 105
on repetitive DNA, 109–110, 211
on restriction enzymes, 75
on revolutionizing biology, 83, 150, 319
on sequencing, 71, 74, 80–81
cDNA, 136–137, 139
technology for, 71, 74, 142–144
on STS markers, 123–127, 195
on technology development
importance of, 75, 146
outlook for, 82
for pattern recognition and image analysis, 146
for sequencing, 71, 74, 142–144
on technology transfer, 84
telomere discovered by, 63
on tools for scientific community, 79, 82, 84
vita, 180–181, 301

mRNA. *See* Messenger RNA

Muller, Hermann Joseph, 28, 33

Multifactorial disorders, defined, 26

Multigenic disorders, defined, 26

Multigenic-trait analysis, Human Genome Project goals, 78–80, 84, 320–322, 328

Multiplex sequencing, 144

Muscular dystrophy, 27, 50, 77–78

Mus musculus
fibroblast of, 6
hybrid-cell lines, 235
karyotype of, 11
See also Mus musculus genome

Mus musculus genome
development of mice and, 167
genetic-linkage mapping of, 137, 141
human genome and, 65, 136–137, 139, 167
immune receptor loci, sequencing regions for, 81, 139
number of chromosomes, 12
physical mapping of, 141

Mutagens, defined, 334

Mutations
causes of, 3, 33, 334

defined, 3, 29, 334
frequency of, 33
penicillin as negative selection factor for, 76
role of, 29, 36
sequencing DNA and, 61
See also Aberrations
Myers, E., 275
Myotonic dystrophy, 212

N
Nadeau, J., 266
*Nae*I, 238
National Gene Library Project. *See* National Laboratory Gene Library Project
National Institutes of Health
Assessing Genetic Risks study, 311–312
cystic fibrosis pilot studies, 178–179, 311–312
ELSI and, 167, 304, 318–319
five-year plan for Human Genome Project, 74
funding for Human Genome Project, 82, 85, 141
inaccessibility of data at, 160–161
number of genome centers, 83
sequencing without doing biology and, 81
National Laboratory Gene Library Project, 114, 184, 236
National Research Council, committee on Human Genome Project, 71
Needleman, S., 274
Negative supercoiling, 175–176
Nematode genome. *See Caenorhabditis elegans* genome
Nematodes
defined, 334
development of, 166–167
See also Caenorhabditis elegans
Networks. *See* Computer networks
Neurofibromatosis, 26, 74, 77, 86, 212, 317
Neurological disorders, 74
Neuronal ceroid lipofuscionosis, juvenile-onset, 185
Neurospora crassa, 37
Nhe, 243
Nirenberg, Marshall Warren, 44, 48
Nitrocellulose filters, 63
Nocardia otidis. *See Not*I
Nondisjunction, defined, 30, 31
Non-sense strands. *See* Template strands

Norum disease, 185
*Not*I, 54, 57–58, 120–121, 223, 243
NP-complete problems, 162–163
NTPs (ribonucleoside triphosphates), 46
Nucleases, defined, 54
Nucleic acids, defined, 335. *See also* DNA; RNA
Nuclein, 16
Nucleolus, defined, 8
Nucleosome core particles, 170–172, 175
Nucleosomes, 170–175
Nucleotides
defined, 40, 335
DNA replication and, 42–43
illustrated, 40–41
protein synthesis and, 48
single-molecule-detection method, 145, 280–296
See also Ribonucleotides
Nucleus
defined, 8
discovery of, 5
Nutter, Harvey L., 280–285

O
Oak Ridge Laboratory, 137, 162
Oculocutaneous tyrosinemia II, 185
Offspring
defined, 17
genetic uniqueness of, 13, 16, 31, 32
Okazaki fragments, 42
Oligonucleotide ligase assay (OLA), 126–127
Oligonucleotides, defined, 128, 335
Olson, Maynard V.
on genetic-linkage mapping, 71
on molecular biology, 76
on physical mapping, 71, 103, 104–110, 135, 140
on sequencing, 71, 103
on sequencing cDNA, 137, 139
on STS markers, 123–125, 195
on technology development, 75–76, 147, 149–150
vita, 181
One gene–one enzyme hypothesis, 37
On the Origin of Species (Darwin), 25
Oogonium, meiosis of, 15
Open reading frames, 276
-O-P-O- bridges
breaking with restriction enzymes, 52, 54
formation of, 43, 46
Optical microscopes. *See* Microscopes

Optimization approach, for contig assembly, 118, 192, 263–269
Organelles, defined, 8
Orgel, L. E., 211
Origins of replication, defined, 168, 224
Orphan gene identification, Human Genome Project goals, 79

P
Painter, Theophilus Shickel, 36
Palindromes, defined, 223
Pangenesis, 3, 28
Paracelsus, 3
Parasitic DNA. *See* Repetitive DNA
Pardue, Mary Lou, 81
Parental generation, defined, 17
Parents, genetic uniqueness of offspring, 13, 16, 31, 32
Partial digestion, defined, 223, 233
Patenting DNA sequence fragments, 139, 163
Pattern recognition algorithms, 162, 256, 257
Pauling, Linus Carl, 39
PCR. *See* Polymerase chain reaction
Pea, garden. *See Pisum sativum*
Pearson, W., 275
Peierls, R., 294
Penicillin, as negative selection factor for mutants, 76
Pentanucleotide repeats, 186
Peptide bonds, protein synthesis and, 47
Perutz, Max, 107
Phage Group, 37–38
Phages. *See* Bacteriophages; λ phages
Phenotypes
defined, 17–19, 22, 335
independent inheritance of, 21
introduction of term "phenotype," 18
key to differences in, 64
probability of, 20
wildtype, 29, 324, 337
Phenylalanine, codons for, 48
Phosphate groups, of DNA, 38, 40–41
Physical mapping, 98–99, 103–122
ACEDB, 266
chromosome-specific libraries and, 133, 242–243
complexity of, 122, 262–263
defined, 98–99, 103, 221, 257, 335
diversity of techniques for, 111
Encyclopedia of the Mouse, 265–266
fitness criterion for, 263

Physical mapping (*continued*)
  high-resolution contig maps, 98–99,
    103–104, 108–110, 113–122
    branching contigs, 109, 122
    for *Caenorhabditis elegans*, 106–109,
      184–185, 334
    for chromosome 16, 131, 132–133,
      185–206
    collecting clones for, 114–115
    constructing maps
      incremental approach, 108–109,
        115–121, 185–206, 263
      optimization approach, 118, 192,
        263–265, 268–269
      with SIGMA (system for integrated
        genome map assembly), 265,
        267–269
    with cosmid clones, 103–105, 111,
      119, 125, 184–206
    defined, 98, 103, 104, 113, 331
    disconnected contigs, 103–104, 108,
      119–122, 196–203
    disease-gene isolation and, 74, 76–78,
      98–99, 106, 111, 204–206
    for *Escherichia coli*, 121, 184–186
    fitness criterion for, 263
    gap closure
      by fingerprinting, 119, 121
      by walking, 121–122, 143, 195,
        234–235, 265
      with YACs, 103–104, 132–133,
        195–203, 206, 243
    genetic-linkage mapping and, 98–99,
      111, 120, 126, 142, 202–206
    illustrated, 99, 113, 119–120
      for chromosome 16, 191–192, 194,
        200–202, 205
    with λ-phage clones, 103–104
    overlap detection
      overview of, 103
      repetitive-sequence fingerprints and,
        109–110, 186, 188–193
      restriction-fragment fingerprints
        and, 57, 108, 110, 115–119,
        125, 186
      STS markers and, 110, 122–123,
        125, 131–133, 135, 195
    problems with, 103, 104, 105, 108,
      109, 122
    for *Saccharomyces cerevisiae*, 106–
      109, 119–121, 123–124, 184–186
    time required for, 103, 108–109, 122,
      186

    verifying, 120–121, 193–194, 200–
      201, 203–204
    with YAC clones
      cosmid clones and, 104, 111
      gap closure and, 103–104, 195–
        203, 206, 243
      importance of, 103–104, 110
      improving YAC cloning techniques
        and, 195–196
      problems with, 105
      size of, 103–105, 110, 122
      STS markers and, 132–133, 135
Human Genome Project goals
  disease-gene isolation, 74, 76–79, 98–
    99, 106
    emphasis on, 71, 74, 76, 78, 79, 82,
      140, 141, 221
    process described, 98–99, 103–111
    STS markers, 123, 125, 132
  importance of, 98–99, 104–105
  information management for, 161–163,
    257, 260–262, 265–269
  interface software for, 262
  low-resolution
    for chromosome 5, 111, 206, 216–
      217, 242
    for chromosome 16, 193, 194, 202–
      206
    cytogenic breakpoint (hybrid-cell)
      maps, 193–194, 202–205
    cytogenic maps, 202–205
    in-situ hybridization and, 104, 112–
      113, 125, 206
    radiation-hybrid mapping, 216
    STS-content mapping, 125, 195, 206,
      216–217
  for model organisms, 77–78, 141
  motivation for, 105–108
  of *Mus musculus* genome, 141
  problems with, 103–105, 108–109,
    122
  restriction-site maps, 57, 108, 119, 120,
    123–124
  and revolutionizing biology, 78–79
  SCORE program and, 190, 258–261
  SIGMA system, 265–269
  specializing in, 110, 140, 149
  speeding up, 109–110
  technology for, 82, 184
  theoretical approaches to, 149
  time required for, 103, 108–109, 122
  universal language for, 123
  See also specific chromosomes

Physics, Human Genome Project and, 146,
  149
PIC (polymorphism information content),
  98, 100–102, 134
Pisum sativum
  Mendelian experiments, 17–25
  number of chromosomes, 12
PKD1 (polycystic kidney disease), 26, 185,
  207, 307
Plant cells, components of, 8
Plaque (phage), 226
Plasmids
  cloning with, 58–60, 220, 224–226, 232
  defined, 58, 220, 224, 335
  libraries of, 224–226, 247
Plato, 3
Pol II, 64
Polyacrylamide gel, 55, 153, 157, 158
Poly A site, 64
Polycystic kidney disease (PKD1), 26, 185,
  207, 307
Polymerase chain reaction (PCR), 128–134
  cheapest method for recognizing unique
    landmarks, 123
  cloning vs., 60, 128
  date of development of, 58
  defined, 60, 128–131, 335
  Human Genome Project and, 128
  illustrated, 129
  inter-Alu PCR, 133, 196, 198–201,
    203–204
  STS markers and, 110, 123–126, 130–
    135
  YAC library pooling scheme and, 132–
    133, 135, 197
Polymerases, defined, 335. *See also* DNA
  polymerase; RNA polymerase
Polymorphic DNA markers, 94–99
  acceleration of search for, 99, 133–134
  automated techniques for, 126–127
  base-sequence variation and, 94–96
  defined, 73–74, 94, 335
  development of, 73, 94
  disease-gene isolation and, 73–74, 76–
    79, 94–99, 111, 142, 204–206, 256
  finding, 96, 126–127
  genetic-linkage map construction and,
    97, 112–113
  Human Genome Project goals, 74, 97–
    99, 126
    atlas of chromosome maps, 256
    emphasis on, 71, 74, 76, 78–79, 82,
      97

kit of 150 polymorphic markers, 84, 127

polymorphic DNA markers with STSs, 74, 97, 99, 126, 140–141

importance of, 73–74, 76–79, 94, 97

informativeness of, 98, 100–102, 134

kit of 150 markers, 84, 127

restriction fragment length polymorphisms (RFLPs), 96, 97

STS markers and, 74, 97, 99, 126–127, 133–134, 140, 141

Polymorphism information content (PIC), 98, 100–102, 134

Polymorphisms, defined, 73–74, 94, 324

Polypeptide chains

defined, 335

one gene-one enzyme hypothesis and, 37

Polytene chromosomes, 36

Pooling, YAC clone libraries for PCR-based screening, 132–133, 135, 197

Postmeiotic phase, defined, 15

Potato, selective breeding of, 17

Preformation theory, 4

Premeiotic phase, defined, 15

Privacy, genetic, 304, 308–309, 312, 318, 326–327

Probability, Mendelian genetics and, 18–25

Probes

defined, 62–63, 233, 335

hybridization and, 61–63, 112, 335

polymerase chain reaction and, 128

single-copy, 239

STS markers and, 131

for variable-loci detection, 73–74, 94

Prokaryotes

circularity of DNA molecules in, 33, 330

defined, 5, 335

eukaryotes vs., 45–47, 49, 334

gene isolation in, 276–277

protein synthesis in, 45–47

repetitive DNA in, 50

Proline, codons for, 48

Prometaphase, defined, 14

Prometaphase I, 15

Prometaphase II, 15

Promoters, 46, 64, 164–165, 335–336

Prophase, defined, 14

Prophase I, defined, 15

Prophase II, defined, 15

Proteinase K, 247

Proteins

amino acids and

codon preference rules, 276–278

codons for, 44–45, 48, 64

defined, 330

listed, 48

protein structure and, 39, 44, 165

protein synthesis and, 45–48

cDNA and, 136–139, 220

as chromosome component, 10, 169–170

collinearity hypothesis, 45

defined, 336

eukaryotic protein genes

anatomy of, 64

defined, 65

exons, 45, 64, 80, 137, 276, 278, 332

folding problem, 165

functions of, 71, 77, 79–80, 136, 165, 278–279

gene isolation for, 276–279

genetic information flows from DNA to RNA to, 45–46

as genetic material, early support for, 38

introns, 45, 64, 80, 278, 334

percentage of human genome that codes for, 80

signal sequence, 74

structure of, 39, 44, 136, 165, 278–279

synthesis of

cDNA and, 136, 138–139

codon preference rules, 276–278

defined, 45–48, 64

DNA and, 38–40, 44–47

endoplasmic reticulum and, 8, 74

genetic code and, 45–46, 48

illustrated, 45–47

one gene-one enzyme hypothesis, 37

regulatory mechanisms, 164–165

RNA and, 44–47, 137

translocation of, 74–75, 186

See also Enzymes; Histones

Protein scaffold, of chromosomes, 169–170

Proteinuria, with unesterified hypercholesterolemia, 185

p28^{sis}, 256, 257

Public databases. See Databases

Public education, about genetic information, 167, 178, 304, 311, 312, 313

Pulsed-field gel electrophoresis, 55, 56, 58, 104, 184

Pyrophosphate group, DNA replication and, 43

R

Racial discrimination, genetic information and, 306–307

Radiation-hybrid mapping, 111, 216

Rapid DNA sequencing. See Single-molecule-detection sequencing method

Ratliff, Robert R., 280–285

Reading frames, 276–277

Rearrangements, of chromosomes, 36. See also Mutations

Recessive alleles, 19–20, 22, 336

Reciprocal breeding, defined, 29

Recombinant clones

defined, 220, 336

selection of, 225

Recombinant DNA molecules

cloning and, 58–60, 114–115, 195–196, 220, 222–232

defined, 54, 58, 114, 220, 336

first, 75, 223

Recombination

antibiotic resistance and, 232

beginning of recombinant-DNA revolution, 49, 54, 75, 220–221, 223

by crossing over. See Crossing over

defined, 32, 38

historical background, 54, 75, 220–224

overview of progress in, 49–50

safety of, 232

techniques for, 49–53, 57–62. See also specific techniques

transduction and, 38, 76

Recombination events, defined, 88

Recombination fractions

defined, 31–32, 89

first measurement of, 33

genetic distance and, 31–35, 91–92

genetic-linkage mapping and, 88–92

measuring, 34–35, 90

Redgrave, C., 273

Red-green color blindness, 26

Reeders, Steve, 207

Region methods, 278

Regulation, of genes, 64–65, 79–80, 164–166, 177, 276, 332–333

Reichelt, Richard, on ELSI, 302–313

Renaturation, defined, 51–52

Renaturation kinetics, 51–52

Repetitive DNA, 50–52, 109–110, 186–187

amount of, 50, 211

on chromosome 16, 182–183, 186–187, 203–204, 206, 211–213

classes of, 186–187

defined, 50–51, 109–110, 211, 336

discovery of, 51

Repetitive DNA (*continued*)
diseases and, 211–212
function of, 65, 109, 211, 336
renaturation and, 51–52
Repetitive-sequence fingerprints, physical
mapping and, 109–110, 186, 188–
192, 193
Replicating DNA
defined, 39, 42–43, 332
histone acetylation and, 171, 175
illustrated, 42–43
interphase and, 9
lysine acetylation and, 171
nucleosome supercoil and, 174
origins-of-replication base sequence and,
42
semiconservative nature of, 39
See also Amplifying
Replicons, defined, 224
Repressors, defined, 64
Research training, Human Genome Project
goals, 141
Resting phase. *See* Interphase
Restriction enzymes
*Bam*HI, 54, 225, 226, 238
*Cla*I, 206, 230, 243
defined, 52–54, 114, 221–223, 336
discovery of, 75
*Eag*I, 243
*Eco*RI
defined, 52–54, 221–223
repetitive-sequence fingerprints, 188–
191
restriction-fragment fingerprints, 57,
116–119, 186
restriction-site maps, 57, 119, 123–
124
star activity and, 247
*Hae*III, 54
*Hin*dII, 54
*Hin*dIII, 56, 188, 189, 190, 191
importance of, 54, 75, 221
infrequent cutters, 58
*Mbo*I, 54, 95–96
methyltransferases and, 221, 232
*Nae*I, 238
Nhe, 243
*Not*I, 54, 57–58, 120–121, 223, 243
plasmids and, 224
*Sau*3AI, 238
*Sfi*I, 120–121
staggered cuts of, 54
star activity, 247

sticky ends and, 53–54, 59, 221–223
*Taq*I, 54
types of, 54, 223
Restriction-fragment fingerprints, physical
mapping and, 57, 108, 110, 115–119,
125, 186
Restriction-fragment-length polymorphisms
(RFLPs), defined, 96–97, 336
Restriction fragments, defined, 95–96, 336
Restriction-site maps, 57, 108, 119–120,
123–124
Restriction sites, 52, 114–115, 123, 223,
336
Retinoblastoma, 86
Retrotransposons, class II, 187
Retroviruses, reverse transcription and, 46,
138
Reverse transcriptase, defined, 138, 187,
336
Reverse transcription, defined, 46, 138, 336
RFLPs (restriction-fragment-length poly-
morphisms), defined, 96–97, 336
Ribonucleic acid. *See* RNA
Ribonucleoside triphosphates (NTPs), 46
Ribonucleotides
defined, 42–43
DNA replication and, 42–43
protein synthesis and, 45–48
Ribosomal RNA (rRNA)
as catalyst, 47
defined, 46, 336
synthesis of, 8
Ribosomes
defined, 46, 336
illustrated, 8, 47
protein synthesis and, 46, 47
Ribozymes, defined, 332
Richner–Hanhort syndrome, 185
Rine, Jasper, 78
RNA (ribonucleic acid)
codons for amino acids, 48
defined, 44, 336
DNA compared to, 44
DNA replication and, 42–43
genetic information flows from DNA to
RNA to protein, 45, 46
non-protein, isolating genes coding for,
276
probes, 233
protein synthesis and, 44–47
ribosomal (rRNA), 8, 46–47, 336
ribozymes, 332
7SL, 186

structure of, 42–44
uracil and, 44–45
See also Messenger RNA (mRNA);
Transfer RNA (tRNA)
RNA polymerases, 46, 64, 335
T7, 230, 231
RNA splicing, 45, 46, 64, 139, 336
Robotics
hybridization gridding device, 199, 218–
219, 246
need for, 146
for oligonucleotide ligase assay, 127
for sequencing, 143–144
for Southern hybridization, 140
for YAC library pools, 135
rRNA. *See* Ribosomal RNA
Rubinstein–Taybi syndrome (RTS), 185,
206, 208

S
Saccharomyces cerevisiae
as host cell, 218–219, 232
illustrated, 218–219
origins of replication, 42
spheroplasts, 242–243
See also Saccharomyces cerevisiae ge-
nome; YACs (yeast artificial
chromosomes)
Saccharomyces cerevisiae genome
physical mapping of, 106–109, 119–121,
123–124, 184–186
sequencing of, 151, 252
Safety, of recombinant organisms, 232
Sample preparation, for DNA, 50, 58
Sanger (dideoxy chain termination)
sequencing method, 151–153, 156–
158, 232, 247–248, 254
Sanger, Fredrick, 151, 254
Satellite repeats, 186–191, 193, 211, 336.
See also GT repeats
*Sau*3AI, 238
Scicillano, Michael, 198
SCORE, 190, 258–262
Sc1 and Sc2, 170
Screening
DNA libraries, 221, 232–235, 246
genetic, 178–179, 308–309, 311–312,
326–327
Sears Roebuck of molecular biology, 124
Selective breeding, Mendelian experiments
in, 17–25
Selfing, defined, 18
Selfish DNA. *See* Repetitive DNA

Self-pollination, 18

Sense strands
  defined, 45, 48, 64, 276
  illustrated, 45–46, 64

Sequences, defined, 332, 336

Sequence-tagged sites. *See* STSs

Sequencing DNA, 60–61, 151–159
  assembly problem, 162–163
  and biological analysis of sequences, 81–82
  cDNA, 136–139
  complementary sequences, 40, 331
  completely sequenced genomes, 272
  cost of, 61, 139, 151, 159, 252–253, 281
  databases for, 163, 254–255, 266, 270–276
  defined, 60–61, 151–159
  dynamic-programming algorithm, 274–275
  error rate for, 143–144, 151, 158
  first published sequence, 254
  homologous sequences, 333
  Human Genome Project goals
    long-term goals, 70, 72, 142–143, 151, 255
    model organisms, 77, 78, 81, 141
    short-term goals, 71, 79, 81–82, 141, 256
    technology development, 74, 80, 82, 141–145
  hybridization method, 61–63, 145
  large-scale sequencing, 142–145
  length of sequences published, 254
  long sequences, 144, 158
  mass-spectrometry method, 145
  Maxam-Gilbert method, 152–155, 158, 254
  for model organisms, 77–78, 81, 141
  M13 and, 152, 156, 231–232, 235, 247–248, 284
  patenting sequence fragments, 139, 163
  pattern recognition and, 162, 256, 257
  percentage of human genome sequenced, 253
  polyacrylamide gel and, 55, 153, 157–158
  polymerase chain reaction and, 128
  published sequence data, 151, 254
  random ("shotgun") vs. directed strategies, 144, 158
  rapid sequencing, 145, 280–296
  rate of sequence-data accumulation, 254–255

and revolutionizing biology, 142

Sanger (dideoxy chain termination) method, 151–153, 156–158, 232, 247–248, 254
  similarity analysis and, 164, 274–276, 317
  single-molecule-detection method, 145, 280–296
  software for, 137, 144, 162–163, 256
  technology development for
    automation, 110, 143–144, 148, 158–159
    back-end analysis, 143–144, 159
    basis for all current methods, 151
    front-end preparation, 143–144, 159
    Human Genome Project goals, 74, 80, 82, 141–145
    limitations of present technology, 71, 74, 80–81, 142, 151
    outlook for, 75, 82, 142–145
    time required for, 144, 151, 159, 254, 281, 282, 285
  for well-studied organisms, 272
  whole vs. part of human genome
    economics of, 80, 139
    meaninglessness of argument, 139
    stupidity of sequencing whole, 71, 78, 317–318
    technological limitations on sequencing whole, 71, 80, 142–143, 151
    value of sequencing part, 81, 139, 142
    value of sequencing whole, 80–81, 151, 252–253

Serine, codons for, 48

Sex chromosomes, defined, 11–12, 336–337. *See also* X chromosome

Sex selection, ethics of, 311, 322, 327

Sexual reproduction, meiosis and, 13, 15. *See also* Asexual reproduction

Seysenegg, Erich Tschermak von, 16

*Sfi*I, 120–121

Shape, of chromosomes, defined, 33

Shera, E. Brooks
  on rapid DNA sequencing, 280–285
  on single-molecule spectroscopy in solution, 286–296
  vita, 301

Sickle-cell anemia, 26–27, 39, 44, 306, 307

SIGMA (system for integrated genome map assembly), 265–269

Signal sequence, 74

Similarity analysis, for sequences, 164, 274–276, 317

Simpson, Daniel J., 280–285

Singer, Maxine, 277

Single-molecule-detection sequencing method, 145, 280–296

Single-molecule spectroscopy in solution, 286–296

Singletons, defined, 193

Sirotkin, K., 278

Sister-chromatid pairs, 14–15, 168–169, 174, 337

Skolnick, Marik, 94

7SL, 186

Smith, Cassandra, 184

Smith, Hamilton, 75

Smith, Lloyd, 143, 148

Smith, T., 278

Social implications. *See* ELSI

Soderlund, C., 278

Software
  Annotator's WorkBench, 271
  BLAST (basic local alignment search tool), 275–276
  for cosmid overlap detection, 190–191
  database. *See* Databases
  Electronic Data Publishing, 271–272
  FASTA, 275
  GCAA (genetic contig assembly algorithm), 192, 263–265
  GeneID, 278
  GM (gene modeler), 278
  GRAIL (neural nets), 137
  Human Genome Project goals, 141
  interface software, 262, 265
  Map_ed (GCAA interface), 265
  SCORE (Southern Blot scoring), 190, 258–262
  for sequencing, 137, 144, 162–163, 256
  SIGMA (system for integrated genome map assembly), 265, 267–269
  See also Computation

Solanum tuberosum, selective breeding of, 17

Somatic-cell hybrid panels, 235

Somatic cells
  defined, 5, 337
  division of. *See* Mitosis

Soper, Steven A.
  on rapid DNA sequencing, 280–285
  on single-molecule spectroscopy in solution, 286–296

Sorensen, Doug, 263

Southern hybridization
  defined, 61–62, 63, 337

Southern hybridization (*continued*)
   robots for, 140
   SCORE program, 258–261, 262
   uses for, 61–62, 95–96, 190
Sperm. *See* Gametes
Spermatogonium, meiosis of, 15, 265
Spermidine, 243
Spermine, 243
S phase, of interphase, 9, 14
Spheroplasts, 242–243
Spinal muscular atrophy, 212
Splicing, RNA, 45, 46, 64, 139, 336
Stadler, Lewis John, 33
Staff
   of Human Genome Project, 319–320
   of Los Alamos National Laboratory
      Human Genome Center, 297–301
Staggered cuts, 54
Stallings, Raymond L.
   on chromosome 16 repetitive DNA, 211–
      215
   on SCORE, 258–261
   vita, 301
Star activity, 247
START codon, 48, 64, 331
Statistics, of Mendelian genetics, 18–25
Stent, Gunther, 75
Stereoscopic image of DNA, 67
Sticky ends, 53–54, 59, 221–223
STOP codons, 48, 276, 331
Storing
   clones, 124, 126, 131
   DNA libraries, 241–242, 247
Structural biology, 165, 168
STS-content mapping, 125, 195, 206, 216–
   217
STSs (sequence-tagged sites), 123–126,
   130–134
   from cDNA, 136–139
   chromosome 5 mapping and, 206, 216–
      217
   chromosome 16 mapping and, 131–133,
      135, 195–197
   cost of, 125
   cross-species, 136
   defined, 110, 123, 130, 337
   disease-gene isolation and, 124, 126
   example of, 133
   generating, 125, 131–132, 216
   genetic-linkage mapping and, 126–127,
      133–134, 141
   Human Genome Project goals, 123, 125,
      130–132, 141
   importance of, 110, 122–123, 130

libraries for constructing, 195, 247–248
physical mapping and
   contig overlap detection, 110, 122–
      123, 125, 131–133, 135, 195
   STS-content mapping, 125, 195, 206,
      216–217
   polymerase chain reaction and, 110, 123,
      124–126, 130–135
   polymorphic, 126–127, 133–134
   time required to generate, 125
   as universal language, 123
   YACs and, 125, 132–133, 135, 195–197,
      206, 216–217
Students. *See* Graduate students
Studier, Bill, 143
Sturtevant, Alfred Henry, 28, 33
Subtelomeric repeats, 186–187
Sulston, John, 106–108
Supercoiling, 172–176
Sutherland, Grant, 133, 193
Sutherland, Robert, 262
Sutton, Walter Stanborough, 28
Swammerdam, Jan, 4
Synthesizing DNA. *See* Amplifying
System for integrated genome map assem-
   bly (SIGMA), 265, 267–269
Szilard, Leo, 149

T

Tandem repeats, 51, 186–188, 211–212
*Taq*I, 54
Taq polymerase, 130
TATA box, 64
TAT deficiency, 185
Tatum, Edward Lawrie, 37
Tay-Sachs disease, 26–27, 306
T-cell receptor genes, sequencing of, 81
Technology development
   automation of procedures
      need for, 146, 150
      for polymorphic DNA markers, 126–
         127
      for sequencing, 110, 143–144, 148,
         158–159
   biological advances and, 75
   biological information signal processing
      (BISP) chip, 275
   for cloning, 221
   computers and, 150
   engineering component, 147
   funding for, 141
   Human Genome Project goals
      automation, 127, 146, 150

      cloning, 221
      interdisciplinary challenges, 146–150,
         160–163
      mapping, 74, 140, 149
      outlook for, 75, 82, 141
      sequencing, 74, 80, 82, 141–145
   interdisciplinary challenge of, 146–150,
      160–163
   for mapping, 82, 184
   outdated technology, 146
   outlook for, 75, 82, 141
   physicists and, 146, 149
   robotics
      hybridization gridding device, 199,
         218–219, 246
      need for, 146
      for oligonucleotide ligase assay, 127
      for sequencing, 143–144
      for Southern hybridization, 140
      for YAC library pools, 135
   for sequencing
      automation, 110, 143–144, 148, 158–
         159
      back-end analysis, 143–144, 159
      basis for all current methods, 151
      front-end preparation, 143–144, 159
      Human Genome Project goals, 74, 80–
         82, 141–145
      limitations of present technology, 71,
         74, 80, 81, 142
   spin-offs from, 84, 164
   tools for scientific community, 84, 127,
      141, 150, 160
   See also Computation; Databases;
      Software
Technology transfer, Human Genome Project goals, 84, 127, 141, 150
Telomerase, 186
Telomere repeats, 186–187, 211
Telomeres
   defined, 40, 63, 80, 168–169, 337
   discovery of, 63
   repetitive DNA sequences of, 186–187,
      211
   replication of, 42
   vertebrates share same telomeric
      sequence, 63
Telophase, defined, 14
Telophase I, 15
Telophase II, 15
Template strands, defined, 44–45, 64
Test cross
   defined, 33, 73, 86
   example of, 87–91

Testing, genetic, 178–179, 308–309, 311–312, 326–327
Tetracycline-resistant genes, 223, 225–226
Tetrahymena thermophila, rRNA as catalyst and, 47
Tetranucleotide repeats, 186
Thalassemia, 165, 185
*Thermus aquaticus. See Taq*I; *Taq* polymerase
Thierry-Mieg, J., 266
Thin-gel technology, 143
Threonine, codons for, 48
Thymine
    DNA and, 38–41, 48
    RNA and, 44–45
Topoisomerase II, 170
Torney, David
    clone overlap identification algorithm of, 110, 117, 162, 190
    on informativeness of polymorphic DNA markers, 100–101
    on YAC library pooling scheme, 133, 135, 197
Tourette syndrome, 305–306
Traits
    defined, 17, 19
    Mendelian traits, 25, 73
    variable, 73–74, 78–79, 320–326
Trans-acting transcription factors, 64
Transcription
    defined, 44–46, 64, 337
    histone acetylation and, 171, 175
    illustrated, 46, 64
    lysine acetylation and, 171
    nucleosome supercoil and, 174
    reverse, 46, 138, 336
Transcription factors, 252
Transduction
    defined, 37–38, 58, 76, 337
    discovery of, 37–38, 76
Transfer RNA (tRNA)
    defined, 46, 337
    gene isolation for, 276
    length of genes for, 50
    protein synthesis and, 46–47
Transformation, defined, 59, 220, 224–225, 337
Translation, defined, 44–47, 337
Translocations
    defined, 36, 337
    protein, 74–75, 186
Trinucleotide repeats, 186, 212
tRNA. *See* Transfer RNA
Troup, Charles D., 267–269

Tryptophan, codon for, 48
T7 RNA polymerase, 230, 231
Tumor-suppressor gene, 208
Type II restriction endonucleases. *See* Restriction enzymes
Tyrosine, codons for, 48

U
Uniqueness, genetic, 13, 16, 31, 32
University of California at San Francisco, physical mapping projects, 111
Upstream, defined, 64
Uracil, 44–45, 48
Urolithiasis, 185

V
Vacuoles, defined, 8
Valine, codons for, 48
Variable-trait analysis, Human Genome Project goals, 73–74, 78–79, 320–326
Vectors. *See* Cloning vectors
Violence, XYY males and, 310
Virchow, Rudolph, 5
Viruses
    defined, 37, 337
    repetitive DNA in, 50
    retroviruses, reverse transcription and, 46, 138, 336
    See also Bacteriophages; Cytomegalovirus genome
Vitalism, 3
Vries, Hugo De, 16

W
Wagner, Robert P.
    on informativeness of polymorphic DNA markers, 100–101
    on inheritance, 1–66
    vita, 66
Walking, 121–122, 143, 195, 234–235, 265
Wallace, Alfred Russel, 25, 28
Washington University, physical mapping projects, 111, 195
Wasmuth, John, 206, 216
Waterman, Michael, 162, 186, 193
Watson, James Dewey
    on disease-gene isolation, 329
    DNA structure discovered by, 38–39
    on ELSI, 167, 321–323, 325–326, 328
    on revolutionizing biology, 325
    on role in Human Genome Project, 319–320
Weismann, August Friedrich Leopold, 16

Wexler, Nancy S.
    on benefits of Human Genome Project, 84, 179
    on ELSI
        cystic-fibrosis pilot studies, 179
        education, 167, 313
        insurance industry, 167, 178
        international issues, 329
        overview of, 167, 178, 304, 321, 324–325
        privacy issues, 326–327
    on genetic-linkage maps, 126
    on informatics, 160
    on interdisciplinary nature of Human Genome Project, 146–147
    on physical mapping, 105
    vita, 181
White, Raymond L., 94, 127
Wild type, defined, 29, 324, 337
Wilkerson, Charles W., 280–285
Wilkins, Maurice Hugh Frederick, 39
Wilson, Edmund Beecher, 16, 38
Wolff, Caspar Friedrich, 4
Wollman, Elie Leo, 37
Woo, Debra, 307
Wunsch, C., 274

X
X chromosome
    defined, 12
    diseases and, 211–212
    femaleness and, 12
    fragile site on, 211
    micrographs of, 11
    physical mapping of, 111
X-linked traits
    Drosophila melanogaster eye color, 29
    Mendelian disorders, 26–27
X rays
    chromosome aberrations and, 36
    gene mutations and, 33
XYY males, violence and, 310

Y
YACs (yeast artificial chromosomes)
    chimeric, 105, 195–196, 231–232, 243–245, 247
    cloning with, 195–196, 228–232, 235, 247
    contig maps
        high-resolution
            gap closure, 103–104, 132–133, 195–203, 206, 243
            importance of, 103–104, 110

YACs (yeast artificial chromosomes)
 (*continued*)
  improving YAC cloning techniques
   and, 195–196
  problems with, 105
  size of, 103–105, 110, 122
  STS markers and, 132–133, 135
 low-resolution, 125, 195, 206, 216–
   217
 cosmids and, 104, 111
 defined, 42, 58–59, 195, 228–229, 337
 host cells for, 232
 libraries of
  average insert size, 231
  chimeras in, 231
  for chromosome 16, 132–133, 135,
   184, 195–196, 206, 242–243,
   246
  for chromosome 21, 195–196, 243

 from flow-sorted chromosomes, 133,
   195–196, 242–246
 overview of, 184, 228–231
 pooling scheme for PCR-based screening, 132–133, 135, 197
 storing, 247
 STS markers and, 125, 132–133, 135,
   195–197, 206, 216–217
Yanofsky, Charles, 45
Y chromosome, 11–12
Yeast. *See Saccharomyces cerevisiae*
Yeast artificial chromosomes. *See* YACs
Yeast genome. *See Saccharomyces cerevisiae* genome
Yungnickel, D., 135

Z
Zea mays
 chromosome 9 knob, 33

metaphase chromosomes, 10
selective breeding of, 17
Zinder, Norton D.
 on benefits of Human Genome Project,
  74–75
 on disease-gene isolation, 72–74
 on goals of Human Genome Project, 82
 on informatics, 160–161
 on physical mapping, 109, 110–111
 on sequencing cDNA, 137, 139
 on STS markers, 124, 126
 on student interest in genome field, 84
 on technology development, 75–76, 149
 vita, 181
Zola, Irving, 307
Zygotes
 chance and, 19–20
 defined, 18, 337